KU-450-799

Stroke Recovery with Cellular Therapies

CURRENT CLINICAL NEUROLOGY

Daniel Tarsy, MD, SERIES EDITOR

Stroke Recovery with Cellular Therapies

Edited by

Sean I. Savitz, MD

University of Texas-Houston Medical School, Houston, TX

and

Daniel M. Rosenbaum, MD

SUNY Downstate Medical Center, Brooklyn, NY

HUMANA PRESS ✸ TOTOWA, NEW JERSEY

© 2008 Humana Press
999 Riverview Drive, Suite 208
Totowa, New Jersey 07512

humanapress.com

All rights reserved. No part of this book may be reproduced, stored in a retrieval system, or transmitted in any form or by any means, electronic, mechanical, photocopying, microfilming, recording, or otherwise without written permission from the Publisher.

All papers, comments, opinions, conclusions, or recommendations are those of the author(s), and do not necessarily reflect the views of the publisher.

Due diligence has been taken by the publishers, editors, and authors of this book to assure the accuracy of the information published and to describe generally accepted practices. The contributors herein have carefully checked to ensure that the drug selections and dosages set forth in this text are accurate and in accord with the standards accepted at the time of publication. Notwithstanding, as new research, changes in government regulations, and knowledge from clinical experience relating to drug therapy and drug reactions constantly occur, the reader is advised to check the product information provided by the manufacturer of each drug for any change in dosages or for additional warnings and contraindications. This is of utmost importance when the recommended drug herein is a new or infrequently used drug. It is the responsibility of the treating physician to determine dosages and treatment strategies for individual patients. Further it is the responsibility of the health care provider to ascertain the Food and Drug Administration status of each drug or device used in their clinical practice. The publisher, editors, and authors are not responsible for errors or omissions or for any consequences from the application of the information presented in this book and make no warranty, express or implied, with respect to the contents in this publication.

This publication is printed on acid-free paper. ∞
ANSI Z39.48-1984 (American Standards Institute) Permanence of Paper for Printed Library Materials.

Cover illustration: Fig. 2, chap. 3; *see* complete caption on p. 44.

Cover design by: Nancy K. Fallatt

Production Editor: Tara Bugg

For additional copies, pricing for bulk purchases, and/or information about other Humana titles, contact Humana at the above address or at any of the following numbers: Tel.: 973-256-1699; Fax: 973-256-8314; or visit our Website: http://humanapress.com

Photocopy Authorization Policy:

Authorization to photocopy items for internal or personal use, or the internal or personal use of specific clients, is granted by Humana Press Inc., provided that the base fee of US $30.00 per copy, plus US $30.00 per page, is paid directly to the Copyright Clearance Center at 222 Rosewood Drive, Danvers, MA 01923. Fort hose organizations that have been granted a photocopy license from the CCC, a separate system of payment has been arranged and is acceptable to Humana Press Inc. The fee code for users of the Transactional Report-ing Service is: [978-1-58829-732-7/08 $30.00 + $30.00].

Printed in the United States of America. 10 9 8 7 6 5 4 3 2 1
eISBN 978-1-60327-057-1

Library of Congress Control Number: 2007930162

Series Editor's Foreword

Stroke Recovery with Cellular Therapies by Drs. Savitz and Rosenbaum is a brave look into the future, focusing on the possibility of "neurorestorative" therapy for stroke. Restoring brain function after the destructive effects of stroke has been regarded as a lofty goal well out of reach of conventional treatments. To date, attention has centered on stroke prevention, the use of thrombolytic agents to treat acute stroke, and a search for "neuroprotective" agents to minimize ischemic brain injury. Thrombolytic therapy has greatly impacted the approach to acute stroke care in the emergency room setting but, at the present time, has been available to relatively few patients because of narrow therapeutic windows and logistical issues. Unfortunately, although a large number of "neuroprotective" treatments, which intervene at various steps in the cascade of ischemic brain injury, have appeared promising in the laboratory, they have to date shown little or no useful clinical effect in patients.

The concept of brain tissue transplantation has inherent appeal for patients living in an era of dramatic and sometimes lifesaving developments in the field of peripheral organ and tissue transplantation. Transplantation of fetal tissue substantia nigra dopamine neurons into the striatum has been carried out in Parkinson's disease in several multicenter clinical trials with technical success but disappointing clinical benefit. Laboratory investigations into stem cell transplantation in animal models of Parkinson's disease are now ongoing but progress is slow. However, by contrast with progressive neurological disorders, the challenges for cellular transplantation in stroke appear to be more formidable. As pointed out in the chapter by Savitz and Caplan, the brain is a functionally and anatomically heterogeneous organ, which may not lend itself to a neuronal replacement approach in the chronic setting. However, as pointed out in the chapter by Dr.Chopp, in the acute setting it is possible that tissue transplantation may turn out to help by providing trophic supports, thereby enhancing angiogenesis, synaptogenesis, gliogenesis, and perhaps even neurogenesis. To this end, several sources of cellular support currently under active investigation are described by the authors in this volume including bone marrow, umbilical cord blood, and adipose tissue. As explored in Dr. Mehler's chapter, the latter research may even lead to new multipronged approaches to enhance tissue repair, which may obviate the need for exogenous cell transplantation.

Daniel Tarsy MD
Beth Israel Deaconess Medical Center
Harvard Medical School
Boston MA

Preface

1. HISTORICAL BACKGROUND

During the past decade, the field of stroke has emerged from an era of therapeutic nihilism to a speciality that offers timely therapies to reperfuse the ischemic brain. While there has been limited success with thrombolytic agents for acute stroke, few patients receive these medications because of the narrow therapeutic time window. Despite immediate medical attention, many patients still have disabling deficits. Once damage from stroke has plateaued, little can be done to recover premorbid function. As the leading cause of adult disability, stroke poses substantial economic and psychological burdens on populations around the world. Surveys show that healthy people prefer death rather than suffer a stroke *(1)*. Against this dismal backdrop, several novel "neurorestorative" approaches are being investigated as adjunctive treatments to physiotherapy. This book discusses the promising investigations around world on cell-based therapies to enhance recovery from stroke.

Cell transplantation as a strategy to improve neurological deficits and relieve disability is being pursued in a number of neurological disorders. Stem cell therapy has raised particular interest among investigators in Parkinson's disease, stroke, and multiple sclerosis. In the laboratory, neurons and glia have successfully been generated from stem cells in culture. In addition, the identification, proliferation, migration, and differentiation of endogenous stem cells in the embryonic and adult brain have suggested that the brain retains an intrinsic capacity of self-repair, which may be too limited to promote meaningful recovery from neurological disease. It is therefore hoped by many that the exogenous application or endogenous stimulation of stem cells will provide an inexhaustible supply of neurons, glia, and endothelia for cell and segmental replacement in disorders of the brain and spinal cord.

Parkinson's disease, which causes the destruction of nigrostrial dopaminergic neurons, was one of the first neurological disorders for which cell transplantation was considered. Clinical trials on transplanted human fetal dopaminergic neurons have shown improvement in some patients with early Parkinson's disease. The success of these trials has fueled interest in pursuing cell-based therapies for patients with other neurological disorders such as stroke.

2. RATIONALE OF CELL THERAPY FOR STROKE

Admittedly, ischemic stroke is far from an ideal neurological condition for which transplant therapy should be considered. In Chapter 9, Dr. Louis Caplan discusses some of the unique conditions stroke poses that will impact the potential success of transplantation to enhance recovery. In contrast to Parkinson's disease, ischemic stroke destroys a highly complicated architecture of glia, microglia, endothelia, and neurons along with their segmental connections. How will transplanted cells bring about a reconstitution of the neuronal network lost or damaged in stroke? Can transplanted cells differentiate into all the necessary cellular components in the right proportions and in the right topographic layout that duplicates the complex tapestry of the brain? These questions raise the central issue: what is the goal behind cell transplantation in stroke? The ultimate goal of transplantation in the future might be to replace dead neurons, remyelinate axons, and repair damaged neural circuits. However, this is not realistic at the present time. It is possible that certain transplanted cell types might differentiate into interneurons that support lost segmental connections. Alternatively, transplanted cells may serve as a source of trophic support, enhancing endogenous self-repair mechanisms such as neurogenesis, angiogenesis, and synaptogenesis. As discussed in Chapter 2 by Dr. Michael Chopp, transplants could also attenuate gliosis and scar formation after a stroke. Depending on the time course of transplantation, cells administered to the brain might also prevent the ongoing damage by inhibiting cell death or reducing inflammation.

A tantalizing new concept to explain some of the effects of transplanted cells is cell fusion. Studies from the laboratory of Dr. Alvarez-Buylla provide evidence that transplanted cells may fuse with host mature cells within individual organs. He has shown that bone marrow cells fuse spontaneously with neural stem cells in cell culture, and bone marrow transplantation leads to the fusion of marrow cells with cardiomyoctes in the heart, hepatocytes in the liver, and Purkinje cells in the brain (2). Whether there is fusion of transplanted cells with endogenous stem or mature cells in the brain after a stroke is unknown, and the mechanisms of how cell fusion would affect recovery from stroke is purely speculative. In addition, we do not know whether other types of donor cells besides bone marrow undergo fusion when transplanted.

3. CRITERIA FOR TRANSPLANTATION AND AVAILABLE CELL TYPES

What do we need to design a safe and effective cell-based therapy for stroke? First, we need a reliable and readily available source of cells. The cells should be proliferative to allow for ex vivo production of high numbers. Second, there should be adequate differentiation into all desired cell types, but some daughter cells may need to retain the properties of stem cells. Third, once transplanted, the cells should localize to sites of injury to exert a functional effect. Fourth, transplanted cells should remain viable, not be rejected by the immune system, and withstand the adverse environment of the damaged brain. Finally, transplants should pose no untoward effects such as tumor formation or seizures. We are a long way from achieving these goals.

4. VARIOUS TYPES OF CELLS UNDER INVESTIGATION

Many types of adult, fetal, and embryonic stem cells might be suitable to meet these criteria, but extensive work lies ahead to better understand stem cell biology. Some have argued, and with good reason, that the biology of stem cells should be better characterized before embarking on their application as therapeutics for neurological disorders. Given the ethical and political considerations and limited supply of human fetal tissue, there is little work on human embryonic stem cells and human fetal neural stem cells in stroke. Other sources of stem cells with potential to differentiate into neurons have been investigated, including bone marrow, umbilical cord, and adipose tissue. Dr. Chopp and his colleagues discuss their extensive work on bone marrow stromal cells. Drs. Alison Willing and Paul Sanberg present their work on umbilical cord stem cells and Dr. Henry Rice discusses the use of stromal cells from adipose tissue as another potential source of stem cell therapy for stroke.

An alternative approach is to use immortalized human cells with neural stem cell properties. Dr. Lawrence Wechsler discusses his center's trial experience with the Layton Bioscience (LBS) neurons, a cell line that was originally derived from a testicular teratochorio-carcinoma. This cell line, the NT-2 cells, possesses the properties of neural stem cells: after exposure to retinoic acid, they can differentiate into various types of neurons capable of forming dendrites and synapses. Another cell line that has recently emerged is CTX0E03 designed by investigators at ReNeuron Inc., derived from human fetal brain tissue and immortalized with the c-mycER(TAM) gene, allowing for controlled clonal expansion and differentiation under the regulation of tamoxifen.

5. ALTERNATIVE APPROACHES, MODELS, AND ANCILLARY TESTING

Rather than exogenous cell transplantation, in Chapter 7 Dr. Mark Mehler from Albert Einstein College of Medicine argues for a multi-factorial augmentation of the endogenous neural stem cell response to ischemic stroke. Dr. Mehler lays out a vision of enhancing the brain's self-repair mechanism, including stem cell activation, expansion, migration, differentiation, and neural network remodeling.

In addition to ischemic stroke, cell-based therapies are also being pursued in other causes of stroke. Dr. Jae-Kyu Roh and his colleagues have been investigating the effects of transplanted neural stem cells in animal models of intracerebral hemorrhage. They find that intracerebral or systemic delivery of transplanted cells accelerates recovery in rats. This is encouraging data that suggest we may in the future be able to use cell-based therapies for other types of stroke.

Throughout the book, many chapters detail the potential benefits of various types of cells and approaches for ischemic and hemor-rhagic stroke, and all studies rely upon traditional histological and functional outcomes. A major step forward in our understanding of cell-based therapies for neurological disorders will come from the ability to observe transplanted cells in the brain. Dr. Mathias Hoehn in Chapter 5 discusses cutting edge work from his laboratory and others on novel imaging methods to monitor implanted cells. This work raises hope that we will one day be able to track transplanted cells in stroke patients.

While there is much enthusiasm for cell-based approaches to enhance recovery, stem cell research continues to be a politically and ethically charged topic in the United States. Dr. Ruth Macklin, an internationally renowned bioethicist, addresses the ethical considera-tions surrounding stem cell research in Chapter 8 and discusses the recent political debates on the president's position and federal laws limiting stem cell research.

We hope this book provides an overview of the field, stimulates ideas for further research, will help serve as a foundation on which cell-based therapies can move forward as a viable approach for stroke recovery in the future. There is much hype and hope about cell therapy for stroke and stem cells in general, but we believe cell transplantation holds potential to advance stroke recovery.

Sean I. Savitz, MD
Daniel M. Rosenbaum, MD

References

1. Matchar DB, Duncan PW, Samsa GP et al. The Stroke Prevention Patient Outcomes Research Team. Goals and methods. Stroke 1993;24:2135–2142.
2. Alvarez-Dolado M, Pardal R, Garcia-Verdugo JM, et al. Fusion of bone-marrow-derived cells with Purkinje neurons, cardiomyocytes and hepatocytes. Nature 2003;425:968–973.

Contents

Contributors

LOUIS CAPLAN, MD • Department of Neurology, Beth Israel
  Deaconess Medical Center, Harvard Medical School, Boston, MA
NING CHEN • Center of Excellence for Aging & Brain Repair and
  Departments of Neurosurgery, University of South Florida,
  Tampa, FL
MICHAEL CHOPP, PhD • Department of Neurology, Henry Ford Health
  Sciences Center, Detroit, MI, Department of Physics, Oakland
  University, Rochester, MI, and Department of Neurology, Henry
  Ford Health Sciences Center, Detroit, MI
KON CHU, MD • Stroke and Neural Stem Cell Laboratory, Clinical
  Research Institute, Stem Cell Research Center, Department
  of Neurology, Seoul National University Hospital, Seoul,
  Republic of Korea
MAXIM D. HAMMER, MD • Stroke Institute, University of Pittsburgh
  Medical School, Pittsburgh, PA
MATHIAS HOEHN, PhD • Max-Planck-Institute for Neurological
  Research, Cologne, Germany
KEUN-HWA JUNG, MD • Stroke & Neural Stem Cell Laboratory,
  Clinical Research Institute, Stem Cell Research Center, Department
  of Neurology, Seoul National University Hospital, Seoul,
  Republic of Korea
DOUGLAS KONDZIOLKA, MD • Department of Neurological Surgery,
  University of Pittsburgh Medical Center, Pittsburgh, PA
YI LI, PhD • Department of Neurology, Henry Ford Health Sciences
  Center, Detroit, Michigan, Department of Physics, Oakland
  University, Rochester, MI, and Department of Neurology, Henry
  Ford Health Sciences Center, Detroit, MI
RUTH MACKLIN, PhD • Department of Epidemiology and Population
  Health, Albert Einstein College of Medicine Bronx, NY
MARK F. MEHLER, MD • Institute for Brain Disorders and Neural
  Regeneration, Departments of Neurology, Neuroscience and
  Psychiatry and Behavioral Sciences, the Rose F. Kennedy Center
  for Research in Mental Retardation and Developmental Disabilities
  and the Einstein Cancer Center, Albert Einstein College of
  Medicine, Bronx, NY
KEITH R. PENNYPACKER • Department of Pharmacology and
  Molecular Therapeutics, University of South Florida, Tampa, FL

HENRY E. RICE, MD • Department of Surgery, Duke University Medical Center, Durham, NC

JAE-KYU ROH, MD • Stroke & Neural Stem Cell Laboratory, Clinical Research Institute, Stem Cell Research Center, Department of Neurology, Seoul National University Hospital, Seoul, Republic of Korea

KRISTINE M. SAFFORD • Department of Surgery, Duke University Medical Center, Durham, NC

PAUL R. SANBERG, PhD • Center of Excellence for Aging & Brain Repair & Department of Neurosurgery, University of South Florida, Tampa, FL

SEAN I. SAVITZ, MD • Department of Neurology, University of Texas-Houston Medical School, Houston, TX

LIHONG SHEN, PhD • Department of Neurology, Henry Ford Health Sciences Center, Detroit, MI, Department of Physics, Oakland University, Rochester, MI, and Department of Neurology, Henry Ford Health Sciences Center, Detroit, MI

LAWRENCE R. WECHSLER, MD • Stroke Institute, University of Pittsburgh Medical School, Pittsburgh, PA

SUSANNE WEGENER, PhD • University of California San Diego Center for Functional MRI, San Diego, CA

A. E. WILLING, PhD • Center of Excellence for Aging & Brain Repair & Departments of Neurosurgery, University of South Florida, Tampa, FL

Color Plates

Color Plates follow p. 78.

the T2-weighted images; the T2* presentation (**C**) is rather insensitive to the depiction of the ischemic lesion on the right hemisphere. Groups of migrating cells are marked by blue arrows while stem cells in the perilesional target zone are indicated by red arrows. Cells having reached the ischemic boundary zone from the cisterna magna (**A**) are marked by white arrows, showing the cell persistence for at least 5 weeks after injection. ((**A**) courtesy of Michael Chopp, Detroit; (**B**) courtesy of Mike Modo, London.

Color Plate 6   Correlation between histology (left) and luciferase bioluminescence imaging (right). Neural progenitor cells, transfected to stably express β-galactosidase and luciferase, were injected into the left, normal hemisphere of a mouse following stroke induction on the right hemisphere. In the first two animals, cells were injected into the parenchyma (white arrow on histological section). In the third animal, cells were intraventricularly injected. In the case of the infarcted animals (first animal and third animal), cells were found at the ischemic lesion periphery at 21 days after implantation. In the sham-operated animal (second animal), cells have not migrated away from the primary implantation site. (Taken with permission from 69.)

Safety and Efficacy of Transplanting Immortalized Neural Stem Cells in Stroke Patients

Maxim D. Hammer, MD, Douglas Kondziolka, MD and Lawrence R. Wechsler, MD

1. INTRODUCTION: STROKE, DISABILITY, AND THE NEED FOR REPAIR STRATEGIES

Since the publication of the National Institute of Neurological Disorders and Stroke (NINDS) tissue plasminogen activator (tPA) trial in 1995 *(1)*, the management of ischemic stroke has been focused on acute therapy. Even so, relatively few stroke patients receive intravenous tPA *(2)* or other forms of acute treatment. The natural history of stroke is such that only approximately 25% of victims survive with minimal deficits, while most of the remainder suffer disabling weakness or cognitive deficits, and in fact, comprise the largest cause of long-term disability in the USA *(2)*.

A neuronal repair therapy is being sought for the growing number of permanently disabled stroke survivors. This would fundamentally require the replacement of lost neurons in a self-sustainable tissue milieu. Furthermore, it would necessitate the reintegration of the replacement cells into networks involving unaffected brain, in order to ultimately restore functions that have been lost. It is hoped that transplantation of multipotent progenitor cells, along with adequate trophic support, may accomplish these goals.

From: *Current Clinical Neurology: Stroke Recovery with Cellular Therapies*
Edited by: Sean I. Savitz and Daniel M. Rosenbaum © Humana Press Inc., Totowa, NJ

2. NEUROTRANSPLANTATION

2.1. Precedent for Neurotransplantation

   Cell therapies for Parkinson's disease (PD) have been the frontier of neurotransplantation. Transplantation of neural stem cells into the substantia nigra was first reported by Bjorklund in 1971 *(3)* and has been achieved in multiple animal and human studies since then *(4)*. The animal studies collectively suggested at least temporary graft survival and improvement of function. The two human trials, which were both randomized, double-blinded, and sham-controlled studies, were unable to demonstrate an overall benefit *(5,6)*. However, there was significant and long-lasting benefit among the younger patients in both studies. The high incidence of adverse effects, along with the emergence of promising alternative treatments such as deep brain stimulation, has shifted the focus away from fetal cell transplantation for PD. Nevertheless, the wealth of research data acquired over the last 25 years suggests at least a potential for success of transplantation in restoring lost neurologic function, in the setting of chronic neurodegenerative disease.

2.2. Sources of Transplant Cells

   Stem cells must possess two characteristics: they must be able to replicate and they must have the capacity for differentiation into multiple cell lines *(7)*. Stem cells vary in their degree of potential for differentiation. Totipotent cells can form the embryo, as well as any cell line. Pluripotent cells cannot form an embryo, but can differentiate into cells of multiple different tissue cell lines. Multipotent cells can only produce a limited set of cell lines, appropriate for a given tissue environment. Unipotent cells can only generate one cell type.
   Thus, fetal tissue can possibly yield pluripotent stem cells and certainly generate organ-specific multipotent stem cells. Of course, the use of human fetal tissue is controversial for ethical reasons and limited (in the USA) by recent legislative restrictions. Other potential sources for stem cells exist. Multipotent stem cells have been identified within adult tissue, including brain, although not in sufficient numbers to be reasonably extracted for clinical use *(8)*. In some organs, notably the bone marrow, multipotent cells have shown a capacity to "change their minds" and transdifferentiate into lineages of other organs, including neural cells *(9,10)*. There is evidence that human umbilical cord blood

cells (HUBCs) may also manifest transdifferentiation *(11)*. Finally, tumor cell lines occasionally yield lines of immortal, organ-specific, multipotent stem cells.

An example of a tumor cell line that may prove useful in neurotransplantation is the Ntera 2/cl.D12 (NTs) human embryonic carcinoma-derived cell line *(12)*. These cells replicate and differentiate into human neuronal cells *(13,14)*. Thus, NTs have the characteristics of multipotent neural stem cells.

When transplanted, these neuronal cells survive, extend processes, express neurotransmitters, form functional synapses, and integrate with the host. The final cells appear virtually indistinguishable from terminally differentiated, postmitotic neurons. The cells are capable of differentiation to express different neuronal markers characteristic of mature neurons. Their neuronal phenotype makes them a promising candidate for replacement in central nervous system disorders, as a virtually unlimited supply of pure, postmitotic, terminally differentiated human neuronal cells.

2.3. Multipotent Cell Transplants in Animal Models of Stroke

In 1998, Borlongan et al. showed that transplants of LBS-neurons could reverse the deficits caused by a stroke *(15)*. They used a rat model of permanent focal ischemia. At 1 month postischemia surgery, they selected all rats that showed significant behavioral deficits and randomized this group to receive transplantation either of fetal rodent striatal cells ($n = 8$) or human embryonic carcinoma-derived (hNT) neurons ($n = 14$). They had an existing set of 22 control rats that received transplants of either cerebellar cell or cell medium. They tested all animals at 1, 2, 3, and 6 months after surgery, having noted previously that ischemic animals continue to display significant deficits for >3 months postischemia. They used the passive avoidance test (the same test used to identify rats with significant deficits poststroke) and the elevated body swing test (EBST), a measure of motor asymmetry. The rats who received either striatal fetal cells or hNT neurons significantly outperformed the controls; rats receiving hNT had a significantly earlier recovery of behavioral deficits compared to those who received the striatal fetal cells. Similarly, rats who received hNT neurons recovered motor symmetry significantly faster than those receiving striatal fetal cells, while both of these groups significantly outperformed the controls. Immunohistochemical staining done on treatment rats showed that there was survival of the grafted cells after 6 months.

2.4. Cell Transplants in Human Stroke

The transplantation of hNT neurons into the brains of humans with stroke has now undergone Phase I and Phase II trials, with promising results.

The first clinical study of transplantation of the immortalized line of hNT cells into human stroke victims was conducted at the University of Pittsburgh. The goal was to demonstrate the safety and feasibility of the neuronal cell implantation procedure. The study was an open-label trial with observer-blinded neurologic evaluation of patients with stroke who received stereotactic implants of human neuronal cells.

Patients with basal ganglia infarcts and stable motor deficits were enrolled. They had to have had strokes between 6 months and 6 years prior to transplantation. The mean time since onset of the stroke was actually 27 months (range 7 to 55). Cells were delivered stereotactically via three 20-μl injections along a single trajectory through the infarct. The first four patients received 2 million cells via single-pass injections into the area of infarction. The next eight patients were randomized to receive either 2 or 6 million cells (three separate stereotactic trajectories with three injections each around the stroke). Because of concerns for cell rejection, the patients were given intravenous methylprednisolone during the procedure, followed by cyclosporine-A administration beginning 1 week before surgery and for 8 weeks following.

Patients were evaluated for safety and efficacy at ten intervals over the 52 weeks following surgery. Disability was assessed using the National Institutes of Health Stroke Scale (NIHSS), European Stroke Scale (ESS), and Barthel Index (BI). Positron emission tomography using fluorodeoxyglucose (FDG-PET) and magnetic resonance imaging (MRI) scans were obtained at baseline; MRI was repeated at weeks 4 and 24, while PET was repeated at weeks 24 and 52.

The goals of demonstrating safety were met, with no adverse events related to implantation. One patient developed renal insufficiency attributed to the cyclosporine-A. One patient, whose infarct involved temporal lobe cortical tissue, had a generalized seizure 6 months after the surgery and was treated successfully with anticonvulsant medication. One patient had a subsequent stroke, remote from the site of neuronal transplantation, 6 months after the surgery. No malignancies, deaths, or cell-related adverse events occurred in the follow-up period.

Although the study was not designed as an efficacy study, the functional outcomes suggested clinical benefit. The ESS, which had been stable between the preoperative evaluation and the day of surgery, improved in 6 of the 12 patients, remained unchanged in 3, and deteriorated in 3, compared with baseline scores. The mean improvement in ESS from baseline to week 24 was 2.9 points, achieving significance ($p = 0.046$). Motor improvement accounted for much of the clinical improvement in the ESS in the patients enrolled in this first study. The NIHSS seemed to improve overall in the group, without achieving significance: eight patients had improved, one was unchanged, and three deteriorated at the 24-week follow-up. The BI did not change significantly.

Serial MRI scans showed no changes in the brain after the surgery when compared with baseline. The serial PET scans, however, manifested differences between the baseline and follow-up studies done 6 months later. There was an increase in $\geq 15\%$ in the relative uptake of FDG within the transplant site, in 6 of 11 patients. This increased metabolic activity suggests the return of viable neurons to the areas of infarction. While an inflammatory response could produce such findings, there was no sign of inflammation on serial MRI.

The suggestion of cell survival in the serial PET studies was corroborated by some pathological data. One of the patients, a 71-year-old man, died of a presumed myocardial infarction 27 months following the transplantation surgery. He was one of the patients who demonstrated no motor recovery. Histochemical stains of his brain demonstrated a population of neurons at the graft site. Many of these were NF protein immunoreactive, suggesting that they were nNT neurons. This was confirmed with a special single chromosome 21-specific probe (specific for hNT neurons) that detected multiple signals in nuclei within the area of the graft.

Therefore, in the Phase I study, transplantation of the hNT neurons into areas of stroke was shown to be both safe and feasible. The transplant cells survived, and there was even a suggestion of clinical benefit. A Phase II dose–response trial was undertaken at two centers (University of Pittsburgh and Stanford University). Patients were randomized. The first seven of these received 5 million cells along five trajectories with five injections each (i.e., one million cells per trajectory), while another seven patients received 10 million cells, along five trajectories and with five injections each. There were four control patients. All patients received cyclosporine for 6 months as well as focused stroke rehabilitation. The primary outcome was the motor ESS at 6 months. NIHSS, ESS, and MRI were done on routine follow-up.

The safety results of the Phase II trial were similar to the those of Phase I, with no major medical complications of the procedure and no lasting effects due to implantation or cyclosporine administration. One patient experienced a syncopal episode, 1 month following surgery. One patient experienced a seizure 1 day after surgery. One patient, who was on aspirin and clopidogrel combination therapy, underwent surgical drainage of a chronic subdural hematoma, 1 month following transplant.

Two of the four control patients experienced improvements in their motor ESS scores after 6 months of physical therapy. The range of change on this scale was −0.5 to +3.5 points. Of the transplant group, 8 of the 14 improved after 6 months, and the range was −5.5 to +14.5. Overall, the transplant group had a statistically insignificant improvement in motor ESS over the control group ($p = 0.148$). However, the relatively large degree of improvement of some of the transplant patients was notable.

Unexpected improvements were also noted in some of the secondary outcome measurements. For example, there seemed to be a trend toward improvement in the treatment group with respect to hand and wrist movement. Interestingly, there were significant improvements in certain neuropsychological measurements, such as visuospatial construction and retention, and nonverbal memory, in the treatment group compared with the controls. These results were recently published *(16,17)*.

From these first two trials, it is inferred that stereotactic cell implantation of immortalized multipotent neural stem cells, derived from a tumor cell line, is relatively safe and devoid of delayed cell-related adverse effects; the transplanted cells survive in vivo; and some patients that received cell transplants showed motor and cognitive improvements. Future trials using this cell line will have to address optimal patient selection, timing of surgery, number of cells needed, optimal implant location, and the need for immunosuppression.

2.5. Possible Mechanisms

It remains unclear exactly how hNT neuron transplants exert their effects in animal stroke models and their possible effects in humans with stroke. There is suggestive evidence that the transplanted cells do survive. It remains to be proven whether they also integrate into the existing neural network that surrounds them, although the surprising improvement in cognition that was observed in some of the transplant patients, if attributable to the transplant, implies that function is being restored.

There must also be other mechanisms involved. The improvements noted in the bone marrow stromal cell *(18)* pilot trial (BMSC, refer to chapter 3) and in the HUBC animal models *(19)* (refer to chapter 4) occurred too soon to be attributable to neuronal integration. Perhaps, the transplanted cells induced a host response, such as the secretion of neurotrophic factors, which independently promoted recovery. BMSCs are known to secrete interleukins (IL)-6, IL-7, IL-8, IL-12, IL-14, IL-15, along with macrophage stimulating factor, Flt-3 ligand, and stem cell factor *(20)*. These cytokines have been identified as promoters of growth and survival for mouse hippocampal neuron progenitor cells *(21)*. BMSCs also release neurotransmitters which can supplement for lost neurons after ischemia. It is therefore possible that these or other trophic factors could perhaps stimulate synaptic sprouting in damaged brain tissue.

3. CONCLUSION

Stroke is a major cause of disability, and a repair strategy needs to be developed. Cell therapies have the potential for providing a means of repairing brain tissue that has been permanently injured by stroke.

There are several sources of neuronal progenitor cells that are under investigation. In animal models, it has been successfully shown that fetal cell transplants are able to survive and convey functional recovery. BMSCs and HUBCs seem to be able to transdifferentiate into neuronal cells and survive in the brains of animals with stroke. On the other hand, further research is required to determine the functional significance of this mode of transplantation. Implanted tumor-derived neuronal progenitor cells (hNT neurons) survive and convey functional improvement in animals. There is promising preliminary evidence that the same holds true for humans.

Once a source of neuronal progenitor cells can be found that can consistently differentiate into viable neuronal cells and then survive within stroke-injured brain tissue, further research will then be able to refine the process. Future research would then focus on determining the ideal timing of transplantation, selection of the best size and location of the cellular implant, and possibly even optimizing the cellular environment by controlling local trophic factor concentrations. The goal is to replace lost neurons in a self-sustainable tissue milieu, and reintegrate the replacement cells into existing neural networks, in order to ultimately restore functions that have been lost.

REFERENCES

1. Tissue plasminogen activator for acute ischemic stroke. The National Institute of Neurological Disorders and Stroke rt-PA Stroke Study Group. *N Engl J Med* 1995;333(24):1581–1587.
2. American Heart Association. 2004.
3. Bjorklund A, Steveni U. Growth of central catecholamine neurones into smooth muscle grafts in the rat mesencephalon. *Brain Res* 1971;31(1):1–20.
4. Roitberg B, Urbaniak K, Emborg M. Cell transplantation for Parkinson's disease. *Neurol Res* 2004;26(4):355–362.
5. Freed CR, Greene P, Breeze RE, et al. Transplantation of embryonic dopamine neurons for severe Parkinson's disease. *N Engl J Med* 2001;344(10):710–719.
6. Olanow CW, Goetz C, Kordower JH, et al. A double-blind controlled trial of bilateral fetal nigral transplantation in Parkinson's disease. *Ann Neurol* 2003;54(3):403–414.
7. Preston SL, Alison M, Forbes SJ, Direkze NC, Poulsom R, Wright NA. The new stem cell biology: something for everyone. *Mol Pathol* 2003;56(2):86–96.
8. Gu W, Brannstrom T, Wester P. Cortical neurogenesis in adult rats after reversible photothrombotic stroke. *J Cereb Blood Flow Metab* 2000;20:1166–1173.
9. Sanchez-Ramos J, Song S, Cardozo-Pelaex F. Adult bone marrow stromal cells differentiate into neural cells in vitro. *Exp Neurol* 2000;164:247–256.
10. Woodbury D, Schwarz EJ, Prockop DJ, Black IB. Adult rat and human bone marrow stromal cells differentiate into neurons. *J Neursci Res* 2000;61:364–370.
11. Sanchez-Ramos JR, Song S, Kamath SG. Expression of neural markers in human umbilical cord blood. *Exp Neurol* 2001;171:109–115.
12. Kleppner SR, Robinson KA, Trojanowski JQ, Lee VM. Transplanted human neurons derived from a teratocarcinoma cell line (NTera-2) mature, integrate, and survive for over 1 year in the nude mouse brain. *Comp Neurol* 1995;357(4):618–632.
13. Trojanowski JQ, Mantione JR, Lee JH, et al. Neurons derived from a human teratocarcinoma cell line establish molecular and structural polarity following transplantation into the rodent brain. *Exp Neurol* 1993;122(2):283–294.
14. Pleasure SJ, Lee VM. NTera 2 cells: a human cell line which displays characteristics expected of a human committed neuronal progenitor cell. *J Neursci Res* 1993;35(6):585–602.
15. Borlongan CV, Tajima Y, Trojanowski JQ, Lee VM, Sanberg PR. Transplantation of cryopreserved human embryonal carcinoma-derived neurons (NT2N cells) promotes functional recovery in ischemic rats. *Exp Neurol* 1998;149(2):310–321.
16. Kondziolka D, Steinberg GK, Wechsler LR, et al. Neurotransplantation for patients with subcortical motor stroke: a phase 2 randomized trial. *J Neurosurg* 2005;103(1):38–45.
17. Stilley CS, Ryan CM, Kondziolka D, Bender A, Decesare S, Wechsler LR. Changes in cognitive function after neuronal cell transplantation for basal ganglia stroke. *Neurology* 2004;35:585–602.
18. Bang OY, Lee JS, Lee PH, Lee G. Autologous mesenchymal stem cell transplantation in stroke patients. *Ann Neurol* 2005;57:874–882.

19. Chen J, Sanberg PR, Li Y, et al. Intravenous administration of human umbilical cord blood reduces behavioral deficits after stroke in rats. *Stroke* 2001;32(11):2682–2688.
20. Eaves CJ, Cashman JD, Kay RJ, Dougherty GJ, Otsuka T, Gaboury SL, Gerson SL. Mechanisms that regulate the cell cycle status of very primitive hematopoietic cells in long-term human marrow cultures: analysis of positive and negative regulators produced by stromal cells within the adherent layer. *Blood* 1991;78:110–117.
21. Mehler MF, Rozental R, Dougherty M, Spray DC, Kessler JA. Cytokine regulation of neuronal differentiation of hippocampal progenitor cells. *Nature* 1993;362:62–65.

2

Transplantation of Bone Marrow Stromal Cells for the Treatment of Stroke

Michael Chopp, Yi Li and Lihong Shen

1. INTRODUCTION

We focus on data generated in our laboratory using bone marrow stromal cells (BMSCs) in rodents for the treatment of stroke. BMSCs obtained from donor rats, mice, or humans have been transplanted into the rodent central nervous system (CNS) via local and systemic routes. BMSCs selectively target damaged tissue, promote neurological functional recovery, and remodel brain architecture. Although some BMSCs express proteins phenotypic of neural cells, it is highly unlikely that benefit is derived by replacement of damaged tissues and rewiring brain with transdifferentiated BMSCs. The far more likely explanation is that BMSCs secrete and induce within host parenchymal cells expression of growth or trophic factors that activate endogenous restorative processes, e.g., angiogenesis, synaptogenesis, gliogenesis, and neurogenesis (Fig. 1).

The brain after stroke or neural injury responds by necrotic and apoptotic cell death in damaged areas and reverts to a quasi-developmental state in perilesional areas. This developmental state is recognized at the molecular level. Embryonic and developmental proteins and genes are expressed in adult damaged brains. Proteins such as nestin *(1,2)*, growth-associated protein-43 (GAP-43) *(3,4)*, cyclin D1*(4)*, synaptophysin *(5)*, vascular endothelial growth factor (VEGF) *(6)* that promote neurogenesis, synaptogenesis, and angiogenesis are profusely expressed in the region of tissue adjacent to the ischemic lesion. Within the ischemic boundary tissue having quasi-developmental characteristics, we hypothesized that stem and progenitor cells in the subventricular zone (SVZ) respond to and affect

From: *Current Clinical Neurology: Stroke Recovery with Cellular Therapies*
Edited by: Sean I. Savitz and Daniel M. Rosenbaum © Humana Press Inc., Totowa, NJ

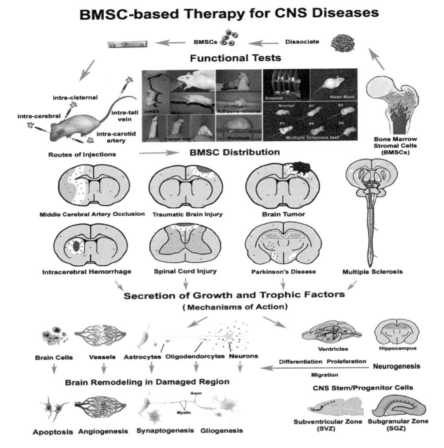

Fig. 1. Illustration of our experimental studies supporting the potential treatment of central nervous system (CNS) disorders with bone marrow stromal cells (BMSCs). BMSCs are extracted, separated, and cultured. They are then injected via different local or systemic routes into the animal with CNS diseases. A battery of neurological functional tests are performed, such as the mNSS (e.g., raising the rat tail shows forepaw flexes for motor test, closing the rat to an object shows no vision for sensory test, and beam balance test), adhesive-removal test (A-R test, time of removal of a sticky tab from the paw), corner test (turning in one versus the other direction while the vibrissae are stimulated), footfault test (the foot falls while walking on a grid), rotarod test (the duration of persisting on an accelerating treadmill), water maze test (learning and memory), and specific grading 0–5 score for multiple sclerosis test. BMSCs selectively migrate and survive in the damaged tissue and the perilesion areas in the animals with stroke, traumatic brain injury, intracerebral hemorrhage, spinal cord injury, brain tumor, and multiple sclerosis. An array of restorative events are mediated by BMSC and possibly by parenchymal cell secretion of cytokines, growth

this developmental microenvironment. These molecular alterations of the ischemic boundary zones occur at a time at which there is enhanced neurogenesis in the SVZ *(7,8)*. These two remodeling events may act synergistically to promote repair of brain and recovery of neurological function. Adult brain is a highly dynamic structure *(9)*. The adult brain has the ability to repair itself with its endogenous pool of parenchymal cells; however, the supply of such pools is limited. Novel strategies for the treatment of stroke and other CNS disorders are needed in order to enhance the recovery process.

Bone marrow is composed of nonadherent hematopoetic and adherent stromal cell compartments. BMSCs provide a stromal microenvironment for hematopoiesis, including stem-cell factor (SCF), granulocyte colony-stimulating factors (G-CSF), macrophage colony-stimulating factors (M-CSF), granulocyte-macrophage colony-stimulating factor (GM-CSF), tumor necrosis factors, interferon-gamma (IFN-gamma), and interleukins (IL)-6 and IL-7 *(10,11)*. Some of the cytokines have been reported to exert influence on proliferation and differentiation of cells. These data indicate that BMSCs supply autocrine, paracrine, and juxtacrine factors that influence the cells of the marrow microenvironment itself *(10)*. In addition to cytokines, BMSCs express factors associated with bone formation such as bone morphogenetic proteins (BMPs) *(11)*, which define patterning and morphogenesis, and play a regulatory role during differentiation of embryonic cells, by modifying mesodermal and neuroectodermal pathways *(12)*. BMSCs also secrete neurotrophins that are target-derived soluble factors required for neuronal survival, including nerve growth factor (NGF) and brain-derived neurotrophic factor (BDNF) *(11)*.

2. TREATMENT OF CNS DISEASES WITH BMSCS

We have performed therapeutic interventions with bone marrow cells for experimental stroke *(7,13–20)*, traumatic brain injury, intracerebral hemorrhage, spinal cord injury, Parkinson's disease, multiple

Fig. 1. *(Continued)* factors, and trophic factors, e.g., NGF, BDNF, bFGF, VEGF, and IGF. These factors may decrease apoptosis, increase angiogenesis, gliogenesis, synaptogenesis, and neurogenesis for brain remodeling and may enhance neuroprotective and neurorestorative mechanisms to improve functional recovery. (*See* Color Plate 1 following p. 78.)

sclerosis, and brain tumors in more than 6,000 rodents. Our data reveal an obvious reduction of neurological deficits with BMSCs for all studies; efficacy is dependent upon the strain of animal, cell origin, cell preparation and purification, route of administration, therapeutic window, as well as short-term or long-term observations.

The principal hypothesis was that these bone marrow cells promote functional recovery. A complete neurological examination was employed in our studies for stroke and traumatic brain injury (Figure 1, Neurological Functional Tests), referred to as the modified neurological severity score (mNSS). This test provides an index of motor, sensory, balance, and reflex. Additional tests were performed for stroke and other CNS disorders: adhesive-removal somatosensory test, corner test, footfault test, rotarod test, water maze test, and grading 0–5 multiple sclerosis score. A sophisticated integrated outcome analysis, call the "global test," was performed to measure the BMSC effect on functional recovery.

3. STROKE

Stroke is characterized by extensive tissue injury in the territory of an affected vessel. We have induced stroke by insertion of a nylon suture *(13)* or an embolus into the internal carotid artery to block the middle cerebral artery in the male and female *(7)* young adult (2–3 months), and retired breeder (10–12 m) rats *(18)*, as well as mice. After onset of cerebral ischemia, brain cells die by necrosis or apoptosis *(21–23)*. The ischemic boundary zone (the penumbra of infarct) is a metabolically, biochemically, and molecularly active region where a variety of mutagens, trophic factors, adhesion molecules, and intra- and extracellular matrix molecules, among others, are uniquely elaborated in the stroke brain *(24–28)*.

Relying on the hypothesis that BMSCs promote functional recovery after stroke, we were confronted with an array of options of implementing preclinical cellular therapy protocols. Among questions to address were "when and where to implant the cells?" We initially elected to treat the rodent 1 day after middle cerebral artery occlusion (MCAo) *(14,20)*. This time point is clinically reasonable. If deficits persist for 1 day after a stroke, then the event is classified as a stroke and not as a transient ischemic attack (TIA). We expanded the time window from 7 days *(13)* until 1 month. The most direct route of placement of cells into damaged brain is intracerebral surgical transplantation *(14)* and intracisternal cell injection *(29)* (Figure 1, Routes of intra-cerebral, intra-cisternal, intra carotidartery, and intra-tail vein Injections). The success of the direct implantation of BMSCs into the brain prompted experiments on a less invasive, vascular route of administration. The carotid artery ipsilateral to the ischemic hemisphere was cannulated for injection of BMSCs *(15)*. Then, a more clinically relevant venous route was used for BMSC administration *(13)*. As described above, rats were subjected to a battery of neurological outcome measures and exhibited significant functional improvement on these tests after treatment with BMSCs. However, dead BMSCs *(19)* and liver fibroblasts showed no therapeutic benefit above that of phosphate-buffered saline (PBS)-treated control animals.

One question addressed with histological analysis was whether BMSCs differentiate into brain parenchymal cells. It is necessary to mark the injected BMSCs, so that they can be identified in tissue. BMSCs prelabeled with bromodeoxyuridine (BrdU, a thymidine analog, which is incorporated into newly formed DNA) *(12,18)* or male derived BMSCs injected into female rats and the sex Y-chromosome identified by in situ hybridization *(5)* or human cells were injected into rats and specific anti-human antibodies (e.g., MAB1281) were employed *(14)*. BMSCs selectively target injured tissue. In all the studies, therapeutic benefit became evident within days of transplantation. Yet, the numbers of BMSCs transplanted are miniscule compared to the approximately 35–39 % of the hemispheric brain tissue infarcted after induction of MCAo. For example, at 14 days after MCAo in rats with 3×10^6 BMSC intravenous (IV) administration, approximately $3.2 \times 10^4 \pm 0.8 \times 10^4$ BMSCs survive (approximately 12 % of transplanted BMSCs) *(14)*, of which a small percentage of cells express neural proteins (approximately 1 % neuronal nuclear marker, NeuN; approximately 2 % neuronal cytoplasm marker, MAP-2; and approximately 5 % astrocytic marker, GFAP) in the injured brain, far too few to even potentially replace the infarcted tissue. Very few (approximately 0.01–0.5 %) injected BMSCs were also found in the host bone marrow, muscle, spleen, kidney, lung, and liver. Most BMSCs encircle vessels in these organs, with few cells located in parenchyma. Injected BMSC expression of brain cell phenotypic markers does not indicate true differentiation and neuronal or glial cell function.

4. MECHANISMS OF ACTION

BMSCs administered to animals with various CNS diseases provide significant functional benefit. There are multiple basic questions to address, including why the BMSCs survive in the injured brain? What mechanisms target these cells specifically to sites of injury? How do BMSCs provide their benefit? Is there any significance to the lesion-site localization of these BMSCs and to the distance-site of the germinal areas—the SVZ and SGZ? How do the BMSCs affect the brain and thereby promote restorative processes? The most interesting question is how these effects translate into therapeutic benefit?

4.1. Immune Priority of Both Brain and BMSCs

For any new treatment, safety issues must be addressed first. The immune reaction of syngeneic and allogeneic rat (r)BMSCs in rodents were investigated in stroke rats *(30)*. Wistar rats were intravenously injected with allogeneic ACI- or syngeneic Wistar-rBMSCs at 24 h after MCAo and sacrificed at 28 days. Significant functional recovery was found in both cell-treated groups compared to PBS controls, but no difference was detected between allogeneic and syngeneic cell-treated rats. T cells from mesenteric and cervical lymph nodes of syn-rBMSC or allo-rBMSC-treated rats were evaluated by T-cell activation to antigens by the one-way mixed lymphocyte reaction (MLR) assay. Rats were bled at sacrifice, and their sera were evaluated for antibodies specific for rBMSCs by flow cytometry. There was no significant difference between the two treatment groups compared with the control PBS group, indicating that syn-rBMSCs and allo-rBMSCs did not elicit immune response. Our findings of allogeneic "immune privilege" of BMSCs in the rat model suggest that the animals may have been tolerized to ACI alloantigens by the rBMSC injection. No evidence of T-cell priming or humoral antibody production to rBMSCs was found in recipient rats after treatment with allogeneic cells. Human (h)BMSCs were also injected intravenously into rats 1 day after MCAo *(16,17)*. Effective functional improvement was found after hBMSC treatment in stroke rats. T lymphocytes are implicated as an initiator of graft-versus-host fatal iatrogenic disease. Graft-versus-host T-cell response was measured using a ^{51}Cr assay to determine the lytic effect. We neither observe any indication of immunorejection nor any obvious increase in inflammatory response to hBMSCs. Additional support for the absence of rejection was obtained from evaluation of splenic cell proliferation and cytotoxic T-lymphocyte (CTL) responses of exposed splenic cells. These data indicate that although hBMSCs are capable of inducing a primary proliferative response in the rat splenic lymphocytes, the administration of hBMSCs to the rats fails to sensitize lymphocytes in vivo for a secondary in vitro proliferative response. In addition, hBMSCs failed to induce a CTL response in the rat spleen cells.

Immune monitoring studies demonstrated that syn-rBMSC and allo-rBMSC or hBMSC treatment after stroke in rats improved neurological recovery, with no indication of T-cell sensitization or antibody production in immunocompetent recipients. These findings are in agreement with previous reports showing that BMSCs do not stimulate division of allogeneic T cells in vitro, probably due to active suppressive mechanisms *(31,32)*. hBMSCs have been employed to treat patients with cancer *(33,34)*, multiple sclerosis *(35)*, and stroke *(36)*. Thus, safety data in humans are available. It is possible that, allogeneic cells, and not autologous cells, may be used to treat patients.

4.2. Targeting BMSCs to Sites of Cerebral Damage

Where do the injected cells migrate, especially after the more clinically relevant IV injection? Damaged brain appears to attract BMSCs (Figure 1, BMSC Distribution-BMSCs selectively target damaged tissue.), with the majority of these cells congregating in the perilesional areas, and many cells present adjacent to or within vessels. Signals that target inflammatory cells to injured tissue likely direct BMSCs to injury sites. Using a microchemotaxis Boyden chamber, an in vitro assay was performed for cell migration between an upper chamber and a lower chamber separated by a permeable membrane *(37)*. BMSCs are placed in the upper chamber. Chemotactic molecules macrophage such as inflammatory protein-1 (MIP-1), monocyte chemoattractant protein-1 (MCP-1), IL-8, or adhesion molecules, such as intercellular adhesion molecule-1 (ICAM-1), which attract inflammatory cells into brain tissue were placed into the lower chamber. A dose-dependent effect of chemotactic molecules on BMSC migration into the lower chamber was found. The enhanced migration was effectively blocked by placement against antibodies to these molecules into the lower chamber. This suggests that BMSCs respond to chemotactic factors as do inflammatory cells. Instead of specific chemotactic or adhesion agents, brain tissue from injured and stroke brain placed in the lower chambers also significantly increased BMSC migration *(37,38)*. These data provide insight into how the cells assume an inflammatory-like cell identity, and how they "know" to target specifically injured tissue. Thus, any brain damage, which may have an inflammatory response, including neurodegenerative processes, may guide BMSCs to the affected sites. The dependence of guidance on the degree of injury also provides a form of titration of "effective" dose of BMSCs. The more severe the injury and concomitant inflammatory response, the greater the numbers of BMSCs recruited to the site.

4.3. Secretion of Trophic Factors and Brain Remodeling

Secretion by BMSCs of an array of cytokines and trophic factors from BMSCs may activate restorative mechanisms (Figure 1, Secretion of Growth and Trophic Factors, Mechanisms of Action – Interwoven Events). BMSCs behave as small molecular "factories." We and others have demonstrated that BMSCs induce significant increases in injured brain of various trophic and growth factors, such as HGF, NGF, BDNF, VEGF, basic fibroblast growth factor (bFGF), and insulin-like growth factor 1 (IGF-1), among many others in animals *(9,39,40)*. In addition, BMSCs secrete many of these factors in vitro *(41,42)*. A very important observation is that BMSCs when cultured under different ionic microenvironments, e.g., calcium, respond to the cues of the ionic microenvironment by adjusting growth factor expression. Thus, the degree of tissue injury and the corresponding disruption of the ionic environment may dictate the secretion levels of trophic factors. It is the dynamic effect of this variety of factors secreted by BMSCs and not the single bullet of a particular growth factor that facilitates the beneficial effect. Given the assumption that BMSCs selectively enter injured brain and secrete growth and trophic factors in a tissue feedback loop, the question remains how these factors possibly alter brain to promote therapeutic benefit? We speculate that the process that promotes restoration of function is not a single modification of tissue. Therapeutic benefit is induced by a set of events associated with brain plasticity. This includes but is not restricted to a reduction of apoptosis and glial scarring, and an increase in angiogenesis, synaptogenesis, gliogenesis, reconstruct glial-axonal architectures; and within the germinal SVZ and SGZ, an increase in neurogenesis followed by cell proliferation, migration, and differentiation.

4.4. Apoptosis Versus Cell Survival

Apoptosis is an ongoing process that persists for months after stroke *(22,23)*. The perilesioned area is highly susceptible to apoptotic cell death *(22,23)*. Cell death or survival is mediated by the production of growth factors, such as NGF, within the injured brain. The reduction of apoptosis within this region may sustain cerebral rewiring. We demonstrated that treatment of stroke with BMSCs significantly reduces apoptosis within the perilesioned area after MCAo in the rat. Apoptosis is present in many cells in brain, including neurons, astrocytes, and endothelial cells after stroke. Astrocytes are the most numerous cells in the brain, and astrocytes are known to provide structural, trophic, and metabolic support for neurons. Thus, astrocytes are critical for neural survival postischemia. In our in vitro studies, we investigated the influence of BMSCs on rat astrocytic apoptosis and survival postischemia employing an anaerobic chamber. Our data indicate that BMSCs reduce apoptotic cell death and increase the DNA proliferation rate in astrocytes postischemia. MEK/Erk and PI3K/Akt pathways are involved in cell survival. Western blot showed that BMSCs activate these two pathways in astrocytes postischemia and upregulate total Erk 1/2 and Akt. BMSCs increase astrocyte survival via upregulation of PI3K/Akt and MEK/Erk pathways and stimulate astrocyte trophic factor gene expression after anaerobic insult. Since astrocytes produce various neurotrophic factors, we performed reverse transcriptase-polymerase chain reaction (RT-PCR) to investigate BMSC effect on astrocyte growth factor gene expression postischemia. We observed that BDNF, VEGF, and bFGF gene expression was enhanced by BMSC coculture. These data suggest that BMSCs increase astrocytic survival postischemic injury, which may involve the activation of MEK/Erk and PI3K/Akt pathways and upregulation of BDNF, VEGF, and bFGF.

4.5. Angiogenesis and Brain Repair

We tested the effect of BMSCs or supernatant from BMSCs on the induction of angiogenesis both in vitro and in vivo. Rats were subjected to MCAo and were injected intravenously with BMSCs at 24 h later. To examine cerebral microvessels, rats were injected intravenously with fluorescein isothocyanate (FITC)-dextran 5 min before sacrifice. Vascular structure was measured in three dimensions using quantitative laser scanning confocal microscopy. VEGF and bFGF are potent angiogenic agents *(43,44)*. Immunohistochemistry was used to identify BrdU and VEGF expression. The BMSC treatment group revealed a significant increase in total surface area of vessels in the ipsilateral hemisphere compared with PBS-treated animals. Microvessels were enlarged and exhibited a significant increase in BrdU$^+$ endothelial cells compared with PBS-treated rats. BMSC treatment promoted VEGF expression in the ischemic boundary zone. In vitro, the secretion of VEGF by BMSCs was measured using enzyme-linked immunosorbent assay (ELISA). BMSC-conditioned medium was tested by measuring the formation of capillary-like tubes from brain microvascular endothelial cells. BMSC supernatant significantly induced capillary-like tube formation compared with regular medium. BMSCs secrete and induce the expression of VEGF in vitro and in vivo, respectively, and promote endothelial cell proliferation and angiogenesis after stroke. The classic vascular corneal assay was also employed as an additional in vivo assay *(45)*. A surgical incision forms a pocket in the cornea, into which a collagen wafer coated with BMSC supernatant is placed, or alternatively BMSCs are directly placed within the pocket *(46)*. Our data demonstrated rapid and robust corneal angiogenesis in the wafer loaded with BMSC supernatant. The induction of angiogenesis is more robust with the BMSC supernatant than with the direct use of VEGF, suggesting that the supernatant is a highly effective source of angiogenic factors. Although the induction of angiogenesis does not directly translate into promotion of function, we have previously demonstrated that treatment of stroke with VEGF one or more days after stroke significantly enhances functional recovery and enhances angiogenesis *(47,48)*.

4.6. Synaptogenesis and Synaptic Modification

Though neurotrophins were initially characterized for their roles in promoting neuronal survival and differentiation, they also participate in many aspects of synapse function. Growth factors, such as BDNF and NGF, play an important role in synaptogenesis in the developing brain. A current hypothesis proposed that plasticity, and therefore, learning new skills, is based on changes in synaptic function. Synapse formation and stabilization in the CNS is a dynamic process, requiring bidirectional communication between pre- and postsynaptic partners. It is necessary for mature neurons to sprout and establish new synaptic connections in the CNS during adult life because of changes in circuitry resulting from environmental changes or cell death *(49)*. Astrocytes and possibly oligodendrocytes contribute to activity-dependent structural plasticity in the adult brain *(50)*. The powerful transport function of astrocytes helps terminate the postsynaptic action of neurotransmitters released presynaptically and the replenishment of the neurotransmitter pool. An alteration of these two processes could cause severe neuronal dysfunction and neuronal death. A significant increase of the synapse maker synaptophysin immunoreactivity was detected in rats subjected to MCAo with BMSC treatment compared with nontreated animals. The BMSC-mediated increased synapse activity may enhance functional benefit of the treatment of CNS diseases with BMSCs. This effect is mediated directly by BMSC secretion of neurotrophins or indirectly through astrocyte-related microenvironment plasticity.

4.7. Gliogenesis and Glial-Axonal Remodeling

Communication between neurons and glia is essential for axonal conduction, synaptic transmission, and information processing and is required for normal functioning of the nervous system during development and throughout adult life *(51)*. There are two types of neuronal degeneration, anterograde and retrograde degeneration, with both types of degeneration affecting the synapse. Axonal sprouting is supported by astrocytes; however, it is inhibited under some conditions by the astrocytic scar. The white matter contains large amounts of the insulating material, myelin. After stroke, myelin repair is evident in the brain *(52)*. Microglia release compounds that affect the inflammatory and immune reactions of the CNS *(53)*. Investigation of glial-axonal remodeling after CNS damage may provide insight into restorative processes after stroke. Retired breeder rats were subjected to MCAo and injected intravenously with BMSCs at 7 days and sacrificed at 4 months *(18)*. Concomitant with neurological benefit, BMSC treatment significantly decreased the thickness of the scar wall and reduced the numbers of microglia/macrophages within the scar wall. Double staining showed increased expression of an axonal marker (GAP-43), among reactive astrocytes in the scar boundary zone and in the SVZ in the treated rats. BrdU in cells preferentially colocalized with markers of astrocytes (GFAP) and oligodendrocytes (RIP) in the ipsilateral hemisphere, and gliogenesis was enhanced in the SVZ of the rats treated with BMSCs. BrdU in cells colocalized with NG-2 (oligodendrocyte precursors and/or new $NG-2^+$ glia), and RIP (early oligodendrocyte differentiation), in the SVZ and in the striatum, corpus callosum, and cingulum of the white matter. This study demonstrates that brain tissue repair is an ongoing chronic process with reactive glial-axonal remodeling.

4.8. Neurogenesis with Proliferation, Migration, and Differentiation

The CNS can partially self-repair from injury *(54–57)*. A significant increase in new cell numbers identified by BrdU$^+$ and Ki67$^+$ immunoreactivity was measured in the SVZ after stroke *(58–61)*. Many of these cells expressed progenitor-like molecular markers, such as nestin, TUJ-1, and NG-2, indicative of the activation of adult cerebral tissue into a quasi-developmental state after brain injury *(2,19)*. BMSCs amplify neurogenesis within the SVZ after MCAo. Our traumatic brain injury data confirm BMSC administration promotes endogenous cellular proliferation in rats. Newly generating cells were mainly present in the SVZ, SGZ, and boundary zone of contusion *(62)*. Induction of cell proliferation and differentiation by means of BMSCs may contribute to functional improvement after brain injury.

The presence of factors secreted from BMSCs appears to promote the rapid induction and migration of new cells from a primary source within the SVZ into the injured brain. For example, we tested the hypothesis that IV injection of BMSCs promotes bFGF secretion and SVZ cell migration in vitro and in vivo after stroke in rats subjected to 2 h MCAo and sacrificed at 14 days *(7)*. Immunohistochemistry staining of bFGF and doublecortin (DCX, a neuronal migration marker) was employed. To test whether BMSCs secrete bFGFs which promote neuronal migration, SVZ explants were extracted from rats 7 days after MCAo and cultured with supernatant of BMSCs or bFGF. The lengths of SVZ cell migration from the explant were measured in vitro. Morphological analyses revealed significant increases in the density of bFGF$^+$ cells in the ischemic boundary zone in rats with BMSC treatment compared with control. In addition, treatment with BMSCs after stroke significantly increased DCX. In vitro, SVZ explant migration was significantly enhanced by BMSC supernatant and bFGF alone compared with normal control medium. The neutralizing antibody to bFGF significantly inhibited BMSC supernatant-induced SVZ explant migration. Thus, bFGF plays an important role in neuronal migration induced by BMSC treatment after stroke. The migration of these new cells into the damaged cerebral tissue may be guided by astrocytic-like projections emanating from the SVZ *(16)*, resembling morphogenesis within the developing brain.

5. FROM BENCH TO BED

We seek to fully develop BMSC-based therapies in experimental models of CNS diseases in animals to prepare the groundwork for cell administration to the patient. As we look back at the discoveries made in the animals, one finding that stands out is that the transplanted BMSCs enhance functional recovery. Thus, BMSC transplantation appears to be a strong candidate for cell-based neurorestorative therapy. The basic biologic profiles for BMSC transplantation remain to be demonstrated, and the dynamics of affected growth factor and corresponding receptors also need to be measured. The subsequent events induced by secretions of BMSCs also require further investigation. Studies using transgenic animals are useful to tease out the role for specific growth factors. BMSCs have been employed for patients with cancer patients *(33,34)*, multiple sclerosis *(35)*, and stroke *(36)* with autologous cells. The basic and preclinical studies described in this review indicate that treatment of CNS diseases with BMSCs may provide a viable and highly effective restorative therapy. Thus, clinical studies to bring this therapeutic procedure to patients are warranted.

6. CONCLUSIONS

We have demonstrated a significant improvement in functional outcome after stroke with BMSC treatment. Mechanisms that enhance recovery from stroke have been widely studied at cellular and molecular levels. BMSC therapy can enhance the endogenous restorative mechanisms of the injured brain, assisting in its returns to a "developmental" state and supporting the processes of angiogenesis, synaptogenesis, gliogenesis, and neurogenesis, and ultimately neural reorganization. It is anticipated that cellular therapy, in combination with standard rehabilitation therapy, can improve functional outcomes following CNS diseases.

REFERENCES

1. N. Duggal, R. Schmidt-Kastner and A. M. Hakim, Nestin expression in reactive astrocytes following focal cerebral ischemia in rats, *Brain Res* 768, 1–9 (1997).
2. Y. Li and M. Chopp, Temporal profile of nestin expression after focal cerebral ischemia in adult rat, *Brain Res* 838, 1–10 (1999).
3. R. P. Stroemer, T. A. Kent and C. E. Hulsebosch, Neocortical neural sprouting, synaptogenesis, and behavioral recovery after neocortical infarction in rats, *Stroke* 26(11), 2135–2144 (1995).

4. Y. Li, N. Jiang, C. Powers and M. Chopp, Neuronal damage and plasticity identified by microtubule-associated protein 2, growth-associated protein 43, and cyclin d1 immunoreactivity after focal cerebral ischemia in rats, *Stroke* 29(9), 1972–1980 (1998).
5. L. H Shen, Y. Li, J. Chen, J. Zhang, P. Vanguri, J. Borneman and M. Chopp, Intracarotid transplantation of bone marrow stromal cells increases axonmyelin remodeling after stroke, *Neuroscience* 137, 393–399 (2006).
6. Z. Zhang and M. Chopp, Vascular endothelial growth factor and angiopoietins in focal cerebral ischemia, *Trends Cardiovasc Med* 12(2), 62–66 (2002).
7. J. Chen, Y. Li, M. Katakowski, X. Chen, L. Wang, D. Lu, M. Lu, S. C. Gautam and M. Chopp, Intravenous bone marrow stromal cell therapy reduces apoptosis and promotes endogenous cell proliferation after stroke in female rat, *J Neurosci Res* 73(6), 778–786 (2003).
8. R. Zhang, Z. Zhang, L. Wang, Y. Wang, A. Gousev, L. Zhang, K. L. Ho, C. Morshead and M. Chopp, Activated neural stem cells contribute to stroke-induced neurogenesis and neuroblast migration toward the infarct boundary in adult rats, *J Cereb Blood Flow Metab* 24(4), 441–448 (2004).
9. G. Kempermann, H. van Praag and F. H. Gage, Activity-dependent regulation of neuronal plasticity and self repair, *Prog Brain Res* 127, 35–48 (2000).
10. S. E. Haynesworth, M. A. Baber and A. I. Caplan, Cytokine expression by human marrow-derived mesenchymal progenitor cells in vitro: Effects of dexamethasone and il-1 alpha, *J Cell Physiol* 166(3), 585–592 (1996).
11. S. P. Dormady, O. Bashayan, R. Dougherty, X. M. Zhang and R. S. Basch, Immortalized multipotential mesenchymal cells and the hematopoietic microenvironment, *J Hematother Stem Cell Res* 10(1), 125–140 (2001).
12. J. Rohwedel, K. Guan, W. Zuschratter, S. Jin, G. Ahnert-Hilger, D. Furst, R. Fassler and A. M. Wo-bus, Loss of beta1 integrin function results in a retardation of myogenic, but an acceleration of neuronal, differentiation of embryonic stem cells in vitro, *Dev Biol* 201(2), 167–184 (1998).
13. J. Chen, Y. Li, L. Wang, Z. Zhang, D. Lu, M. Lu and M. Chopp, Therapeutic benefit of intravenous administration of bone marrow stromal cells after cerebral ischemia in rats, *Stroke* 32(4), 1005–1011 (2001).
14. J. Chen, Y. Li, L. Wang, M. Lu, X. Zhang and M. Chopp, Therapeutic benefit of intracerebral transplantation of bone marrow stromal cells after cerebral ischemia in rats, *J Neurol Sci* 189, 49–57 (2001).
15. Y. Li, J. Chen, L. Wang, M. Lu and M. Chopp, Treatment of stroke in rat with intracarotid administration of marrow stromal cells, *Neurology* 56(12), 1666–1672 (2001).
16. Y. Li, J. Chen, X. G. Chen, L. Wang, S. C. Gautam, Y. X. Xu, M. Katakowski, L. J. Zhang, M. Lu, N. Janakiraman and M. Chopp, Human marrow stromal cell therapy for stroke in rat: Neurotrophins and functional recovery, *Neurology* 59(4), 514–523 (2002).
17. J. Chen, Y. Li, R. Zhang, M. Katakowski, S. C. Gautam, Y. Xu, M. Lu, Z. Zhang and M. Chopp, Combination therapy of stroke in rats with a nitric oxide donor and human bone marrow stromal cells enhances angiogenesis and neurogenesis, *Brain Res* 1005, 21–28 (2004).

18. Y. Li, J. Chen, C. L. Zhang, L. Wang, D. Lu, M. Katakowski, Q. Gao, L. H. Shen, J. Zhang, M. Lu and M. Chopp, Gliosis and brain remodeling after treatment of stroke in rats with marrow stromal cells, *Glia* 49(3), 407–417 (2005).

19. Y. Li, J. Chen and M. Chopp, Adult bone marrow transplantation after stroke in adult rats, *Cell Transplant* 10(1), 31–40 (2001).

20. Y. Li, M. Chopp, J. Chen, L. Wang, S. C. Gautam, Y. X. Xu and Z. Zhang, Intrastriatal transplantation of bone marrow nonhematopoietic cells improves functional recovery after stroke in adult mice, *J Cereb Blood Flow Metab* 20(9), 1311–1319 (2000).

21. J. H. Garcia, Y. Yoshida, H. Chen, Y. Li, Z. G. Zhang, J. Lian, S. Chen and M. Chopp, Progression from ischemic injury to infarct following middle cerebral artery occlusion in the rat, *Am J Pathol* 142(2), 623–635 (1993).

22. Y. Li, V. G. Sharov, N. Jiang, C. Zaloga, H. N. Sabbah and M. Chopp, Ultrastructural and light microscopic evidence of apoptosis after middle cerebral artery occlusion in the rat, *Am J Pathol* 146(5), 1045–1051 (1995).

23. Y. Li, M. Chopp, N. Jiang, F. Yao and C. Zaloga, Temporal profile of in situ DNA fragmentation after transient middle cerebral artery occlusion in the rat, *J Cereb Blood Flow Metab* 15(3), 389–397 (1995).

24. Y. Li, M. Chopp, J. H. Garcia, Y. Yoshida, Z. G. Zhang and S. R. Levine, Distribution of the 72-kd heat-shock protein as a function of transient focal cerebral ischemia in rats, *Stroke* 23(9), 1292–1298 (1992).

25. Y. Li, M. Chopp, Z. G. Zhang, C. Zaloga, L. Niewenhuis and S. Gautam, P53-immunoreactive protein and p53 mrna expression after transient middle cerebral artery occlusion in rats, *Stroke* 25(4), 849–855 (1994).

26. Y. Li, M. Chopp, C. Powers and N. Jiang, Immunoreactivity of cyclin d1/cdk4 in neurons and oligodendrocytes after focal cerebral ischemia in rat, *J Cereb Blood Flow Metab* 17(8), 846–856 (1997).

27. R. L. Zhang, M. Chopp, Y. Li, C. Zaloga, N. Jiang, M. L. Jones, M. Miyasaka and P. A. Ward, Anti-icam-1 antibody reduces ischemic cell damage after transient middle cerebral artery occlusion in the rat, *Neurology* 44(9), 1747–1751 (1994).

28. Z. G. Zhang, M. Chopp, F. Bailey and T. Malinski, Nitric oxide changes in the rat brain after transient middle cerebral artery occlusion, *J Neurol Sci* 128(1), 22–27 (1995).

29. Z. G. Zhang, L. Zhang, Q. Jiang and M. Chopp, Bone marrow-derived endothelial progenitor cells participate in cerebral neovascularization after focal cerebral ischemia in the adult mouse, *Circ Res* 90(3), 284–288 (2002).

30. Y. Li, K. McIntosh, J. Chen, C. Zhang, Q. Gao, J. Borneman, K. Raginski, L. H. Shen, J. Zhang, D. Lu, and M. Chopp, Allogeneic bone marrow stromal cells promote glial-axonal remodeling without immuologic sensitization after stroke in rats, *Exp Neurol* 198, 313–325.

31. K. R. McIntosh, K. Beggs, R. Dodds, A. Lyubimov, A. Bartholomew, C. Cobbs, A. Smith and A. Moseley, High dose administration of allogeneic mesenchymal stem cells to immunocompetent baboons. *Suppl Bone Marrow Transplant* 29, S38 (Abstract) (2002).

32. W. T. Tse, J. D. Pendleton, W. M. Beyer, M. C. Egalka and E. C. Guinan, Suppression of allogeneic t-cell proliferation by human marrow stromal cells: Implications in transplantation, *Transplantation* 75(3), 389–397 (2003).

33. O. N. Koc, S. L. Gerson, B. W. Cooper, S. M. Dyhouse, S. E. Haynesworth, A. I. Caplan and H. M. Lazarus, Rapid hematopoietic recovery after coinfusion of autologous-blood stem cells and culture-expanded marrow mesenchymal stem cells in advanced breast cancer patients receiving high-dose chemotherapy, *J Clin Oncol* 18(2), 307–316 (2000).

34. O. N. Koc and H. M. Lazarus, Mesenchymal stem cells: Heading into the clinic, *Bone Marrow Transplant* 27(3), 235–239 (2001).

35. P. Mandalfino, G. Rice, A. Smith, J. L. Klein, L. Rystedt and G. C. Ebers, Bone marrow transplantation in multiple sclerosis, *J Neurol* 247(9), 691–695 (2000).

36. O. Y. Bang, J. S. Lee, P. H. Lee and G. Lee, Autologous mesenchymal stem cell transplantation in stroke patients, *Ann Neurol* 57(6), 874–882 (2005).

37. L. Wang, Y. Li, J. Chen, S. C. Gautam, Z. Zhang, M. Lu and M. Chopp, Ischemic cerebral tissue and mcp-1 enhance rat bone marrow stromal cell migration in interface culture, *Exp Hematol* 30(7), 831–836 (2002).

38. L. Wang, Y. Li, X. Chen, J. Chen, S. C. Gautam, Y. Xu and M. Chopp, Mcp-1, mip-1, il-8 and ischemic cerebral tissue enhance human bone marrow stromal cell migration in interface culture, *Hematology* 7(2), 113–117 (2002).

39. A. Mahmood, D. Lu and M. Chopp, Intravenous administration of marrow stromal cells (MSCs) increases the expression of growth factors in rat brain after traumatic brain injury, *J Neurotrauma* 21(1), 33–39 (2004).

40. J. Zhang, Y. Li, J. Chen, M. Yang, M. Katakowski, M. Lu and M. Chopp, Expression of insulin-like growth factor 1 and receptor in ischemic rats treated with human marrow stromal cells, *Brain Res* 1030(1), 19–27 (2004).

41. X. Chen, Y. Li, L. Wang, M. Katakowski, L. Zhang, J. Chen, Y. Xu, S. C. Gautam and M. Chopp, Ischemic rat brain extracts induce human marrow stromal cell growth factor production, *Neuropathology* 22(4), 275–279 (2002).

42. X. Chen, M. Katakowski, Y. Li, D. Lu, L. Wang, L. Zhang, J. Chen, Y. Xu, S. Gautam, A. Mahmood and M. Chopp, Human bone marrow stromal cell cultures conditioned by traumatic brain tissue extracts: Growth factor production, *J Neurosci Res* 69(5), 687–691 (2002).

43. Y. Tamada, C. Fukiage, D. L. Boyle, M. Azuma and T. R. Shearer, Involvement of cysteine proteases in bfgf-induced angiogenesis in guinea pig and rat cornea, *J Ocul Pharmacol Ther* 16(3), 271–283 (2000).

44. K. Hamano, T. S. Li, T. Kobayashi, S. Kobayashi, M. Matsuzaki and K. Esato, Angiogenesis induced by the implantation of self-bone marrow cells: A new material for therapeutic angiogenesis, *Cell Transplant* 9(3), 439–443 (2000).

45. G. A. Fournier, G. A. Lutty, S. Watt, A. Fenselau and A. Patz, A corneal micropocket assay for angiogenesis in the rat eye, *Invest Ophthalmol Vis Sci* 21(2), 351–354 (1981).

46. M. Chopp and Y. Li, Treatment of neural injury with marrow stromal cells, *Lancet Neurol* 1(2), 92–100 (2002).

47. Z. G. Zhang, L. Zhang, W. Tsang, H. Soltanian-Zadeh, D. Morris, R. Zhang, A. Goussev, C. Powers, T. Yeich and M. Chopp, Correlation of VEGF and angiopoietin expression with disruption of blood-brain barrier and angiogenesis after focal cerebral ischemia, *J Cereb Blood Flow Metab* 22(4), 379–392 (2002).

48. Z. G. Zhang, W. Tsang, L. Zhang, C. Powers and M. Chopp, Up-regulation of neuropilin-1 in neovasculature after focal cerebral ischemia in the adult rat, *J Cereb Blood Flow Metab* 21(5), 541–549 (2001).

49. S. Cohen-Cory, The developing synapse: Construction and modulation of synaptic structures and circuits, *Science* 298(5594), 770–776 (2002).
50. T. Theodosis and D. A. Poulain, *Contribution of astrocytes to activity-dependent structural plasticity in the adult brain*, pp. 175–182 Kluwer Academic/Plenum Publishers, New York (1999).
51. R. D. Fields and B. Stevens-Graham, New insights into neuron-glia communication, *Science* 298(5593), 556–562 (2002).
52. J. Fok-Seang, N. A. DiProspero, S. Meiners, E. Muir and J. W. Fawcett, Cytokine-induced changes in the ability of astrocytes to support migration of oligodendrocyte precursors and axon growth, *Eur J Neurosci* 10(7), 2400–2415 (1998).
53. N. G. Gourmala, S. Limonta, D. Bochelen, A. Sauter and H. W. Boddeke, Localization of macrophage inflammatory protein: Macrophage inflammatory protein-1 expression in rat brain after peripheral administration of lipopolysaccharide and focal cerebral ischemia, *Neuroscience* 88(4), 1255–1266 (1999).
54. V. Darsalia, U. Heldmann, O. Lindvall and Z. Kokaia, Stroke-induced neurogenesis in aged brain, *Stroke* 36(8): 1790–1795 (2005).
55. R. J. Lichtenwalner and J. M. Parent, Adult neurogenesis and the ischemic forebrain, *J Cereb Blood Flow Metab* Advance online publication 15 June (2005).
56. P. M. Rossini and G. Dal Forno, Neuronal post-stroke plasticity in the adult, *Restor Neurol Neurosci* 22(3–5), 193–206 (2004).
57. S. B. Frost, S. Barbay, K. M. Friel, E. J. Plautz and R. J. Nudo, Reorganization of remote cortical regions after ischemic brain injury: A potential substrate for stroke recovery, *J Neurophysiol* 89(6), 3205–3214 (2003).
58. Y. Li, J. Chen and M. Chopp, Cell proliferation and differentiation from ependymal, subependymal and choroid plexus cells in response to stroke in rats, *J Neurol Sci* 193(2), 137–146 (2002).
59. R. L. Zhang, Z. G. Zhang, L. Zhang and M. Chopp, Proliferation and differentiation of progenitor cells in the cortex and the subventricular zone in the adult rat after focal cerebral ischemia, *Neuroscience* 105(1), 33–41 (2001).
60. R. L. Zhang, L. Zhang, Z. G. Zhang, D. Morris, Q. Jiang, L. Wang, L. J. Zhang and M. Chopp, Migration and differentiation of adult rat subventricular zone progenitor cells transplanted into the adult rat striatum, *Neuroscience* 116(2), 373–382 (2003).
61. R. Zhang, Z. Zhang, C. Zhang, L. Zhang, A. Robin, Y. Wang, M. Lu and M. Chopp, Stroke transiently increases subventricular zone cell division from asymmetric to symmetric and increases neuronal differentiation in the adult rat, *J Neurosci* 24(25), 5810–5815 (2004).
62. S. C. Cramer and M. Chopp, Recovery recapitulates ontogeny, *Trends Neurosci* 23(6), 265–271 (2000).

3

Cord Blood Cells as a Treatment for Stroke

Alison E. Willing, Ning Chen, Keith R. Pennypacker and Paul R. Sanberg

1. WHAT DOES A STROKE THERAPY NEED TO TREAT?

The unfortunate history in the development of new treatments for stroke is that many therapeutics show such promise in experimental animal models but fail utterly when translated into the clinical setting. Tissue plasminogen activator (rtPA) and other clot busters have been rare exceptions to this general rule. Even so, not all patients receive treatment, either because they do not receive medical attention within the narrow treatment window for this drug or because they have a hemorrhagic stroke which would exacerbate tPA treatment.

Part of the reason for this failure in translating experimental therapies from the bench to the bedside is that as researchers we are not considering important variables in dealing with human patients as opposed to rodent patients. Neuroprotective therapies may work well in rats or mice where we can administer them just before or immediately after the stroke, but as yet, doctors cannot predict when their soon-to-be patients are going to have a stroke and thereby pre-empt the dire consequences of neural injury by treating them immediately after the event. Such prescience is in the realm of science fiction. Yet as researchers, we still focus on these early interventions.

Current thinking is that there are three stages of stroke (*1,2*). The underlying physiological processes in each of these stages may be different. The initial stage is characterized predominantly by excitotoxicity and peri-infarct depolarizations. During the second phase

From: *Current Clinical Neurology: Stroke Recovery with Cellular Therapies*
Edited by: Sean I. Savitz and Daniel M. Rosenbaum © Humana Press Inc., Totowa, NJ

Table 1
Putative Mechanisms of Cord Blood-Induced Brain Repair after Stroke

Mechanism		Phase of recovery	References
Neural reconstruction	Differentiate into neurons, astrocytes, oligodendrocytes	Long term	
Neuroprotective Trophic support	Prevent degeneration; stimulate remaining cells (neuritic outgrowth; protein production)	Initial—long term	*(33)*
Antiapoptotic	Prevent degeneration through interruption of the apoptotic cascade	Initial—secondary	*(30)*
Angiogenesis	↑ revascularization delivering nutrients to brain ↓ cellular and molecular infiltration of the brain by reestablishing the BBB	Secondary—long term	*(94)*
Neurogenesis	↑ generation, migration, and integration of new neurons, astrocytes, or oligodendrocytes	Secondary—long term	*(94)*
Anti-inflammatory	↓ astrocytic and microglia proinflammatory responses ↑ astrocytic and microglial anti-inflammatory responses ↓ peripheral immune cell infiltration into the brain	Secondary—long term	*(29,30,32)*

which may occur within hours to days, inflammation is the primary player that may contribute to further enlargement of the stroke lesion. During this time, cells within the penumbral region surrounding the core die through apoptotic mechanisms. The third phase involves the secondary degeneration, scar formation, and repair/regeneration responses, occurring over weeks. It is with these three very different phases of injury and the underlying processes occurring in each that we must focus on if we are to develop effective therapies for stroke or any other brain injury or disease. These considerations must also dictate the testing paradigm we employ. If we want to develop good candidate therapies that will have an impact on the stroke patient, we must carefully design our studies to mimic the clinical situation. The promise of human umbilical cord blood (HUCB) cells as a treatment for stroke is that unlike many putative therapies, these cells can target the second inflammatory phase of stroke injury.

It is not just in the realm of stroke treatments that the viewpoint on drug discovery and therapy development is changing. The standard in developing pharmacologics has been to focus on a single molecular target. However, the underlying degenerative process in stroke or any other neurologic disease involves an intertwining of many different processes, and treating one will not necessarily change the outcome of the disease. The current focus is shifting to a multifunctional approach in which a single pharmacologic has multiple molecular or biochemical targets and can therefore treat the disease or consequences of injury more fully *(3)*. From this perspective, HUCB is a multifunctional biologic therapy. The cells modify more than one physiological process to induce recovery (*see* Table 1). The more we have studied these cells, the more our understanding of the possible mechanisms of action of these cells has expanded as well as our appreciation of their potential. In the following pages, we retrace the journey from the first use of these cells in experimental models of stroke to the current understanding of how these cells work as a therapeutic agent and how they meet the objective of any stroke therapy—decreasing neurodegeneration and increasing the therapeutic window.

2. HUCB AS A SOURCE OF STEM CELLS

Initially, our excitement and optimism over the HUCB cells hinged on the presence of a stem cell population within the circulating mononuclear cell fraction. The concept of treating stroke through administration of HUCB was born at a time when researchers were beginning to think that adult stem cells could exhibit much more plasticity than originally believed. With the right environment and stimuli, it was believed that resident stem cells from anywhere in the body could become cells from anywhere else. For example, bone marrow has both hematopoietic stem cells responsible for repopulating the immune system and non-hematopoietic or mesenchymal stem cells, which have been shown to give rise to connective tissue throughout the body. While the mesenchymal stem cell from bone marrow was known to differentiate into adipocytes *(4)*, fibroblasts, smooth muscle cells, endothelial cells, and osteoblasts *(5)*, these were cells that shared the same mesodermal origin. It was much more startling when reports began to emerge that marrow-derived cells could be observed expressing neural antigens in the brain *(6–11)*. Soon reports emerged that the opposite was also true—neural stem cells can produce nonneural hematopoietic cells *(12)*.

Against this background, there was great hope that HUCB, which is a rich source of hematopoietic stem cells, could also be coaxed to differentiate into neurons, astrocytes, and oligodendrocytes. It is estimated that approximately 2 % of the HUCB cells are stem cells capable of reconstituting blood lineages; this is similar to the percentage observed in bone marrow *(13–16)*. These hematopoietic stem cells have been used to reconstitute bone marrow and blood cell lineages; outcome as defined by engraftment and relapse rate was comparable to outcome after bone marrow transplantation, although graft versus host disease (GVHD) occurred less often and was less severe if it did occur [*see (17)* for a review of the field].

In a series of in vitro experiments, we have shown that, similar to mesenchymal cells from bone marrow, HUCB-derived mononuclear cells can also be induced to express neural proteins *(18)*. These observations have been replicated by other groups as well. Bicknese et al. *(19)* and Buzanska et al. *(20)* demonstrated the induction of class III β-tubulin (TuJ1), a neural filament-associated protein, glial fibrillary acidic protein (GFAP) which is associated with astrocytes, and galactocerebroside (GalC) a glycolipid found in the cell membrane of oligodendrocytes. Similarly, a third group *(21)* showed that these cells can express microtubule-associated protein 2 (MAP-2) (a marker of more mature neurofilament) using immunohistochemistry and reverse transcriptase-polymerase chain reaction (RT-PCR).

It is not clear, however, which are the progenitor cells that give rise to these "neural" cells. In the study by Buzanska et al. *(20)*, the mononuclear fraction was first depleted of the CD34[+] hematopoietic stem cells. In another study, the mononuclear fraction underwent immunomagnetic sorting for CD133, a more primitive cell-surface antigen than even CD34 and it is found on hematopoietic stem cells and neural stem cells *(22)*. Only in the CD133[+] cultures was there significant expression of stem cell markers such as ABCG2 and nestin as determined using RT-PCR. When these cells were treated with retinoic acid, the cord blood-derived cells then expressed basic helix loop helix (bHLH) transcription factors associated with neurogenesis, including Pax6, Wnt1, Olig2, NeuroD1, Otx2, and Hash1; only the last two were expressed in nonretinoic acid-exposed CD133$^+$ cells. It may not be surprising then that neural filament (light, medium, and heavy chain), GFAP, and myelin basic protein, synaptophysin, CNPase, neuronal specific enolase, and TuJ1 were also expressed in these cells.

Our approach to characterization of the HUCB-derived mononuclear cells has been based on adhesion properties. This cellular fraction is a mixed cell population that separates into two main populations, one that adheres to the plastic cultureware and one that remains floating *(23)* (*see* Fig. 1). The adherent population is a mixed population composed of large round egg-shaped cells, bi- or multipolar cells, and small round cells. In the cultures examined, none of the cells expressed CD133 or the c-kit receptor for stem cell factor (CD117), whereas approximately 3% of the cells from the floating fraction expressed these antigens. There were more glial antigens expressed by cells in the adherent fraction and more neuronal antigens expressed by cells within the floating fraction.

While these in vitro results were suggestive, the tissue culture dish is an artificial environment where the cells can behave in ways unrelated to their function within the body. This was particularly highlighted in two recent studies with bone marrow in which it was shown that cellular toxicity can produce cells in the culture dish that adopt a neuronal morphology and express neurofilament proteins *(24)*. Upon closer examination, however, toxicity within the culture dish induced cellular remodeling and retraction of processes *(25)*. A subsequent study by Buzanska's group is suggestive that HUCB-derived cells can give rise to neuronal like cells *(26)*. Using their nonimmortalized HUCB cell line, derived from CD34$^-$ and CD45$^-$ cells, and then further selected from the nonadherent proliferating cells in these cultures, they showed that these cells not only expressed multiple neurotransmitters and their receptors, but they also had inward and outward rectifying potassium channels that responded to the application of dopamine, serotonin, γ-aminobutyric acid (GABA), and acetylcholine. While gene array analysis suggested that the differentiated cells also had sodium channels, they did not observe a tetrodotoxin-sensitive sodium channel, even though a rapid depolarization similar to an action potential was observed using whole cell patch clamp. Therefore, to truly demonstrate that the HUCB cells can

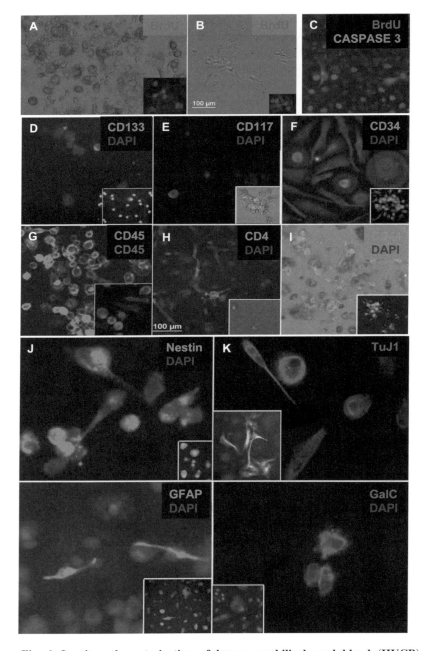

Fig. 1. In vitro characterization of human umbilical cord blood (HUCB) cells. HUCB cells were cultured for 18 days in serum-containing medium. The nonadherent, floating fraction was then collected and replated for 2 h prior to

become neurons, it is essential to demonstrate both neuronal phenotype in vivo and neuronal function.

The major issue with these studies is that these cells may display neuronal morphology, but it is not clear whether they are functional. As a first step to examine these cells in vivo, we have examined the differentiation potential of the HUCB cells in the live animal. We transplanted the HUCB cells into the anterior subventricular zone (SVZ) of the neonate, a region in which neurogenesis occurs throughout life. At this age when proliferative and differentiative signals are still strong as the young brain develops, we demonstrated that at least some of the HUCB cells differentiated into neuronal and glial phenotypes within this neurogenic region (*16*), regardless of whether they were cultured in advance with Dulbecco's modified Eagle's medium (DMEM) with fetal bovine serum (FBS) or with media supplemented with retinoic acid and nerve growth factor (NGF). Although phenotypically similar to neurons, their functionality was still a question.

Fig. 1. *(Continued)* performing immunohistochemistry. Cells in both the adherent fraction (**A**) and the floating, nonadherent fraction (**B**) incorporated bromodeoxyuridine (BrdU) as shown in these combined phase-contrast/epifluorescence images. Insets show fluorescent BrdU labeling alone. The BrdU$^+$ cells in the adherent fraction remained small and round, while those in the floating fraction began to differentiate after replating. Scale bar $= 20\,\mu$m. (**C**) Few of the BrdU$^+$ cells expressed caspase 3 and therefore were not undergoing DNA repair or cell death processes. (**D**) Few CD133$^+$ cells were found in the adherent fraction; more were observed in the floating fraction (inset). (**E**) CD117$^+$ cells were rarely found in the adherent fraction, but they were observed in nonadherent fraction (*green*, inset). (**F**) CD34$^+$ cells (*green*) were present in both fractions. (**G**) Both fractions had a large number of cells with the CD45 marker on the cell surface. (**H**) A small number of CD4$^+$ cells were observed in both fractions with irregular cell morphology. (**I**) CD44 antigen (hematopoietic cellular adhesion molecule) was present in both fractions, but especially in the adherent fraction. In addition to hematopoietic antigens, these cells also express neural antigens. The nonadherent cells were replated for 10 days in serum-containing medium and compared to the adherent fraction at the same time point. (**J**) Nestin-positive cells (*green*) were observed in both fractions. The inset is the replated nonadherent fraction. (**K**) Only a few of cells expressed the early neuronal antigen TuJ1 (*red*) in either the adherent or replated nonadherent fraction culture (*bright*, inset). (**L**) The expression of glial antigens in both fractions (*green*). Inset shows replated nonadherent fraction. (**M**) Both fractions in cultured HUCBmnf express GalC, a typical marker for oligodendrocytes. Blue DAPI counterstaining was used for visualization of nuclei of cultured cells. (*See* Color Plate 2 following p. 78.)

3. HUCB PRODUCE RECOVERY AFTER STROKE

The first demonstration that there may be therapeutic utility in treating stroke with HUCB cells was presented in 2001 (27), when undifferentiated HUCB cells were intravenously injected into rats that had undergone a middle cerebral artery occlusion (MCAO) (27) either 24 h or 7 days previously. Those animals that received the cells performed significantly better on a battery of neurologic indicators as well as on the rotorod test of motor coordination, especially when cells were administered at 24 h post-MCAO. Further, HUCB cells were observed in the infarcted hemisphere but not within the normal hemisphere. Some of these surviving cells even expressed neural antigens such as NeuN, MAP-2, and GFAP. This was a significant demonstration that not only neurogenic regions, but also the injured brain could provide instructive signals that help these cells differentiate into a neural phenotype.

We have continued to explore the ability of the HUCB cells to improve outcome after a stroke. Using a permanent MCAO model in rats, we have explored issues of route of delivery, cell dosing, and window of treatment efficacy, with interesting and controversial results. The first surprise was the demonstration that HUCB cells were more effective at improving motor function when administered intravenously (28). While recovery of function was similar between intravenous and local, intraparenchymal HUCB delivery out to 1 month post-MCAO, performance deteriorated thereafter in the local intrastriatal delivery group to the point that on the step test, this group was performing worse than even the untreated MCAO-only control. In the intravenous group, in contrast, motor function was stable for 2 months. This study was the first to suggest that immune/inflammatory modulation is one of the ways that HUCB cells induced recovery. The cellular infiltrate in those animals treated with HUCB cells was minimal, although in vitro studies using a two-chamber migration system suggested that signals are generated by the damaged brain that establish a positive chemotactic gradient that causes migration of the cells toward the injured brain (29). In fact, examining the extent of HUCB migration over time after the stroke predicted the optimal therapeutic window (30) obtained in our later studies.

HUCB-induced behavioral recovery is also dependent on the number of cells administered (31). Using a similar battery of behavioral tests (spontaneous activity, elevated body swing test, and step test) and delivering cells 24 h after the stroke, we found that motor function improved as the number of HUCB cells implanted increased from 10^4 to 5×10^7 cells. One million cells was the threshold dose for observing statistical significance. However, optimal recovery of function occurred with the 10^7 cells. Furthermore, infarct volume was minimal at this dose of cells.

Once dosage and route of administration were established, we examined efficacy of HUCB treatment as a function of time of delivery. The HUCB cells were administered from 3 h to 30 days post-MCAO and performance was measured on multiple tests of motor function. Whereas all previous studies had been conducted with administration 24 h post-MCAO, the best time to administer the cells was at 48 h after the stroke *(30)*. Even more amazing, in many of the animals treated at this time, there was limited damage in the stroked hemisphere. Cellular infiltrates were minimal, GFAP labeling was less than in all other groups, and Ox-6-labeled microglia were rare. These data provided more evidence that HUCB cells may be acting directly on immune cells to decrease the inflammatory response that occurs at more delayed time points poststroke.

4. DO THE HUCB CELLS INDUCE RECOVERY THROUGH NEURAL DIFFERENTIATION?

The observation that some HUCB-derived cells survived in the brain and expressed neural antigens *(27)* and also induced behavioral recovery led us to speculate that HUCB cells induced recovery by restoring neural circuitry. However, in subsequent studies, which examined recovery for 1 to 2 months post-HUCB administration, it became clear that few of these cells may survive in the brain long term, and few of those that do survive become neurons and astrocytes. At 1 month posttransplant, it is possible to find human DNA within the stroked hemisphere of the brain *(31)*; however, immunohistochemical analysis did not demonstrate many cells and those that were observed tended to be associated with the vasculature. At 2 months posttransplant, we did not observe any HUCB cells within the damaged hemisphere using immunohistochemistry *(28)*, and yet recovery of function on our battery of behavioral tests was stable at this time after systemic delivery of the cells.

5. ARE HUCB CELLS NEUROPROTECTIVE?

Measurements of infarct volume demonstrates that HUCB cell administration is preventing cell death within the damaged hemisphere. The question is whether this neuroprotection or rescue of neurons is a function of a direct neuroprotective effect or simply a consequence of other processes, such as an inhibition of inflammation. We initiated investigations to examine whether HUCB cells can influence neuronal survival in two separate in vitro models *(32)*. In the first, we used an organotypic hippocampal culture system in which the slices were exposed to oxygen and glucose deprivation for 3 days and cell death was measured with propidium iodide uptake. In some cultures, HUCB cells were added to inserts that were placed in the culture dish with the slice. In these cultures exposed to HUCB cells, there was much less propidium iodide uptake, particularly in the dentate gyrus. This is especially interesting since this is one of the regions in the adult brain in which neurogenesis occurs throughout life. In the second study, we exposed primary cultures to 16 h of hypoxia followed by 24 h of normoxia. Using lactate dehydrogenase (LDH) production as an index of cell death, cultures treated with HUCB cells immediately after hypoxia had less LDH production than cultures without HUCB cells.

Together, these observations would suggest that the HUCB cells are having a neuroprotective effect, but they do not of themselves show that the HUCB cells or a factor released by these cells are directly interacting with neurons. Both culture systems have multiple cell types present that HUCB cells could be impacting. To truly determine where the cells are having their effects, it is necessary to examine the response of neurons, astrocytes, oligodendrocytes, and microglia to hypoxia when they are cultured with or without HUCB cells.

These results do, however, suggest that there is an HUCB-produced factor that is directly responsible for the improvements in functional outcome after transplantation. In the organotypic cultures, there was no direct contact between the hippocampal slice and the HUCB cells; therefore, any effect had to be mediated by a factor released by the cells.

A recent study examined whether growth factors had a role in the recovery of function and infarct volume after HUCB cell administration *(33)*. When subthreshold numbers of cells were administered either with or without a blood–brain barrier (BBB) permeabilizer (mannitol), the HUCB cells reduced the size of the infarct and improved the performance on the elevated body swing test of motor asymmetry and the passive avoidance test of learning and memory. While the cells were not detected in the brain even after 3 days, there were elevated levels of glial-derived neurotrophic factor (GDNF) that were measurable in the blood of only the HUCB$^+$ mannitol group. The addition of the mannitol should have enhanced the entry of the cells into the brain over intravenous administration of HUCB cells alone and could thereby enhance the therapeutic benefit of the less than optimal number of cells that were delivered either by direct provision of growth factors to the damaged brain or by stimulating the local astrocytes or microglia to release GDNF. Incubating the HUCB cells with neutralizing antibodies to GDNF, brain-derived neurotrophic factor (BDNF), and NGF prior to transplantation eliminated the therapeutic benefits of the cells.

There are multiple growth factors that are expressed by cells within the cord blood. While most of them have a role in the maintenance and function of hematopoiesis and blood lineages, others have broader roles in immune modulation. Transforming growth factor (TGF-β1) and GDNF are present in a putative stem cell population within the mononuclear fraction that is lineage negative for hematopoietic markers *(34)*. Both of these growth factors are neuroprotective in stroke *(35,36)*. Similarly, stromal-derived factor-1 (SDF-1) is expressed by $CD34^+$ stem cells *(37)*. Other growth factors that are detectable in cells of the HUCB mononuclear fraction include stem cell factor *(38)*, NGF and BDNF transcripts *(39)*, fibroblast growth factor-2 (FGF-2) *(40)*, and vascular endothelial growth factor (VEGF) *(41)*. Clearly, these cells are capable of producing a cocktail of factors supportive of neuroprotection and repair.

6. HUCB CELLS REDUCE APOPTOSIS

Based on the current understanding of cell death in response to acute insults in the brain, delivering the cells 48 h after the stroke should not have been able to rescue the neurons within the core of the infarct and yet infarct volume was approximately 3 % of hemispheric volume. Therefore, the core of the infarct is smaller than initially anticipated, with cell death predominantly occurring through apoptotic mechanisms in the penumbra. When we examined the evolution of infarct volume, it took 4 days for infarct volume to stabilize. After 48 h, infarct volume was 20 % of intact tissue, while at 96 h it was closer to 50 % *(30)*. Administering the HUCB cells at 48 h prevented any further enlargement in infarct volume. Clearly, the majority of cells compromised at 48 h can be rescued. We then examined whether there was a change in apoptotic cell death over this 7-day time period poststroke using TUNEL to label apoptotic cells. Extensive TUNEL labeling was observed from 24 h to 7 days poststroke in the MCAO-only group;

HUCB cell delivery at 48 h almost eliminated the apoptosis. Where and how these cells are interrupting the apoptotic cascade is not yet clear. One possible explanation is that HUCB cells inhibit proapoptotic transcription factors such as bax or bad. Alternatively, the cells may stimulate antiapoptotic, survival factors such as bcl2 or bcl-x_L. For a review of the role of bcl2 family proteins in apoptosis and ischemia, *see* Love (2003) *(42)*. It is also possible that decreased cell death is a secondary consequence of HUCB modulation of another process. From these studies, the core is significantly smaller than anticipated, and more cells can be rescued at delayed time points. Further investigation is needed to address these issues.

7. HUCB CELLS HAVE ANTI-INFLAMMATORY PROPERTIES

In addition to the primary insult that occurs with stroke, there is a secondary inflammatory response that may contribute to the overall outcome of the patient *(43,44)*. The more severe the inflammatory response, the worse the prognosis of the patient *(45)*. The cascade of inflammatory events can be broken down into two phases. In the acute phase, microglia remove dead cells and debris. In the second phase, microglia produce proinflammatory cytokines that can contribute to expansion of the infarct *(1)*. The cytokines include tumor necrosis factor-alpha (TNF-α) and interleukin-1 beta (IL-1β).

In addition to activation of microglia, the peripheral immune system also becomes activated after a stroke. After the ischemic event, there is an influx of antigen nonspecific leukocytes, a breakdown in the BBB, and hyperthermia *(46)*. Neutrophils are one of the early cells to arrive at the site of damage; they produce reactive oxygen species, nitric oxide, and proinflammatory cytokines that can potentiate the injury response. Other species of immune cell are also found within the brain after stroke, including T cells, B cells, natural killer (NK) cells, and granulocytes *(47,48)*. Further, there is ample evidence that these cells are lateralized to the damaged hemisphere *(49)*. This situation is associated with a permanent dysregulation of peripheral immune function, suggesting that the stroke is able to modulate the peripheral immune response. It has been shown that there is a change in the profile of immune cells in peripheral blood after a stroke *(50–52)*. Given the alterations in immune function after stroke, it is plausible that the hematopoietic HUCB cells modulate the ongoing inflammatory response to stroke.

The observation that immune cells migrate to the brain suggests that signals are generated within the brain that attract them. After MCAO, there is an increase in the number of chemokines present around the infarct that are known to modulate migration and cell fate of hematopoietic cells. SDF-1 expression is upregulated in astrocytes in the penumbral region around the infarct by 24 h after stroke *(53)*. CXCR4 (SDF-1 receptor) expression on cerebral vessels in both the infarct core and penumbra increases. SDF-1 is important in leukocyte adhesion to endothelial cells during inflammation. Monocyte chemoattractant protein-1 (MCP-1) which attracts monocytes, memory T cells, and NK cells in in vitro assays *(54)* and permeabilizes the BBB *(55)* is also increased 24–48 h after stroke *(54)*. We have shown that MCP-1 is elevated during the period that HUCB cells are effective at inducing behavioral recovery *(29)*. Using DNA array technology, macrophage inflammatory protein-1 (MIP-1) was shown to increase 77-fold after stroke *(56)*. The increase in MIP-1α began in microglia as early as 1 h poststroke and peaked at 8–16 h poststroke *(57,58)*. Such inflammatory signals would attract not only endogenous immune cells, but also transplanted HUCB cells. Indeed, in vitro migration assays using extracts of stroked brains demonstrate that the stroked brains have potent chemoattractant signals that cause HUCB migration *(29)*. The time course of migration corresponds to the therapeutic window of efficacy for cellular administration.

Clearly, there are significant inflammatory responses that occur after the stroke. It is therefore not surprising that numerous studies have employed anti-inflammatory agents in attempts to reduce the severity of postischemic injury. But do HUCB cells modulate this response? First, we used fluorescent-activated cell sorting (FACS) to examine the effect of HUCB administration on infiltration of rat leukocytes into the brain *(32)*. After MCAO, there was a significant increase in infiltrating T cells, B cells, and neutrophils in addition to a change in the monocyte/microglial/macrophage population in the brain. Administering the HUCB cells 24 h poststroke significantly decreased the number of infiltrating B cells and CD11b+ monocytes, microglia, or macrophage by fivefold. Similarly, using esterase0-staining techniques to identify granulocytes and monocytes, there was a decrease in the number of these cells within the treated brains.

The microglial population is the primary cell responsible for the inflammatory response in the brain and is the main source of inflammatory cytokines such as TNF-α and IL-1β *(59)* along with infiltrating leukocytes *(60)*. It was not surprising, therefore, that TNF-α concentrations in the brain increased after MCAO. TNF-α decreased significantly at both the mRNA and protein level after intravenous HUCB delivery. Similarly IL-1β protein concentrations also decreased. These decreases were associated with decreased binding of the transcription factor nuclear factor-κB (NF-κB). TNF-α as well as other inflammation-associated genes, is a major gene target of NF-κB transcription factor.

The role of NF-κB in repair and regeneration of the damaged or diseased brain is still controversial. Activation of NF-κB transcription factor is a crucial step in the immune response where NF-κB-regulated genes play a dominant role in inflammation and host defense *(61)*. The NF-κB/Rel transcription factors have been shown to regulate a number of genes in response to pathogenic stimulation or injury, leading to increased inflammation, cell survival, and proliferation *(62)*. Dysregulation of NF-κB activity is a critical factor in pathological states such as arthritis, cancer, chronic inflammation, asthma, and heart disease *(63–69)*. The discrepancies in the literature as to whether NF-κB activation is neuroprotective may be a function of the time points postinjury at which NF-κB activation has been studied. Early activation of NF-κB may be directly associated with injury-induced repair mechanisms, while activation at later time points are linked with reactive microglia and are detrimental *(70)*. There is evidence that at early time points, NF-κB is activated in neurons whereas at later times, activation occurs in microglia *(71,72)*.

Consistent with this assertion is the observation in a 6-hydroxydopamine (6OHDA) model of parkinsonism in which the 6OHDA was administered into the striatum of animals fed either a control diet or one rich in anti-oxidants *(73)*. At one week postinjection, the area of damage in the striatum was similar across groups, while the number of Ox-6+ [major histocompatibility complex (MHC) II] microglia in the blueberry-treated group was significantly elevated. By 1 month postinjury, the amount of damage in the striatum was significantly less in the blueberry-fed animals compared to control, and the number of Ox-6+ microglia was significantly less. This suggests that the early microglial response was neuroprotective, while the later response was detrimental. While this is a neurotoxicity model, it is conceivable that similar processes occur in other injury or disease models.

At the immunohistological level, we can see changes in the local response of microglia to the stroke when HUCB cells are administered *(30)* *(see* Fig. 2). Delivery of the HUCB cells 48 h after the MCAO almost eliminated the Ox-6 (MHC-II) labeling of activated microglia. This is very consistent with the FACS data demonstrating a decrease in CD11b$^+$ cells.

As well as the changes in the microglial responses, there is also a change in another local cell population. Astrocytes, which account for 50% of total brain volume *(74)*, are essential to the normal functioning of neurons. Through potassium and hydrogen buffering, uptake and release of glutamate, water transport, free radical scavenging, and growth factor and cytokine production, these cells provide critical trophic, nutritive, and structural support to neurons. Astrocytes are activated in response to brain injury, a process referred to as astrocytosis or astrogliosis in which several markers of astrocytes are elevated and the cells undergo hypertrophy *(75)*. During excitotoxicity, extracellular glutamate increases; the glutamate transporters may not be able to clear all the excess glutamate and may actually contribute to excitotoxicity by reversing uptake *(76)* and releasing glutamine *(77)*. Further, GFAP expression increases over the first 24 h poststroke and remains elevated for at least a week. Similarly, the expression of S-100β, a cytosolic calcium-binding protein, is also increased in the astrocytes. The result of this astrocytic activation is increased nitric oxide, TNF-α, and IL-1β expression *(78,79)*, which may exacerbate the ongoing inflammatory response. After HUCB administration, the GFAP expression that is normally elevated after stroke is decreased in the injured brain *(see* Fig. 2).

The in vivo studies all point to a very potent effect of HUCB cells on reducing the inflammation in the brain after a stroke, but the mechanism underlying this effect is not yet clear. In addition to decreasing proinflammatory cytokines, there is increased expression of anti-inflammatory cytokines such as IL-10 or IL-4 after HUCB administration. There was a significant decrease in the mRNA for both of these after stroke. Protein levels of both tended to increase after HUCB administration. IL-10 has been found to inhibit NF-κB after lung injury *(80)* as well as preventing IFNγ induction of ICAM-1 in monocytes by modulating NF-κB-binding activity in the ICAM-1 promoter *(81)*. IL-10, however, may not be the only factor responsible for modulating NF-κB activity. The HUCB cells express many

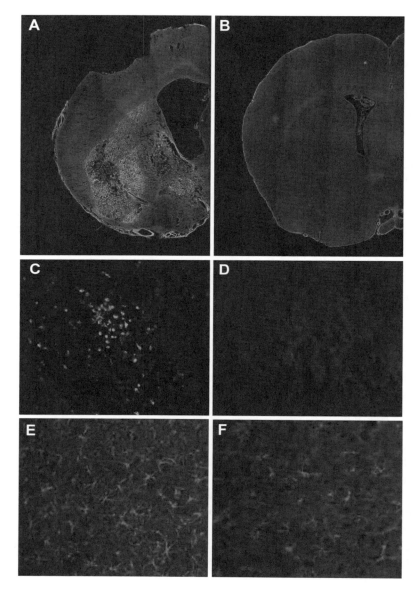

Fig. 2. Cord blood treatment at 48 h decreases the inflammatory response after stroke. (**A**) A montage showing degenerating cells within the brain after middle cerebral artery occlusion (MCAO) visualized with Fluorojade histology. (**B**) Injecting human umbilical cord blood (HUCB) cells 48 h post-MCAO consistently decreases the number of dying cells (montage). (**C**) Ox-6-labeled microglia within the infarcted hemisphere of an MCAO-only animal. These activated microglia consistently have a rounded morphology associated with phagocytic activity.

cytokines *(82,83)*, chemokines *(84)*, and growth factors *(85,86)* that may modulate NF-κB signaling.

8. STIMULATION OF ENDOGENOUS REPAIR MECHANISMS

Neurogenesis occurs in the SVZ and dentate gyrus throughout life. One proposed mechanism of endogenous repair that occurs after a stroke is an upregulation of neurogenesis *(87–92)*. Most of these studies utilize bromodeoxyuridine (BrdU) incorporation into cells with active DNA synthesis. The issue with this technique is that a damaged cell can make an aborted attempt to repair its DNA by re-entry into the cell cycle. Therefore, not only are newly generated cells labeled, but dying cells are as well. The critical demonstration is that BrdU$^+$ cells are not also co-labeled with apoptotic markers. Further, the newly generated neurons, astrocytes, or oligodendrocytes must integrate into the normal neural circuitry and mature.

The idea that neurogenesis may be enhanced through transplantation of hematopoietic cells was originally proposed with regard to transplantation of bone marrow stromal cells after stroke *(93)*. To date, only one group has examined this issue for HUCB cells *(94)*. In mice in which the distal portion of the left MCA was permanently ligated and were then transplanted with CD34$^+$ HUCB cells, there was an increase in the number of cells that expressed polysialylated neuronal cell-adhesion molecule (PSA-NCAM). PSA-NCAM is only found within migrating neuronal progenitor cells. These cells were found migrating away from the SVZ toward the damaged cortex. Further, only in the mice with CD34$^+$ HUCB transplants, there was a significant increase in the number of NeuN$^+$, BrdU$^+$ cells.

An interesting observation is that this change in neurogenesis appears to be correlated with revascularization of the damaged brain. Revascularization within the ischemic zone would itself be beneficial by restoring delivery of blood and nutrients to this compromised region. However, when revascularization is blocked through administration of endostatin, which inhibits proliferation of endothelial cells,

---

Fig. 2. *(Continued)* **(D)** In the HUCB animals treated at 48 h, few Ox-6-labeled microglia were observed. **(E)** There was extensive labeling of astrocytes with glial fibrillary acidic protein (GFAP) in the MCAO-only animals. **(F)** Less GFAP labeling was found in HUCB-treated animals injected at 48 h. (*See* Color Plate 3 following p. 78.)

neurogenesis is impaired. Indeed, the expression of VEGF by mononuclear cells would enhance angiogenesis *(41)*. Taguchi et al. *(94)* found
increased angiogenesis around the infarcted cortex 35 days after HUCB
treatment of stroked animals.

9. IS AN HUCB-BASED THERAPY LIMITED TO ISCHEMIC STROKE?

All our studies have been carried out using the MCAO model
of ischemic stroke. Fully 85 % of strokes are ischemic *(95)*. In this
model, we get consistent improved outcome. It is in embolic stroke that
rTPA therapy is indicated. However, 15 % of strokes are hemorrhagic
strokes for which rTPA treatment would exacerbate the underlying
bleeding. Unlike rTPA treatment, HUCB cell therapy can be used
regardless of the etiology of the stroke. Intravenous administration
of HUCB mononuclear cells 24 h after a hemorrhagic stroke in rats,
improved functional outcome after the stroke as measured with the
neurological severity test, step test, and elevated body swing test *(96)*.
The wider applicability of HUCB therapy would increase the probability of receiving timely treatment regardless of the form of stroke.
Further, the neuroprotective and anti-inflammatory properties would
also be beneficial for treating hemorrhagic stroke.

10. CONCLUSION

From the data presented in this chapter, it is clear that in experimental models of stroke, the HUCB cells have an amazing ability
to rescue injured neural cells to produce functional recovery. These
cells appear to do this through multiple channels—interrupting the
apoptotic cascade, providing neuroprotection, modulating the inflammatory response, and enhancing angiogenesis and neurogenesis. The
cells induce their effects after systemic delivery, which suggests that an
HUCB-derived transplantation therapy that is the equivalent of a blood
transfusion could be developed. Further, their therapeutic benefits are
not limited to the immediate excitotoxic stage of the ischemic incident
but occur at delayed time points. Such a non-invasive approach to
treatment that could be delivered at delayed time points when patients
are more likely to present for treatment would make this a therapeutic
option that could be available in most, if not all, hospital emergency

rooms to all stroke patients. Before this can occur, however, future studies will be necessary to ascertain the predominant mechanism of action of the cells and the potential therapeutic window in humans.

REFERENCES

1. Dirnagl U, Iadecola C, Moskowitz MA. Pathobiology of ischaemic stroke: an integrated view. Trends in Neurosciences 1999;22(9):391–7.
2. Dirnagl U, Priller J. Focal cerebral ischemia: the multifaceted role of glial cells. In: Kettenmann H, Ransom BR, editors. Neuroglia. 2nd ed. New York: Oxford University Press; 2005. pp. 511–520.
3. Youdim MBH, Buccafusco JJ. Multi-functional drugs for various CNS targets in the treatment of neurodegenerative disorders. Trends in Pharmacological Sciences 2005;26(1):27–35.
4. Ahdjoudj S, Lasmoles F, Holy X, Zerath E, Marie PJ. Transforming growth factor beta2 inhibits adipocyte differentiation induced by skeletal unloading in rat bone marrow stroma. Journal of Bone & Mineral Research 2002;17(4):668–77.
5. Dennis JE, Charbord P. Origin and differentiation of human and murine stroma. Stem Cells 2002;20(3):205–14.
6. Brazelton TR, Rossi FM, Keshet GI, Blau HM. From marrow to brain: expression of neuronal phenotypes in adult mice. Science 2000;290(5497):1775–9.
7. Eglitis MA, Mezey E. Hematopoietic cells differentiate into both microglia and macroglia in the brains of adult mice. Proceedings of the National Academy of Sciences of the United States of America 1997;94(8):4080–5.
8. Eglitis MA, Dawson D, Park KW, Mouradian MM. Targeting of marrow-derived astrocytes to the ischemic brain. Neuroreport 1999;10(6):1289–92.
9. Kopen GC, Prockop DJ, Phinney DG. Marrow stromal cells migrate throughout forebrain and cerebellum, and they differentiate into astrocytes after injection into neonatal mouse brains. Proceedings of the National Academy of Sciences of the United States of America 1999;96(19):10711–6.
10. Mezey E, Chandross KJ, Harta G, Maki RA, McKercher SR. Turning blood into brain: cells bearing neuronal antigens generated in vivo from bone marrow. Science 2000;290(5497):1779–82.
11. Prockop DJ. Marrow stromal cells as stem cells for nonhematopoietic tissues. Science 1997;276 (5309):71–4.
12. Bjornson CRR, Rietze R, Reynolds BA, Magli MC, Vescovi AL. Turning brain into blood: a hematopoietic fate adopted by adult neural stem cells in vivo. Science 1999;283(5401):534–537.
13. Bender JG, Unversagt KL, Walker DE, Lee W, Van Epps DE, Smith DH, et al. Identification and comparison of CD34-positive cells and their subpopulations from normal peripheral blood and bone marrow using multicolor flow cytometry. Blood 1991;77:2591.
14. Ho AD, Young D, Maruyama M, Corringham RET, Mason JR, Thompson P, et al. Pluripotent and lineage-committed CD34+ subsets in leukapheresis products mobilized by G-CSF, GM-CSF versus a combination of both. Experimental Hematology 1996;24(13):1460–1468.

15. Wu AG, Michejda M, Mazumder A, Meehan KR, Menendez FA, Tchabo JG, et al. Analysis and characterization of hematopoietic progenitor cells from fetal bone marrow, adult bone marrow, peripheral blood, and cord blood. Pediatric Research 1999;46(2):163–169.

16. Zigova T, Song S, Willing AE, Hudson JE, Newman MB, Saporta S, et al. Human umbilical cord blood cells express neural antigens after transplantation into the developing rat brain. Cell Transplantation 2002;11(3):265–74.

17. Sirchia G, Rebulla P. Placental/umbilical cord blood transplantation. Haematologica 1999;84(8): 738–47.

18. Sanchez-Ramos JR, Song S, Kamath SG, Zigova T, Willing A, Cardozo-Pelaez F, et al. Expression of neural markers in human umbilical cord blood. Experimental Neurology 2001;171(1):109–15.

19. Bicknese AR, Goodwin HS, Quinn CO, Henderson VC, Chien SN, Wall DA. Human umbilical cord blood cells can be induced to express markers for neurons and glia. Cell Transplantation 2002;11(3):261–4.

20. Buzanska L, Machaj EK, Zablocka B, Pojda Z, Domanska-Janik K. Human cord blood-derived cells attain neuronal and glial features in vitro. Journal of Cell Science 2002;115:2131–2138.

21. Ha Y, Choi DH, Yeon DS, Lee JJ, Kim HO, Cho YE. Neural phenotype expression of cultured human cord blood cells in vitro. NeuroReport 2001;12(16): 3523–3527.

22. Jang YK, Park JJ, Lee MC, Yoon BH, Yang YS, Yang SE, et al. Retinoic acid-mediated induction of neurons and glial cells from human umbilical cord-derived hematopoietic stem cells. Journal of Neuroscience Research. 2004;75(4): 573–84.

23. Chen N, Hudsion JE, Walczak P, Misiuta I, Garbuzova-Davis S, Jiang L, et al. Human umbilical cord blood progenitors: The potential of these hematopoietic cells to become neural. Stem Cells 2005;23:1560–70.

24. Lu P, Blesch A, Tuszynski MH. Induction of bone marrow stromal cells to neurons: Differentiation, transdifferentiation, or artifact? Journal of Neuroscience Research 2004;77:174–191.

25. Neuhuber B, Gallo G, Howard L, Kostura L, Mackay A, Fischer I. Reevaluation of in vitro differentiation protocols for bone marrow stromal cells: disruption of actin cytoskeleton induces rapid morphological changes and mimics neuronal phenotype. Journal of Neuroscience Research 2004;77:192–204.

26. Sun W, Buzanska L, Domanska-Janik K, Salvi RJ, Stachowiakc MK. Voltage-sensitive and ligand-gated channels in differentiating neural stem-like cells derived from the nonhematopoietic fraction of human umbilical cord blood. Stem Cells 2005;23:931–945.

27. Chen J, Sanberg PR, Li Y, Wang L, Lu M, Willing AE, et al. Intravenous administration of human umbilical cord blood reduces behavioral deficits after stroke in rats. Stroke 2001;32:2682–8.

28. Willing AE, Lixian J, Milliken M, Poulos S, Zigova T, Song S, et al. Intravenous versus intrastriatal cord blood administration in a rodent model of stroke. Journal of Neuroscience Research 2003;73(3):296–307.

29. Newman MB, Willing AE, Manresa JJ, Davis-Sanberg C, Sanberg PR. Stroke induced migration of human umbilical cord blood: Time course and cytokines. Stem Cells and Development 2005;14:576–86.

30. Newcomb JD, Ajmo CT, Davis Sanberg C, Sanberg PR, Pennypacker KR, Willing AE. Timing of cord blood treatment after experimental styroke determines therapeutic efficacy. Cell Transplantation 2006;15(3):213–23.
31. Vendrame M, Cassady CJ, Newcomb J, Butler T, Pennypacker KR, Zigova T, et al. Infusion of human umbilical cord blood cells in a rat model of stroke dose-dependently rescues behavioral deficits and reduces infarct volume. Stroke 2004;35:2390–5.
32. Vendrame M, Gemma C, de Mesquita D, Collier L, Bickford PC, Davis Sanberg C, et al. Anti-inflammatory effects of human cord blood cells in a rat model of stroke. Stem Cells and Development 2005;14:595–604.
33. Borlongan CV, Hadman M, Davis Sanberg C, Sanberg PR. CNS entry of peripherally injected umbilical cord blood cells is not required for neuroprotection in stroke. Stroke 2004;35(10):2385–9.
34. McGuckin CP, Forraz N, Allouard Q, Pettengell R. Umbilical cord blood stem cells can expand hematopoietic and neuroglial progenitors in vitro. Experimental Cell Research 2004;295(2):350–9.
35. Buisson A, Lesne S, Docagne F, Ali C, Nicole O, MacKenzie ET, et al. Transforming growth factor-beta and ischemic brain injury. Cellular and Molecular Neurobiology 2003;23(4–5):539–50.
36. Harvey BK, Hoffer BJ, Wang Y. Stroke and TGF-beta proteins: glial cell line-derived neurotrophic factor and bone morphogenetic protein. Pharmacology and Therapeutics 2005;105(2):113–25.
37. Giron-Michel J, Caignard A, Fogli M, Brouty-Boye D, Briard D, van Dijk M, et al. Differential STAT3, STAT5, and NF-kappaB activation in human hematopoietic progenitors by endogenous interleukin-15: implications in the expression of functional molecules. Blood 2003;102(1):109–17.
38. Welker P, Grabbe J, Gibbs B, Zuberbier T, Henz BM. Human mast cells produce and differentially express both soluble and membrane-bound stem cell factor. Scandinavian Journal of Immunology 1999;49:495–500.
39. Tam SY, Tsai M, Yamaguchi M, Yano K, Butterfield JH, Galli SJ. Expression of functional TrkA receptor tyrosine kinase in the HMC-1 human mast cell line and in human mast cells. Blood 1997;90(5):1807–20.
40. Kanbe N, Kurosawa M, Nagata H, Yamashita T, Kurimoto F, Miyachi Y. Production of fibrogenic cytokines by cord blood-derived cultured human mast cells. Journal of Allergy and Clinical Immunology 2000;106(1 Pt 2):S85–90.
41. Cao J, Papadopoulou N, Kempuraj D, Boucher WS, Sugimoto K, Cetrulo CL, et al. Human mast cells express corticotropin-releasing hormone (CRH) receptors and CRH leads to selective secretion of vascular endothelial growth factor. Journal of Immunology 2005;174(12):7665–75.
42. Love S. Apoptosis and brain ischaemia. Progress in Neuro-Psychopharmacology and Biological Psychiatry 2003;27:267–82.
43. Sairanen T, Ristimaki A, Karjalainen-Lindsberg ML, Paetau A, Kaste M, Lindsberg PJ. Cyclooxygenase-2 is induced globally in infarcted human brain. Annals of Neurology 1998;43(6):738–47.
44. DeGraba TJ. The role of inflammation after acute stroke: utility of pursuing anti-adhesion molecule therapy. Neurology 1998;51(3 Suppl 3):S62–8.
45. Stoll G, Jander S, Schroeter M. Inflammation and glial responses in ischemic brain lesions. Progress in Neurobiology 1998;56:149–71.

46. Becker K. Targeting the central nervous system inflammatory response in ischemic stroke. Current Opinion in Neurology 2001;14:349–53.

47. Schroeter M, Jander S, Witte OW, Stoll G. Local immune responses in the rat cerebral cortex after middle cerebral artery occlusion. Journal of Neuroimmunology 1994;55(2):195–203.

48. Stevens SL, Bao J, Hollis J, Lessov NS, Clark WM, Stenzel-Poore MP. The use of flow cytometry to evaluate temporal changes in inflammatory cells following focal cerebral ischemia in mice. Brain Research 2002;932(1–2):110–9.

49. Tarkowski E, Blomstrand C, Tarkowski A. Stroke induced lateralization of delayed-type hypersensitivity in the early and chronic phase of the disease: a prospective study. Journal of Clinical and Laboratory Immunology 1995;46(2):73–83.

50. Sancesario G, Pietroiusti A, Cestaro B, Fusco FR, Magrini A, Patacchioli FR, et al. Mild brain ischemia increases cerebral lipid peroxidation and activates leukocytes in the peripheral blood of rats. Functional Neurology 1997;12(5): 283–91.

51. Molchanov VV. [Quantitative characteristics of the state of the T- and B-systems of immunity in the peripheral blood of patients with cerebrovascular disorders]. Zhurnal Nevropatologii i Psikhiatrii Imeni S-S-Korsakova. 1983;83(9): 1299–306.

52. Fiszer U, Korczak-Kowalska G, Palasik W, Korlak J, Gorski A, Czlonkowska A. Increased expression of adhesion molecule CD18 (LFA-1beta) on the leukocytes of peripheral blood in patients with acute ischemic stroke. Acta Neurologica Scandinavica. 1998;97(4):221–4.

53. Hill WD, Hess DC, Martin-Studdard A, Carothers JJ, Zheng J, Hale D, et al. SDF-1 (CXCL12) is upregulated in the ischemic penumbra following stroke: association with bone marrow cell homing to injury. Journal of Neuropathology and Experimental Neurology 2004;63(1):84–96.

54. Chen Y, Hallenbeck JM, Ruetzler C, Bol D, Thomas K, Berman NE, et al. Overexpression of monocyte chemoattractant protein 1 in the brain exacerbates ischemic brain injury and is associated with recruitment of inflammatory cells. Journal of Cerebral Blood Flow and Metabolism 2003;23(6):748–55.

55. Stamatovic SM, Keep RF, Kunkel SL, Andjelkovic AV. Potential role of MCP-1 in endothelial cell tight junction 'opening': signaling via Rho and Rho kinase. Journal of Cell Science 2003;116 (Pt 22):4615–28.

56. Kim Y-D, Sohn NW, Kang C, Soh Y. DNA array reveals altered gene expression in response to focal cerebral ischemia. Brain Research Bulletin 2002;58(5):491–8.

57. Gourmala NG, Limonta S, Bochelen D, Sauter A, Boddeke HW. Localization of macrophage inflammatory protein: macrophage inflammatory protein-1 expression in rat brain after peripheral administration of lipopolysaccharide and focal cerebral ischemia. Neuroscience. 1999;88(4):1255–66.

58. Takami S, Nishikawa H, Minami M, Nishiyori A, Sato M, Akaike A, et al. Induction of macrophage inflammatory protein MIP-1alpha mRNA on glial cells after focal cerebral ischemia in the rat. Neuroscience Letters 1997;227(3):173–6.

59. Stoll G, Jander S, Schroeter M. Detrimental and beneficial effects of injury-induced inflammation and cytokine expression in the nervous system. Advances in Experimental Medicine and Biology 2002;513:87–113.

60. Smyth MJ, Johnstone RW. Role of TNF in lymphocyte-mediated cytotoxicity. Microscopy Research and Technique 2000;50(3):196–208.
61. Li Q, Verma IM. NF-kappaB regulation in the immune system. Nature Reviews: Immunology 2002;2:724–34.
62. Baeuerle PA, Baltimore D. NF-kappa B: ten years after. Cell 1996;87(1):13–20.
63. Cechetto D. Role of nuclear factor kappa B in neuropathological mechanisms. Progress in Brain Research 2001;132:391–404.
64. Foxwell B, Browne K, Bondeson J, Clarke C, deMartin R, Brennan F, et al. Efficient adenoviral infection with IkappaB alpha reveals that macrophage tumor necrosis factor alpha production in rheumatoid arthritis is NF-kappaB dependent. Proceedings of the National Academy of Sciences of the United States of America 1998;95:8211–15.
65. Gilmore T, Koedood M, Piffat K, White D. Rel/NF-kappaB/I kappaB proteins and cancer. Oncogene 1996;13:1367–78.
66. Neve BP, Fruchart JC, Staels B. Role of the peroxisome proliferator-activated receptors (PPAR) in atherosclerosis. Biochemical Pharmacology 2000;60(8):1245–50.
67. Mou SS, Haudek SB, Lequier L, Pena O, Leonard S, Nikaidoh H, et al. Myocardial inflammatory activation in children with congenital heart disease. Critical Care Medicine 2002;30(4):827–32.
68. Makarov SS. NF-kappaB as a therapeutic target in chronic inflammation: recent advances. Molecular Medicine Today 2000;6(11):441–8.
69. Grabellus F, Levkau B, Sokoll A, Welp H, Schmid C, Deng MC, et al. Reversible activation of nuclear factor-kappaB in human end-stage heart failure after left ventricular mechanical support. Cardiovascular Research 2002;53(1):124–30.
70. Mattson MP, Camandola S. NF-κB in neuronal plasticity and neurodegenerative disorders. The Journal of Clinical Investigation 2001;107(3):247–54.
71. Cheng B, Christakos S, Mattson MP. Tumor necrosis factors protect neurons against metabolic-excitotoxic insults and promote maintenance of calcium homeostasis. Neuron 1994;12:139–53.
72. Yu ZF, Zhou D, Bruce-Keller AJ, Kindy MS, Mattson MP. Lack of the p50 subunit of NF-κB increases the vulnerability of hippocampal neurons to excitotoxic injury. Journal of Neuroscience 1999;19:8856–65.
73. Stromberg I, Gemma C, Vila J, Bickford PC. Blueberry- and spirulina-enriched diets enhance striatal dopamine recovery and induce a rapid, transient microglia activation after injury of the rat nigrostriatal dopamine system. Experimental Neurology 2005;196:298–307.
74. Tower DB, Young OM. The activities of butyrylcholinesterase and carbonic anhydrase, the rate of anaerobic glycolysis, and the question of a constant density of glial cells in cerebral cortices of various mammalian species from mouse to whale. Journal of Neurochemistry 1973;20:269–78.
75. O'Callaghan JP, Jensen KF, Miller DB. Quantitative aspects of drug and toxicant astrogliosis. Neurochemistry International 1995;26(2):115–24.
76. Seki Y, Feustel PJ, Keller RWJ, Tranmer BI, Kimelberg HK. Inhibition of ischemia-induced glutamate release in rat striatum by dihydrokinate and an anion channel blocker. Stroke 1999;30:433–40.
77. Bradford HF, Ward HK, Thomas AJ. Glutamine–a major substrate for nerve endings. Journal of Neurochemistry 1978;30:1453–9.

78. Emerich DF, Dean RL, III, Bartus RT. The role of leukocytes following cerebral ischemia: pathogenic variable or bystander reaction to emerging infarct? Experimental Neurology 2002;173(1):168–81.

79. Pennypacker KR, Kassed CA, Eidizadeh S, Saporta S, Sanberg PR, Willing AE. NF-kappaB p50 is increased in neurons surviving hippocampal injury. Experimental Neurology 2001;172(2):307–19.

80. Fan J, Ye RD, Malik AB. Transcriptional mechanisms of acute lung injury. American Journal of Physiology Lung Cellular and Molecular Physiology 2001;281(5):L1037–50.

81. Song S, Ling-Hu H, Roebuck KA, Rabbi MF, Donnelly RP, Finnegan A. Interleukin-10 inhibits interferon-g – induced intercellular adhesion molecule-1 gene transcription in human monocytes. Blood 1997;89(12):4461–9.

82. Cohen SB, Madrigal JA. Immunological and functional differences between cord and peripheral blood. Bone Marrow Transplantation 1998;21(Suppl 3):S9–12.

83. Ferrarese C, Mascarucci P, Zoia C, Cavarretta R, Frigo M, Begni B, et al. Increased cytokine release from peripheral blood cells after acute stroke. Journal of Cerebral Blood Flow and Metabolism 1999;19:1004–9.

84. Kostulas N, Kivisakk P, Huang Y, Matusevicius D, Kostulas V, Link H. Ischemic stroke is associated with a systemic increase of blood mononuclear cells expressing interleukin-8 mRNA. Stroke 1998;29(2):462–6.

85. Bracci-Laudiero L, Celestino D, Starace G, Antonelli A, Lambiase A, Procoli A, et al. CD34-positive cells in human umbilical cord blood express nerve growth factor and its specific receptor TrkA. Journal of Neuroimmunology 2003;136 (1–2):130–9.

86. Schipper LF, Brand A, Reniers NC, Melief CJ, Willemze R, Fibbe WE. Effects of thrombopoietin on the proliferation and differentiation of primitive and mature haemopoietic progenitor cells in cord blood. British Journal of Haematology 1998;101(3):425–35.

87. Liu J, Solway K, Messing RO, Sharp FR. Increased neurogenesis in the dentate gyrus after transient global ischemia in gerbils. Journal of Neuroscience 1998;18(19):7768–78.

88. Parent JM, Vexler ZS, Gong C, Derugin N, Ferriero DM. Rat forebrain neurogenesis and striatal neuron replacement after focal stroke. Annals of Neurology 2002;52(6):802–13.

89. Jiang W, Gu W, Brannstrom T, Rosqvist R, Wester P. Cortical neurogenesis in adult rats after transient middle cerebral artery occlusion. Stroke 2001;32(5):1201–7.

90. Arvidsson A, Kokaia Z, Lindvall O. N-methyl-D-aspartate receptor-mediated increase of neurogenesis in adult rat dentate gyrus following stroke. European Journal of Neuroscience 2001;14(1):10–8.

91. Jin K, Minami M, Lan JQ, Mao XO, Batteur S, Simon RP, et al. Neurogenesis in dentate subgranular zone and rostral subventricular zone after focal cerebral ischemia in the rat. Proceedings of the National Academy of Sciences of the United States of America 2001;98(8):4710–5.

92. Kee NJ, Preston E, Wojtowicz JM. Enhanced neurogenesis after transient global ischemia in the dentate gyrus of the rat. Experimental Brain Research 2001;136(3):313–20.

93. Chen J, Li Y, Katakowski M, Chen X, Wang L, Lu D, et al. Intravenous bone marrow stromal cell therapy reduces apoptosis and promotes endogenous cell proliferation after stroke in female rat. Journal of Neuroscience Research 2003;73(6):778–86.

94. Taguchi A, Soma T, Tanaka H, Kanda T, Nishimura H, Yoshikawa H, et al. Administration of CD34+ cells after stroke enhances neurogenesis via angiogenesis in a mouse model.[see comment]. Journal of Clinical Investigation 2004;114(3):330–8.

95. Smith WS, Johnston SC, Easton JD. Cerebrovascular diseases. In: Kasper DL, Fauci AS, Hauser SL, Longo DL, Jameson JL, Isselbacher KJ, editors. Harrison's Prinicipals of Internal Medicine. 16th ed. McGraw-Hill; 2005.

96. Nan Z, Grande A, Sanberg CD, Sanberg PR, Low WC. Infusion of human umbilical cord blood ameliorates neurologic deficits in rats with hemorrhagic brain injury. Annals of the New York Academy of Sciences 2005;1049:84–96.

4

Adipose-Derived Stem Cells as a Potential Therapy for Stroke

Henry E. Rice and Kristine M. Safford

1. INTRODUCTION

Reservoirs of stem and progenitor cells have been shown to exist in several types of adult tissue, including skin, muscle, bone marrow, and fat *(1–4)*. Growing evidence suggests that these cells may retain multilineage potential and are capable of giving rise to cells with properties that differ from those of the resident tissue. Although whether adult cells can actually undergo reprogramming from one cell lineage to another remains controversial, this reprogramming is termed "transdifferentiation" *(5,6)*. The possibilities raised by transdifferentiation are exciting for several reasons. First, the traditional concept that cells in adult tissue cannot change their developmental fate may not be absolute. Second, the use of adult stem cells would circumvent the ethical and logistic concerns associated with the use of embryonic stem (ES) cells. Third, adult stem cells present an easily accessible, abundant, and replenishable source of cells for use in clinical applications.

Recent discoveries in the area of neural transdifferentiation are especially interesting given the limited capacity of neurons for regeneration *(7,8)*. Neuronal transdifferentiation is difficult to demonstrate, and evidence of transdifferentiation is generally based on genetic analysis of transdifferentiated cells, immunocytochemistry for the presence of neuronal markers and the absence of non-neuronal markers, as well as demonstration of neuronal function *(7,8)*. Initial work in the field of neuronal differentiation of mesenchymal cells was observed with bone marrow stroma, first demonstrating in vitro expression of

From: *Current Clinical Neurology: Stroke Recovery with Cellular Therapies*
Edited by: Sean I. Savitz and Daniel M. Rosenbaum © Humana Press Inc., Totowa, NJ

neural markers, followed by in vivo studies of transplantation and animal models of neural injuries and disease *(9–13)*.

The capacity of adipose-derived stem cells (ASCs) for neural differentiation has been the subject of a number of recent investigations, opening up the possibility of using these cells in the treatment of various neurologic disorders. This review examines recent studies on the uses of ASCs for neuronal therapies, particularly for recovery from cerebral ischemia.

2. SOURCES OF STEM CELLS

A long-standing pillar of developmental biology continues to be challenged, namely that a cell committed to a specific phenotype cannot change its destiny. Recent studies have demonstrated the conversion of cells between lineages, even between different germ layers *(14–16)*. This concept of transdifferentiation has been challenged by explanations other than lineage switching, such as the presence of contaminating cells from a different lineage or cell fusion *(17,18)*. To help develop new therapeutic options for neuronal diseases, it is essential to understand both the potentials and the limitations of various stem cell populations.

A stem cell is defined by its capability both to self-renew and to generate multiple differentiated progeny. The prototypical stem cell is the totipotent egg, and many critical advances in developmental biology have benefited from the study of ES cells. ES cells can differentiate into various cell lineages in vivo and in vitro, including neuronal tissue *(19–21)*. Both fetal and adult neuronal stem cells (NSCs) can differentiate into neurons and glia in vitro and in vivo *(21–26)*. However, the clinical use of both ES and NSC cells is encumbered by numerous logistic and ethical constraints.

3. MESENCHYMAL STEM CELLS

Increasing recognition is being made of the plasticity of stromal cells within bone marrow, termed mesenchymal stem cells (MSCs) *(27)*. MSCs can differentiate into multiple mesodermal lineages, including bone, fat, and cartilage, as well as cells that are not part of their normal repertoire, including hepatocytes as well as skeletal and cardiac muscle *(28–31)*. In addition to mesenchymal lineages, MSCs have been reported to differentiate into cells with neuronal characteristics in vitro. Verfaille has identified a rare cell within marrow, termed a multipotent adult progenitor cell, which can differentiate into all three germ layers, including neurons *(30)*. Both Eglitis and Woodbury have shown that MSCs can differentiate into neurons in vitro *(9,13)*.

Several common themes have emerged from these studies. First, the isolation of a homogeneous population of MSCs results from the adherence of stromal cells to plastic, which depletes hematopoietic progenitors and other cells. Second, culture cocktails used to induce neuronal differentiation generally require agents such as retinoic or valproic acid, growth factors, antioxidants, demethylating agents, or compounds that increase intracellular cAMP. Other studies have shown a role for genetic inducers of neuronal differentiation, including *Noggin* and *Notch* *(32,33)*. The findings of differentiation induced by these approaches have been challenged by a number of groups *(34)*.

In addition to in vitro studies, in vivo studies have suggested that MSCs are capable of neuronal differentiation. Following transplantation in animal models, MSCs assume a neuronal phenotype, migrate in central nervous system (CNS), and restore function following CNS injury *(35–40)*. These findings raise intriguing questions about plasticity across lineage boundaries and suggest that similar approaches may be applicable to other stem cell sources.

4. ADIPOSE TISSUE AS AN ALTERNATIVE SOURCE OF STEM CELLS

Recently, adult adipose tissue has become recognized as an alternative and rich source of stem cells *(41–46)*. Observations of ectopic bone formation in patients suffering from progressive osseus heteroplasia and the expansion in adipocyte numbers seen in obesity both support the idea that a pool of multipotent cells exists within adipose tissue. The isolation of progenitor cells from rodent adipose tissue was described by Rodbell *(47)*, followed later by reports of similar procedures to isolate progenitors from human adipose tissue *(48,49)*. In 2001, Halvorsen et al. and Zuk et al. *(43,46)* both published modifications of existing isolation methods using liposuction waste as a starting material, demonstrating the potential of adipose tissue for clinical therapies.

Current methods for isolating ASCs vary among investigators, but generally rely on enzymatic digestion of adipose tissue followed by centrifugal separation to isolate the stromal/vascular cells from primary adipocytes. The stromal/vascular fraction contains blood cells, fibroblasts, pericytes, and endothelial cells. Following plating of the stromal/vascular fraction on plastic tissue culture dishes, adherent stromal cells separate from non-adherent hematopoietic and other contaminating cells. The final population of adherent cells can be maintained in an undifferentiated state for extended periods. These cells have been called several names by various groups, including adipose-derived stromal cells, preadipocytes, and processed lipoaspirate *(43,46,50)*. Given the variety of terminology, investigators in this field have reached consensus on nomenclature, and these cells have been termed ASCs *(51)*.

ASCs display a fibroblast-like morphology and lack intracellular lipid droplets seen in adipocytes. After expansion in culture, ASCs display a distinct phenotype based on cell-surface protein expression and cytokine expression *(52)*. This phenotype is similar to that described for marrow-derived stromal cells and skeletal muscle-derived stem cells *(52–54)*. Adipose tissue is a rich source of stem cells, as the frequency of stem cells within adipose tissue ranges from 1:100 to 1:1500 adherent cells, which far exceeds the frequency of MSCs in bone marrow *(55,56)*.

5. DIFFERENTIATION OF ASCs INTO NON-NEURAL LINEAGES

Under specific culture conditions, ASCs can be induced to differentiate into various mesenchymal and endothelial lineages *(43,45, 46,50)*. Under adipogenic conditions, ASCs demonstrate perinuclear lipid droplets and expression of differentiation selective genes. Under osteogenic conditions, ASCs loaded onto a hydroxyapaptite/tricalcium biomatrix form bone when implanted in mice. Under chondrogenic conditions, ASCs express cartilage matrix molecules. Human ASC-derived chondrocytes maintain a chondrogenic phenotype after implantation in nude mice *(57)*. In addition to the in vitro characterization of the ASC mesenchymal differentiation, various lines of study are underway to explore bone and cartilage replacement strategies for these cells.

6. NEURONAL DIFFERENTIATION OF ASCs

The success of mesenchymal differentiation of ASCs has led to interest in ASCs for neuronal differentiation. Several groups have reported the differentiation of ASCs into neuron-like cells *(45,58–62)*. Although each laboratory has based their studies on different methods for neuronal induction of ASCs, in general they suggest that adipose tissue may contain a group of cells that may be able to be induced toward neuronal/glial lineages, and that these cells may represent a promising alternative strategy for CNS repair.

Neuronal differentiation of ASCs has been achieved by a variety of techniques, but generally involves exposing ASCs to a cocktail of specific induction agents. Several groups have based their media on agents known to induce cellular differentiation, including butylated hydroxyanisole, valproic acid, and forskolin *(45, 58–61)*. Butylated hydroxyanisole is an antioxidant known to promote neural stem cell (NSC) survival after ischemic injury. Valproic acid is a branch-chained fatty acid whose mechanism is not fully known, but is involved in the blockade of voltage-dependent sodium channels and the potentiation of GABAergic transmission. Forskolin is a neural stimulus involved in the regulation of neurotransmitter transporters and ion channels. These induction cocktails are modifications of previously published neuronal induction protocols developed for bone marrow-derived stromal cells *(12,13)*.

Other groups examining neuronal differentiation of ASCs use alternative approaches. Kang et al. *(59)* first exposed the ASCs to 5-azacytidine, a demethylating agent capable of affecting gene expression. Further differentiation is achieved by maintaining the cells in neurobasal medium containing B27 supplement. Ashjian et al. *(62)* treated ASCs with indomethacin, isobutylmethylxanthine, and insulin to induce neural differentiation. Isobutylmethylxanthine is a phosphodiesterase inhibitor, resulting in an elevation of intracellular cyclic adenosine monophosphate (cAMP), which acts as a neural stimulus for several cell types.

Reports of neural differentiation of ASCs have generally based their findings on cell morphology and protein expression seen in ASCs after culture for various periods of time under defined conditions. Most groups have shown that within several hours to days under defined conditions, select cells display retraction of cytoplasm toward the nucleus and formation of compact cell bodies with cytoplasmic extensions. Similar among these studies is the finding of cells that become spherical and refractile, exhibiting a perikaryal appearance, suggestive of a primitive neuronal/glial phenotype. However, whether these changes simply represent non-specific cytoskeletal responses to these induction agents remains a challenge to these studies.

In terms of protein expression, both immunohistochemistry and Western blot analysis have shown that a variety of neuronal and glial markers can be expressed by ASCs (Table 1).T1 We have found that ASCs after exposure to neuronal induction media begin to express glial markers including GFAP, vimentin, and S100 by immunocyto-chemistry *(60,61)*. Expression of the oligodendrocyte marker O4 has not been seen on neuronally induced ASCs in vitro. The fraction of ASCs expressing neuronal phenotypic markers in vitro is relatively high, with some markers such as NeuN seen in approximately 80% of neuronally induced ASCs. The co-expression of NeuN and GFAP in some cells suggests that at least in short-term culture, some ASCs may retain the potential for neuronal as well as glial development.

The expression of neuronal and glial markers on ASCs has been examined in more detail by other groups using Western blot and polymerase chain reaction (PCR) analysis. Zuk et al. *(46)* found nestin expression both in undifferentiated ASCs and in ASCs exposed to neuronal induction media for 9 h. No GFAP expression was found in either group of cells. Another group also found nestin expression in undifferentiated cells *(59)*. We found that after neuronal induction, ASCs displayed increased nestin expression, as well as MAP2 expression *(60,61)*.

In toto, these studies suggest that under specific culture conditions, there appear to be a population of cells within adipose tissue that can adopt several morphologic and phenotypic characteristics of neuronal or glial tissue. Whether these findings can be extended toward more rigorous studies of cell differentiation, including analysis of genetic switching, clonal analysis, or functional studies, remain unclear and are crucial to forward this technology. As well, common shortcomings of these studies include imprecise quantification of cells committed to neuronal or glial lineages, as well as inconsistent results among various laboratories.

7. FUNCTION OF ASCs IN VITRO

Several groups have described a neuronal/glial protein expression profile of ASCs exposed to neuronal induction agents in vitro. However, the functional capabilities of ASCs have been more difficult to establish. We have made initial attempts at determining whether the ASCs possess any functional potential using immunohistochemistry for markers of more mature neuronal function, including neurotrans-mitter, neurotransmitter precursor, and neural protein markers *(61)*. We found that a small portion of ASCs express markers of both GABA and glutamate pathways. Also, select ASCs express subunits

Table 1
A Comparison of the Phenotype of ASC Neuronal/Glial Differentiation In Vitro

	Murine Safford et al. (2004) (*61*)	Safford et al. (2002) (*60*)	Fujimura et al. (2005) (*58*)	Human Safford et al. (2002) (*60*)	Kang et al. (2003) (*59*)	Ashjian et al. (2003) (*62*)	Zuk et al. (2002) (*45*)
Nestin	+	+	+	+			
NSE						+	
Neu N	+	+		+		+	+
MAP 2		+		+	+		–
Beta-III tubulin	+						
Trk-A						+	
NF-70			+	+			
IF-M						–	
Tau	+						
GFAP	+	+	+		+	–	–

Adopted from Fujimura et al. BBRC 2005;333:116–121.

of the glutamate NMDA receptor, synapsin I, the α-1 calcium channel marker, or GAP-43, suggesting that some neuronally induced ASCs may have the potential to respond to neuronal agonists *(61)*.

Although this immunocytochemical data is significant, it does not confirm that ASCs are capable of any neuronal functional activity. Using indirect measures of neuronal function, we have shown that ASCs demonstrate an excitotoxic response to NMDA, with a loss of cell viability, suggesting that ASCs can be induced to form functional NMDA receptors *(61)*. Zuk et al. *(45)* have shown in limited studies that ASCs are capable of conducting an action potential using electrophysiology. These researchers found that induced ASCs display a delayed rectifier K$^+$ current, suggesting the presence of voltage-dependent K$^+$ channels. They hypothesize that the expression of these channels, which precede Na$^+$ and Ca^{2+} channels, correlates to the temporal development of ion channels in maturing neurons *(62)*. However, these limited studies have not been replicated, and further confirmatory studies are necessary to demonstrate that ASCs can be induced to neuronal functions.

8. IN VIVO TRANSPLANTATION USING ASCs

The success of in vitro studies of ASCs has led to the fundamental question of whether these cells are capable of survival and function after transplantation into the CNS. We have observed that neuronally induced ASCs can survive after stereotactic transplantation into the dentate gyrus of the intact mouse brain *(63)*. Preliminary results from our model suggest that neuronally induced ASCs, but not undifferentiated ASCs, can survive in vivo to at least 12 weeks after transplantation. Surviving ASCs migrated up to 2.0 mm from the injection site similar to other studies of marrow stromal cells and adult neural progenitor cells, with migration along the corpus callosum and around the rostrocaudal axis within the striatum. Select surviving ASCs maintain the expression of a neuronal phenotype. These findings are similar to observations of transplanted neural progenitor cells, which survive and migrate in response to local in vivo cues *(64,65)*. Markers of mature neurotransmitter function were not seen. In these experiments, in vitro exposure of ASCs to induction agents appears to be necessary for their survival within a neuronal microenvironment.

In a comparable study, Kang et al. *(59)* found survival and migration of human ASCs that were transplanted into rats by the intracerebrovascular route. This group cultured ASCs in neurobasal medium with B27 supplement, 5-azacytidine, and the growth factors BDNF, bFGF, and nerve growth factor. After transplantation into the lateral ventricle of the rat brain, ASCs survived and migrated to multiple areas of the brain. ASCs that were transplanted into animals with focal ischemia from middle cerebral artery occlusion migrated into the injured area of the cortex, suggesting that ischemia-induced factors facilitate donor cell migration *(59)*. Finally, behavioral testing demonstrated that ASCs improved functional recovery after MCA occlusion, with additional benefit seen when ASCs were transfected with BDNF prior to transplantation.

9. TRANSDIFFERENTIATION

Much debate has centered on the mechanisms involved in the transdifferentiation of adult cells. Although controversial, the process is theorized to occur primarily through DNA transcriptional activation and repression from chromatin structure modifications, which are determined by intrinsic and extrinsic growth factors *(66,67)*. No single unifying model describing this process has yet emerged, a result of the complexity of the mechanisms involved.

Both in vitro and in vivo studies of ASC differentiation outlined above provide some insights to the potential of using ASCs for neuronal therapies and raise additional questions about the transdifferentiation potential of adult stem cells. It is relatively clear that ASCs are able to survive and migrate after transplantation into the CNS and may even improve behavioral outcomes after cerebral ischemia. However, it remains unclear whether ASCs are able to express a full profile of neuronal and glial markers in vivo. Furthermore, it remains unclear the extent to which the phenotypic fate of ASCs was determined in vitro prior to transplantation, or whether the final fate is altered by the local microenvironment. The neuronal differentiation of ASCs may result from a complex series of mechanisms, including interactions of local cells, cytokine modification, and changes in intercellular signals *(66)*.

Can the findings of these in vitro and in vivo studies be explained by mechanisms other than transdifferentiation? Several reports have suggested that the transdifferentiation seen with ASCs is the result of the fusion of donor and host cells in vivo *(34,68–71)*. Increasing skepticism of studies of transdifferentiation has begun to question whether the adult cells are capable of changing their phenotype, or whether cell fusion can explain all of the findings seen from transplantation studies. In contrast to studies involving the transplantation of marrow stromal cells or ES cells into mitotically active host tissues such as liver, the limited proliferative capacity of the brain may restrict fusion events in the CNS. Kang et al. *(59)* suggest that the percentage of engrafted donor cells expressing neural markers is too great to be explained by the low frequency of cell fusion events. Future studies are required to clarify the presence of cell fusion after ASC transplantation.

Another criticism of ASC differentiation studies results from the ASC cell population itself. ASC isolation involves the use of an unpurified population of adherent stromal cells. Critics suggest that even a low fraction of contaminating hematopoietic cells could be the source of the differentiation seen in the ASC experiments. However, flow cytometry data refute that claim by demonstrating that ASCs cells do not express the hematopoietic markers CD11b or CD45 *(61)*. In addition, recent clonal analysis has demonstrated ASC multilineage differentiation, including neuronal differentiation, from clones derived from single-cell clones of human ASCs *(72)*.

Assuming that cell fusion or contamination is not the primary reason for the results seen in the in vivo studies of ASCs, additional proof is needed before ASCs can be labeled as transdifferentiated. For instance, the behavioral improvement seen by Kang et al. *(5)* in rats undergoing ASC transplantation after ischemic injury can be explained by many other mechanisms other than the transdifferentiated of donor cells into neurons. The transplanted cells may release cytokines and trophic factors that act on surviving host cells and produce functional improvement *(5)*. As well, donor cells can be examined for the expression of molecules necessary for synaptic transmission, neurotransmitter synthesis, and neurotransmitter release. More convincing evidence for the neuronal transdifferentiation of ASCs is required to establish this mechanism, such as in vivo analysis of donor cell neuronal function, including electrophysiologic studies. However, even if all ASCs cannot fully differentiate, it is of great interest to see whether ASCs can survive within the CNS, as repair processes may be possible even without complete differentiation, as is seen with other cell types.

10. CONCLUSIONS

Over the past few years, the discovery of NSCs has redefined the previous belief that the nervous system was incapable of regeneration or repair. The interaction of donor NSCs and the CNS microenvironment has raised questions about the use of stem cells for gene therapies, cellular therapies, neuroprotection, and neural repair. Equally as important is the growing evidence that select cells within adult non-CNS tissues retain a certain amount of plasticity, allowing them to undergo a reprogramming from the lineage of their native tissue. Experiments using stem cells derived from bone marrow have already shown potential in models of stroke, traumatic brain injury, spinal cord injury, and Parkinson's disease.

Adipose tissue represents an accessible and replenishable source of multipotent progenitor cells with stem cell properties. Although much more work is required to define the mechanisms behind the neuronal differentiation of ASC, the potential of these cells for use for neurological diseases and injuries may add to the limited repertoire of therapies for these conditions. The promise of ASCs for the treatment of neural diseases and injuries warrants committed exploration and may offer insights not only into stem cell biology, but the use of donor cells from a variety of tissues for CNS therapies.

REFERENCES

1. Adachi N, Sato K, Usas A, et al. Muscle derived cell based ex vivo gene therapy for the treatment of full thickness articular cartilage defects. J Rheumatol 2002;29:1920–3.
2. Nicholl SB, Wedrychowska A, Smith NR. Modulation of proteoglycan and collagen profiles in human dermal fibroblasts by high density micromass culture and treatment with lactic acid suggests change to a chondrogenic phenotype. Connective Tissue Research 2001;42:59–69.
3. Weissman IL, Anderson DJ, Gage F. Stem and progenitor cells: origins, phenotypes, lineage commitments, and transdifferentiations. Annual Review of Cell and Developmental Biology 2001;17(1):387–403.
4. Young HE, Duplaa C, Young TM, et al. Clonogenic analysis reveals reserve stem cells in postnatal mammals: I. Pluripotent mesenchymal stem cells. Anatomical Record 2001;263(4):350–60.
5. Jin K, Greenberg DE. Tales of transdifferentiation. Experimental Neurology 2003;183:255–7.
6. Sanchez-Ramos JR. Neural cells derived from adult bone marrow and umbilical cord blood. Journal of Neuroscience Research 2002;69:880–93.
7. Gage FH. Neurogenesis in the adult brain. Journal of Neuroscience 2002;22:612–3.
8. Strelau J, Unsicker K. Neuroregeneration. Philadelphia: Lipincott Williams and Wilkins; 2003.
9. Eglitis MA, Mezey E. Hematopoietic cells differentiate into both microglia and macroglia in the brains of adult mice. Proceedings of the National Academy of Sciences USA 1997;94(8):4080–5.

10. Kohyama J, Abe H, Shimazaki T, et al. Brain from bone: efficient "meta-differentiation" of marrow stroma-derived mature osteoblasts to neurons with Noggin or a demethylating agent. Differentiation 2001;68:235–44.

11. Reyes M, Verfaillie CM. Characterization of multipotent adult progenitor cells, a subpopulation of mesenchymal stem cells. Annals of the New York Academy of Sciences 2001;938:231–5.

12. Sanchez-Ramos J, Song S, Cardozo-Pelaez F, et al. Adult bone marrow stromal cells differentiate into neural cells in vitro. Journal of Experimental Neurology 2000;164(2):247–56.

13. Woodbury D, Schwarz EJ, Prockop DJ, Black IB. Adult rat and human bone marrow stromal cells differentiate into neurons. Journal of Neuroscience Research 2000;61:364–70.

14. Ferrari G, Cusella-De Angelis G, Coletta M, et al. Muscle regeneration by bone marrow-derived myogenic progenitors. Science 1998;279:1528–30.

15. Gussoni E, Soneoka Y, Strickland CD, et al. Dystrophin expression in the mdx mouse restored by stem cell transplantation. Nature 1999;401:390–4.

16. Rao MS. Multipotent and restricted precursors in the central nervous system. Anatomic Record 1999;257:137–48.

17. Lee SH, Lumelsky N, Auerbach JM, McKay RD. Efficient generation of midbrain and hindbrain neurons from mouse embryonic stem cells. Nature Biotechnology 2000;18:675–9.

18. Reh T. Neural stem cells: form and function. Nature Neuroscience 2002;5(5):392–4.

19. Kim J-H, Auerbach JM, Rodriguez-Gomez JA, et al. Dopamine neurons derived from embryonic stem cells function in an animal model of Parkinson's disease. Nature 2002;418:50–6.

20. Snyder EY, Daley GQ, Goodell M. Taking stock and planning for the next decade: realistic prospects for stem cell therapies for the nervous system. Journal of Neuroscience Research 2004;76:157–68.

21. Wichterle H, Lieberam I, Porter JA, Jessell TM. Directed differentiation of embryonic stem cells into motor neurons. Cell 2002;11(3):385–97.

22. Gage FH, Coates PW, Palmer TD. Survival and differentiation of adult neuronal progenitor cells transplanted to the adult brain. Proceedings of the National Academy of Sciences, USA 92 1995;92:11879–83.

23. Gage FH. Mammalian neural stem cells. Science 2000;287:1433–8.

24. Johansson CB, Momma S, Clarke DL, Risling M, Lendahl U, Frisen J. Identification of a neural stem cell in the adult mammalian central nervous system. Cell 1999;96:25–34.

25. Kordover J, Freeman, T., Chen, E., Mufson, E., Sanberg, P., Hauser, R., Snow, B., Olanow, C. Fetal nigral grafts survive and mediate clinical benefit in a patient with Parkinson's disease. Movement Disorders 1998;13:383–93.

26. Snyder EY, Yoon C, Flax JD, Macklis JD. Multipotent neural precursors can differentiate toward replacement of neurons undergoing targeted apoptotic degeneration in the adult mouse neocortex. Proceedings of the National Academy of Sciences, USA 1997;94:11163–8.

27. Pittenger MF, McacKay AM, Beck SC, et al. Multilineage potential of adult human mesenchymal stem cells. Science 1999;284:143–7.

28. Bruder SP, Jaiswal N, Ricalton NS, Mosca JD, Kraus KH, Kadiyala S. Mesenchymal stem cells in osteobiology and applied bone regeneration. Clinical Orthopaedics and Related Research 1998;355S:S247–56.

29. Caplan AI, Bruder SP. Mesenchymal stem cells: building blocks for molecular medicine in the 21st century. Trends in Molecular Medicine 2001;7(6):259–64.

30. Jiang Y, Jahagirdar BN, Reinhardt RL, et al. Pluripotency of mesenchymal stem cells derived from adult marrow. Nature 2002;418:41–9.

31. Potten C. Stem cells in gastrointestinal epithelium: numbers, characteristics, and death. Philosophical Transactions of the Royal Society of London 1998;353: 821–30.

32. Dezawa M, Kanno H, Hoshino M, et al. Specific induction of neuronal cells from bone marrow stromal cells and application for autologous transplantation. The Journal of Clinical Investigation 2004;113(12):1701–10.

33. Neuhuber B, Gallo G, Howard L, Kostura L, Mackay A, Fischer I. Reevaluation of in vitro differentiation protocols for bone marrow stromal cells: Disruption of actin cytoskeleton induces rapid morphological changes and mimics neuronal phenotype. Journal of Neuroscience Research 2004;77(2):192–204.

34. Liu Y, Rao MS. Transdifferentiation-fact or artifact. Journal of Cellular Biochemistry 2003;88:29–40.

35. Azizi SA, Stokes D, Augelli BJ, DiGirolamo C, Prockop DJ. Engraftment and migration of human bone marrow stromal cells implanted in the brains of albino rats-similarities to astrocyte grafts. Proceedings of the National Academy of Sciences, USA 1998;95:3908–13.

36. Borlongan CV, Koutouzis TK, Poulos SG, Saporta S, Sanberg PR. Bilateral fetal striatal grafts in the 3-nitropropionic acid-induced hypoactive model of Huntington's disease. Cell Transplantation 1998;7:131–5.

37. Brazelton TR, Rossi FMV, Keshet GI, Blau HE. From marrow to brain: expression of neuronal phenotypes in adult mice. Science 2000;290:1775–9.

38. Kopen GC, Prockop DJ, Phinney DG. Marrow stromal cells migrate throughout the forebrain and cerebellum, and they differentiate into astrocytes after injection into neonatal mouse brains. Proceedings of the National Academy of Sciences, USA 1999;96:10711–6.

39. Li Y, Chopp M, Chen J, et al. Intrastriatal transplantation of bone marrow nonhematopoietic cells improves functional recovery after stroke in adult mice. Journal of Cerebral Blood Flow and Metabolism 2000;20(9):1311–20.

40. Mahmood A, Lu D, Yi L, Chen JL, Chopp M. Intracranial bone marrow transplantation after traumatic brain injury improving functional outcome in adult rats. Journal of Neurosurgery 2001;94(4):683–5.

41. Gimble JM, Robinson CE, Wu X, Kelly KA. The function of adipocytes in the bone marrow stroma: an update. Bone 1996;19(5):421–8.

42. Gimble JM, Youkhana K, Hua X, et al. Adipogenesis in a myeloid supporting bone marrow stromal cell line. Journal of Cellular Biochemistry 1992;50(1): 73–82.

43. Halvorsen YD, Bond A, Sen A, et al. Thiazolidinediones and glucocorticoids synergistically induce differentiation of human adipose tissue stromal cells: biochemical, cellular, and molecular analysis. Metabolism 2001;50(4): 407–13.

44. Halvorsen YC, Wilkison WO, Gimble JM. Adipose-derived stromal cells–their utility and potential in bone formation. International Journal of Obesity and Related Metabolic Disorders 2000;24 Suppl 4:S41–4.

45. Zuk P, Zhu M, Ashjian P, et al. Human adipose tissue is a source of multipotent stem cells. Molecular Biology of the Cell 2002;13:4279–95.

46. Zuk PA, Zhu M, Mizuno H, et al. Multilineage cells from human adipose tissue: Implications for cell-based therapies. Tissue Engineering 2001;7(2):211–28.

47. Rodbell M. Effects of hormone on fat metabolism and lipolysis. The Journal of Biological Chemistry 1964;239:375–80.

48. Hauner H, Entenmann G, Wabitsch M. Promoting effect of glucocorticoids on the differentiation of human adipocyte precursor cells cultured in a chemically defined medium. The Journal of Clinical Investigation 1989;84:1663–70.

49. Lalikos JF, Li YQ, Roth TP. Biochemical assessment of cellular damage after adipocyte harvest. The Journal of Surgical Research 1997;70:95–100.

50. Gimble JM, Guilak F. Adipose-derived adult stem cells: isolation, characterization, and differentiation potential. International Society for Cellular Therapy 2003;5:362–9.

51. Zuk P. Signal transduction pathways involved in ADSC lineage commitment and differentiation. In: International Fat Applied Technology Society; 2004; Pittsburgh; 2004.

52. Gronthos S, Franklin DM, Leddy HA, Robey PG, Storms RW, Gimble JM. Surface protein characterization of human adipose tissue-derived stromal cells. Journal of Cellular Physiology 2001;189(1):54–63.

53. Williams SK, Rose DG, Jarrell BE. Liposuction derived human fat used for vascular sodding contains endothelial cells and not mesothelial cells as the major cell type. Journal of Vascular Surgery 1994;19:916–23.

54. Young HE, Steele TA, Bray RA, et al. Human pluripotent and progenitor cells display cell surface cluster differentiation markers CD10, CD13, CD56 and MHC Class I. Proceedings of the Society of Experimental Biology and Medicine 1999;221:63–71.

55. De Ugarte DA, Morizono K, Elbarbary A, et al. Comparison of multi-lineage cells from human adipose tissue and bone marrow. Cells Tissues Organs 2003;174(3):101–19.

56. Kral JG, Crandall DL. Development of a human adipocyte synthetic polymer scaffold. Plastic and Reconstructive Surgery 1999;104(6):1732–8.

57. Erickson GR, Gimble JM, Franklin DM, Rice HE, Awad H, Guilak F. Chondrogenic potential of adipose tissue-derived stromal cells in vitro and in vivo. Biochemical and Biophysical Research Communications 2002;290(2):763–9.

58. Fujimura J, Ogawa R., Mizuno H., Fukunaga Y., Suzuki H. Neural differentiation of adipose-derived stem cells isolated from GFP transgenic mice. Biochemical and Biophysical Research Communications 2005;333:116–21.

59. Kang SK, Lee DH, Bae YC, Kim HK, Baik SY, Jung JS. Improvement of neurological deficits by intracerebral transplantation of human adipose tissue-derived stromal cells after cerebral ischemia in rats. Experimental Neurology 2003;183(2):355–66.

60. Safford KS, Hicok KC, Safford SD, et al. Neurogenic differentiation of murine and human adipose-derived stromal cells. Biochemical and Biophysical Research Communications 2002;294:371–9.

61. Safford KS, Safford SD, Gimble JM, Shetty AK, Rice HE. Characterization of neuronal/glial differentiation of murine adipose-derived adult stromal cells. Experimental Neurology 2004;187:319–28.
62. Ashjian PH, Elbarbary AS, Edmonds B, et al. In vitro differentiation of human processed lipoaspirate cells into early neural progenitors. Plastic and Reconstructive Surgery 2003;111(6):1922–31.
63. Rice HE, Hsu EW, Sheng H, et al. MR-guided transplantation of SPIO-labeled adipose-derived stem cells in MCAO-injured mice. American Journal of Roentgenology (in press).
64. Fricker RA, Carpenter MK, Winkler C, Greco C, Gates MA, Bjorklund A. Site-specific migration and neuronal differentiation of human neural progenitor cells after transplantation in the adult rat brain. Journal of Neuroscience 1999;19(14):5990–6005.
65. Gage FH, Ray J, Fisher LJ. Isolation, characterization, and use of stem cells from the CNS. Annual Review of Neuroscience 1995;18:159–92.
66. Cova L, Ratti A, Volta M, et al. Stem cell therapy for neurodegenerative diseases: the issue of transdifferentiation. Stem Cells and Development 2004;13:121–31.
67. Tada T, Tada M. Toti/pluripotential stem cells and epigenetic modifications. Cell Structure and Function 2001;26:149–60.
68. Dahlke MH, Popp FC, Larsen S, Schlitt HJ, Rasko JE. Stem cell therapy of the liver–fusion or fiction? Liver Transplantation 2004;10(4):471–9.
69. Lagasse E, Connors H, Al-Dhalimy M, et al. Purified hematopoietic stem cells can differentiate into hepatocytes in vivo. Nature Medicine 2000;6(11):1229–34.
70. Terada N, Hamazaki T, Oka M, et al. Bone marrow cells adopt the phenotype of other cells by spontaneous cell fusion. Nature 2002;416(6880):542–5.
71. Ying QL, Nichols J, Evans EP, Smith AG. Changing potency by spontaneous fusion. Nature 2002;416:545–8.
72. Lott KE, Awad HA, Gimble JM, Guilak F. Clonal analysis of the multipotent differentiation of human adipose-derived adult stem cells. In: Transactions of the Orthopedic Research Society; 2004; San Francisco; 2004. p. 162.

5

Novel Imaging Modalities to Monitor Implanted Embryonic Stem Cells in Stroke

Susanne Wegener and Mathias Hoehn

1. INTRODUCTION

In vitro studies of stem cells demonstrating their potential to differentiate into various cell types have raised expectations for therapeutical application of these cells in stroke. Until recently, once stem cells were implanted into the host organ, they were beyond direct monitoring capacity for the scientist. Today, in vivo imaging of implanted stem cells has become possible and has enabled a whole new perspective on stem cell research in stroke.

In principle, in vivo imaging has the potential to answer the following questions:

1. How many cells were implanted into the tissue?
2. How many cells survive in vivo and for how long?
3. Where are cells localized? Do they migrate?
4. Do implanted cells differentiate and integrate into the host tissue?
5. What is the impact of implanted stem cells on the lesion and the host tissue?

Obviously, addressing these issues by histological analysis is tedious, time consuming, and difficult: It requires sacrifice of animals or tissue biopsies and can therefore only grant a snapshot insight into the complex fate of the implanted cells. In vivo imaging techniques that allow longitudinal monitoring of stem cells in the brain noninvasively have emerged and are increasingly applied today. Of several imaging modalities, magnetic resonance imaging (MRI) has been the

From: *Current Clinical Neurology: Stroke Recovery with Cellular Therapies*
Edited by: Sean I. Savitz and Daniel M. Rosenbaum © Humana Press Inc., Totowa, NJ

mainstay for tracking implanted stem cells in vivo *(1–4)* due to its superior spatial resolution and cell/tissue contrast. Based on the present preponderance of MRI literature for this application, the focus of this chapter will be on novel MR imaging approaches. Other interesting in vivo imaging strategies, such as optical imaging or positron emission tomography (PET), are discussed later in this chapter.

2. METHODOLOGICAL CHALLENGES

2.1. Generating Cell Contrast on MR Images

Although powerful high-resolution MRI can discriminate signal within volume elements (voxels) of a few tens of a micron in live animals, intrinsic contrast of cells against a host tissue is currently not sufficient for visualization by MRI. The primary issue is therefore how cells can stand out from the surrounding tissue for in vivo imaging.

The MR signal is based on the detection of field fluctuations from protons aligning with a magnetic field, a process usually referred to as relaxation. Depending on the interaction between these protons and other molecules, such as proteins, the relaxation rates of different tissues will be distinguishable. The relaxation constants T1 and T2 are the source of contrast in MR images. T1 is the "longitudinal" relaxation time and reflects relaxation along the main magnetic field in the magnet. The T1 of water at a field strength of 3T is about 3 s, whereas with 1.3 s the T1 of gray matter is considerably shorter. Another important magnetization component is the "transverse" relaxation time T2, which arises after the magnetic field has been systematically perturbed by a radiofrequency pulse, tipping proton magnetization 90° into the transverse plane. The signal induced in this process decays away with the time constant T2, about 10 times smaller than T1. In practice, the signal decays even faster than would be anticipated by the tissue T2. This is reflected by the T2* relaxation mechanism, which describes the portion of T2 that is influenced not by the composition of the tissue, but by magnetic field inhomogeneities.

The acquisition parameters of an MR image can be adjusted to bring out specific tissue relaxation time differences of interest (e.g., by T1 or T2 weighting). Besides, MR relaxation times can be reduced in a targeted and localized fashion to generate contrast for implanted stem cells. Paramagnetic contrast agents possess unpaired electrons and create a fluctuating magnetic field in their vicinity, thereby reducing T1. The most commonly used paramagnetic contrast agents contain the lanthanide metal ion gadolinium (Gd). Gd compounds injected into the blood are confined to the intravascular space, as long as the blood–brain barrier is intact. In pathological states, such as in tumors or subacute ischemic lesions, the agent leaks into the extravascular space and thus (reducing T1) enhances the signal on T1-weighted images. Another useful feature of Gd agents was discovered in the late 1980s *(5)*: their ability to alter local magnetic susceptibility. Magnetic susceptibility describes the magnetization of a material in response to a magnetic field and is a common source of MR image artifacts (especially at interfaces of air and bone). These susceptibility changes can be picked up on T2*-weighted images. For cell labeling, paramagnetic compounds can both reduce T1 and create a hyperintensity on T1-weighted images and also shorten T2 and T2*, resulting in a hypointense signal on T2/T2*-weighted images.

Superparamagnetic particles, such as iron oxide nanoparticles, have an even stronger effect on magnetic susceptibility (T2/T2* shortening) and have been the most commonly used cell-labeling substances so far. These agents come in different formulations, such as superparamagnetic particles (SPIOs) with a diameter above 50 nm, ultrasmall superparamagnetic particles (USPIOs), about 10–20 nm in diameter, or micron-sized iron oxide particles (MPIOS).

2.2. Optimization of the Imaging Modality

The traceability of implanted stem cells can be improved, if the signal-to-noise ratio (SNR) of an image is high. This, to a large extent, depends on the MR scanner hardware (field strength, gradient strength, and RF=radiofrequency coil diameter) and image acquisition parameters, such as the voxel size or the number of scans averaged. In general, a higher SNR can be achieved at the cost of a lower image resolution and a longer image acquisition time. As mentioned before, even with an optimized MR protocol for highest SNR, intrinsic cell contrast needs to be enhanced with a contrast agent.

Contrast that is visually apparent is defined by a contrast-to-noise ratio (CNR) >5, with CNR$= (I_A - I_B)N^{-1}$, with I_A and I_B the signal intensities of two adjacent regions and N the noise level.

The potential of different agents to generate MR contrast is expressed by their relaxivity (R). Paramagnetic substances predominantly influence T1, while superparamagnetic substances mainly affect T2 and T2*. The higher the relaxivity for T1 or T2 ($R1$ or $R2$), the fewer ions need to be incorporated into the cell for the same contrast. Higher ion concentrations as well as larger particle size result in larger $R2/R2^*$ relaxivity *(6)* (Fig. 1). At some point, with increasing $R2/R2^*$ relaxivity of an agent, the signal will be completely quenched (saturated), which means that further loading with particles is not beneficial *(7)*. On the contrary, from the biological point of view, one would try to minimize the concentration of contrast agent to avoid any influence on the cell, which could range from slowing of cell metabolism to toxicity.

The T2* effects of superparamagnetic iron oxides (such as ultrasmall dextran-coated iron oxide particles, USPIOs) are larger than the $R1$ of paramagnetic manganese or lanthanide-chelates, because, in order to generate T1 contrast, water molecules are required in close proximity to the paramagnetic center of the compound *(8)*. Therefore, the choice of the contrast agent should not be based on SNR considerations alone, as will be set forth in the next paragraphs.

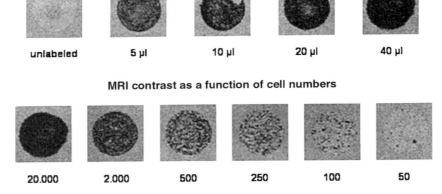

Fig. 1. T2*-weighted magnetic resonance (MR) image at 7 T of an agarose phantom with iron oxide nanoparticle-labeled embryonic stem (ES) cells in each hole. Cells in the upper row were incubated in the medium with increasing amounts of the lipofection agent Metafectene® and 10 mg SINEREM®, a contrast agent consisting of ultrasmall iron oxide nanoparticles (USPIOs). In the lower row, a constant amount of metafectene was used, but the cell number was titrated down from 20,000 to 50 cells per microliter. Clearly visible is the increasing contrast with higher iron amounts incorporated into the cells, due to the more effective lipofection-mediated incorporation of contrast agent (upper row), while the cell titration experiment demonstrates that even small numbers of cells can be detected and are actually represented by individual dark spots (lower row).

2.3. Labeling of Cells for Contrast Generation

Contrast agents can be attached to the cell surface or internalized, and this can in principle happen in vitro or in vivo. Labeling in vitro has the advantage that it can be controlled by the experimenter and targeted to cells with high specificity. The downside of this approach is that cells have to be somehow brought into the brain. In vivo labeling for MRI has the inherent risk of labeling other cells (low specificity), not enough cells (low sensitivity), and being more variable depending on host characteristics that are not under the experimenter's control.

For external labeling, receptor-mediated *(9,10)* or antibody-mediated *(11)* delivery is possible. The disadvantage of these methods is that labeling might be unspecific or the label might detach. A promising approach for external labeling was recently introduced by Zheng and colleagues, allowing detectability of implanted pancreatic islet cells in the mouse for up to 2 weeks: a macrocyclic lanthanide Gd chelate, which is very lipophilic, was spontaneously incorporated into the intact plasma membrane *(12)*.

Due to the anticipated higher stability of the label when incorporated inside the cell, in vitro labeling strategies with internalized contrast agents are the most prevalent in the stem cell MRI literature to date and will be reviewed in more detail. The simplest way to bring a label into a cell is by endocytosis, the ability of a cell to engulf the agent with its cell membrane and package it into lysosome vesicles. How well this works depends on size and polarity of the agent as well as on the particular cell type (e.g., it is very efficient in phagocytic cells (phagocytosis). Co-incubation with MPIOS has been shown to result in very efficient (>90%) labeling of mesenchymal stem cells without evidence of toxicity *(6)*.

The uptake of contrast agents can be further facilitated through lipofection, a technique originally developed to transfect cells with DNA. In lipofection, cationic lipids complex with the extracellularly present contrast agent and form a liposome with a positive net charge, which then associates well with the negative net charge of the cell membrane *(13)* (Fig. 2). A similar transfection tool is the magneto-dendrimer, consisting of iron oxide particles coated with carboxylated dendrimers *(14)*. Transfection agents have been shown to increase labeling efficiency without impacting cell viability *(15,16)* and have been used in studies of in vivo stem cell tracking *(2,17)*. Nevertheless, effects of the transfection agent on cell proliferation and viability

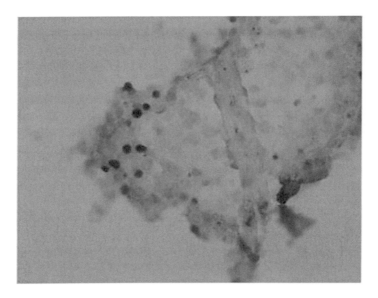

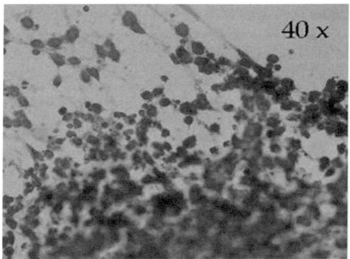

Fig. 2. Diaminobenzidine (DAB)-enhanced Prussian blue staining of embryonic stem (ES) cells in culture after incubation with ultrasmall iron oxide nanoparticles (USPIOs). Upon spontaneous endocytosis of USPIOs (top), the cells show only slight brown coloring, while incubation of the cells with USPIOs in the presence of lipofection agent (bottom) leads to much stronger staining, indicating a much more effective contrast agent incorporation into the cells. Magnification: 40× for both panels. (*See* Color Plate 4 following p. 78.)

have been reported and should always be carefully excluded before implantation *(16)*.

This caution also applies to another transfection strategy, adopted from molecular biology: electroporation. By applying an electrical field pulse, the permeability of the plasma membrane is increased for a short period of time to allow entry of molecules through the enlarged pores into the cell. Daldrup-Link and colleagues showed that after electroporation, natural killer cells were immediately loaded with iron oxides, but needed extended recovery time in cell culture, because significantly less (about 80 %) cells were still viable *(18)*. Others have implemented electroporation for iron oxide labeling of stem cells without harmful effects on the cells *(19)*.

Yet another route to shuttle contrast agents through the cell membrane is via conjugation to small membrane-permeable molecules, such as polyarginine *(20,21)* or polylysine *(22)*. Why and how these compounds are incorporated into the cell is still not known. Kayyem and colleagues were even able to demonstrate efficient delivery of contrast agent as well as DNA into cells in culture; unfortunately, this proved to be impractical for use in whole animals. The Weissleder group has developed a method for cell labeling, by which the HIV-tat peptide that carries a transmembrane and nuclear localization signal in its sequence can translocate exogenous molecules into cells *(23–25)*. As a viral vector for SPIO delivery into cells, the hemagglutinating virus of Japan envelope (HVJ-E) was suggested by Miyoshi and colleagues and shown to be superior to lipofection regarding labeling efficiency *(26)*.

2.4. Tolerance of Label and Labeling Procedure

For in vivo stem cell tracking, two aspects of toxicity have to be considered when planning an experiment: toxicity for the labeled cells as well as harmful effects for the host after cells have been implanted. Viability assays and growth studies in cell culture will easily reveal obvious toxic effects of the label and/or labeling method. Long-term effects and subtle changes in cell differentiation or migration potential will be more difficult to assess, especially since not all of these factors can be fully simulated in vitro. Furthermore, the labeling method itself has the potential to be detrimental for the cells.

Both free iron and Gd ions are toxic for the cells and the host organism; therefore, the active contrast-generating ions are chelated and/or coated. Although iron is naturally occurring in the body, concentrations of free iron are extremely low in the healthy organism. Iron ions can catalyze the conversion of hydrogen peroxide to free radical ions, which can damage membranes and other cellular structures *(27)*. Iron chelators or antioxidants may attenuate the oxidative stress *(27,28)*. Iron oxide compounds have been observed to dose dependently effect proliferation, but not differentiation of mesenchymal stem cells *(29)*, or change the expression patterns of surface antigens in dendritic cells *(11)*. High concentrations of (U)SPIOs (up to 2 mg/iron/ml) have been shown to slow down proliferative rate and even induce cell death *(15)*. However, most groups have reported no impact on cell viability, proliferation, or differentiation with iron oxide incorporation in their experimental models *(1,2,4,24,26,30,31)*.

To avoid toxic effects of lanthanide contrast agents, chelates have been used and their safety has been evaluated *(32)*. Gd dextrans are well tolerated in vivo *(1,33)*. As the use of cellular contrast agents is approaching the clinical stage, more studies are needed to assess and verify the safety of these substances for patients. Fortunately, formulations containing Gd or iron oxide particles are already part of clinical routine MRI applications *(34,35)*.

2.5. Quantification of Cells Before and After Implantation

Quantification of labeled cells and correlation of MR contrast to cell number can be easily achieved in vitro with agarose phantoms *(2)*. By titrating increasing numbers of labeled cells into the phantom, the MRI detection limits can be tested. Several groups have demonstrated the in vitro detection of even single cells loaded with iron oxide particles (SPIOs) at higher (7–14 T) and lower (1.5 T) field strengths *(6,24,36,37)*. Very recently, single cells loaded with iron oxide particles could be visualized in vivo, too *(38,39)*. In order to achieve an optimal imaging resolution and sensitivity for detection of single cells labeled with SPIOs, MRI sequence parameters were adjusted and tested in an earlier work by Heyn and colleagues *(40)*. They studied the effects of MR sequence parameters determining resolution as well as the effects of the SPIO loading (especially compartmentalization) on contrast and derived an expression for the prediction of the minimum SPIO load necessary for single-cell detection. With image resolution of about 100 μm and an SNR of 60, they calculated that subpicomolar concentrations of SPIOs would be a sufficient loading dose. Shapiro and colleagues worked with higher

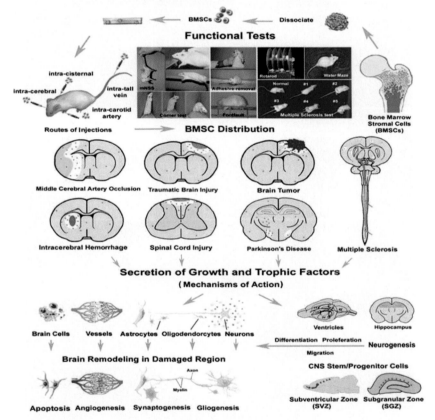

Color Plate 1. Illustration of our experimental studies supporting the potential treatment of central nervous system (CNS) disorders with bone marrow stromal cells (BMSCs). (*See* discussion on p. 11.)

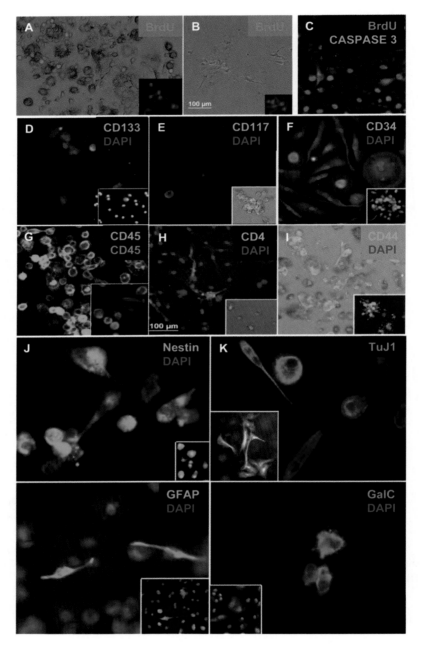

Color Plate 2. In vitro characterization of human umbilical cord blood (HUCB) cells. (*See* complete caption on p. 35 and discussion on p. 33.)

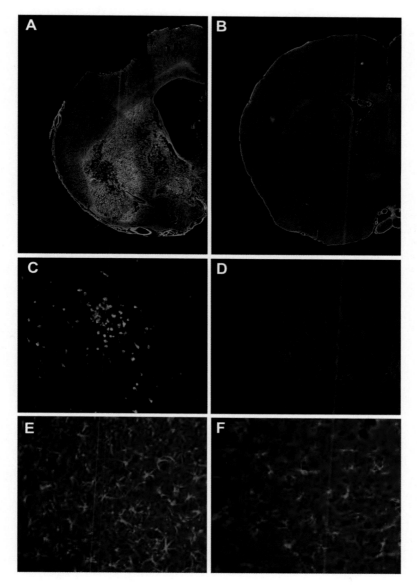

Color Plate 3. Cord blood treatment at 48 h decreases the inflammatory response after stroke. (*See* complete caption on p. 44 and discussion on p. 43.)

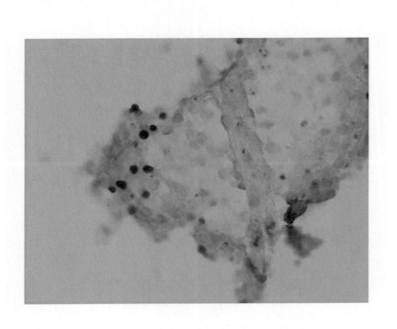

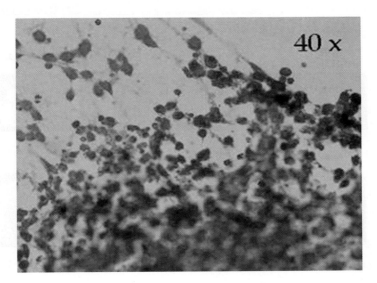

Color Plate 4. Diaminobenzidine (DAB)-enhanced Prussian blue staining of embryonic stem (ES) cells in culture after incubation with ultrasmall iron oxide nanoparticles (USPIOs). Upon spontaneous endocytosis of USPIOs (facing page), the cells show only slight brown coloring, while incubation of the cells with USPIOs in the presence of lipofection agent (above) leads to much stronger staining, indicating a much more effective contrast agent incorporation into the cells. Magnification: 40× for both panels. (*See* discussion on p. 75.)

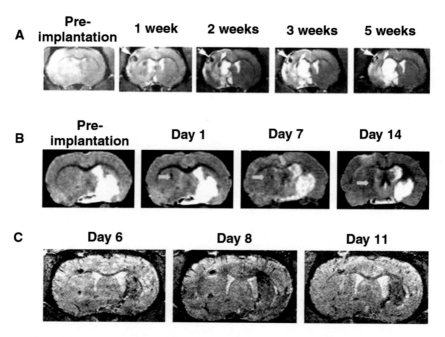

Color Plate 5. Combination of in vivo magnetic resonance (MR) image sequences after implantation of labeled embryonic stem (ES) cells into the ischemic rat brain. Iron oxide-labeled cells were either implanted into the cisterna magna (**A**) or directly into the parenchyma (**B, C**) on the hemisphere contralateral to the lesion (primary implantation sites are indicated by yellow arrows). In studies (**A**) and (**B**), T2-weighted imaging was used, while T2* weighting was applied in (**C**) for increased detection sensitivity of labeled cells. The ischemic lesion is visualized as hyperintense areas on the T2-weighted images; the T2* presentation (**C**) is rather insensitive to the depiction of the ischemic lesion on the right hemisphere. Groups of migrating cells are marked by blue arrows while stem cells in the perilesional target zone are indicated by red arrows. Cells having reached the ischemic boundary zone from the cisterna magna (**A**) are marked by white arrows, showing the cell persistence for at least 5 weeks after injection. ((**A**) courtesy of Michael Chopp, Detroit; (**B**) courtesy of Mike Modo, London.) (*See* discussion on p. 79.)

β-gal staining

In vivo BLI
of luciferase

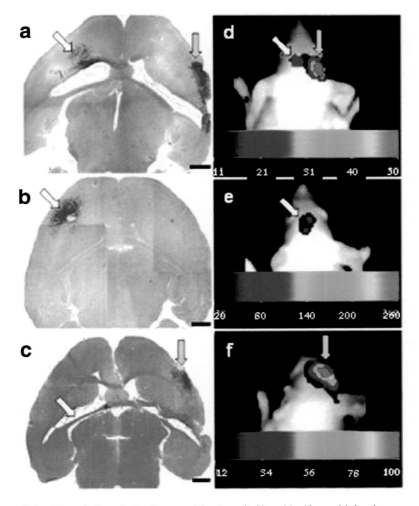

Color Plate 6. Correlation between histology (left) and luciferase bioluminescence imaging (right). Neural progenitor cells, transfected to stably express β-galactosidase and luciferase, were injected into the left, normal hemisphere of a mouse following stroke induction on the right hemisphere. In the first two animals, cells were injected into the parenchyma (white arrow on histological section). In the third animal, cells were intraventricularly injected. In the case of the infarcted animals (first animal and third animal), cells were found at the ischemic lesion periphery at 21 days after implantation. In the sham-operated animal (second animal), cells have not migrated away from the primary implantation site. (Taken with permission from 69.) (*See* discussion on p. 87.)

concentrations of iron oxide (>50 pg of iron per cell) in the form of MPIOs (1.63 μm in diameter) to visualize single cells. Although the iron load was comparatively high with their approach, it was well tolerated by the cells due to a protective polymer coating *(39)*. Another advantage of MPIOs is that their large size and magnetic moment allow detection even with lower resolution (300 μm slice thickness in Shapiro's study), which can substantially save scan time. Besides, dilution of the label does not become a problem; even after 1 year, these particles can still be detected within a cell *(6,29,41)*.

For Gd^+-based contrast agents, single-cell detection has not yet been achieved in vitro or in vivo. In principle, with known relaxivities of the compounds, local concentrations can be predicted by measuring T1 relaxation values *(42)*. However, this quantification approach is not straightforward, especially when concentrations of Gd chelates are increased above 0.1 μmol/mg protein *(33)*, possibly due to competing $T2^*$ effects under those conditions.

3. CURRENT IMAGING-BASED STUDIES IN STROKE RESEARCH

3.1. Cell Labeling and Route of Application in Stroke Research

For a successful MRI delineation of implanted stem cells in host tissue, the labeling strategy needs to be tailored to the application. This applies to the choice of the label (endogenous tissue contrast) as well as to the amount of label and its route of uptake. For cells that are labeled in vitro and expected to undergo several cell divisions, as is the case for stem cells, dilution of the label can become a problem. Therefore, a higher label load would be desirable. If an important part of the study involves a combined in vivo and postmortem histological analysis, dual-labeling approaches for MRI and histology (e.g., with fluorescent probes) may be preferred *(1)*. Here again, iron-based contrast agents may interfere with fluorescence analysis due to fluorescent quenching, which would then make Gd compounds the label of choice *(43)*.

Most studies attempting in vivo stem cell tracking in stroke models to date have been based on iron oxide labels *(2,44,45)*, while one group used Gd compounds, but again relied on $T2^*$-weighted signal decreases on MRI *(1)* (Fig. 3). The most commonly chosen route of cell delivery into the brain so far has been intracerebral implantation *(1,2,44)*, since this places cells closest to the ischemic lesion and can therefore be

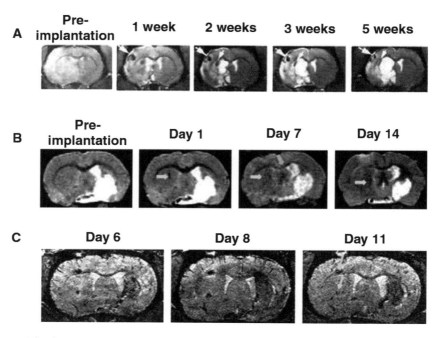

Fig. 3. Combination of in vivo magnetic resonance (MR) image sequences after implantation of labeled embryonic stem (ES) cells into the ischemic rat brain. Iron oxide-labeled cells were either implanted into the cisterna magna (**A**) or directly into the parenchyma (**B, C**) on the hemisphere contralateral to the lesion (primary implantation sites are indicated by yellow arrows). In studies (**A**) and (**B**), T2-weighted imaging was used, while T2* weighting was applied in (**C**) for increased detection sensitivity of labeled cells. The ischemic lesion is visualized as hyperintense areas on the T2-weighted images; the T2* presentation (**C**) is rather insensitive to the depiction of the ischemic lesion on the right hemisphere. Groups of migrating cells are marked by blue arrows while stem cells in the perilesional target zone are indicated by red arrows. Cells having reached the ischemic boundary zone from the cisterna magna (**A**) are marked by white arrows, showing the cell persistence for at least 5 weeks after injection. ((**A**) courtesy of Michael Chopp, Detroit; (**B**) courtesy of Mike Modo, London.) (*See* Color Plate 5 following p. 78.)

expected to yield the highest number of cells reaching the target site. In some studies, cells were injected into the cisterna magna (*45,46*). Sykova and colleagues tested systemic (i.v.) administration of stem cells and first detected these cells at the lesion area about 1 week after injection (*3*). The systemic administration of the cells would be highly desirable for future patient therapies, but requires a permeable blood–brain barrier, which, although usually part of the ischemic injury in stroke patients, would have to be detected and "timed" with the cell administration.

3.2. Detectability

Immediately after implantation of 1,000–30,000 labeled stem cells, areas of signal extinction can be readily detected at the implantation site on T2*-weighted images *(1,2)*. When implanting higher cell concentrations (120,000 cells) into the rat striatum at 7 T, Stroh and colleagues found labeled cells distributed throughout a wide area of the ipsilateral hemisphere *(4)*. In animals with ischemic lesions, the MRI patterns of the stem cell depots changed over the next 14 days: within a few days to a week, the signal loss on T2*-weighted images was either unchanged or diminished—Modo and colleagues described it as more "patchy" around the injection tract *(1–3)*. At the same time, dark lines of contrast were discernable in the corpus callosum, indicating transcallosal migration of stem cells to the infarct on the contralateral hemisphere *(2)*. This interpretation of the in vivo MRI data was corroborated using histology *(1,3)*. Over the next 1–2 weeks, cell accumulation at the lesion borderzone was observed, while some contrast still remained at the primary injection site *(1–3)*. Zhang and colleagues, who injected cells into the contralateral cisterna magna, reported an increase in contrast close to the lesion, which was obvious after 1 week and remained conspicuous until their last observation time point at 5 weeks. About 15 % of the label had moved with an average speed of about 65 μm/h toward the lesion, which is about double the speed estimated for endogenous stem cell migration along the rostral migratory stream in healthy brains *(45)*.

These observations were the first exciting hint for a directed migration of implanted stem cells toward an ischemic lesion. They suggest that at least some of the implanted cells had retained vitality and were able to respond to intrinsic signals of the injured host brain.

3.3. Specific Challenges for Cell Tracking in Ischemia

The background (host) tissue contrast has a major impact on the detection of labeled cells. This has been a particular challenge for stem cell tracking in ischemic tissue. In ischemic brains, specific changes in background MR contrast have to be considered depending on lesion type and pathophysiological developments at the time of observation, such as vasogenic edema (T1 and T2 increase) or hemorrhage. Acute hemorrhage and late vascular degradation can be part of the transformation of ischemic lesions into a fibrotic tissue scar. Blood leads to a signal decrease on T2/T2*-weighted MR images, because the iron contained in erythrocytes causes susceptibility-related nonuniformities of the magnetic field. Intact blood vessels appear dark (hypointense) on T2/T2*-weighted images for the same reason, but it is possible to identify them by following their course, especially on three-dimensional imaging data. Adjusting the inhalation gas mixture during anesthesia has further helped to overcome problems in differentiating contrast originating from blood vessels from contrast that stems from implanted cells *(47)* (Fig. 4 top).

Delayed vascular degradation in T2*-weighted MR imaging

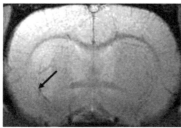 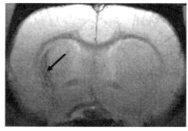

Modulation of inhalation gas for assignment of vascular origin BOLD effect

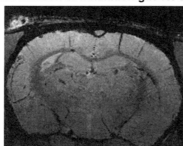 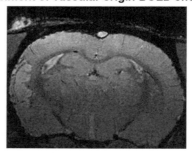

Fig. 4. T2*-weighted images of a rat brain after induction of stroke in the left hemisphere. Top: at 2 weeks after stroke, a discrete line in the ischemic striatum reflects a major vessel (arrow). At 10 weeks after stroke induction, this has changed into a diffuse widespread hypointense area due to delayed vascular degradation with consequent erythrocyte leakage into the adjacent parenchyma. Bottom: during normal 30 % oxygen breathing, dark lines appear in the brain tissue, in particular, radially in the cortex. These reflect vessels due to the Blood Oxygenation level dependent (BOLD) effect induced by deoxyhemoglobin. When allowing the animal to breathe a mixture of 95 % O_2 and 5 % CO_2, the small vessel contrast completely disappears, while the major vessels become much thinner and fade against the tissue. (Images: courtesy of Ralph Weber and Uwe Himmelreich, Cologne.)

However, while late vascular degradation can be distinguished from post-stroke hemorrhage by a specific constellation of MR parameters *(48)*, it remains difficult to separate these conditions from susceptibility effects induced by iron oxide-loaded stem cells (Fig. 4 bottom).

4. FUTURE PERSPECTIVES

4.1. New MR Labeling Strategies

Intrinsic contrast from iron-containing blood in vasculature, hemorrhages, or iron-loaded macrophages has been a drawback of stem cell tracking in stroke up to today, but new labeling options have appeared on the horizon. In a recent study, Anderson and colleagues introduced a Gd fullerene compound that does not cause T2 signal extinction, but an increase of T1, which would create a more obvious and specific contrast of labeled cells *(49)*. It consists of a Gd^{3+} ion wrapped in a 60- or 82-carbon fullerene cage, making it insensitive to steric changes or sequestration that may have hampered earlier attempts to apply Gd compounds in vivo to track cells based on T1 contrast *(1)*. The Gd fullerene proved to have high relaxivity, was well tolerated, and allowed tracking of mesenchymal stem cells in the mouse muscle.

Silvio Aime's group has performed extensive work on the use of Gd compounds to generate cellular T1 contrast *(50)*. They co-incubated the commercially available Gd chelate GdHPDO3A with blood-derived endothelial progenitor cells, injected them subcutaneously into mice, and detected them as hyperintense regions on T1-weighted images. They thus convincingly demonstrated the usefulness of Gd chelates for in vivo imaging. For a dual MR and fluorescent probe, they proposed the application of another lanthanide ion, europium (Eu), as a chelate together with Gd, because of its excellent fluorescent properties, and provided evidence for the feasibility of this idea *(51)*. Another new class of contrast agents that was exploited by this group are PARACEST agents (paramagnetic metal complexes for chemical exchange saturation transfer) *(52)*. These agents contain mobile protons, which can transfer saturated magnetization to the bulk water signal upon selective rf-irradiation. They can act as negative contrast agents (T2 shortening) if the rf-irradiation frequency is set to their proton-absorption frequency. With this label, one could acquire a "standard" MR image and then switch the excitation frequency to detect the labeled cells exclusively. A similar strategy without paramagnetic ions (CEST) has already yielded promising results in vitro *(53)*.

Contrast agents are typically packaged into a cell to constitutively produce the MRI contrast. However, most biological applications, including stem cell tracking in stroke, would hugely benefit from information about the physiological and metabolic status of the labeled cells. "Responsive" or "smart" contrast agents have dynamic relaxation properties that can be switched on in response to a change in the environment or the activity of a particular enzyme *(54)*. These agents are based on Gd chelates and obtain dynamic properties through changes in the coordination number of water molecules with contact to the paramagnetic ion, with more coordination sites blocked during the inactive state. When water molecules are excluded from the inner sphere of the complex, the effect on the water T1 relaxation time is less pronounced. As a way to monitor enzyme activity (and thus gene expression) in vivo, Meade and coworkers developed a complex in which all potential coordination binding sites for water are shielded by a sugar molecule. When the enzyme β-galactosidase is expressed, it cleaves the sugar from the chelate, thus permitting water to get access to the Gd ion and, in consequence, T1 contrast increases *(55)*. A Gd chelate which is originally insoluble but becomes water soluble (and thereby contrast active) by enzymatic cleavage of lipophilic side chains has recently been applied for the selective detection of dendritic cells after their implantation into the intact rat brain (Fig. 5).

Other contrast agents allowed to sense intracellular changes in the second messenger calcium *(56)*, changes in the tissue oxygenation state *(57,58)*, or in pH *(59)*. As a pH responsive agent, a Gd chelate is used containing a sulfonamide nitrogen that is protonated at low pH. In the protonated state, it is unable to chelate the Gd ion and allows access of water to the complex, thus increasing the contrast on T1-weighted images.

Moving closer to imaging molecular processes, Weissleder and his group developed superparamagnetic nanoparticles that allowed the detection of target oligonucleotides and the DNA cleaving compounds *(60)*. Upon hybridization of the nanoparticles with complementary oligonucleotides, stable assemblies are formed that decrease the T2 relaxation times of neighboring water protons.

Incorporation of responsive contrast agents into stem cells for the purpose of in vivo cell tracking in stroke has still to be accomplished. Potentially, these agents can aid in reporting on the functional status of the cells as well as of the tissue the cells were engrafted in. Changes in pH, pO_2, and calcium concentrations are common consequences of

Dendritic cells with responsive contrast agent

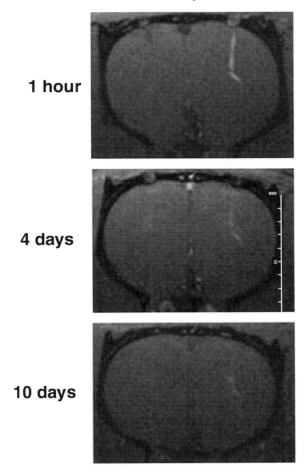

1 hour

4 days

10 days

Fig. 5. Dendritic cells with gadolinium (Gd) chelate labeling after intracerebral implantation into the rat. Cells were incubated for 24 h in the presence of 10 mM Gd-DTPA-FA, a responsive contrast agent that is activated selectively by enzymatic activity of lipase. Cells were stereotactically grafted into the cortex of the rat brain. T1-weighted images (FLASH; TR/TE: 80/5 ms; flip angle 65°) were acquired at 1 h, 4 days, and 10 days after implantation of 100,000 cells, suspended in 2 μl. (Courtesy Uwe Himmelreich, Cologne.)

ischemia, and therefore interesting aspects of the host tissue for stem cell survival.

Complementary to smart contrast agents, "smart cells" could be synthesized to activate or deactivate a contrast agent or even produce their own contrast depending on transcription of certain genes *(61)*.

4.2. Other Imaging Modalities

MRI is more and more taking the lead in clinical and experimental stroke imaging. The high spatial resolution and unlimited repeatability of imaging are some of the prominent advantages of MRI explaining this development. MR sequences such as diffusion-weighted imaging have allowed insights into acute processes in stroke that had till then been inaccessible. It is conceivable in this context that tracking implanted stem cells has been mainly attempted within the well-established MRI stroke imaging routines. However, other imaging modalities have the potential and may even be superior in some particular context to image cells in vivo. In the following paragraph, we therefore weigh the potential of other molecular imaging modalities for the purpose of stem cell monitoring.

4.2.1. PET and SPECT

The radionuclide imaging methods PET and single-photon emission tomography (SPECT) have been previously applied to the characterization of gene expression in cancer cells *(62)*. Although their spatial resolution is considerably lower, a variety of very sensitive and specific radioligands for cell imaging are available for these techniques. Due to the high sensitivity (nanomolar concentrations of a target substance), very small amounts of injected tracer are sufficient for detection of the target. Knowledge about safety of radiolabeled probes has already been gathered, since these agents have been applied in the clinical setting, e.g., to follow macrophages or dendritic cells injected to attack tumors *(63)*. But long-term toxicity from the exposure to radio-isotopes remains a caveat.

For cell labeling, different strategies are possible for PET and SPECT: pre-labeling with rather long-lived isotopes (similar to in vitro labeling with MR contrast agents) and the construction of stably expressed receptor genes in cells that can be visualized with radio-labeled probes. While pre-labeling is limited by dilution and decay of the label as well as toxicity considerations, introducing reporter genes into cells is a potent method to track cells with radionuclide imaging. Useful marker genes could be receptors, transporters, or enzymes. As an example, the mutant herpes simplex type 1 thymidine kinase (TK) gene can be expressed in stem cells, and after periodic injection of its radiolabeled substrate ^{18}FHBG, cells can be followed over the course of months *(64)*. In addition to localizing cells, genetically engineered receptor genes can be turned off and thereby identify cells that have died. [For a review on available reporter genes for cell tracking with PET and SPECT see 65.] Interestingly, PET imaging was conducted in the first human neuroimplantation trial for stroke. Meltzer and colleagues characterized the cerebral metabolic response to the implantation using serial [^{18}F]fluorodeoxyglucose PET. They described changes in metabolic activity that correlated with motor performance tests. But it must be noted that the implanted cells were not visualized in this study *(66)*.

The increasing availability of rodent PET scanners (microPET) with an improved spatial resolution (<2 mm) can be expected to motivate more intensive research in cellular PET imaging *(67)*.

4.2.2. Optical Imaging

Optical imaging methods can be categorized as being based on either fluorescence (a high-energy photon is absorbed and a lower energy photon with longer wavelength is emitted) or bioluminescence (emission of light by a living organism not requiring external illumination). In bioluminescence imaging (BLI), photons are emitted through the energy (ATP) and oxygen-dependent action of a luciferase enzyme. Luciferase genes can therefore serve as reporters of biological function. Cells can be pre-labeled via transfection with a luciferase reporter gene before implantation. With the help of a highly sensitive CCD camera, the emitted photons can be counted and mapped longitudinally and noninvasively *(68)*. In a mouse model of ischemic stroke, Kim and colleagues demonstrated the applicability of BLI for tracking stem cell recruitment to the infarct *(69)*. They implanted 1×10^6 stem cells into the healthy, contralateral hemisphere of nude mice and visualized their transhemispheric migration toward the ischemic lesion (Fig. 6).

In two aspects, BLI outperforms MRI for cell tracking in stroke: the inherent information that cells are alive and the lack of confounding host tissue contrast (excellent specificity). On the other hand, the spatial resolution of BLI is very poor, and signal detection is hampered in thicker tissues (greater than a few mm) due to substantial absorption

β-gal staining   In vivo BLI
of luciferase

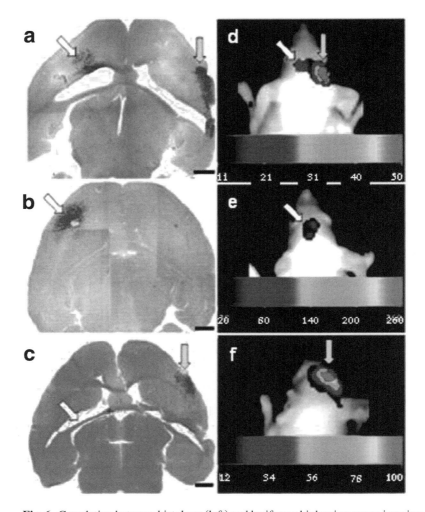

Fig. 6. Correlation between histology (left) and luciferase bioluminescence imaging (right). Neural progenitor cells, transfected to stably express β-galactosidase and luciferase, were injected into the left, normal hemisphere of a mouse following stroke induction on the right hemisphere. In the first two animals, cells were injected into the parenchyma (white arrow on histological section). In the third animal, cells were intraventricularly injected. In the case of the infarcted animals (first animal and third animal), cells were found at the ischemic lesion periphery at 21 days after implantation. In the sham-operated animal (second animal), cells have not migrated away from the primary implantation site. (Taken with permission from 69.) (*See* Color Plate 6 following p. 78.)

and light scattering. These latter aspects make the translation of BLI for human applications difficult.

The most difficult hurdle for the application of fluorescence imaging to track cells in vivo is the limited penetration of emitted photons through tissues. Near infrared (NIR) light (700–900 nm) has the optimal characteristics for tissue imaging, as it can be detected through 4–10 cm of tissue *(70)*. Optical probes for NIR imaging can be coupled to peptides that are activated by specific enzymes, which then dramatically increases fluorescence at the target site *(71)*. Similar to BLI, fluorescence imaging can transfer information about viability of cells with very low background contamination.

A slightly different imaging approach was chosen by Shichinohe and colleagues to monitor the migration of stromal cells transplanted into mice with experimental stroke: cells were harvested from transgenic mice expressing the green fluorescent protein (GFP). The green light of the transplanted 1×10^5 cells was detected by fluorescent optical imaging through the exposed skull. The same marker (GFP) was then used for immunohistochemical validation of imaging results *(72)*.

4.2.3. Combination of Different Imaging Modalities

Different imaging approaches may, in principle, be combined to achieve a more complex picture of the functional fate of stem cells after implantation into the host brain. Optical methods, through their high specificity, capability to assess viability of cells, and rather low-priced and practicable equipment, appear feasible and very interesting for a combination with high-resolution MRI assessment.

This will be even more promising, if one probe can be detected by different imaging modalities. Aside from the previously mentioned dual MRI/fluorescence probes *(1)*, cells were recently genetically modified to carry simultaneous markers for fluorescence, BLI, and PET *(73)*. This triple-fusion reporter contained a red fluorescent protein, firefly luciferase, and a truncated HSV type 1 TK reporter gene. Stem cells with this construct were not compromised regarding viability or differentiation characteristics and were successfully detected in the hearts of mice.

5. CONCLUSIONS

At present, powerful imaging techniques, such as MRI, have reached a sensitivity that permits detection of stem cells implanted into ischemic brains and monitor their route of migration. Now, the time is ripe to go one step further: explore the feasibility to investigate in vivo the intrinsic properties of stem cell changes, particularly in the ischemic environment. Responsive contrast agents and the combined use of high-resolution MRI with techniques that quickly report changes in the metabolic or gene-expression profile of a cell will provide researchers with the long needed information to conduct controlled therapeutic stem cell implantations.

ACKNOWLEDGMENTS

Support by the European Networks of Excellence EMIL (European Molecular Imaging Laboratories) and DiMI (Diagnostic Molecular Imaging) is gratefully acknowledged.

REFERENCES

1. Modo, M., et al., *Mapping transplanted stem cell migration after a stroke: a serial, in vivo magnetic resonance imaging study.* Neuroimage, 2004. **21**(1): p. 311–7.
2. Hoehn, M., et al., *Monitoring of implanted stem cell migration in vivo: a highly resolved in vivo magnetic resonance imaging investigation of experimental stroke in rat.* Proc Natl Acad Sci USA, 2002. **99**(25): p. 16267–72.
3. Sykova, E. and P. Jendelova, *Magnetic resonance tracking of implanted adult and embryonic stem cells in injured brain and spinal cord.* Ann N Y Acad Sci, 2005. **1049**: p. 146–60.
4. Stroh, A., et al., *In vivo detection limits of magnetically labeled embryonic stem cells in the rat brain using high-field (17.6 T) magnetic resonance imaging.* Neuroimage, 2005. **24**(3): p. 635–45.
5. Villringer, A., et al., *Dynamic imaging with lanthanide chelates in normal brain: contrast due to magnetic susceptibility effects.* Magn Reson Med, 1988. **6**(2): p. 164–74.
6. Hinds, K.A., et al., *Highly efficient endosomal labeling of progenitor and stem cells with large magnetic particles allows magnetic resonance imaging of single cells.* Blood, 2003. **102**(3): p. 867–72.
7. Weissleder, R., et al., *Magnetically labeled cells can be detected by MR imaging.* J Magn Reson Imaging, 1997. **7**(1): p. 258–63.
8. Lauffer, R.B., *Paramagnetic metal complexes as water proton relaxation agents for NMR imaging: theory and design.* Chem Rev, 1987. **87**: p. 901–27.
9. Moore, A., et al., *Human transferrin receptor gene as a marker gene for MR imaging.* Radiology, 2001. **221**(1): p. 244–50.
10. Bulte, J.W., et al., *Neurotransplantation of magnetically labeled oligodendrocyte progenitors: magnetic resonance tracking of cell migration and myelination.* Proc Natl Acad Sci USA, 1999. **96**(26): p. 15256–61.
11. Ahrens, E.T., et al., Receptor-mediated endocytosis of iron-oxide particles provides efficient labeling of dendritic cells for in vivo MR imaging. Magn Reson Med, 2003. **49**(6): p. 1006–13.

12. Zheng, Q., et al., *A new class of macrocyclic lanthanide complexes for cell labeling and magnetic resonance imaging applications.* J Am Chem Soc, 2005. **127**(46): p. 16178–88.
13. Felgner, P.L., et al., *Lipofection: a highly efficient, lipid-mediated DNA-transfection procedure.* Proc Natl Acad Sci USA, 1987. **84**(21): p. 7413–7.
14. Bulte, J.W., et al., *Magnetodendrimers allow endosomal magnetic labeling and in vivo tracking of stem cells.* Nat Biotechnol, 2001. **19**(12): p. 1141–7.
15. van den Bos, E.J., et al., *Improved efficacy of stem cell labeling for magnetic resonance imaging studies by the use of cationic liposomes.* Cell Transplant, 2003. **12**(7): p. 743–56.
16. Arbab, A.S., et al., *Comparison of transfection agents in forming complexes with ferumoxides, cell labeling efficiency, and cellular viability.* Mol Imaging, 2004. **3**(1): p. 24–32.
17. Rudelius, M., et al., *Highly efficient paramagnetic labelling of embryonic and neuronal stem cells.* Eur J Nucl Med Mol Imaging, 2003. **30**(7): p. 1038–44.
18. Daldrup-Link, H.E., et al., *In vivo tracking of genetically engineered, anti-HER2/neu directed natural killer cells to HER2/neu positive mammary tumors with magnetic resonance imaging.* Eur Radiol, 2005. **15**(1): p. 4–13.
19. Walczak, P., et al., *Instant MR labeling of stem cells using magnetoelectroporation.* Magn Reson Med, 2005. **54**(4): p. 769–74.
20. Allen, M.J. and T.J. Meade, *Synthesis and visualization of a membrane-permeable MRI contrast agent.* J Biol Inorg Chem, 2003. **8**(7): p. 746–50.
21. Allen, M.J., et al., *Cellular delivery of MRI contrast agents.* Chem Biol, 2004. **11**(3): p. 301–7.
22. Kayyem, J.F., et al., *Receptor-targeted co-transport of DNA and magnetic resonance contrast agents.* Chem Biol, 1995. **2**(9): p. 615–20.
23. Bhorade, R., et al., *Macrocyclic chelators with paramagnetic cations are internalized into mammalian cells via a HIV-tat derived membrane translocation peptide.* Bioconjug Chem, 2000. **11**(3): p. 301–5.
24. Lewin, M., et al., *Tat peptide-derivatized magnetic nanoparticles allow in vivo tracking and recovery of progenitor cells.* Nat Biotechnol, 2000. **18**(4): p. 410–4.
25. Zhao, M., et al., *Differential conjugation of tat peptide to superparamagnetic nanoparticles and its effect on cellular uptake.* Bioconjug Chem, 2002. **13**(4): p. 840–4.
26. Miyoshi, S., et al., *Transfection of neuroprogenitor cells with iron nanoparticles for magnetic resonance imaging tracking: cell viability, differentiation, and intracellular localization.* Mol Imaging Biol, 2005: **7**(4): 286–295.
27. Emerit, J., C. Beaumont, and F. Trivin, *Iron metabolism, free radicals, and oxidative injury.* Biomed Pharmacother, 2001. **55**(6): p. 333–9.
28. Stroh, A., et al., *Iron oxide particles for molecular magnetic resonance imaging cause transient oxidative stress in rat macrophages.* Free Radic Biol Med, 2004. **36**(8): p. 976–84.
29. Hill, J.M., et al., *Serial cardiac magnetic resonance imaging of injected mesenchymal stem cells.* Circulation, 2003. **108**(8): p. 1009–14.
30. Bos, C., et al., *In vivo MR imaging of intravascularly injected magnetically labeled mesenchymal stem cells in rat kidney and liver.* Radiology, 2004. **233**(3): p. 781–9.

31. Shapiro, E.M., S. Skrtic, and A.P. Koretsky, *Sizing it up: cellular MRI using micron-sized iron oxide particles.* Magn Reson Med, 2005. **53**(2): p. 329–38.
32. Caravan, P., et al., *Gadolinium (III) chelates as MRI contrast agents: structure, dynamics, and applications.* Chem Rev, 1999. **99**: p. 2293–352.
33. Crich, S.G., et al., *Improved route for the visualization of stem cells labeled with a Gd-/Eu-chelate as dual (MRI and fluorescence) agent.* Magn Reson Med, 2004. **51**(5): p. 938–44.
34. Bourrinet, P., et al., *Preclinical safety and pharmacokinetic profile of ferumoxtran-10, an ultrasmall superparamagnetic iron oxide magnetic resonance contrast agent.* Invest Radiol, 2006. **41**(3): p. 313–24.
35. Tombach, B. and P. Reimer, *Soluble paramagnetic chelates and stabilized colloidal particle solutions of iron oxides as contrast agents for magnetic resonance imaging.* Curr Med Chem, 2005. **12**(23): p. 2795–804.
36. Dodd, S.J., et al., *Detection of single mammalian cells by high-resolution magnetic resonance imaging.* Biophys J, 1999. **76**(1 Pt 1): p. 103–9.
37. Foster-Gareau, P., et al., *Imaging single mammalian cells with a 1.5 T clinical MRI scanner.* Magn Reson Med, 2003. **49**(5): p. 968–71.
38. Heyn, C., et al., *In vivo magnetic resonance imaging of single cells in mouse brain with optical validation.* Magn Reson Med, 2006. **55**(1): p. 23–9.
39. Shapiro, E.M., et al., *In vivo detection of single cells by MRI.* Magn Reson Med, 2006. **55**(2): p. 242–9.
40. Heyn, C., et al., *Detection threshold of single SPIO-labeled cells with FIESTA.* Magn Reson Med, 2005. **53**(2): p. 312–20.
41. Shapiro, E.M., S. Skrtic, and A.P. Koretsky, *Long term cellular MR imaging using microsized iron oxide particles.* Proc Int Soc Magn Reson Med, 2004: p. 166.
42. Morawski, A.M., et al., *Targeted nanoparticles for quantitative imaging of sparse molecular epitopes with MRI.* Magn Reson Med, 2004. **51**(3): p. 480–6.
43. Daldrup-Link, H.E., et al., *Cell tracking with gadophrin-2: a bifunctional contrast agent for MR imaging, optical imaging, and fluorescence microscopy.* Eur J Nucl Med Mol Imaging, 2004. **31**(9): p. 1312–21.
44. Jendelova, P., et al., *Magnetic resonance tracking of human CD34+ progenitor cells separated by means of immunomagnetic selection and transplanted into injured rat brain.* Cell Transplant, 2005. **14**(4): p. 173–82.
45. Zhang, Z.G., et al., *Magnetic resonance imaging and neurosphere therapy of stroke in rat.* Ann Neurol, 2003. **53**(2): p. 259–63.
46. Jiang, Q., et al., *Investigation of neural progenitor cell induced angiogenesis after embolic stroke in rat using MRI.* Neuroimage, 2005. **28**(3): p. 698–707.
47. Himmelreich, U., et al., *Improved stem cell MR detectability in animal models by modification of the inhalation gas.* Mol Imaging, 2005. **4**(2): p. 104–9.
48. Weber, R., et al., *MRI detection of macrophage activity after experimental stroke in rats: new indicators for late appearance of vascular degradation?* Magn Reson Med, 2005. **54**(1): p. 59–66.
49. Anderson, S.A., K.K. Lee, and J.A. Frank, *Gadolinium-fullerenol as a paramagnetic contrast agent for cellular imaging.* Invest Radiol, 2006. **41**(3): p. 332–8.
50. Aime, S., et al., *Insights into the use of paramagnetic Gd(III) complexes in MR-molecular imaging investigations.* J Magn Reson Imaging, 2002. **16**(4): p. 394–406.

51. Aime, S., et al., *Targeting cells with MR imaging probes based on paramagnetic Gd(III) chelates*. Curr Pharm Biotechnol, 2004. **5**(6): p. 509–18.

52. Aime, S., et al., *Tunable imaging of cells labeled with MRI-PARACEST agents*. Angew Chem Int Ed Engl, 2005. **44**(12): p. 1813–5.

53. Aime, S., et al., *Iopamidol: Exploring the potential use of a well-established x-ray contrast agent for MRI*. Magn Reson Med, 2005. **53**(4): p. 830–4.

54. Meade, T.J., A.K. Taylor, and S.R. Bull, *New magnetic resonance contrast agents as biochemical reporters*. Curr Opin Neurobiol, 2003. **13**(5): p. 597–602.

55. Louie, A.Y., et al., *In vivo visualization of gene expression using magnetic resonance imaging*. Nat Biotechnol, 2000. **18**(3): p. 321–5.

56. Li, W.H., et al., *Mechanistic studies of a calcium-dependent MRI contrast agent*. Inorg Chem, 2002. **41**(15): p. 4018–24.

57. Burai, L., R. Scopelliti, and E. Toth, *EuII-cryptate with optimal water exchange and electronic relaxation: a synthon for potential pO2 responsive macromolecular MRI contrast agents*. Chem Commun (Camb), 2002. (20): p. 2366–7.

58. Aime, S., et al., *A p(O(2))-responsive MRI contrast agent based on the redox switch of manganese(II / III)–porphyrin complexes*. Angew Chem Int Ed Engl, 2000. **39**(4): p. 747–50.

59. Lowe, M.P., et al., *pH-dependent modulation of relaxivity and luminescence in macrocyclic gadolinium and europium complexes based on reversible intramolecular sulfonamide ligation*. J Am Chem Soc, 2001. **123**(31): p. 7601–9.

60. Perez, J.M., et al., *DNA-based magnetic nanoparticle assembly acts as a magnetic relaxation nanoswitch allowing screening of DNA-cleaving agents*. J Am Chem Soc, 2002. **124**(12): p. 2856–7.

61. Cohen, B., et al., *Ferritin as an endogenous MRI reporter for noninvasive imaging of gene expression in C6 glioma tumors*. Neoplasia, 2005. **7**(2): p. 109–17.

62. Shah, K., et al., *Molecular imaging of gene therapy for cancer*. Gene Ther, 2004. **11**(15): p. 1175–87.

63. Thompson, M., et al., *In vivo tracking for cell therapies*. Q J Nucl Med Mol Imaging, 2005. **49**(4): p. 339–48.

64. Wu, J.C., et al., *Molecular imaging of cardiac cell transplantation in living animals using optical bioluminescence and positron emission tomography*. Circulation, 2003. **108**(11): p. 1302–5.

65. Acton, P.D. and R. Zhou, *Imaging reporter genes for cell tracking with PET and SPECT*. Q J Nucl Med Mol Imaging, 2005. **49**(4): p. 349–60.

66. Meltzer, C.C., et al., *Serial [18F] fluorodeoxyglucose positron emission tomography after human neuronal implantation for stroke*. Neurosurgery, 2001. **49**(3): p. 586–91; discussion 591–2.

67. Kornblum, H.I., et al., *In vivo imaging of neuronal activation and plasticity in the rat brain by high resolution positron emission tomography (microPET)*. Nat Biotechnol, 2000. **18**(6): p. 655–60.

68. Welsh, D.K. and S.A. Kay, *Bioluminescence imaging in living organisms*. Curr Opin Biotechnol, 2005. **16**(1): p. 73–8.

69. Kim, D.E., et al., *Imaging of stem cell recruitment to ischemic infarcts in a murine model*. Stroke, 2004. **35**(4): p. 952–7.

70. Frangioni, J.V. and R.J. Hajjar, *In vivo tracking of stem cells for clinical trials in cardiovascular disease*. Circulation, 2004. **110**(21): p. 3378–83.

71. Shah, K. and R. Weissleder, *Molecular optical imaging: applications leading to the development of present day therapeutics.* NeuroRx, 2005. **2**(2): p. 215–25.
72. Shichinohe, H., et al., *In vivo tracking of bone marrow stromal cells transplanted into mice cerebral infarct by fluorescence optical imaging.* Brain Res Brain Res Protoc, 2004. **13**(3): p. 166–75.
73. Wu, J.C., et al., *Transcriptional profiling of reporter genes used for molecular imaging of embryonic stem cell transplantation.* Physiol Genomics, 2006. **25**(4): 29–38.

6

Cell Transplantation
for Intracerebral Hemorrhage

Kon Chu, Keun-Hwa Jung and Jae-Kyu Roh

1. PATHOPHYSIOLOGICAL ASPECTS
OF INTRACEREBRAL HEMORRHAGE

Our understanding of the pathophysiology of intracerebral hemorrhage (ICH) has changed much in recent years, and the issue remains very much under investigation. What was thought to be a simple and rapid bleeding event is now known to be a dynamic and complex process. The mechanism by which cellular injury occurs during ICH is biphasic. The initial insult is due to direct mechanical forces resulting from an expanding hematoma, which causes local tissue deformation and compression of the surrounding brain and microvasculature (1). And, almost immediately, neurons and myelinated white matter tracts within the hematoma itself are destroyed (2). The pathophysiology of ICH involves not only this mechanical damage, but also edema formation, free radical injury, excitotoxicity, the impairment of local blood flow, and the extravasation of blood, and of its attendant potentially damaging molecules, into the brain parenchyma (3–5). Moreover, inflammatory response, although engaged in the absorption of erythrocytes and other post-hemorrhage debris, contributes to secondary brain injury and swelling (6,7). Experimental studies on ICH provide strong evidence for the presence of robust inflammation in response to ICH, such as, microglial activation, polymorphonuclear leukocyte (PMNL) and macrophage infiltration, the activation of proinflammatory transcription factors, cytokine, and chemokine release, the expressions of inflammatory enzymes and adhesion molecules, complement activation, and astrogliosis (7–12). In addition, plasma, rich in thrombin and other coagulation end-products released by a

From: *Current Clinical Neurology: Stroke Recovery with Cellular Therapies*
Edited by: Sean I. Savitz and Daniel M. Rosenbaum © Humana Press Inc., Totowa, NJ

clotted hematoma, seeps into the surrounding brain tissue and is a primary trigger of the inflammatory process *(11)*. As a result of blood–brain barrier (BBB) disruption during ICH, macrophages and leucocytes adhere to damaged brain endothelia and infiltrate the brain parenchyma, and resident microglia and astrocytes are activated *(7)*. These processes have been proposed to constitute a primary mechanism of cell death. Hemoglobin and its degradation products resulting from the lysis of red blood cells (RBCs) also contribute to delayed brain injury following ICH via free radical reaction *(13)*. The cell death process peaks at 24 h and hematoma resolves at 7 days, and during the following several weeks, a scar forms, and atrophy occurs in the region of the ICH residue. Given the importance of matrix metalloproteinases (MMPs) during inflammation within the brain, it would also be anticipated that ICH-induced MMP expression contributes to tissue destruction, increased capillary permeability, and subsequent brain edema formation or further bleeding *(14,15)*. The appearance of edema, free radical injury, apoptosis, and inflammation in perihematomal brain suggests that these events may be targets for therapeutic intervention. To date, the medical management of ICH has only had a minimal impact on the disease, and the preclinical development of protective strategies has markedly lagged behind that of ischemic stroke.

2. POTENTIAL TARGETS FOR INTERVENTION

2.1. Hematoma Expansion

Recent evidence suggests that clot formation in humans is a gradual process rather than a monophasic event *(1)* and that hematoma volume is a principal determinant of mortality and functional outcome after ICH *(16,17)*. It is also recognized that early hematoma growth is an important cause of neurologic deterioration *(1,18)*. The mechanisms that lead to early hematoma growth during the acute stage of ICH remain unclear. A sudden increase in intracranial pressure (ICP), local tissue distortion, shear forces, and disruption of the normal cerebral anatomy can lead to a multifocal bleeding process *(19)*, and other changes in surrounding tissue, such as vascular engorgement related to a limitation in venous outflow, early transient ischemia, and breakdown of the BBB, and the possible transient creation of a local coagulopathy, might contribute in part to early hematoma growth *(19,20)*. MMP-9 is one of the most important molecules involved in hematoma expansion, and the level of MMP-9 has been shown to increase in experimental

ICH models *(21)*. In a recent phase II trial, recombinant activated factor VIIa (eptacog alfa) reduced hematoma expansion, mortality, and disability when given within 4 h of ICH onset *(22)*, and in a recent study, we found that the NMDA receptor antagonist (memantine, given 2 h after ICH onset) reduced hematoma expansion in an experimental ICH model by inhibiting MMP-9 via the suppression of excitotoxicity and endogenous tissue plasminogen activator (tPA) activation *(23)*. In addition, intervention with the so-called ultra-early hemostatic therapy improved outcomes after ICH by arresting ongoing bleeding and thus minimizing increases in hematoma volume *(20)*.

2.2. Brain Edema

Brain edema is an important complication of ICH and has clear clinical management implications. Perihematomal edema is commonly observed during the acute and subacute stages and is known to exacerbate brain injury. Previous studies on ICH suggest that brain edema increases progressively during the first 24 h, remains stable for several days, and then begins to resolve after 4–5 days *(24)*. A number of mechanisms appear to be involved in edema formation, which can be divided into three phases, an immediate phase (the first several hours) that involves hydrostatic pressure and clot formation, a second phase (first 2 days) involving coagulation cascade activation with thrombin formation, and a third phase (after 3 days) that involves RBC lysis and hemoglobin toxicity *(13,25,26)*. Brain parenchyma inflammatory response plays an important role in the second and third of these phases. Moreover, potential therapeutic strategies have been described to address each of these phases. Thrombin contributes during the early phase of brain edema *(26,27)*; its direct intracerebral infusion was found to cause inflammation, edema, reactive gliosis, apoptosis, and scar formation *(27,28,29)*, and the significance of thrombin during this period of early edema formation is substantiated by the ability of thrombin inhibitors to reduce edema *(26,30)*. Thus, the administration of argatroban, even 6 h after ICH, can reduce ICH-induced edema formation *(31)*, but subsequently, marked BBB disruption underlies delayed edema formation due to the toxic effects of lysed RBCs *(25)*. This delayed edema formation occurs at 3 days after ICH and is associated with the cellular toxicities attributable to hemoglobin and its degradation products *(25)*. Perihematomal edema at 24 h can be reduced by >70 % when the clot is lysed early with tPA and aspirated *(32)* and can be partly prevented by administering the iron chelator deferroxamine *(13)*. It has also been reported that prompt albumin therapy instituted at 60 min after an ICH improves BBB integrity *(33)*, and that atorvastatin, celecoxib, granulocyte colony-stimulating factor (G-CSF), or erythropoietin reduce brain edema due to their putative anti-inflammatory actions *(34–37)*.

2.3. Inflammation

Previous preclinical studies indicate that ICH-induced inflammation is a key factor that leads to secondary brain damage, which suggests that anti-inflammatory approaches may usefully prevent the secondary brain injury that evolves over days after the formation of the primary clot. In general, inflammation is the result of a complex array of enzyme activation, mediator release, fluid extravasation, cell migration, and tissue breakdown and repair, and microglial activation and leukocyte infiltration are important markers of ICH-induced brain inflammation *(7)*. Infiltrating leukocytes could contribute to brain cell injury by releasing cytotoxic enzymes, free oxygen radicals, nitric oxide, and the products of the phospholipid cascade *(7)*. In addition, from 6 h to 3 days after ICH, cyclooxygenase-type 2 (COX-2) proteins are significantly upregulated and appear to play an important role in mediating neuronal damage or brain edema formation *(35)*. Moreover, proteolytic enzymes such as elastase might damage endothelial cell membranes and the basal lamina and alter the BBB and thus lead to brain edema *(38)*. Activated microglia also secretes a number of cytotoxic compounds like interleukins, interferon, and tumor necrosis factor *(39)*. Neutrophil infiltration can be identified by measuring myeloperoxidase (MPO) levels, and activated microglia can be identified by intense OX-42 staining and by morphological changes that include an enlarged size and stout processes *(40)*. Our previous studies indicate that inflammatory response occurs in and around a blood clot after ICH, and that this is marked by the infiltration of MPO-positive neutrophils and OX42-positive activated microglial cells *(23,34–36)*.

Since progressive brain edema formation and brain injury surrounding a hematoma may increase mortality and neurological deficits, anti-inflammation intervention offers a possible means of controlling the injury and its sequelae. The modulation of inflammatory response using the potent immunosuppressant, FK-506, COX-2 inhibitor, celecoxib, 3-hydroxy-3-methyl-glutaryl-coenzyme A (HMG-CoA) reductase inhibitor, atorvastatin, G-CSF, memantine, or erythropoietin has been reported to reduce brain edema and tissue damage and to improve functional outcome in experimental ICH *(23,34–36,41)*.

2.4. Excitotoxicity

The early period of ICH is characterized by perihematomal glutamate accumulation *(42)*, and the resulting overstimulation of *N*-methyl-D-aspartate-type glutamate receptor (NMDAR) induces excito-toxic damage and consequent excessive Ca^{2+} influx, which contributes to a series of detrimental enzymatic reactions, namely, the generation of toxic oxygen- and nitrogen-free radicals and the abundant accumulation of abnormal protein aggregates *(43)*. Glutamate-mediated NMDAR stimulation also results in an increase in glucose metabolism in the perihematomal brain during the early stage, and this may lead to metabolic stress *(44)*. A reproducible hypermetabolic area has been demonstrated in the perihematomal brain after experimental ICH *(44)*, and the direct injection of non-metabolizable glutamate receptor agonists into the striatum induced pronounced hyperme-tabolism, which was blocked by the glutamate receptor antagonists MK-801 or NBQX *(44)*. Moreover, we found that memantine (a moderate-affinity, uncompetitive, open-channel NMDAR antagonist) exerts both anti-inflammatory and anti-apoptotic effects in the hemor-rhagic rat brain *(23)*.

2.5. Apoptosis

Contemporary evidence suggests that apoptosis may be involved in the pathophysiology of cell death after ICH. After ICH induction, significant numbers of TUNEL-positive cells appear within and around the hematoma and are significantly reduced by caspase inhibitor treatment. Apoptotic DNA fragmentation forms 200-bp ladders, as shown by gel electrophoresis, and the caspase substrate gelsolin is much cleaved in the perihematomal brain *(45)*. Although the triggers responsible for initiating the apoptotic cascade after ICH remain to be determined, perihematomal ischemia and inflammatory responses have been suggested to mediate apoptosis *(45)*. Activated blood components induce high levels of extracellular cytokines, and cytokine-mediated signaling has been associated with apoptosis *(46,47)*. Fas and the tumor necrosis factor family of cell-surface receptors represent a major apoptotic signaling pathway *(48)*. Given that Fas ligand and tumor necrosis factor are upregulated after ICH *(48)*, they may play critical roles in mediating cellular apoptosis after ICH. Thrombin, iron/heme, and glutamate are obviously abundant in blood and in the hemorrhagic brain and may also be apoptotic triggers. Moreover, treatments with memantine, atorvastatin, celecoxib, or G-CSF after ICH have been reported to reduce TUNEL-positive cell density and attenuate the expressions of apoptotic molecules *(23,34–36)*.

2.6. Oxidative Stress

Increased free radical and reactive oxygen species (ROS) production may play an important role in the pathogenesis of ICH and perihematomal edema *(49,50)*. Elevated levels of ROS, as measured by protein carbonyl formation in a porcine lobar ICH model, were detected within minutes of autologous blood injection *(51)*, suggesting that oxidative stress may play a pathogenic role immediately after ICH induction. In the presence of free radical scavengers, hemoglobin-induced neuronal damage was less evident, and in rat models of ICH, anti-free radical therapy was demonstrated to improve functional outcome *(49,50)*. Moreover, treatment with disodium 4-[(tert-butylimino)methyl]benzene-1,3-disulfonate *N*-oxide (NXY-059), a free radical trapping agent, improved neurological outcome and reduced neutrophil infiltrate and the number of TUNEL-positive cells after ICH in a rat model *(49)*. Although the precise source of oxidative stress is unknown, hemoglobin released during RBC lysis and/or its breakdown products may be major sources of ROS and pathological process mediation *(13)*. The injection of autologous lysed erythrocytes into rat striatum was found to increase protein carbonyl levels, and this was associated with an increase in the numbers of cells containing damaged DNA *(52)*. Moreover, strategies targeting iron as a potential source of free radicals were demonstrated to limit ICH-induced pathology, i.e., brain edema volume and behavioral dysfunction *(53)*. Thus, pharmacologic evidence suggests that selected approaches targeting ROS may provide useful treatments for ICH.

2.7. Matrix Metalloproteinases

The zinc-dependent endopeptidases, better known as the MMPs, can degrade many components of the extracellular matrix and have received special attention as potential contributors to ICH-induced damage *(21)*. The temporal expression profiles of various MMPs were examined in a rat model of ICH, and MMP-2 and MMP-9 activations were found to be increased at 16–24 h after ICH induction *(54)*. Moreover, BB-1101 and BB-94, synthetic inhibitors of MMP activity, were shown to reduce edema and hemorrhage after ICH induction, which suggests that MMPs play an important role in ICH-induced BBB disruption *(21,55)*. It was also reported that inhibition with the broad-spectrum MMP inhibitor (GM6001) ameliorated dysregulation of gelatinase activity, neutrophil infiltration, and oxidative stress and reduced brain edema and subsequently improved functional deficit *(15)*. In an extension of this work, it was demonstrated that ICH increased not only MMP-2 and MMP-9 levels, but also increased the levels of MMP-3 and MMP-7, and in particular increased MMP-12 mRNA levels. Moreover, a reduction in ICH-induced behavioral deficit and cellular loss after minocycline administration was associated with a robust reduction in MMP-12 mRNA levels, rather than reductions in the expressions of MMP-2, MMP-7, and MMP-9 *(54)*. This inverse association between MMP-12 mRNA expression and ICH-induced damage makes MMP-12 a potentially important target for ICH therapy.

3. STEM CELL TRANSPLANTATION IN ICH

A number of reports have been issued concerning stem cell transplantation in ICH. However, as mentioned above, a detailed knowledge of the target disease and its pathophysiology is a prerequisite of stem cell treatment (vide supra) *(56)*. The categories of stem cells used for ICH treatment are neural stem cells (NSCs) *(57)*, human umbilical cord blood cells (HUCBCs) *(58)*, embryonic stem cells (ESCs) *(59)*, rat mesenchymal stem cells (MSCs) *(60)*, and human bone marrow stromal cells (BMSCs) *(61)*. In the first report issued on this topic, Jeong et al. *(57)* showed that adult human NSCs in an ICH rat model can migrate to the hemorrhagic brain, differentiate into neural cells, and promote functional recovery. NSCs derived from human fetal cortical tissue (gestation week 15, 5 million cells/rat) were administered intravenously 1 day after ICH and were found to home to the hemorrhagic site surrounding the hematoma. In particular, these NSCs migrated to the perihematomal area and populated it in a center-to-periphery pattern. Moreover, rats treated by NSC transplantation recovered from neurological deficits 2 weeks after ICH (rotarod test and modified limb placing test), and these improved functions persisted for 8–12 weeks. Furthermore, it was found that NSCs differentiate into neurons and astroglia in the hemorrhagic brain.

Another group at the University of Minnesota and South Florida investigating HUCBC transplantation in ICH rat models found that intravenous infusions of umbilical cord blood can ameliorate the neurologic deficits associated with hemorrhagic brain injury *(58)*, by using experimental paradigms similar to ours, which involved the transplantation of HUCBCs intravenously at 24 h after ICH, a collagenase model, and 2.4 to 3.2 million cells/rat. In particular, it was found that animals given HUCBCs recovered 6–13 days after ICH (stepping test, neurologic severity scale, and elevated body swing test). They also noted a paucity of human cord blood cells within the perilesional brain parenchyma despite the functional recovery observed. Moreover, scant numbers of cord blood cells were observed in the brain on the injured side even in animals that had received high doses of cord blood cells, which significantly spared host brain tissue. Thus, it appears that HUCBCs need not penetrate the brain parenchyma to induce therapeutic effects. These results suggest that mechanisms other than cell replacement may underlie the restorative effects of cord blood cells.

Researchers at the Nara Medical University, Japan, have been active in the ESC transplantation field *(59)* and found that mouse ESCs differentiated into nestin-positive neural precursors in vitro after all-trans retinoic acid (ATRA) administration. In this study, ATRA-treated ESCs (0.1 million cells/rat) were transplanted into the lateral ventricle in the hemisphere contralateral to the hemorrhage 7 days after collagenase infusion. Donor-derived neurons and astrocytes were observed around brain hematoma cavities in all ten rats that received grafts, and donor-derived neurons were also observed in the subependymal area of the lateral ventricle as cellular nodules. Unfortunately, no functional recovery or cellular integration data were presented. Moreover, one of these ten rats showed uncontrolled ESC-derived astroglial growth, which indicates the possibility of tumorigenesis (donor-derived astrocytic tumor in the host brain or teratoma). Pluripotent ESCs are being intensely investigated in several strategic directions, e.g., ESC cloning, removal of animal gene/protein contamination, refinement of feeder layer cells, safe transplantation issues, differentiation, and the development of individualized genetic disease models *(62)*.

Other researchers also investigated whether rat MSCs administered by intraarterial injection or human BMSCs by intravenous injection can have a beneficial effect on outcome after ICH in rats *(60,61)*. Both transplantations significantly improved neurological function in rats subjected to ICH. This improvement in the treated animals was associated with reduced tissue loss and increased local presence of the transplanted cells, mitotic activity, immature neurons, synaptogenesis, and neuronal migration.

4. SYSTEMIC TRANSPLANTATION OF NEURAL PROGENITOR/STEM CELLS

Neural stem/progenitor cells can be transplanted systemically, i.e., intravenously or intraarterially, and this has been reported by four different laboratories. Target diseases include brain tumor (63), experimental allergic encephalomyelitis (EAE) (64,65), global ischemia (66), focal ischemia (67–70), ICH (57), temporal lobe epilepsy (TLE) (71) and Huntington's disease (HD) model (72,73). The concept of intravascular NSC transplantation originated from the immense amount of clinical and experimental work conducted on hematopoietic stem cells (HSCs) and bone marrow transplantation. HSCs express many surface antigens and receptors. They react to homing signals (chemokines), attach to vascular endothelium (by interacting with adhesion molecules), and migrate to target tissues (e.g., bone marrow). However, unlike the majority of tissues, the brain, like the testes and the placenta, has a very strong barrier, the so-called BBB. Inflammation plays a central role in the pathogenesis of many acute and relapsing–remitting CNS illnesses, and inflammation occurs in the brain endothelium, causing the upregulation of many inflammatory chemokines, cytokines, and adhesion molecules. Moreover, CNS inflammation can be aggravated by infiltrating neutrophils and macrophages, as well as by microglia (74,75), and these infiltrating species share many mechanisms with stem cells which underlie *effective migration* to the diseased brain.

NSCs express many adhesion molecules and chemo/cytokine receptors (64,65,76,77), and this has led many researchers to consider the possibility of systemic NSC transplantation, in the hope that NSCs will act like HSCs or other blood-borne cells. Actually, NSCs do behave like HSCs in the systemic circulation. For example, they react to injury signals, are chemoattracted to diseased endothelia, and attach and further migrate into the CNS; this is referred to as the *chemoattractive hypothesis* (74,75). Using an EAE model, researchers at the University of Milan showed that 2.5–3.5% of infused NSCs home to the brain almost immediately (1 day after infusion) (64,65), whereas others reported that surviving donor cell numbers increased 10-fold at 2 weeks after infusion *(66–68,70)*. These findings suggest two possibilities, i.e., the in situ proliferation of NSCs in the host brain *(68)*, or the persistent homing of the circulating donor cells in host blood *(70)*.

Intravascular NSC transplantation has many advantages. First, the systemic transplantation of NSCs is probably the least invasive method of cell administration. In rodents, in which the majority of experimentation has been done, the brain is comparatively small compared to the immense volume of the human brain. Thus, in human, the local, stereotaxic infusion of NSCs may be severely limited in terms of transplantation foci (spatial), and because the infused cells have to migrate great distances to embrace entire disease sites (temporal). To overcome these obstacles, one must inject NSCs at numerous sites in the diseased brain. In contrast, intravascular injection can disperse NSCs according to natural cues and allow them to migrate along the "chemotactic gradients" of the host *(64,65,68)*.

Second, NSCs in the circulation can interact directly and comprehensively with inflamed, dysfunctional endothelia to cause *microenvironment stabilization (78–80)*. A recent definitive experiment showed that NSCs can be trans-differentiated into endothelial cells (ECs) in vitro and in vivo *(81)*, especially when they are in contact with ECs, and this result was also reported in the setting of cerebral ischemia *(67)*. Moreover, in the transplanted brain, NSCs may stimulate the host brain to stabilize, remodel, and restore the disturbed milieu.

Third, when NSCs have migrated into the diseased brain, they can similarly differentiate into functional neurons with intraparenchymal or intraventricular injections. Jin et al. *(70)* found no relationship between sites of entry of GFP-positive NSCs into the subventricular zone (SVZ) and immunohistochemically detected macrophages, labeled with an antibody against CD68, which contradicts the notion that transplanted cells enter the SVZ at macrophage-associated regions, termed "fractones" *(82)*. In the case of intravenously transplanted cells, it has been suggested that enhanced entry into the ischemic brain may simply reflect altered BBB permeability characteristics; and that NSCs differentiate at similar rates regardless of the method of introduction *(70)*.

Fourth, intravascular transplantation has marked anti-inflammatory and immune-modulatory effects as evidenced by EAE models *(64,65)*. Recent experiments with used syngenic or allogenic mouse NSCs without immune suppression have shown that NSCs induce the apoptosis of blood-borne CNS-infiltrating encephalitogenic T cells in vitro and in vivo *(65)*, and similar findings were reported using human NSCs (human NSCs to mouse, rat, and monkey) *(83,84)*.

Furthermore, NSCs transplanted when EAE remitted, ameliorated intense inflammation in the brain, and stabilized the host CNS microenvironment *(65)*. NSCs may also weakly express major histocompatibility class (MHC) class antigens *(76,83,85,86)*, and MHC expressional suppression in reaction to interferon-gamma using a viral stealth mechanism, which was reported for a human NSC line *(87)*.

5. LIMITATIONS AND QUESTIONS TO BE ANSWERED

Although a great deal of progress has been made, many limitations remain to be overcome and many questions have yet to be answered. Perhaps the most pressing issue concerns the comparative efficacies of the intravascular and intraparenchymal transplantations of NSCs *(70)*. In ICH, similar degrees of sensorimotor recovery were observed for these two methods (5 million cells for intravascular versus 1 million cells for intraparenchymal injection into ipsilateral cortices), when NSCs were injected 1 day after ICH *(88)*. Other researchers have found that various injection sites (ipsilateral hemisphere, contralateral hemisphere, or ventricle) produce somewhat different effects on functional stroke recovery, e.g., more sensorimotor recovery for an intraparenchymal injection versus more cognitive recovery for an intraventricular injection *(89)*.

The second issue is that NSCs in the systemic circulation may react to inflammatory chemokine signals *(90)*. Many factors can affect NSC migration into the brain, for example, BBB leakage *(70)*, although this occurs over a limited period (the first few days) in the ICH or ischemic brain. In view of the fact that BBB leakage is staunched within 7 days of ICH, there must be a specific *time window* for intravascular NSC transplantation *(88)*. According to our experiments, 7 to 10 days post-ICH appears to represent a deadline for the promotion of neurological recovery by intravenously transplanted NSCs. However, when we examined primary outcome using more delicate tests, e.g., the swimming test or fine forelimb coordination test, we found that the effective period may be longer. In contrast, the intraparenchymal injection of NSCs can be effective 4 or 5 weeks after ICH, as determined by conventional asymmetry neurologic testing, e.g., limb placing tests or detailed neurological scale testing.

The third issue, raised by EAE experiments *(65)*, concerns whether the intravascular injection of NSCs is neuroprotective in ischemia and ICH. In terms of the different pathophysiologies and disease courses of stroke and EAE, the neuroprotective effect of NSCs must be proven during the period immediately following the incident, because brain injury in stroke occurs within a few days. Another common question concerns the possibility of infusing NSCs during the first 24 h after stroke, and in view of the immature technological state of *massive stem cell expansion* ex vivo, it would appear that this kind of experiment may be unavailable clinically in the near future. Nevertheless, experimental evidence indicates that NSCs exert their actions on the diseased brain by secreting trophic factors, suppressing inflammation, acting as antioxidants, and by interacting with dysfunctional neurons/glia/endothelia during the acute period of CNS pathologies *(91)*.

The fourth issue concerns the homing of NSCs in the brain. A radioisotope analysis study reported that the proportion of NSCs migrating into the brain by intravascular transplantation is around 3% of cells infused *(65)*. In another report, homing was blocked by pre-culturing NSCs with anti-neutralizing CXCR4 antibody *(77)* or anti-VLA-4 antibody *(65)*, which implies that homing to the CNS may be dependent on stromal cell-derived factor-1α (SDF-1α)–CXC chemokine receptor 4 signaling, or adhesion molecule–receptor signaling. As in the case of HSC homing/engraftment to bone marrow, various strategies may arise, such as the enhancement of the action of SDF-1, the upregulation of CXCR4 on NSCs by chemical or genetic modification, and the co-administration of intervening molecules with stem cells.

In another respect, intravascular transplantation can be performed via two representative routes, i.e., intravenous or intraarterial routes *(92)*. According to experiments and clinical trials performed in a setting of heart ischemia, cardiologists prefer injecting stem cells into coronary arteries rather than intravenously *(93,94)*. Kim et al. *(95)* asserted that only small numbers of intravenously infused cells can reach the coronary circulation, and by utilizing Strauer's calculation *(96)*, it was found that only 3% of cardiac output reaches the coronary circulation, and therefore that fewer than 3% of intravenously infused cells can potentially reach the infarcted myocardium. This figure (<3%) corresponds well with the percentage of NSCs that homed to the brain when NSCs were injected intravenously. However, one study cautioned regarding the risks of intraarterial cell infusion, as acute myocardial ischemia and subacute myocardial microinfarction was noted after the intracoronary arterial injection of MSCs into dogs *(97)*. Accordingly, due caution should be exercised when considering the possibility of clinical trials on the basis of basic transplantation research data.

Fifth, NSCs introduced to the circulation can populate systemic organs, for example, CNS illnesses may influence the whole body, and NSCs may respond accordingly. The roles and actions of NSCs in systemic organs are not known, but laboratory tests and histologic examinations in our laboratory or others have revealed no definite evidence of clinical or microscopic harm, though transplanted HSCs were later found in various organs (brain, kidney, liver, and skin). Moreover, in an experimental setting, problems related to xenotransplantation were found to arise (for a detailed review see ref. 91). It was found that species differences affect the following parameters post-stem cell transplantation: brain and cortex size, blood pH, osmolarity, pO_2, hemoglobin, and cholesterol levels, plasma enzyme activity, and membrane and synaptic properties *(91)*. When we examine transplanted brains at 4–12 weeks, a proportion (20–35%) of the injected stem cells remained in the "undifferentiated" state *(65,67,71)*; some of these cells resided in the host's *stem cell niches*, and some were found at lesion peripheries. These "long-term undifferentiated cells" in the host brain have also been observed by others. In addition, such undifferentiated progenitor cells may act as primary anti-inflammatory effectors or adopt immune-modulating roles.

6. CONCLUSIONS

ICH is a highly complex disorder, and diverse strategies should be prepared for therapeutic interventions that fully consider disease pathogenesis and course. Given that NSCs have many functions and that they intervene in the host's pathology, a dichotomized strategy for stem cell transplantation can be proposed—i.e., one for regeneration (repair, restoration, and replenishment) and the other for neuroprotection; the former targets the latent or subacute period of CNS disease, whilst the latter targets the acute period. This dichotomized approach facilitates the delineation of the roles of NSCs in the treatment of ICH and enhances therapeutic efficacy by encouraging the development of combined tactics, e.g., the use of neuroprotectant(s) plus NSCs, other kinds of stem cells and NSCs, or trophic factor(s) plus NSCs. As discussed in the above paragraphs, a substantial gap remains despite the tantalizing advances made in stem cell biology, and the current paucity of data concerning clinical transplantation in stroke (ICH and ischemia) patients demonstrates that much has yet to be achieved.

ACKNOWLEDGMENTS

This work was supported by a grant (SC3060) from the Stem Cell Research Center of the 21st Century Frontier Research Program funded by the Ministry of Science and Technology, Republic of Korea. The authors thank Professor Seung Up Kim in Gachon University, Incheon, Korea, for his generous offer of human NSCs to our experiments. Space limitations preclude our inserting many references to earlier primary literature, for which we apologize.

REFERENCES

1. Brott T, Broderick J, Kothari R, et al. Early hemorrhage growth in patients with intracerebral hemorrhage. Stroke 1997;28:1–5.
2. Felberg RA, Grotta JC, Shirzadi AL, et al. Cell death in experimental intracerebral hemorrhage: the "black hole" model of hemorrhagic damage. Ann Neurol 2002;51:517–24.
3. Xue M, Del Bigio MR. Acute tissue damage after injections of thrombin and plasmin into rat striatum. Stroke 2001;32:2164–9.
4. Qureshi AI, Ling GS, Khan J, et al. Quantitative analysis of injured, necrotic, and apoptotic cells in a new experimental model of intracerebral hemorrhage. Crit Care Med 2001;29:152–7.
5. Matsushita K, Meng W, Wang X, et al. Evidence for apoptosis after intercerebral hemorrhage in rat striatum. J Cereb Blood Flow Metab 2000;20:396–404.
6. Wu J, Hua Y, Keep RF, et al. Oxidative brain injury from extravasated erythrocytes after intracerebral hemorrhage. Brain Res 2002;953:45–52.
7. Gong C, Hoff JT, Keep RF. Acute inflammatory reaction following experimental intracerebral hemorrhage in rat. Brain Res 2000;871:57–65.
8. Castillo J, Davalos A, Alvarez-Sabin J, et al. Molecular signatures of brain injury after intracerebral hemorrhage. Neurology 2002;58:624–9.
9. Dziedzic T, Bartus S, Klimkowicz A, et al. Intracerebral hemorrhage triggers interleukin-6 and interleukin-10 release in blood. Stroke 2002;33:2334–5.
10. Hickenbottom SL, Grotta JC, Strong R, et al. Nuclear factor-kappaB and cell death after experimental intracerebral hemorrhage in rats. Stroke 1999;30:2472–7.
11. Wagner KR, Xi G, Hua Y, et al. Lobar intracerebral hemorrhage model in pigs: rapid edema development in perihematomal white matter. Stroke 1996;27:490–7.
12. Yang S, Nakamura T, Hua Y, et al. The role of complement C3 in intracerebral hemorrhage-induced brain injury. J Cereb Blood Flow Metab 2006 Mar 22 [Epub ahead of print].
13. Huang F, Xi G, Keep RF, et al. Brain edema after experimental intracerebral hemorrhage: role of hemoglobin degradation products. J Neurosurg 2002;96:287–93.
14. Wang X, Lo EH. Triggers and mediators of hemorrhagic transformation in cerebral ischemia. Mol Neurobiol 2003;28:229–44.

15. Wang J, Tsirka SE. Neuroprotection by inhibition of matrix metalloproteinases in a mouse model of intracerebral haemorrhage. Brain 2005;128:1622–33.

16. Broderick JP, Brott TG, Duldner JE, et al. Volume of intracerebral hemorrhage: a powerful and easy-to-use predictor of 30-day mortality. Stroke 1993;24:987–93.

17. Hemphill JC III, Bonovich DC, Besmertis L, et al. The ICH score: a simple, reliable grading scale for intracerebral hemorrhage. Stroke 2001;32:891–7.

18. Kazui S, Naritomi H, Yamamoto H, et al. Enlargement of spontaneous intracerebral hemorrhage: incidence and time course. Stroke 1996;27:1783–7.

19. Mayer SA. Ultra-early hemostatic therapy for intracerebral hemorrhage. Stroke 2003;34:224–9.

20. Mayer SA, Lignelli A, Fink ME, et al. Perilesional blood flow and edema formation in acute intracerebral hemorrhage: a SPECT study. Stroke 1998;29:1791–8.

21. Rosenberg GA, Navratil M. Metalloproteinase inhibition blocks edema in intracerebral hemorrhage in the rat. Neurology 1997;48:921–6.

22. Mayer SA, Brun NC, Begtrup K, et al. Recombinant activated factor VII for acute intracerebral hemorrhage. N Engl J Med 2005;352:777–85.

23. Lee ST, Chu K, Jung KH, et al. Memantine reduces hematoma expansion in experimental intracerebral hemorrhage, resulting in functional improvement. J Cereb Blood Flow Metab 2006;26:536–44.

24. Xi G, Keep RF, Hoff JT. Erythrocytes and delayed brain edema formation following intracerebral hemorrhage in rats. J Neurosurg 1998;89:991–6.

25. Keep RF, Xi G, Hua Y, et al. The deleterious or beneficial effects of different agents in intracerebral hemorrhage: think big, think small, or is hematoma size important? Stroke 2005;36:1594–6.

26. Lee KR, Colon GP, Betz AL, et al. Edema from intracerebral hemorrhage: the role of thrombin. J Neurosurg 1996;84:91–6.

27. Xi G, Wagner KR, Keep RF, et al. Role of blood clot formation on early edema development after experimental intracerebral hemorrhage. Stroke 1998;29:2580–6.

28. Nishino A, Suzuki M, Ohtani H, et al. Thrombin may contribute to the pathophysiology of central nervous system injury. J Neurotrauma 1993;10:167–79.

29. Lee KR, Betz AL, Keep RF, et al. Intracerebral infusion of thrombin as a cause of brain edema. J Neurosurg. 1995;83:1045–50.

30. Lee KR, Betz AL, Kim S, et al. The role of the coagulation cascade in brain edema formation after intracerebral hemorrhage. Acta Neurochir 1996;138:396–400.

31. Kitaoka T, Hua Y, Xi G, et al. Delayed argatroban treatment reduces edema in a rat model of intracerebral hemorrhage. Stroke 2002;33:3012–8.

32. Wagner KR, Xi G, Hua Y, et al. Ultra-early clot aspiration after lysis with tissue plasminogen activator in a porcine model of intracerebral hemorrhage: edema reduction and blood brain barrier protection. J Neurosurg 1999;90:491–8.

33. Belayev L, Saul I, Busto R, et al. Albumin treatment reduces neurological deficit and protects blood–brain barrier integrity after acute intracortical hematoma in the rat. Stroke 2005;36:326–31.

34. Jung KH, Chu K, Jeong SW, et al. HMG-CoA reductase inhibitor, atorvastatin, promotes sensorimotor recovery, suppressing acute inflammatory reaction after experimental intracerebral hemorrhage. Stroke 2004;35:1744–9.

35. Chu K, Jeong SW, Jung KH, et al. Celecoxib induces functional recovery after intracerebral hemorrhage with reduction of brain edema and perihematomal cell death. J Cereb Blood Flow Metab 2004;24:926–33.
36. Park HK, Chu K, Lee ST, et al. Granulocyte colony-stimulating factor induces sensorimotor recovery in intracerebral hemorrhage. Brain Res 2005;1041:125–31.
37. Lee ST, Chu K, Sinn DI, et al. Erythropoietin reduces perihematomal inflammation and cell death with eNOS and STAT3 activations in experimental intracerebral hemorrhage. J Neurochem 2006;96:1728–39.
38. Hartl RL, Schurer L, Schmid-Schonbein GW, et al. Experimental antileukocyte interventions in cerebral ischemia. J Cereb Blood Flow Metab 1996;16:1108–19.
39. Boje KM, Arora PK. Microglial-produced nitric oxide and reactive nitrogen oxides mediate neuronal cell death. Brain Res 1992;587:250–6.
40. Kato H, Kogure K, Liu XH, et al. Progressive expression of immunomolecules on activated microglia and invading leukocytes following focal cerebral ischemia in the rat. Brain Res 1996;734:203–12.
41. Peeling J, Yan HJ, Corbett D, et al. Effect of FK-506 on inflammation and behavioral outcome following intracerebral hemorrhage in rat. Exp Neurol 2001;167:341–7.
42. Qureshi AI, Ali Z, Suri MF, et al. Extracellular glutamate and other amino acids in experimental intracerebral hemorrhage: an in vivo microdialysis study. Crit Care Med 2003;31:1482–9.
43. Lipton SA, Chen HS. Paradigm shift in neuroprotective drug development: clinically tolerated NMDA receptor inhibition by memantine. Cell Death Differ 2004;11:18–20.
44. Ardizzone TD, Lu A, Wagner KR, et al. Glutamate receptor blockade attenuates glucose hypermetabolism in perihematomal brain after experimental intracerebral hemorrhage in rat. Stroke 2004;35:2587–91.
45. Matsushita K, Meng W, Wang X, et al. Evidence for apoptosis after intercerebral hemorrhage in rat striatum. J Cereb Blood Flow Metab 2000;20:396–404.
46. Zhao X, Zhang Y, Strong R, et al. 15d-Prostaglandin J(2) activates peroxisome proliferator-activated receptor-gamma, promotes expression of catalase, and reduces inflammation, behavioral dysfunction, and neuronal loss after intracerebral hemorrhage in rats. J Cereb Blood Flow Metab 2005 Oct 5 [Epub ahead of print].
47. MacManus JP, Linnik MD. Gene expression induced by cerebral ischemia: an apoptotic perspective. J Cereb Blood Flow Metab 1997;17:815–32.
48. Nagata S, Golstein P. The Fas death factor. Science 1995;267:1449–56.
49. Peeling J, Del Bigio MR, Corbett D, et al. Efficacy of disodium 4-[(tert.-butylimino) methyl] benzene-1,3-dis-ulfonate N-oxide (NXY-059), a free radical trapping agent, in a rat model of hemorrhagic stroke. Neuropharmacology 2001;40:433–9.
50. Peeling J, Yan HJ, Chen SG, et al. Protective effects of free radical inhibitors in intracerebral hemorrhage in rat. Brain Res 1998;795:63–70.
51. Wagner KR, Packard BA, Hall CL, et al. Protein oxidation and heme oxygenase-1 induction in porcine white matter following intracerebral infusions of whole blood or plasma. Dev Neurosci 2002;24:154–60.

52. Wu J, Hua Y, Keep RF, Schallert T, et al. Oxidative brain injury from extravasated erythrocytes after intracerebral hemorrhage. Brain Res 2002;953:45–52.
53. Nakamura T, Keep RF, Hua Y, et al. Deferoxamine-induced attenuation of brain edema and neurological deficits in a rat model of intracerebral hemorrhage. J Neurosurg 2004;100:672–8.
54. Power C, Henry S, Del Bigio MR, et al. Intracerebral hemorrhage induces macrophage activation and matrix metalloproteinases. Ann Neurol 2003;53: 731–42.
55. Lapchak PA, Chapman DF, Zivin JA. Metalloproteinase inhibition reduces thrombolytic (tissue plasminogen activator)-induced hemorrhage after thromboembolic stroke. Stroke 2000;31: 3034–40.
56. Aronowski J, Hall CE. New horizons for primary intracerebral hemorrhage treatment: experience from preclinical studies. Neurol Res 2005;27:268–79.
57. Jeong SW, Chu K, Jung KH, et al. Intravenous human neural stem cell transplantation promotes functional recovery with experimental intracranial hemorrhage in the adult rats. Stroke 2003;34:2258–63.
58. Nan Z, Grande A, Sanberg CD, et al. Infusion of human umbilical cord blood ameliorates neurologic deficits in rats with hemorrhagic brain injury. Ann NY Acad Sci 2005;1049:84–96.
59. Nonaka M, Yoshikawa M, Nishimura F, et al. Intraventricular transplantation of embryonic stem cell-derived neural stem cells in intracerebral hemorrhage rats. Neurol Res 2004;26:265–60.
60. Seyfried D, Ding J, Han Y, Li Y, Chen J, Chopp M. Effects of intravenous administration of human bone marrow stromal cells after intracerebral hemorrhage in rats. J Neurosurg. 2006;104:313–8.
61. Zhang H, Huang Z, Xu Y, Zhang S. Differentiation and neurological benefit of the mesenchymal stem cells transplanted into the rat brain following intracerebral hemorrhage. Neurol Res 2006;28:104–12.
62. Atala A. Recent developments in tissue engineering and regenerative medicine. Curr Opin Pediatr 2006;18:167–71.
63. Aboody KS, Brown A, Rainov NG, et al. Neural stem cells display extensive tropism for pathology in adult brain: evidence from intracranial gliomas. Proc Natl Acad Sci USA 2000;97:12846–51.
64. Pluchino S, Quattrini A, Brambilla E, et al. Injection of adult neurospheres induces recovery in a chronic model of multiple sclerosis. Nature 2003;422: 688–94.
65. Pluchino S, Zanotti L, Rossi B, et al. Neurosphere-derived multipotent precursors promote neuroprotection by an immunomodulatory mechanism. Nature 2005;436:266–71.
66. Chu K, Kim M, Jeong SW, et al. Human neural stem cells can migrate, differentiate and proliferate after intravenous transplantation in the adult rats with transient forebrain ischemia. Neurosci Lett 2003;343:129–33.
67. Chu K, Kim M, Jung KH, et al. Human neural stem cell transplantation enhances neurogenesis and behavioral recovery in adult rats with transient focal cerebral ischemia. Brain Res 2004;1016:145–53.

68. Chu K, Kim M, Chae SH, et al. The distribution and in situ proliferation patterns of intravenously transplanted human neural stem-like cells in rats with focal cerebral ischemia. Neurosci Res 2004;50:459–65.

69. Chu K, Park KI, Lee ST, et al. Combined treatment of vascular endothelial growth factor and human neural stem cells in experimental focal cerebral ischemia. Neurosci Res 2005;53:384–90.

70. Jin K, Sun Y, Xie L, et al. Comparison of ischemia-directed migration of neural precursor cells after intrastriatal, intraventricular, or intravenous transplantation in the rat. Neurobiol Dis 2005;18:366–74.

71. Chu K, Kim M, Jung KH, et al. Human neural stem cell transplantation reduces spontaneous recurrent seizures following pilocarpine-induced status epilepticus in adult rats. Brain Res 2004;1023:213–21.

72. Lee ST, Chu K, Park JE, et al. Intravenous administration of human neural stem cells induces functional recovery in Huntington's disease rat model. Neurosci Res 2005;52:243–9.

73. Lee ST, Park JE, Lee K, et al. Noninvasive Method of neuronal stem cell transplantation in an experimental model of Huntington's disease. J Neurosci Methods 2006;152:250–4.

74. Pluchino S, Zanotti L, Deleidi M, et al. Neural stem cells and their use as therapeutic tool in neurological disorders. Brain Res Rev 2005;48:211–9.

75. Pluchino S, Martino G. The therapeutic use of stem cells for myelin repair in autoimmune demyelinating disorders. J Neurol Sci 2005;233:117–9.

76. Mi R, Luo Y, Cai J, et al. Immortalized neural stem cells differ from nonimmortalized cortical neurospheres and cerebellar granule cell progenitors. Exp Neurol 2005;194:301–19.

77. Imitola J, Raddassi K, Park KI, et al. Directed migration of neural stem cells to sites of CNS injury by the stromal cell-derived factor 1α/CXC chemokine receptor 4 pathway. Proc Natl Acad Sci USA 2004;101:18117–22.

78. Ourednik J, Ourednik V, Lynch WP, et al. Neural stem cells display an inherent mechanism for rescuing dysfunctional neurons. Nat Biotechnol 2002;20:1103–10.

79. Imitola J, Park KI, Teng YD, et al. Stem cells: cross-talk and developmental programs. Philos Trans R Soc Lond B Biol Sci 2004;359:823–37.

80. Snyder EY, Daley GQ, Goodell M. Taking stock and planning for the next decade: realistic prospects for stem cell therapies for the nervous system. J Neurosci Res 2004;76:157–68.

81. Wurmser AE, Nakashima K, Summers RG, et al. Cell fusion-independent differentiation of neural stem cells to the endothelial lineage. Nature 2004;430:350–6.

82. Mercier F, Kitasako JT, Hatton GI. Anatomy of the brain neurogenic zones revisited: fractones and the fibroblast/macrophage network. J Comp Neurol 2002;451:170–88.

83. Parker MA, Anderson JK, Corliss DA, et al. Expression profile of an operationally-defined neural stem cell clone. Exp Neurol 2005;194:320–32.

84. Ourednik V, Ourednik J, Flax JD, et al. Segregation of human neural stem cells in the developing primate forebrain. Science 2001;293:1820–4.

85. Modo M, Rezaie P, Heuschling P, et al. Transplantation of neural stem cells in a rat model of stroke: assessment of short-term graft survival and acute host immunological response. Brain Res 2002;958:70–82.

86. Modo M, Mellodew K, Rezaie P. In vitro expression of major histocompatibility class I and class II antigens by conditionally immortalized murine neural stem cells. Neurosci Lett 2003;337:85–8.

87. Lee EM, Kim JY, Cho BR, et al. Down-regulation of MHC class I expression in human neuronal stem cells using viral stealth mechanism. Biochem Biophys Res Commun 2005;326:825–35.

88. Chu K, Park HK, Jeong SW, et al. Optimal therapeutic time window for human neural stem cell transplantation in experimental intracerebral hemorrhage. Stroke 2004;35:246 [Abstract from International Stroke Conference 2004].

89. Modo M, Stroemer RP, Tang E, et al. Effects of implantation site of stem cell grafts on behavioral recovery from stroke damage. Stroke 2002;33:2270–8.

90. Imitola J, Snyder EY, Khoury SJ. Genetic programs and responses of neural stem/progenitor cells during demyelination: potential insights into repair mechanisms in multiple sclerosis. Physiol Genomics 2003;14:171–97.

91. Ginis I, Rao MS. Toward cell replacement therapy: promises and caveats. Exp Neurol 2003;184:61–77.

92. Li Y, Chen J, Wang L, et al. Treatment of stroke in rat with intracarotid administration of marrow stromal cells. Neurology 2001;56:1666–72.

93. Kang HJ, Kim HS, Zhang SY, et al. Effects of intracoronary infusion of peripheral blood stem-cells mobilised with granulocyte-colony stimulating factor on left ventricular systolic function and restenosis after coronary stenting in myocardial infarction: the MAGIC cell randomised clinical trial. Lancet 2004;363:751–6.

94. Wollert KC, Meyer GP, Lotz J, et al. Intracoronary autologous bone-marrow cell transfer after myocardial infarction: the BOOST randomised controlled clinical trial. Lancet 2004;364:141–8.

95. Kim HS, Kang HJ, Park YB. Stem-cell therapy for myocardial diseases. Lancet 2004;363:1734–5.

96. Strauer BE, Brehm M, Zeus T, et al. Repair of infarcted myocardium by autologous intracoronary mononuclear bone marrow cell transplantation in humans. Circulation 2002;106:1913–18.

97. Vulliet PR, Greeley M, Halloran SM, et al. Intra-coronary arterial injection of mesenchymal stromal cells and microinfarction in dogs. Lancet 2004;363:783–4.

7

Therapeutic Strategies Employing Endogenous Neural Stem Cells in Tissue Remodeling Following Ischemic Injury

The Promise, the Peril and Novel Future Applications

Mark F. Mehler, MD

1. INTRODUCTION

It is well known that stroke is one of the most common causes of morbidity and mortality in adults within industrialized societies. There are approximately 200 new cases of acute cerebrovascular accidents per 100,000 adults per year *(1)*. In the USA, stroke is the most common cause of protracted disability and the third leading cause of death with an incidence of stroke of approximately 750,000 cases per year *(2)*. Most affected individuals survive the initial ictus but are left with significant degrees of sensory, motor, cognitive, and neurobehavioral disabilities.

Recent attempts to reduce the incidence of stroke by better control of acknowledged vascular risk factors have been offset by the cumulative effects of dramatic rises in the incidence of obesity, diabetes mellitus, associated metabolic syndromes, and the progressive aging of the population. Intra-arterial and intravenous thrombolytic therapy is the only currently accepted efficacious therapy for acute stroke, but its use is significantly limited by a narrow therapeutic window of opportunity and by strict exclusion criteria instituted to prevent the risk of hemorrhagic complications. Neuroprotective therapeutic protocols targeted at preventing additional neuronal loss in the ischemic penumbra have been largely futile, and no universally agreed upon neuroprotective agent is currently available for routine clinical use *(3)*.

From: *Current Clinical Neurology: Stroke Recovery with Cellular Therapies*
Edited by: Sean I. Savitz and Daniel M. Rosenbaum © Humana Press Inc., Totowa, NJ

2. SPECTRUM AND PATHOPHYSIOLOGY
OF CEREBROVASCULAR SYNDROMES

Progressive forms of cerebrovascular disease culminating in diverse stroke syndromes are complex pathophysiological entities whose spectrum of disease manifestations is not always readily appreciated *(4–6)*. Stroke may affect any area of the neuraxis and be unifocal or multifocal and extensive or circumscribed.

Clinicopathological evolution may be rapid, stepwise, or slowly progressive. Milder forms of central nervous system (CNS) hypoxia and ischemia may be symptomatic or subclinical and may either promote or protect (ischemic pre-conditioning) against further cerebrovascular insults. Focal ischemia of the middle cerebral artery (MCA) may result in larger divisional infarctions or smaller branch occlusions and may affect both cortical and subcortical structures including stem cell generative zones.

Similarly, occlusion of the internal carotid artery may result in huge anterior and MCA territory infarctions or in unifocal or multifocal areas of ischemia and milder degrees of parenchymal compromise. Within the posterior circulation, different degrees and causes of vertebrobasilar occlusion (thrombosis, embolus, and hypo- perfusion) may target focal or more diffuse areas of the lower and middle brainstem or more global or patchy areas of rostral basilar artery territory including the occipital lobes, the posterior temporal lobes, the diencephalon, and the mesencephalon. Moreover, pre-existing cerebrovascular disease may contribute to different degrees of collateral circulation that may significantly modify the clinicopathological spectrum of acute stroke syndromes. Additional vascular anomalies and persistence of the fetal circulation may further modulate these patterns of CNS dysfunction.

Acute infarction of the anterior spinal artery results in a classical syndrome affecting restricted areas of the spinal cord, and global cerebral ischemia may affect multiple CNS areas in a graded fashion, with a predilection for causing selective delayed loss of hippocampal CA1 pyramidal neurons. Additional forms of arterovenous occlusive disease including venous occlusive disease (venous sinus syndromes and cortical venous infarctions), arterial dissections, cavernous sinus thrombosis, arterovenous malformations, arterial spasm following subarachnoid hemorrhage, and many additional complications of systemic diseases may also result in varying degrees of parenchymal compromise and neuronal dysfunction and death that do not obey classical arterial territories, may evolve over different time scales, and may elicit different forms of injury responses and adaptive mechanisms.

These cumulative considerations suggest that the development of effective broadly based therapeutic applications for preventing irreversible cellular injury and cell death as well as for promoting more enduring degrees of cellular genetic re-programming, tissue remodeling, and ultimate therapeutic cures will require novel strategies employing the targeted activation, expansion, migration, cellular differentiation, and eventual neural network integration of endogenous stem cells present throughout the neuraxis within the adult and even the senescent brain and spinal cord.

3. CHARACTERIZATION AND REGULATION OF ENDOGENOUS STEM AND PROGENITOR CELL SUBPOPULATIONS IN ADULT BRAIN AND SPINAL CORD

Endogenous neural stem cells have been identified throughout the brain and spinal cord of embryonic, postnatal, adult, and aging rodents and primates primarily within discrete paramedian generative zones *(7–12)*. In addition, recent reports have corroborated their presence in humans although with reduced profiles of expression and diminished functional capabilities *(13–16)*. Despite the broad patterns of endogenous neural stem cell expression, areas of ongoing neurogenesis in the adult brain are normally restricted to the cortical subependymal region of the anterior subventricular zone (SVZ) and the subgranular zone (SGZ) of the dentate gyrus of the hippocampus *(17–20)*.

The true identification o endogenous stem cells is still the subject of innumerable debates *(19,20)*. Initial reports attributed stem cell qualities to ciliated ependymal cells lining the ventricular surface and bathed in cerebrospinal fluid *(21,22)*. However, more recent studies have shown that adult neural stem cells reside within the SVZ in microenvironmental niches that provide trophic support to these cells and to their proximate progenitors, radial glia *(23–26)*.

Neural stem cells are capable of long-term self-renewal and exuberant proliferation and give rise to proximate progenitor species that can undergo progressive lineage restriction and can migrate away from the SVZ and progressively differentiate into region-specific neuronal and glial subtypes or remain as pools of lineage-restricted neuronal or glial transit amplifying cells within subcortical or cortical niches where they have the potential to more rapidly respond to environmental perturbations *(16,19,20,25,26)*. In addition, neural stem cell pools have been identified in areas of the subcortical white matter and the neocortex remote from the paramedian SVZ, and these multipotent self-renewing stem cells are normally shielded from premature cellular differentiation by the presence on the cell surface of the polysialyated (embryonic) form of neural cell-adhesion molecule (PSA-NCAM) *(27–29)*. Moreover, there is considerable evidence that adult neuronal and glial progenitor cells may exist in abundance and distinct from the maturational pathways of adult neural stem cells within specialized neocortical and subcortical white matter niches, respectively, as transit amplifying cells that are mitogenic and biased toward specific neural lineages with the unique properties of representing rapid and efficient responders to focal environmental perturbations but with retention of multilineage potential under unusual circumstances *(16)*.

The ability of regional neural stem cells to undergo self-renewal, expansion, survival, cellular migration, and differentiation are modulated by a broad array of growth factors and cytokines including epidermal and fibroblast growth factors, neurotrophins, transforming growth factor α, and the transforming growth factor β superfamily, hemopoietins such as interleukins, colony-stimulating factors, vascular endothelial growth factor (VEGF), neuropoietic and GP 130 subunit-related factors, stem cell factor, erythropoietin, thrombopoietin, flt ligand, chemokines such as interleukin 8, members of the tumor necrosis factor family, and the glial derived neurotrophic factor subfamily *(30–34)*. Additional modulatory influences on progressive neural stem cell activation, expansion, and progressive neural lineage maturation include multiple complex and synergistic hormonal effects, cell–cell interactions particularly those modulated by Notch pathway signaling, integrins and various profiles and permutations of gap junction (connexin protein) expression, neurotransmitter expression and actions including glutamate and glutamatergic receptor subtype signal transduction, gamma amino butyric acid (GABA) and serotonin, extracellular matrix molecules and growth factor activity, and morphogenetic gradient modulators and environmental modifications including enrichment and learning paradigms and specific generalized stressors including seizures *(25,35)*.

4. PERSPECTIVES ON THE EFFICACY
OF ENDOGENOUS STEM CELL THERAPIES
FOR STROKE SYNDROMES

Using endogenous regional neural stem cells for tissue remodeling in stroke therapies has many intrinsic advantages *(36)*. There is no requirement for an external source of cells; no need to pool multiple different embryos; no risk of introducing exogenous pathogens; no risk of inducing cell transformation; no risk of enhanced CNS immune surveillance, inflammatory reactions, or tissue rejection, and the divisiveness of political and ethically issues are effectively bypassed. There are also some potential disadvantages that may limit the wider use of endogenous stem cells in cerebrovascular diseases *(36)*.

Different brain regions may possess divergent degrees of regenerative potential based on local stem cell density, position, differentiation potential, microenvironmental molecular inhibitory constraints, or additional heterogeneous functional properties. The migratory or maturational potential of regional stem cell progeny may be too limited to permit effective repair including appropriate integration into existing regional neural networks, synaptic remodeling, and propagation of appropriate degrees of basal synaptic transmission, cross-modulatory cellular and synaptic interactions, and appropriate profiles of synaptic plasticity.

Further, it may be very challenging to orchestrate the precise profiles of expression and the dynamic interplay between local environmental cues, cell–cell signals, and cell autonomous transcription factor codes required for directed stem cell activation, expansion, survival, differentiation, migration, synaptogenesis, and appropriate neural network integration *(25,26)*. Finally, it may be even more difficult to properly program these stem cell maturational events in response to multifocal, temporally dispersed, and etiologically distinct or complex forms of ischemic injury. Moreover, there is significant experimental evidence that stem cell re-population potential declines precipitously with aging at least, in part, due to the progression of replicative senescence *(11,17,37)*.

5. CONSTITUTIVE AND INDUCED NEUROGENESIS
IN THE ADULT CNS

Studies of the fate of stem and progenitor cells transplanted between normally neurogenic regions in the adult brain, particularly the rostral migratory stream/olfactory bulb and the dentate gyrus of the hippocampus, suggest that local cellular and molecular cues are crucial in determining the fate of neural stem cells and their proximate progenitor species and their ability to integrate into heterotopic brain regions *(38)*. These studies have begun to identify the constellation of multifactorial extracellular matrix factors, guidance cues, soluble signals, autocrine and paracrine signaling pathways, cell–cell modulators, and cell intrinsic transcriptional networks involved in promoting endogenous neural stem cell-mediated tissue remodeling, and neural network integration *(20,25,26,39)*. In contrast to the convincing evidence of adult neurogenesis within the olfactory bulb and the dentate gyrus of the hippocampus, the vast majority of studies suggest that constitutive neurogenesis does not occur at significant levels in the murine or rat cerebral cortex, and more rigorous methods have cast doubt on the presence of neurogenesis in limited areas of the primate cortex *(40–47)*. By contrast, cortical regions undergoing synchronous apoptotic loss of projection neurons can form an instructive environment to guide the progressive maturation of neural precursor or immature neuronal species *(48–52)*.

In addition, studies of laser ablation of corticothalamic neurons in layer 6 of the anterior cortex have demonstrated that endogenous neural progenitor species in situ can be induced to differentiate into cortical neurons, survive for extended periods of time, and form appropriate long-distance connections within the adult mammalian brain *(40)*. These findings definitively show that endogenous neural precursors can be orchestrated to differentiate into neocortical neurons in a region- and layer-specific manner and to reestablish proper corticothalamic connections in normally non-neurogenic regions of the adult brain. Similar results have recently been obtained from regions of the hippocampus and the striatum *(53–55)*. These overall findings suggest that the normal absence of constitutive neurogenesis in non-neurogenic regions of the adult brain does not necessarily reflect an intrinsic lack of regional neural stem cell activation, migratory, or maturation potential but rather reflect the absence of appropriate microenvironmental signals required for neuronal survival, migration, maturation, and progressive neural network integration. These and other studies have affirmed that many adult neural precursor species are capable of undergoing long-distance radial and tangential forms of migration and that these adult neural precursors can extend axons over significant distances within the mature brain.

In an in vivo model of global ischemia, it was recently demonstrated that massive elimination of CA1 pyramidal neurons was followed by large-scale re-population of these neurons by a significant proliferative response within the posterior periventricular zone and that this endogenous neural precursor cell response was dramatically augmented by intraventricular infusion of the stem cell mitogens, epidermal and basic fibroblast growth factors *(53)*. Initial analysis of the changes in gene and protein expression in regions undergoing degeneration of projection neurons indicates that a selective profile of neurotrophins and related neural cytokines are upregulated and that corresponding changes in growth factor receptor expression occur in stem cell generative zones contained within the columnar organization of the lesion site *(56,57)*. Surrounding interneurons and glia are also capable of undergoing significant changes in gene and protein expression of effectors of regional stem cell maturation often in an activity-dependent manner and through the establishment of dynamic autocrine and paracrine signaling circuits *(36,57)*.

6. ENDOGENOUS STEM AND PROGENITOR CELL RESPONSES TO FOCAL AND GLOBAL ISCHEMIA INJURY IN ANIMAL MODELS

Several studies have documented an endogenous neural stem cell response to focal MCA ischemia. In one model of focal ischemia, it was found that there was an increase in proliferating (BrdU$^+$) cells in the SVZ following the ischemic insult with a peak at 7 days postoperatively *(58)*. However, the identity of the SVZ cells was never established, and although some of the proliferating cells expressed the migrating neuroblast marker, PSA-NCAM, none of the cells expressed markers of mature neurons even when assessed after 28 days. Additional studies of focal MCA ischemia have demonstrated that endogenous neural stem cells proliferate and migrate from the SVZ to the striatum where they express markers of striatal GABAergic neurons *(54,55)*. However, in these studies, no proliferating cortical cells could be identified in affected cortical regions, despite a large cortical lesion burden. Only a very small fraction of newborn neurons (0.2 %) survived over time to furnish replacement neurons, and ablation of cell division in the SVZ inhibited the striatal neurogenesis.

Another study of focal ischemia revealed the transitory presence of proliferating cells within the parietal cortex without significant conversion to newly minted mature neurons *(58)*. Using a more limited photothrombotic lesion paradigm, it was shown that a limited subset *(3–6%)* of newborn cells expressed neuronal markers at 30 days postlesion inducement *(59)*. When the same investigators used an intraluminal filament model of focal ischemia leading to a larger cortical and a subcortical infarction, there was still only sparse evidence of newborn cells expressing neuronal markers within distinct cortical layers (two to six) *(60)*. Interestingly, a further study has demonstrated the induction of proliferating newborn cells in both the ipsilateral and the contralateral hemispheres following focal ischemia *(61)*. These studies reveal the absence of a consistent pattern of cortical neurogenesis following the induction of focal ischemia. Possible reasons for the absence of more robust cortical neurogenesis following focal MCA infarction include modulation of a regenerative response as a function of lesion volume or mass, presence of subcortical injury, distance from the appropriate stem cell generative zone, barriers to cell migration in the form of glial scar formation, presence of myelin breakdown products, and alterations in the fidelity and functional profiles of axon guidance cues and chemoattractant and morphogenetic gradients *(35)*.

In a gerbil model of global ischemia, it was revealed that following the ischemic insult, the number of proliferating (BrdU$^+$) cells increased more than 10-fold, with most of the newly born cells turning into mature neurons (60%) and surviving for prolonged time periods (7 months) *(7)*. Interestingly, these newborn cells migrated exclusively to the CA1 region of the hippocampus, and the induction of neurogenesis was independent of CA1-related cell death because the use of ischemic pre-conditioning paradigms prevented CA1 cell loss but did not dampen de novo neurogenesis. Using a rat model of global ischemia, it was demonstrated that the number of proliferating cells increased almost sixfold in the SGZ of experimental animals *(11)*. The proportion of proliferating cells steadily declined within a 1-month interval following the ischemic insult, but the majority of residual cells expressed a mature neuronal marker although the functional role of these newly minted neurons was not properly assessed. These findings are compatible with those of other investigators *(62,63)*.

7. AUGMENTING THE ENDOGENOUS STEM CELL RESPONSE TO ISCHEMIC INJURY

Several investigators have studied the effects of augmenting the endogenous stem cell response to ischemic injury on de novo neurogenesis. In a study of intercisternal administration of basic fibroblast growth factor following permanent MCA occlusion, it was shown that young neuroblasts represented up to 30% of SVZ-labeled cells but that the number of neuroblasts declined to 2% by day 21 poststroke induction *(64)*. These experimental observations suggest that the newborn cells either do not survive or migrate out of the SVZ or rather undergo more long-distance migration; unfortunately, this latter parameter was never properly examined. In a model of transient occlusion of both common carotid arteries inducing global ischemia, it was shown that adenoviral vector induction of basic fibroblast growth factor was superior to intraventricular installation of factor as assessed by more widespread spatial dissemination of fibroblast growth factor expression *(65)*. Under these viral mediated conditions, the number of proliferating cells peaked at 1 week postinfarction and subsided by the end of the second week. There was a modest increase in the number of proliferating cortical cells, although the majority of these cells generated astrocytes, with only 3 and 10% of cells expressing mature neuronal markers in the cortex and hippocampus, respectively. After focal cerebral ischemia, the number of proliferating cells in the SVZ and the SGZ also peaks in the initial week following the insult but remains elevated for up to 1 month *(66)*. The proportion of proliferating cells further increased with intraventricular infusion of insulin-like growth factor I or glial derived neurotrophic factor. However, in this study, the majority of proliferating cells did not express mature neuronal markers and, in fact, the vast majority of proliferating cortical cells expressed microglial or macrophage protein markers rather than neuronal antigens.

Another cautionary note has been sounded by studies of the negative influence of aging on the induction of neurogenesis in response to ischemic injury. In one study, aged (12-month-old) rats were capable of mounting a proliferative stem cell response to an ischemic insult, but the reparative response was not sustained, and almost all cells died within 1 month without exhibiting or sustaining the expression of mature neuronal markers *(4)*. By contrast, similar studies with younger animals (3 months of age) have demonstrated a more protracted period of cell survival following ischemic infarction *(11)*. Studies of primate global ischemia models have revealed a much less robust endogenous stem cell response to the massive global insult with a much lower proportion of proliferating cells induced and a very poor profile of developmental differentiation to mature neurons *(67)*.

On a more optimistic note, selected studies of mitogenic cytokine augmentation of the endogenous stem cell response in a rodent model of global ischemia has convincingly demonstrated robust de novo neurogenesis into a normally non-neurogenic region (CA1 region of the hippocampus) with the induction of synaptogenesis, appropriate connectivity patterns, characteristic electrophysiological signatures, and appropriate amelioration of anatomically linked memory deficits *(53)*. These exciting findings suggest that reestablishment of functional neural networks by de novo neurogenesis following severe brain ischemic damage may contribute directly to improvements in higher intellectual functions.

8. EPILOGUE: INTEGRATED THERAPEUTIC APPROACHES FOR ENHANCING AN ENDOGENOUS STEM CELL RESPONSE TO ISCHEMIC INJURY

A systematic approach to promoting a robust, enduring, and delimited endogenous stem cell response to all of the various permutations of possible ischemic forms of neural cell injury will of necessity be multifactorial and multidisciplinary. First, it will be essential to define the temporal and spatial extent of the ischemic insult, the etiology, the systemic vascular risk factors, and details of the pathological vasculature. Second, it will be crucial to be able to monitor endogenous stem cell activation, expansion, migration, differentiation, and neural network remodeling using appropriate contrast agents and high-field magnetic resonance imaging and other evolving neuroimaging modalities. Third, it will be important to assess the levels of the neuraxis that have already undergone irrevocable cellular dysfunction and death, those that are reversibly injured, and those under threat of impending lesion extension or necrotic or hemorrhagic transformation.

Endogenous stem cell subpopulations representing different levels and intrasegmental microdomains of the neuraxis are under the influence of distinct profiles of growth factors, cytokines, and gradient morphogens for activation, self-renewal, expansion, survival, progressive stages of differentiation, migration, and neural network integration *(19,20,25)*. In addition, progressive stages of regional neural stem cell lineage restriction and lineage maturation are characterized by changing profiles of combinatorial transcription factor codes that successively activate semiautonomous maturational transcription factor cascades *(39,68,69)*. Further, robust profiles of stem cell-mediated developmental specification invariably involves the positive promotion of specific lineage events (i.e., neurogenesis) while simultaneously actively inhibiting other lineage specification processes (i.e., gliogenesis), thus necessitating the concerted actions of complementary cell autonomous and environmental signaling events *(70)*. Moreover, the elaboration of specific regional projection neuronal subtypes is inextricably linked to later dynamic functional interactions with a complex set of complementary modulatory neuronal and glial cell types that must be elaborated in precise temporal register to the primary neuronal subtype *(71)*. Recent studies have begun to define distinct regional subsets of inhibitory interneurons that gate excitatory neurotransmission and distinct regional oligo-dendroglial and astroglial species that enhance neuronal intracellular communications and the efficacy of synaptic transmission and cell viability and other physiological functions, respectively *(72–74)*. These overall experimental observations suggest that targeted activation of endogenous regional neural stem cell pools in response to ischemic injury will require multifactorial manipulations of environmental signals (growth factors, cytokines, and gradient morphogens), cell–cell recognition cues (Notch signaling pathway factors, sequential connexin proteins, integrins, and combinatorial cell identity signatures), and cell autonomous molecular pathways (specific combinatorial patterns of transcription factor codes that may activate multiple self-perpetuating gene cascades).

A novel area of research in the field of ischemic injury-mediated self-repair, tissue remodeling, and cellular genetic re-programming is in the evolving field of epigenomic medicine *(75–78)*. Epige-netic regulation of genome-wide profiles of gene expression involves three interrelated mechanisms that promote the integrated expression of single or multiple linked genes contained within functional gene networks without causing permanent changes in DNA. Epigenetic regulation is orchestrated by DNA methylation, by changes in higher-order chromatin structure through numerous post-translational modifi-cations to the histone code, and by the actions of numerous classes of non-coding RNAs that modulate all aspects of transcriptional-translational coupling and multiple additional aspects of cell function through both nuclear and cytoplasmic processing networks. Epige-netic mechanisms are now known to regulate all aspects of neural stem cell fate, progressive neural maturational decisions, as well as neural network function and plasticity *(75,79–81)*. In fact, epigenetic regulatory processes have already been implicated in neural responses to ischemic injury. For example, DNA methylation through the actions of DNA methyltransferase contributes to delayed ischemic brain injury and inhibition of methyltransferase activity, and addition of a histone deacetylation inhibitor confer significant stroke protection *(82)*. In addition, global ischemic insults have been shown to derepress the neuronal silencer factor, REST/NRSF, in vulnerable CA1 pyramidal neurons destined to die *(83)*.

Acute knockdown of REST expression abrogates the ischemia-induced apoptotic cascade and rescues vulnerable neurons. Interestingly, REST-mediated gene repression in non-neuronal cells including neural stem and progenitor cells is orchestrated by a distinct set of domain-specific epigenetic regulatory mechanisms *(84–86)*. Therefore, the ability to dynamically modulate and selectively sculpt deregulated gene profiles and functional genetic and epigenetic regulatory networks in ischemic injury by a concerted spectrum of epigenetic mechanisms may obviate the need to individually modulate and normalize the expression of complex profiles of stem cell-associated environmental, cell–cell signaling and cell intrinsic cues.

New initiatives in drug discovery are actively compiling a range of novel therapeutic agents to selectively target specific sets of epigenetic regulatory molecules and processes that will be important in promoting a more enduring, robust, and selective regenerative response to different forms of ischemic injury.

9. COMPLEMENTARY THERAPEUTIC APPROACHES FOR MAXIMIZING NEURAL REGENERATIVE INTERACTIONS BETWEEN THE ISCHEMIC INJURY SITE AND PARAMEDIAN STEM CELL GENERATIVE ZONES

In concert with dynamic modulation of the regional endogenous stem cell responses to diverse forms of ischemic injury, it will be important to immediately institute experimental manipulations that can modulate local injury signals and different forms of dynamic and evolving communications between the site of ischemic injury and the contiguous stem cell generative zone.

It is well known that ischemic injury elicits inflammatory and innate and adaptive immune surveillance responses that involve sequential waves of inflammatory and immunomodulatory cytokines and additional soluble and cell–cell-mediated cues that carry both positive and negative modulatory signals for neural stem cell activation and targeted migration and maturation *(32)*. In addition, these progressive perilesional pathological and adaptive events induce excitotoxicity, nitric oxide production, free radical damage, and neural cell apoptosis *(87)*. Further, inhibition of axonal regeneration by factors released following myelin breakdown including Nogo A, oligodendrocyte-myelin glycoprotein, and myelin-associated glyco-protein often occurs prior to the formation or consolidation of glial scarring that also contributes to the inhibition of neural cell migration and axonal pathfinding *(88)*. These axonal inhibitors are located in myelin membranes immediately adjacent to the axon, providing an ideal location to mediate axon–glia interactions. Moreover, these inhibitors all bind to the Nogo receptor, inhibiting axonal outgrowth and further re-myelination while preventing concomitant neuronal recovery *(89)*.

Targeted blockade of the Nogo receptor may permit an enhanced neural regenerative response following ischemic injury, thereby augmenting the mechanisms of de novo neurogenesis. Future research initiatives will require coordinated approaches to modifying the perile-sional environment in concert with directed orchestration of a robust, enduring but delimited regional generative zone-mediated endogenous neural stem cell response to the ischemic insult.

Prior studies have suggested that the site of the ischemic lesion possesses powerful informational signals that have the potential to progressively sculpt an efficacious endogenous stem cell response to combat the ongoing pathological ischemic cascades *(36)*. These informational signals will almost certainly include retrograde cues directed from the injury site to the stem cell generative zones through the mediation of soluble cytokines, gradient morphogens, associated extracellular matrix factors, and cell–cell signaling cues particularly changing profiles of integrins, connexins, and Notch pathway ligands and intracellular transduction cassettes *(25)*.

As with the integrated endogenous stem cell response, an essential therapeutic goal will be to reestablish the primacy of instructive and informational cues contained within the injury response while selectively downregulating or otherwise positively altering the temporal profiles of the inflammatory and immunomodulatory cytokine responses to optimize cross-regulatory complementary and synergistic pathways of neural repair and regeneration. Moreover, the concerted use of advanced therapeutic modalities aimed at providing innovative neuroprotection strategies to vulnerable neurons and glia that have not yet been irrevocably injured and dying in addition to providing environmental enrichment that will further enhance de novo neuro-genesis within a neuroscience-based intensive care unit setting will furnish the ideal multidisciplinary therapeutic portfolio to maximally enhance tissue remodeling and cellular genetic re-programming.

ACKNOWLEDGMENTS

This work was supported by grants from the National Institutes of Health (NS38902, MH66290, and HD01799), the F. M. Kirby Foundation, the Skirball Foundation, the Rosanne H. Silbermann Foundation, and the Leslie and Roslyn Goldstein Foundation.

REFERENCES

1. Davenport R, Dennis M. Neurological emergencies: acute stroke. J Neurol Neurosurg Psychiatry 2000; 68: 277–288.
2. Williams GR, Jiang JG, Matchar DB et al. Incidence and occurrence of total (first-ever and recurrent) stroke. Stroke 1999; 30: 2523–2528.
3. Leker RR, Shohami E. Cerebral ischemia and trauma-different etiologies yet similar mechanisms: neuroprotective opportunities. Brain Res Brain Res Rev 2002; 39: 55–73.
4. de Freitas GR, Bogousslavsky J. Primary stroke prevention. Eur J Neurol 2001; 8: 1–15.
5. Savitz SI, Caplan LR. Vertebrobasilar disease. N Engl J Med 2005; 352: 2618–2626.
6. Brott T, Bogousslavsky J. Treatment of acute ischemic stroke. N Engl J Med 2000; 343: 710–722.
7. Liu J, Solway K, Messing RO et al. Increased neurogenesis in the dentate gyrus after transient global ischemia in gerbils. J Neurosci 1998; 18: 7768–7778.
8. Moskowitz MA, Lo EH. Neurogenesis and apoptotic cell death. Stroke 2003; 34: 324–326.
9. Perfilieva E, Risedal A, Nyberg J et al. Gender and strain influence on neurogenesis in dentate gyrus of young rats. J Cereb Blood Flow Metab 2001; 21: 211–217.
10. Schmidt W, Reymann KG. Proliferating cells differentiate into neurons in the hippocampal CA1 region of gerbils after global cerebral ischemia. Neurosci Lett 2002; 334: 153–156.
11. Yagita Y, Kitagawa K, Ohtsuki T et al. Neurogenesis by progenitor cells in the ischemic adult rat hippocampus. Stroke 2001; 32: 1890–1896.
12. Yagita Y, Kitagawa K, Sasaki T et al. Differential expression of Musashi1 and nestin in the adult rat hippocampus after ischemia. J Neurosci Res 2002; 69: 750–756.
13. Blumcke I, Schewe JC, Normann S et al. Increase of nestin-immunoreactive neural precursor cells in the dentate gyrus of pediatric patients with early-onset temporal lobe epilepsy. Hippocampus 2001; 11: 311–321.
14. Eriksson PS, Perfilieva E, Bjork-Eriksson T et al. Neurogenesis in the adult human hippocampus. Nat Med 1998; 4: 1313–1317.
15. Sanai N, Tramontin AD, Quinones-Hinojosa A et al. Unique astrocyte ribbon in adult human brain contains neural stem cells but lacks chain migration. Nature 2004; 427: 740–744.
16. Goldman S. Stem and progenitor cell-based therapy of the human central nervous system. Nat Biotech 2005; 23: 862–871.

17. Cameron HA, McKay R. Stem cells and neurogenesis in the adult brain. Curr Opin Neurobiol 1998; 8: 677–680.
18. McKay RD. Brain stem cells change their identity. Nat Med 1999; 5: 261–262.
19. McKay R. Stem cells in the central nervous system. Science 1997; 276: 66–71.
20. Gage FH. Mammalian neural stem cells. Science 2000; 287: 1433–1438.
21. Morshead CM, Reynolds BA, Craig CG et al. Neural stem cells in the adult mammalian forebrain: a relatively quiescent subpopulation of subependymal cells. Neuron 1994; 13: 1071–1082.
22. Goldman SA, Zukhar A, Barami K et al. Ependymal/subependymal zone cells of postnatal and adult songbird brain generate both neurons and nonneuronal siblings in vitro and in vivo. J Neurobiol 1996; 30: 505–520.
23. Alvarez-Buylla A, Garcia-Verdugo JM. Neurogenesis in adult subventricular zone. J Neurosci 2002; 22: 629–634.
24. Doetsch F, Petreanu L, Caille I et al. EGF converts transit-amplifying neurogenic precursors in the adult brain into multipotent stem cells. Neuron 2002; 36: 1021–1034.
25. Mehler MF. Mechanisms regulating lineage diversity during mammalian cerebral cortical neurogenesis and gliogenesis. Results Probl Cell Differ 2002; 39: 27–52.
26. Mehler MF. Regional forebrain patterning and neural subtype specification: implications for cerebral cortical functional connectivity and the pathogenesis of neurodegenerative diseases. Results Probl Cell Differ 2002; 39: 157–178.
27. Marmur R, Mabie PC, Gokhan S et al. Isolation and developmental characterization of cerebral cortical multipotent progenitors. Dev Biol 2998; 204: 577–591.
28. Marmur R, Kessler JA, Zhu G et al. Differentiation of oligodendroglial progenitors derived from cortical multipotent cells requires extrinsic signals including activation of gp130/LIFbeta receptors. J Neurosci 1998; 18: 9800–9811.
29. Mehler MF, Gokhan S. Postnatal cerebral cortical multipotent progenitors: regulatory mechanisms and potential role in the development of novel neural regenerative strategies. Brain Pathol 1999; 9: 515–526.
30. Mehler MF, Kessler JA. Hematolymphopoietic and inflammatory cytokines in neural development. Trends Neurosci 1997; 20: 357–365.
31. Mehler MF, Mabie PC, Zhang D et al. Bone morphogenetic proteins in the nervous system. Trends Neurosci 1997; 20: 309–317.
32. Mehler MF, Kessler JA. Cytokine effects on CNS cells: Implications for the pathogenesis and prevention of stroke. In Progress in Inflammation Research: Inflammation and Stroke, Feuerstein GZ (ed), Birkhauser-Verlag, Basel, 2001; 115–140.
33. Tsai PT, Ohab JJ, Kertesz N et al. A critical role of erythropoietin receptor in neurogenesis and post-stroke recovery. J Neurosci 2006; 26: 1269–1274.
34. Schanzer A, Wachs F-P, Wilhelm D et al. Direct stimulation of adult neural stem cells in vitro and neurogenesis in vivo by vascular endothelial growth factor. Brain Pathol 2004; 14: 237–248.
35. Leker RR, McKay RDG. Using endogenous neural stem cells to enhance recovery from ischemic brain injury. Curr Neurovasc Res 2004; 1: 421–427.
36. Mitchell BD, Emsley JG, Magavi SSP et al. Constitutive and induced neurogenesis in the adult mammalian brain: manipulation of endogenous precursors toward CNS repair. Dev Neurosci 2004; 26: 101–117.

37. Kuhn HG, Dickinson-Anson H, Gage FH. Neurogenesis in the dentate gyrus of the adult rat: age-related decrease of neuronal progenitor proliferation. J Neurosci 1996; 16: 2027–2033.

38. Suhonen JO, Peterson DA, Ray J et al. Differentiation of adult hippocampus-derived progenitors into olfactory neurons in vivo. Nature 1996; 383: 624–627.

39. Gokhan S, Marin-Husstege M, Yung SY et al. Combinatorial profiles of oligodendrocyte-selective classes of transcriptional regulators differentially modulate myelin basic protein gene expression. J Neurosci 2005; 25: 8311–8321.

40. Magavi SS, Leavitt BR, Macklis JD. Induction of neurogenesis in the neocortex of adult mice. Nature 2000; 405: 951–955.

41. Gould E, Reeves AJ, Graziano MS et al. Neurogenesis in the neocortex of adult primates. Science 1999; 286: 548–552.

42. Gould E, Vail N, Wagers M et al. Adult-generated hippocampal and neocortical neurons in macaques have a transient existence. Proc Natl Acad Sci USA 2001; 98: 10910–10917.

43. Kaplan MS. Neurogenesis in the 3-month-old rat visual cortex. J Comp Neurol 1981; 195: 323–338.

44. Ehninger D, Kempermann G. Regional effects of wheel running and environmental enrichment on cell genesis and microglia proliferation in the adult murine neocortex. Cereb Cortex 2003; 13: 845–851.

45. Koketsu D, Mikami A, Miyamoto Y et al. Nonrenewal of neurons in the cerebral neocortex of adult macaque monkeys. J Neurosci 2003; 23: 937–942.

46. Kornack DR, Rakic P. Continuation of neurogenesis in the hippocampus of the adult macaque monkey. Proc Natl Acad Sci USA 1999; 96: 5768–5773.

47. Kornack DR, Rakic P. The generation, migration and differentiation of olfactory neurons in the adult primate brain. Proc Natl Acad Sci USA 2001; 98: 4752–4757.

48. Macklis JD. Transplanted neocortical neurons migrate selectively into regions of neuronal degeneration produced by chromophore-targeted laser photolysis. J Neurosci 1993; 13: 3848–3863.

49. Madison R, Macklis JD. Noninvasively induced degeneration of neocortical pyramidal neurons in vivo: selective targeting by laser activation of retrogradely transported photolytic chromophore. Exp Neurol 1993; 121: 153–159.

50. Scharff C, Kirn JR, Grossman M et al. Targeted neuronal death affects neuronal replacement and vocal behavior in adult songbirds. Neuron 2000; 25: 481–492.

51. Sheen VL, Dreyer EB, Macklis JD. Calcium-mediated neuronal degeneration following singlet oxygen production. Neuroreport 1992; 3: 705–708.

52. Sheen VL, Macklis JD. Apoptotic mechanisms in targeted neuronal cell death by chromophore-activated photolysis. Exp Neurol 1994; 130: 67–81.

53. Nakatomi H, Kuriu T, Okabe S et al. Regeneration of hippocampal pyramidal neurons after ischemic brain injury by recruitment of endogenous neural progenitors. Cell 2002; 110: 429–441.

54. Arvidsson A, Collin T, Kirik D et al. Neuronal replacement from endogenous precursors in the adult brain after stroke. Nat Med 2002; 8: 963–970.

55. Parent JM, Vexler ZS, Gong C et al. Rat forebrain neurogenesis and striatal neuron replacement after focal stroke. Ann Neurol 2002; 52: 802–813.

56. Wang Y, Sheen VL, Macklis JD. Cortical interneurons upregulate neurotrophins in vivo in response to targeted apoptotic degeneration of neighboring pyramidal neurons. Exp Neurol 1998; 154: 389–402.

57. Emsley JG, Mitchell BD, Kempermann G et al. Adult neurogenesis and repair of the adult CNS with neural progenitors, precursors, and stem cells. Prog Neurobiol 2005; 75: 321–341.
58. Zhang RL, Zhang ZG, Zhang L et al. Proliferation and differentiation of progenitor cells in the cortex and the subventricular zone in the adult rat after focal cerebral ischemia. Neuroscience 2001; 105: 33–41.
59. Gu W, Brannstrom T, Wester P. Cortical neurogenesis in adult rats after reversible photothrombotic stroke. J Cereb Blood Flow Metab 2000; 20: 1166–1173.
60. Jiang W, Gu W, Brannstrom T et al. Cortical neurogenesis in adult rats after transient middle cerebral artery occlusion. Stroke 2001; 32: 1201–1207.
61. Takasawa K, Kitagawa K, Yagita Y et al. Increased proliferation of neural progenitor cells but reduced survival of newborn cells in the contralateral hippocampus after focal cerebral ischemia in rats. J Cereb Blood Flow Metab 2002; 22: 299–307.
62. Iwai M, Hayashi T, Zhang WR et al. Induction of highly polysialylated neural cell adhesion molecule (PSA-NCAM) in postischemic gerbil hippocampus mainly dissociated with neural stem cell proliferation. Brain Res 2001; 902: 288–293.
63. Kee NJ, Preston E, Wojtowicz JM. Enhanced neurogenesis after transient global ischemia in the dentate gyrus of the rat. Exp Brain Res 2001; 136: 313–320.
64. Wada K, Sugimori H, Bhide PG et al. Effect of basic fibroblast growth factor treatment on brain progenitor cells after permanent focal ischemia in rats. Stroke 2003; 34: 2722–2728.
65. Matsuoka N, Nozaki K, Takagi Y et al. Adenovirus-mediated gene transfer of fibroblast growth factor 2 increases Brdu-positive cells after ischemia in gerbils. Stroke 2003; 34: 1519–1525.
66. Dempsey RJ, Sailor KA, Bowen KK et al. Stroke-induced progenitor cell proliferation in adult spontaneously hypertensive rat brain: effect of exogenous IGF-1 and GDNF. J Neurochem 2003; 87: 586–597.
67. Tonchev AB, Yamashima T, Zhao L et al. Differential proliferative response in the postischemic hippocampus, temporal cortex, and olfactory bulb of young adult macaque monkeys. Glia 2003; 42: 209–224.
68. Jessell TM. Neuronal specification in the spinal cord: inductive signals and transcriptional codes. Nat Rev Genet 2000; 1: 20–29.
69. Dasen JS, Tice BC, Brenner-Morton S et al. A Hox regulatory network establishes motor neuron pool identity and target-muscle connectivity. Cell 2005; 123: 477–491.
70. Mehler MF, Mabie PC, Zhu G et al. Developmental changes in progenitor cell responsiveness to bone morphogenetic proteins differentially modulate progressive CNS lineage fate. Dev Neurosci 2000; 22: 74–85.
71. Yung SY, Gokhan S, Jurcsak J et al. Differential modulation of BMP signaling promotes the elaboration of cerebral cortical GABAergic neurons or oligodendrocytes from a common sonic hedgehog-responsive ventral forebrain progenitor species. Proc Natl Acad Sci USA 2002; 99: 16273–16278.
72. Xu Q, Cobos I, De La Cruz F et al. Origins of cortical interneuron subtypes. J Neurosci 2004; 24: 2612–2622.
73. Kessaris N, Fogarty M, Iannarelli P et al. Competing waves of oligodendrocytes in the forebrain and postnatal elimination of an embryonic lineage. Nat Neurosci 2006; 9: 173–179.

74. Richardson WD, Kessaris N, Pringle N. Oligodendrocyte wars. Nat Rev Neurosci 2006; 7: 11–18.
75. Hsieh J, Gage FH. Epigenetic control of neural stem cell fate. Curr Opin Genet Dev 2004; 14: 461–469.
76. Bjornsson HT, Fallin MD, Feinberg AP. An integrated epigenetic and genetic approach to common human disease. Trends Genet 2004; 20: 350–358.
77. Costa FF. Non-coding RNAs: new players in eukaryotic biology. Gene 2005; 357: 83–94.
78. Mattick JS, Makunin IV. Small regulatory RNAs in mammals. Hum Mol Genet 2005; 14: R121–132.
79. Davies W, Isles AR, Wilkinson LS. Imprinted gene expression in the brain. Neurosci Biobehav Rev 2005; 29: 421–430.
80. Klein ME, Impey S, Goodman RH. Role reversal: the regulation of neuronal gene expression by microRNAs. Curr Opin Neurobiol 2005; 15: 507–513.
81. Colvis CM, Pollock JD, Goodman RH et al. Epigenetic mechanisms and gene networks in the nervous system. J Neurosci 2005; 25: 10379–10389.
82. Endres M, Meisel A, Biniszkiewicz D et al. DNA methyltransferase contributes to delayed ischemic brain injury. J Neurosci 2000; 20: 3175–3181.
83. Calderone A, Jover T, Noh KM et al. Ischemic insults derepress the gene silencer REST in neurons destined to die. J Neurosci 2003; 23: 2112–2121.
84. Kuwabara T, Hsieh J, Nakashima K et al. A small modulatory dsRNA specifies the fate of adult neural stem cells. Cell 2004; 116: 779–793.
85. Lee MG, Wynder C, Cooch N et al. An essential role for CoREST in nucleosomal histone 3 lysine 4 demethylation. Nature 2005; 437: 432–435.
86. Wynder C, Hakimi MA, Epstein JA et al. Recruitment of MLL by HMG-domain protein iBRAF promotes neural differentiation. Nat Cell Biol 2005; 7: 1113–1117.
87. Abrahams JM, Gokhan S, Flamm S et al. De novo neurogenesis and acute stroke: are exogenous stem cells really necessary? Neurosurgery 2004; 54: 150–156.
88. Domeniconi M, Cao Z, Spencer T et al. Myelin-associated glycoprotein interacts with the Nogo66 receptor to inhibit neurite outgrowth. Neuron 2002; 35: 283–290.
89. Kruger GM, Morrison SJ. Brain repair by endogenous progenitors. Cell 2002; 110: 399–402.

8

Ethics and Stem Cell Research

Ruth Macklin

The announcement in November 1998 that researchers had succeeded in deriving human embryonic stem cells (hereinafter, HESCs) was hailed as a stunning scientific achievement. Not only was the scientific achievement itself noteworthy, but it held the promise for dramatic therapeutic applications in the future. It was not long, however, before the discovery raised ethical questions in the minds of some people because the stem cells are derived from living human embryos. What quickly followed was the beginning of a national debate about the ethics of stem cell research and the intertwining of ethical, legal, and political issues that have not abated at the time of this writing. On the day that James A. Thomson, an embryologist at the University of Wisconsin, and his colleagues published their findings in *Science*, Rick Weiss wrote in the Washington Post: "...in the political arena, the new work has reignited a smoldering debate over a four-year-old congressional ban on the use of federal funds for human embryo research. With the therapeutic potential of embryonic cells suddenly very real, advocates are calling for a reexamination of that ban, saying the development of lifesaving applications will be hindered if federal dollars remain off-limits" *(1)*.

What ethical issues does stem cell research raise, and are those issues limited to the concerns about research on human embryos? That question is often posed in the following form: "Isn't the real issue regarding stem cells whether it is ethical to kill human embryos in order to derive the stem cells?" A reply to this formulation of the question states that there is not just one "real" issue. It is true that for some people, the chief—or even the only—ethical concern regarding stem cell research is the destruction of human embryos that results from the derivation of the stem cells. For others, however, the moral

From: *Current Clinical Neurology: Stroke Recovery with Cellular Therapies*
Edited by: Sean I. Savitz and Daniel M. Rosenbaum © Humana Press Inc., Totowa, NJ

status of a several-day-old human embryo is far from clear. According to some religious viewpoints, a fertilized egg has all the rights of a living human being. According to others—both religious and secular— an entity at the blastocyst stage of development has no moral status. It is abundantly clear that in the USA and elsewhere in the world, there is no consensus regarding at what stage developing human life acquires moral status and therefore, a "right to life."

The stark opposition between these two viewpoints emerges with startling clarity in two letters to the editor that appeared in the *New York Times* on the same day. One letter said: "Embryonic stem cell research means the killing of a human being to extract the embryonic stem cells. . . . We must begin to show respect for human life at all stages of development" *(2)*. The other letter said: "Mr. Bush and the religious right believe that life begins at conception and, as such, creating human embryos with the intent of therapeutic cloning amounts to the destruction of a human life. The reality is that stem cells are derived not from a human being but from a microscopic ball of cells" *(3)*. Although the debate over stem cell research that revolves around the destruction of human embryos is not the only ethical issue, it has certainly occupied center stage since Dr Thomson's announcement in *Science* and the subsequent reports in the popular press.

1. POLITICS, LAW, AND ETHICS INTERTWINED

It is a peculiarity of laws in the USA that federal funds may not be used for some activities even if those same activities are not prohibited by federal law. For example, under current law, no federal funds may be used for abortions except when the pregnancy endangers a woman's life or results from rape or incest. Although individual states have passed a variety of restrictive laws (typically restricting the rights of adolescents), abortion nevertheless remains a constitutionally protected right. The same conditions obtain in the case of human embryo research according to a law passed by Congress in 1996. According to this law (known as the Dickey– Wicker Amendment), no funds from the Department of Health and Human Services (DHHS), of which the NIH is a branch, can be used to "create a human embryo or embryos for research purposes; or for research in which a human embryo or embryos are destroyed, discarded or knowingly subjected to risk of injury or death.' Perhaps paradoxically, however, there are no laws in the USA governing the disposal of unused embryos resulting from in vitro fertilization (IVF) carried out in fertility clinics. Couples who do not intend to implant their embryos leftover from IVF in the future, to donate them to other couples, or to donate them for non-federally funded research may choose to have the embryos destroyed. From the moment that Thomson and colleagues succeeded in the derivation of HESCs, fertility clinics were recognized as a likely source of embryos for stem cell research. Nevertheless, the fact that such embryos were slated for destruction was not sufficient to overcome the barrier of using federal funds to conduct stem cell research.

1.1. NIH and National Bioethics Advisory Commission (NBAC)

So who would pay for the research, if not the federal government? Private industry has not rushed to fill the vacuum created by the ban on government funds, most likely because there is not a definable product from which profits can be derived. The NIH has been eager to fund stem cell research since the announcement of Thomson's achievement. The NIH director quickly empanelled experts in science, public policy, and bioethics to propose guidelines. In the meantime, the general counsel for the DHHS, Harriet Raab, had been hard at work crafting a legal opinion that would allow NIH (federal) funds to be used in some manner for the support of stem cell research. In a memorandum to Harold Varmus, who was the NIH director at the time, Raab stated that "Pluripotent stem cells are not organisms and do not have the capacity to develop into an organism that could perform all the life functions of a human being . . . They are, rather, human cells that have the potential to evolve into different types of cells such as blood cells or insulin producing cells" *(4)*. The point of making this distinction was to permit the use of federal funds for stem cell research once the cells had been derived from human embryos, even though the activity of deriving the cells could not use federal funds because that activity causes the destruction of the embryos. The panel of experts invited by Varmus accepted this analysis and in the initial report that NIH issued, the proposed guidelines relied on the distinction between deriving the stem cells from embryos and using the stem cells for research once they had been derived using non-federal funds.

However, the distinction was not accepted either by pro-life Congressional opponents of stem cell research or by the members of the NBAC, a body that issued a subsequent report on the ethics of stem cell research *(5)*. The Congressional opponents contended that it "would violate both the letter and the spirit of the Federal law' *(6)*. The

NBAC report rejected Raab's distinction as "legalistic' and recommended a change in the current federal law that would allow the use of federal funds to derive stem cells as well as to use the derived cells for research. However, the NBAC report remained conservative on one major point. Although it recommended the use of existing frozen embryos that would otherwise be discarded, it did not take the bolder step of permitting the creation of embryos for the purpose of deriving stem cells for research. NBAC's recommendation 2 stated:

> Research involving the derivation and use of human ES cells from embryos remaining after infertility treatments should be eligible for federal funding. An exception should be made to the present statutory ban on federal funding of embryo research to permit federal agencies to fund research involving the derivation of human ES cells from this source under appropriate regulations that include public oversight and review (5, at 4).

Both the pro-life critics of Counsel Raab's distinction and the more liberal NBAC position rejected the idea that it is legally or ethically defensible to separate the derivation of stem cells from their use in research.

The NIH went ahead and wrote new guidelines based on Raab's distinction and intended to begin funding research using stem cells that had been derived with non-federal funds. But all that took time, and in the delay that ensued, the administration in Washington changed. The new secretary of DHHS, Tommy Thompson, ordered the NIH to postpone a meeting scheduled for April 2001 that NIH had scheduled to begin to review grant proposals for the research. Only a few months later, President George W. Bush issued his restrictive ruling on the use of HESCs for research.

1.2. The Bush Ruling

On August 9, 2001, Bush announced that federal funds could be used to support HESC research but only on stem cell lines that were in existence prior to the date of that announcement. There was both uncertainty and disagreement about just how many cell lines existed at that point. Regardless of the number, there were also scientific assessments that questioned the value and suitability of those cell lines for subsequent research. One key factor was that the existing cell lines had been nurtured using mouse cells, which would have rendered them problematic, if not altogether unacceptable, for later therapeutic research applications.

In any case, from an ethical standpoint, it is reasonable to wonder what would be the difference between using stem cells from embryos that had already been destroyed and deriving cells from embryos that would be destroyed in the future, according to the plans of their progenitors. Is it that the government (or the taxpayers) had no say in the destruction of the embryos in the past but they would be complicit, somehow, in the destruction of any embryos destroyed with the aid of federal funds in the future? One speculation was that allowing the future destruction of embryos would somehow induce women to donate them for stem cell research rather than implant the embryos or donate them to another couple. However, this possibility exists anyway since what is at stake is not the stem cell research but the use of federal funds for that research. Any women or couple so eager to donate their frozen embryos for research could do so in the private sector; it would hardly matter to the women who would be paying for the derivation of the embryos. Nevertheless, there is no evidence that the potential long-range benefits of stem cell research would change the decisions that couples make regarding disposition of unwanted embryos. Although some Congressional leaders, including members of the President's own party, were eager to move the debate forward toward eventual legislation, scarcely a month after Bush's announcement events were overtaken by the attack on September 11, 2001.

In January 2002, Bush announced the members of his newly created President's Council on Bioethics, with Dr Leon R. Kass, a known opponent of research on human embryos, as its chair. Although the Clinton-appointed NBAC had already issued a report on the ethics of stem cell research, the new Bioethics Council undertook that mission anew. The Council issued several other reports (including one on cloning) before the first of its two reports on stem cell research. That first report *(7)* was described by Kass as follows: "Stem cell research has been of interest to, and associated in the public mind with, this Council since its creation. Taking up the charge given to us by President Bush in his August 9, 2001, speech on stem cell research, the Council has from its beginnings been monitoring developments in this fast-paced and exciting field of research. . . . The present monitoring report . . . is in the spirit of an "update" and contains no recommendations for policy' *(8)*.

In its report entitled *White Paper*, issued about a year and a half later, this same committee laid out what it considered to be ethically superior alternatives to the derivation of stem cells from embryos, since the alternatives would not allegedly requiring destroying any embryos *(9)*. The four alternatives described in the *White Paper* are: (i) deriving stem cells from dead embryos, (ii) nonharmful biopsy, (iii) altered nuclear transplantation, and (iv) dedifferentiation.

According to the first alternative, any ethical problems with the use of embryos are eliminated since the embryos from which the stem cells would be derived are already dead. The concept of "death" in this situation is "organismic death," which means that the embryo has irreversibly lost the capacity for continued and integrated cellular division, growth, and differentiation. Scientific and conceptual questions linger, however. Can the concept of organismic death be meaningfully applied to organisms at the very beginning of life when they consist only of a few cells? Since the two standard criteria for determining death in human beings—brain death and cessation of heart and lung functions—are inapplicable to embryos, how can death properly be diagnosed? *(10)*.

The second alternative in the *White Paper* is "nonharmful biopsy." On this alternative, a single cell is removed from an early embryo without destroying it, and that cell is used to create the cell line. Although the same technique is used in prenatal genetic diagnosis (PGD), there are no long-term safety studies. Members of the President's Council objected to this proposal on the grounds that a perfectly healthy embryo would be used for a biopsy that would remove the cell for research. Those who object to any action that would harm embryos found this option unacceptable, especially since these embryos would not be slated for destruction but rather, implanted. In that case, it could very likely lead to the birth of a child, and it is unknown whether that child would be harmed as a result of the procedure carried out when it was at the embryonic stage. The council also suggested that "there might be a strong moral argument against biopsy on the grounds that the embryo is being treated merely as a means to another's ends (10, at 25)." It should be clear, however, that this latter objection already construes the embryo as a living human being having moral status. The prohibition against using any human being as a "mere means" to the ends of others is a strong moral principle based on the writings of the philosopher, Immanuel Kant. But it is a principle that applies to human beings whose moral status is unquestioned. It begs the very question at issue in embryo research to use a moral principle designed for individuals who are unquestionably persons and apply it to the few living cells that constitute a human embryo.

The third alternative, altered nuclear transplantation, would use the technique of somatic cell nuclear transfer (SCNT), commonly known as "cloning." But instead of transplanting a normal nucleus, this technique would involve a defective nucleus, one in which some developmental genes in the somatic cell nucleus would be silenced prior to transfer and then reinserted after the cells were extracted. The point of this maneuver is that the intended product could never develop into a viable human being, so no embryo with moral status was being created. This novel idea is not only untested, but scientists contended that it would be much more complicated than the technique of SCNT, which is difficult enough to accomplish. Numerous objections were made against this bizarre alternative, one of which was quoted in *Science* magazine: "It will be a sad day when scientists use genetic manipulations to deliberately create crippled embryos to please the Church" (10, at 26).

These proposals of the President's Council were attempts to enter this politically charged arena in a way that could please both proponents and opponents of stem cell research. The strongest opposition to the research had come from political conservatives—usually aligned with what has become known in the USA as the "religious right." They are opposed to the destruction of human life "from the moment of fertilization." These opponents include religious spokespersons and some members of Congress, among the many public and private citizens who have weighed in on the matter. One of the most vocal spokespersons from the religious community has been Richard M. Doerflinger, who is deputy director of the Secretariat for Pro-Life Activities, U.S. Conference of Catholic Bishops. Doerflinger has been one of the leading opponents of stem cell research and has argued that adult stem cells could be equally efficacious so there is no need to destroy embryos in order to obtain human stem cells for research—a position that most scientists have emphatically disputed. The chief Congressional opponent of stem cell research has been Senator Sam Brownback from Kansas. The senator's website includes this statement about the ethics of stem cell research:

> Clearly, we must to continue to work to find cures for diseases, and to alleviate suffering. However, it has never been acceptable to deliberately kill one innocent human being in order to help another. Life begins at the beginning at conception. Human beings develop from the one-celled stage onward, and deserve respect because of the dignity they have as human beings *(11)*.

Proponents of stem cell research have included not only scientists, members of various advocacy groups for diseases such as Parkinson's and diabetes, and figures from the entertainment world (such as the actors, Michael J. Fox and Christopher Reeve, afflicted with conditions for which the applications of stem cell research offer some hope), but also other members of Congress, even some who oppose abortion. Those politicians, as well as other opponents of abortion, contend that their position is not inconsistent. One such individual is Senator Orrin Hatch, a long-standing foe of abortion. In a press release issued in connection with his sponsorship of a bill in the Senate, Hatch said: "Now, the last time we introduced this bill, there was interest in the fact that I, as a strongly pro-life senator, would be the lead sponsor. I think we have put that issue behind us, as more pro-life lawmakers have expressed their support for this research. The fact is, I have never believed that life begins in a Petri dish" *(12)*. This remark seeks to justify the apparent inconsistency of opposing abortion but supporting stem cell research by drawing a distinction between fetuses in utero and extracorporeal embryos.

Another distinction that could support stem cell research but not abortion points to the difference between a several-day-old blastocyst consisting of a few cells, and a later-stage fetus, especially after the development of the nervous system. The one move that has been rejected by pro-life spokespersons is the argument that stem cell research will likely yield such overwhelmingly positive contributions to human health that the benefits outweigh the harms caused by destroying embryos. The latter is known as "utilitarian reasoning" and is criticized by those who (mistakenly) believe that utilitarianism is a pernicious ethical perspective that allows the "ends" to justify unacceptable "means."

2. ETHICAL ARGUMENTS

In order to understand the ethics of stem cell research, we must leave politics behind. Setting aside the three alternatives proposed in the *White Paper* issued by the President's Council on Bioethics, there are three main ethical positions on the use in research of HESCs (with subvariations), each of which has implications for public policy: the "absolute prohibition," which holds that no embryonic stem cell research—even using existing cell lines—is ethically permissible; the "future prohibition," which disallows any future derivation of stem cells (this position is identical to the Bush position but without the peculiarity and complication that limits only federal funding but not the use of private funds); the "NBAC position," permitting future stem cell research on embryos slated for destruction and prohibiting the creation of new embryos for the purpose of research; the "non-cloning permissive position," allowing the creation of embryos for stem cell research through IVF but not by means of SCNT; and a variation on the last position, the "cloning permissive position," which would permit the creation of embryos for stem cell research through SCNT. These different positions are discussed in turn below.

2.1. The Absolute Prohibition

This view maintains that no research that involves derivation of stem cells from embryos is acceptable because it results in the destruction of the embryos. The extreme version would disallow the "Bush position" because using existing cell lines derived from human embryos makes the researchers "complicit" in the past events that destroyed the embryos. This view rests on a fundamental view of the moral status of embryos: they are human beings, with all the rights accorded living human beings, especially the "right to life." But why would it be unacceptable to use embryonic stem cell lines that already exist, since it would not involve the destruction of any future embryos? According to this view, if some good is allowed to result from past evil actions, that could lead people to believe that the actions were not so evil after all, since they brought about the eventual good results. This is one form of argument that leads some people to be critical of utilitarian ethical reasoning.

Although few people have taken seriously this specific argument regarding stem cell research, an interesting analogy exists in the debate over the use of data obtained from the horrific experiments conducted by physicians in Nazi Germany. In that debate, some have argued that if the data could be used by current scientists in fruitful ways, it should be permitted. Others contend that use of the Nazi data by reputable scientists could only serve to validate in some way what the German doctors did, and that would be utterly unacceptable.

Whether or not this form of argument is sound, the "absolutist" prohibition rests on the view that extracorporeal embryos have a right to life equal to that of postnatal human beings. That is the fundamental premise that supporters of stem cell research reject, but it is also a premise that the Bush position shares. The key feature of this view is that a human embryo, regardless of its location, has a right to life.

2.2. The Future Prohibition Position

This position holds that stem cell research is permissible only on existing cell lines because the embryos from which the cells were derived are already dead. Any future destruction of embryos in order to derive stem cells would be ethically unacceptable because it involves killing "a living human being." As noted above, Senator Orrin Hatch makes a distinction between extracorporeal human embryos and implanted embryos, holding that the existence of the former "in a Petri dish" removes the characteristic that confers on fetuses in utero a right to life. The extracorporeal embryo is a result of fertilization of an ovum by a sperm, but that (apparently) does not yield an entity that has a right to life.

Senator Brownback would prohibit stem cell research because, as he says (rather infelicitously), "Life begins at the beginning at conception." But this formulation could be consistent with permitting stem cell research because according to the medical definition of *conception,* it is a process that begins with fertilization and ends with implantation. Since extracorporeal embryos are obviously not implanted, Brownback's formulation, if taken in its strictly medical meaning, would allow stem cell research. That is certainly not what he intended. Had he used the term "fertilization," his statement would have the intended result.

Gilbert Meilaender, a professor of Christian Ethics, criticizes the utilitarian argument he accuses some defenders of stem cell research to be making. He writes:

> We might be convinced that the goal of relieving suffering offers a straightforward justification of sacrificing embryos in research. Or we might hold that although embryos merit our respect, the greater good to be achieved by destroying them, the more respect must give way to research. Or, if we take the notion of respect seriously, we might find that relieving suffering is a real but not supreme imperative (13, at 9).

Meilander's critique of utilitarian reasoning comes through clearly in his statement urging a ban on embryonic stem cell research: "isn't [it], in fact, why we sometimes need a ban—precisely to prohibit an unacceptable means to otherwise desirable ends?" (13, at 9). However, this view misconstrues the fundamental premise of proponents of stem cell research: they do not hold the "means"—that is, the destruction of human embryos—to be unacceptable. It is not the form of reasoning that marks the difference between the ethical views of proponents and opponents of stem cell research. It is, rather, the disagreement over the moral status of the embryo that constitutes their divergent ethical views.

Consider this. Suppose it were the case, contrary to fact, that the only way human stem cells could be derived would be to kill a child or adult human being. Only a few would have to be killed in order to create the stem cell lines that could result in future health and life-saving benefits for hundreds of thousands, even millions of future patients. It is absurd to think that those who use utilitarian reasoning would sanction those "unacceptable means" to achieve the enormous potential benefits that might accrue in the future. What makes the means—destroying embryos—acceptable to some and unacceptable to others is their divergent views about the moral status of the several-day-old extracorporeal human embryo.

2.3. The NBAC Position

The report of the NBAC permitted HESC research, subject to certain restrictions. The chief restriction is the use of only those embryos leftover from the clinical practice of IVF that would otherwise be destroyed. In the nature of its work, the NBAC had to couch its recommendations in terms of whether federal funding should or should not be permitted for stem cell research, and under what specific conditions. However, stripped of the language of using federal funds, the main recommendations of NBAC's report are: stem cell research involving the destruction of human embryos that would otherwise be discarded is permissible; the creation of embryos for the explicit purpose of conducting stem cell research should not be permitted; research involving the derivation or use of HESCs from embryos created by means of SCNT into oocytes should not be permitted. NBAC imposed the limitation on this last technique saying that it might nevertheless be acceptable in the future; but at the time the report was issued (September 1999), the commission held that scientific achievements were not sufficiently advanced to warrant approval of research on embryos created through SCNT.

NBAC's conclusions appear eminently reasonable to many people, including those who would refuse to sanction the creation of embryos for the purpose of conducting stem cell research. That is because the leftover embryos in infertility clinics would be discarded anyway, so what would be the ethical problem of destroying them for a potentially beneficial purpose? Additional conditions suggested in the NBAC and other reports included the following restrictions: both members of the couple whose gametes were used to create the embryos would have to give their informed consent for the use of their embryos in stem cell research; the timing of their consent to use the embryos in research should come *after* their decision to destroy remaining unwanted embryos; and commercial transactions involving embryos for stem cell research are prohibited.

The NBAC position can appeal to people who have ethical discomfort over the idea of killing embryos but who remain realistic in recognizing that it makes no sense to allow for the destruction of embryos but to prohibit the use of those embryos for research. Thus, the NBAC position can be acceptable to those on both sides of the fence: people who lament the destruction of embryos but realize that it takes place anyway in infertility clinics; and those who have no moral objection to the destruction of human embryos.

2.4. The "Non-Cloning" Permissive Position

A more permissive stance on the use of embryos for research would divide those who could agree on the NBAC position into two camps. This next position is the view that stem cell research is permissible using embryos that are created for the express purpose of conducting stem cell research. Yet, even this view allows for nuances and differences in the way embryos are construed. One example is the statement by the letter-writer to the *New York Times* quoted earlier: "The reality is that stem cells are derived not from a human being but from a microscopic ball of cells' *(3)*. This is an unequivocal statement about the nature of the entity from which the stem cells are taken and likens the embryo to, say, dead human skin cells that have no moral worth whatsoever.

But other writers consider this characterization of embryos to be too extreme, arguing that even though it is permissible to destroy embryos for the purpose of deriving stem cells, embryos nevertheless have "some moral status" and are "worthy of some moral respect" *(14,15)*. It is difficult for some people to accept the seemingly contradictory view that there are entities that have moral worth and deserve respect, but at the same time it is ethically acceptable to destroy such entities. However, the writers who have articulated this intermediate position provide reasons in support of their view, one of which is the need to move away from what they see as the rigid dogmatism of the two extremes.

One further variation divides this position into two possibilities: one that would disallow the use of stem cells derived from embryos created through SCNT and one that would permit that variation. The view that disallows SCNT has different possible justifications. One is "proceed with caution." Because SCNT is a new and complicated procedure that is difficult to achieve and may have uncertain consequences, it is better to wait until there is more scientific knowledge and technical experience with the technique. The ethical principle that supports this view is known as the "precautionary principle."

A second justification for prohibiting the creation of embryos through SCNT in order to do stem cell research relies on the "slippery slope" argument. The argument is that so-called "therapeutic" cloning (the use of SCNT to create embryos for research designed to develop therapies) will inevitably lead to "reproductive cloning" (the creation of embryos by SCNT with the aim of implanting them in a woman's womb to make a baby that is genetically identical to a living person). The huge public, governmental, and international outcry calling for a ban on reproductive cloning has been unremitting ever since Ian Wilmut reported that he had cloned Dolly, the sheep. Those who uncritically accept the validity of slippery slope arguments contend that if SCNT is permitted to create embryos for the purpose of research, it is only a matter of time before reproductive cloning will find wide acceptance. This type of argument ignores the many situations in which governmental regulations and restrictions are put in place for some types of activities, and law-abiding citizens adhere to and do not seek to overturn or bypass them.

2.5. The "Cloning" Permissive Position

Since 1990, the United Kingdom has adopted the most liberal policies for any embryo research, allowing the creation of embryos specifically for research. Once that was already in place, it required no additional steps to authorize the creation of embryos specifically for stem cell research. The United Kingdom has an oversight body, the Human Fertilisation and Embryo Authority (HFEA), which monitors and regulates assisted reproduction in the therapeutic area, as well as all research involving human embryos. In 2004, the HFEA granted a license to allow researchers to use SCNT cloning for embryonic stem cell research and in 2005 Sweden specifically approved the production of embryonic stem cell lines using SCNT. It is likely that other countries will follow suit, despite a lack of agreement among countries in the European Union regarding the permissibility of any research involving human embryos (Germany remains staunchly opposed). At the time of this writing, many scientists in the USA are concerned that the USA will be left behind in the international scientific arena as experience grows and striking advances begin to be made in HESC research.

3. RECENT DEVELOPMENTS

Despite the existing ban in the USA on federal funding for HESC research, that research is proceeding (albeit somewhat slowly) with the use of private funds and money from some states that have passed legislation with specific authorizations supporting the research. With no regulation, and in the absence of federal or even state oversight bodies, it increasingly became evident that some guidance was needed for scientists and the institutions in which they work to ensure proper ethical and procedural conduct of stem cell research. Accordingly, the National Research Council and the Institute of Medicine of the National Academies of Science appointed a panel of experts to deliberate and issue such guidance. The resulting document, *Guidelines for Human Embryonic Stem Cell Research*, was published in 2005 *(16)*.

These guidelines rest on the presumption that HESC research is ethically permissible. As a result, they do not address the ethical question of whether it is permissible to destroy embryos in order to derive stem cells. Instead, the guidelines address a range of other ethical concerns including informed consent, payment to donors for embryos, directed donation, oversight of research, and related matters. A key feature is the recommendation that Embryonic Stem Cell Research Oversight (ESCRO) committees be established to monitor the research. These committees would not replace the existing Institutional Review Boards (IRBs) that are required in every institution that receives federal funds; instead, they would add another layer of oversight to ensure that researchers and institutions adhere to provisions in the guidelines.

Among the specific provisions are the requirement to obtain informed consent from the donors of embryos for the specific purpose of stem cell research, and assurance of the right of the donors to withdraw their consent at any time before the research begins. Donors should also be informed that their names and other information about them might be known by the researchers working with the stem cells but that every effort will be made to keep their identities and other information confidential. The guidelines specify other elements that must be disclosed in the informed consent process and document: that cells might be manipulated genetically or transplanted into animals for preclinical testing; that although research involving the donors' stem cells may have commercial potential, they (the donors) will not share in any financial benefit. Payments to donors are strictly prohibited, and a number of provisions are designed to prevent conflicts of interest. One such provision prohibits stem cell researchers from attempting to influence any decisions by couples to create embryos for the purpose of stem cell research or more embryos than they would otherwise seek to create for their own reproductive purposes.

The most striking recent development at the time of this writing is the evolving story of the fabrication of results of research results by Hwang Woo-suk, a leading Korean investigator, who reported several breakthroughs in stem cell research and SCNT. In an article published in *Science* in 2005, Hwang claimed to have developed stem cell lines derived from embryos that were produced by somatic SCNT from 11 different patients. These results were questioned when some Korean scientists and journalists identified discrepancies in photos and other data. This led to a detailed inquiry, a call for retraction of the paper in *Science*, and the eventual charge of fabrication of data. Hwang and his colleagues had published earlier groundbreaking papers, including a report on the first successful attempt to clone human embryos and extract stem cells from them, and the first successful cloning of a dog. The veracity of the earlier reports was called into question once it became clear that data in the most recent published article were fabricated. The episode is still under investigation at the time of this writing, and scientists around the world have expressed concerns that it could be a setback for stem cell research and so-called therapeutic cloning.

Just before the story broke of Hwang's falsification of research results, he faced a different sort of accusation regarding the ethics of his conduct in the research. Hwang had earlier claimed that no one in his laboratory had been the source of the eggs used for creation of the embryos used in his research. It later emerged that two of the women who worked in his laboratory had provided their eggs. It was also revealed that women were paid money for the eggs that were used in the research, a practice that some people object to on ethical grounds. Dr Hwang himself did not pay the women, but a physician who was obtaining the eggs for Hwang's research made the payments—US\$1400 to about 20 women—presumably without informing Hwang about the payments.

The bioethics community in the USA is divided on the issue of payment to egg donors *(17)*. Some countries prohibit payment to egg donors whose oocytes are sought by infertility clinics for use by clinicians when women seeking assisted reproduction lack oocytes of their own. There is no prohibition against paying egg donors (who should properly be termed "vendors") in the USA, and there were no laws or regulations to that effect at the time of Hwang's research in Korea. However, in January 2005, Korea enacted a law that banned commercial trading in human oocytes.

In light of the serious charges of scientific misconduct against Hwang and his colleagues, the earlier criticisms regarding the source of eggs and payment to egg donors are minor transgressions, if they constitute ethical lapses at all. While investigations of Hwang's work are ongoing and will no doubt continue for some time, the episode clearly demonstrates the need for oversight and vigilance in this rapidly moving and promising area of research. At the same time, there is a danger of the promise of stem cell research turning hope into hype. One unfortunate example is the introduction of the term, "therapeutic cloning," at a time when HESC research is still in its infancy. While it is true that phrase was introduced to distinguish the purpose of SCNT in stem cell research from that of "reproductive" cloning, use of the term "therapeutic" is premature. One has only to look at gene-transfer research—termed "gene therapy"—from the moment this technique was first employed in humans in 1990. Fifteen years later, gene-transfer research has yielded no proven therapy, and relatively few clinical trials have even reached phase III. There is every good reason to promote stem cell research and attempts to use SCNT to create embryos for the eventual purpose of therapeutic applications. With appropriate ethical guidelines and a robust mechanism for oversight and monitoring, stem cell research should proceed, even in the absence of federal funding, in the USA.

REFERENCES

1. Weiss R. A crucial human cell isolated, multiplied. *Washington Post* November 6, 1998: A01.
2. Houk RC. Letter to the editor, Road to cloning: caution ahead. *New York Times* February 17, 2004. Available at http://query.nytimes.com/gst/fullpage.html?res=9900E7D8143DF934 A25751C0A9629C8B63. Accessed January 5, 2006.
3. Hadjiargyrou M. Letter to the editor, Road to cloning: caution ahead. *New York Times* February 17, 2004. Available at http://query.nytimes.com/gst/fullpage.html?res=9F03E7D8143DF934 A25751C0A9629C8B63. Accessed January 5, 2006.
4. Raab H. Memorandum to Harold Varmus, MD, Director, NIH. Federal funding for research involving human pluripotent stem cells. January 15, 1999.

5. National Bioethics Advisory Commission, *Ethical Issues in Human Stem Cell Research* (Rockville, Maryland, September 1999).
6. Wade N. Ruling in Favor of Stem Cell Research Draws Fire of Seventy Lawmakers. *New York Times* February 17, 1999: A12.
7. The President's Council on Bioethics, *Monitoring Stem Cell Research* (Washington, D.C., January 2004). Available at http://www.bioethics.gov/reports/stemcell.Accessed December 17, 2005.
8. Kass LR. Preface. *Monitoring Stem Cell Research.* Available at http://www.bioethics.gov/reports/stemcell/preface.html. Accessed December 17, 2005.
9. President's Council on Bioethics. *White Paper: Alternative Sources of Pluripotent Stem Cells* (Washington, D.C., May 2005).
10. Steinbock B. Alternative sources of stem cells. Hastings Center Report 2005;35(4):24–26.
11. Brownback S. Embryonic stem cell research. Available at http://brownback.senate.gov/LIStemCell.cfm.Accessed December 26, 2005.
12. Hatch O. *The Senator's Press Releases.* August 21, 2005. Available at http://hatch.senate.gov/index.cfm?FuseAction=PressReleases.Detail&PressRelease_id=1329&Month=4&Year=2005. Accessed December 26, 2005.
13. Meilaender G. The point of a ban: or, how to think about stem cell research. Hastings Center Report 2001;31(1):9–16.
14. Meyer MJ and Nelson LJ. Respecting what we destroy: reflections on human embryo research. Hastings Center Report 2001;31(1):16–23.
15. Warren MA. *Moral Status: Obligations to Persons and Other Living Things.* Oxford: Oxford University Press, 1997.
16. Committee on Guidelines for Human Embryonic Stem Cell Research. Guidelines for Human Embryonic Stem Cell Research. National Academies Press, 2005. Available at http://www.nap.edu/books/0309096537/html. Accessed December 28, 2005.
17. Cohen C (ed.). *New Ways of Making Babies: The Case of Egg Donation.* Bloomington: University of Indiana Press, 1996.

Special Conditions in the Design of Clinical Stroke Trials for Cell Transplantation

Sean I. Savitz, MD and Louis Caplan, MD

1. INTRODUCTION

Compared with neurodegenerative disease, stroke poses special conditions that impact the potential success of cell transplantation to enhance neurological recovery. The anatomy and recovery phase of the stroke will likely be critical factors. The vascular supply raises questions about adequacy of tissue perfusion to sustain a transplant. There is considerable debate about the appropriate site in the brain for implantation, and it is unclear which type of ischemic stroke patients should be enrolled in clinical trials. These issues are discussed below.

2. ANATOMY

In contrast to a neurodegenerative disorder such as Parkinson's disease, which destroys a relatively homogenous population of neurons, strokes affect multiple different neuronal phenotypes. For example, a posterior circulation infarct might involve the thalamus, hippocampus, and striate visual cortex, affecting three or more very different neuronal populations. Specific types of transplanted cells with restricted fates may limit their use as potential sources for implantation in stroke. Moreover, neurons are not the only cell type damaged. Oligo-dendrocytes, astrocytes, and endothelial cells are also affected. Reconstitution of the complex and widespread neuronal–glial–endothelial interrelationships may require access to a broader array of lineage species than more committed phenotypes. Cells for transplant may need to initially remain immature and phenotypically plastic to differentiate

From: *Current Clinical Neurology: Stroke Recovery with Cellular Therapies*
Edited by: Sean I. Savitz and Daniel M. Rosenbaum © Humana Press Inc., Totowa, NJ

into appropriate neural, glial, and endothelial cell types depending on the ectopic site. Strokes also affect the white matter in addition to gray matter. If white matter is destroyed in a stroke, cell implants may not produce functional connections with axons that can penetrate through the scar tissue of a chronic infarct.

A stroke can disrupt various neuroanatomical pathways including motor, sensory, cerebellar, and visual tracts as well as the distributed networks for attention, language, and praxis, to name just a few cortical functions. The clinical features of stroke are, therefore, variable, whereas many of the neurodegenerative conditions cause well-defined collections of impairments.

Which stroke lesions are amenable to cell transplantation? Most preclinical ischemia studies involve intrastrial implantation. Studies of the middle cerebral artery (MCA) rodent model have shown that the striatum is the primary site of damage, and many believe that the resulting deficits in memory, leaning, and motor behavior are directly associated with striatal injury. The striatum and the rest of the basal ganglia are anatomically well defined and stereotactically accessible by following a trajectory under the sylvian fissure. Cortical lesions also may be accessible to transplantation, but infarcts involving the white matter are more problematic. A proliferation of transplanted cells in the cortex may not repair underlying axonal damage. There is even less rationale for neuronal transplants with pure white matter infarcts, which require an entirely different therapeutic strategy.

Finally, the size and extent of infarction involving major arterial territories will play a significant role in patient selection. Ideally, a limited number of cells will reasonably cover the involved area. In patients with widespread damage, however, the number of cells potentially needed to restore function is entirely unknown at the present time.

3. TIMING

The appropriate time to transplant after a stroke is unknown. In the acute setting, release of excitotoxic neurotransmitters, free radicals, and proinflammatory mediators might threaten new tissue introduced into the periinfarct region *(1)*. Ischemic injury may also be an ongoing process. Cells may be dying by apoptosis in the penumbra for several weeks after stroke *(2)*. Furthermore, inflammation leading to microglial activation may inhibit endogenous neurogenesis and may thereby suppress the growth and survival of transplanted cells *(3,4)*. On the other hand, it may be better to take advantage of local repair processes, including the release of neurotrophic factors from the intrinsic milieu and the host environment during the early recovery phase to facilitate implant growth, survival, differentiation, and/or integration. The ischemic environment also promotes the generation of new neurons in periventricular regions and in the cerebral cortex *(5,6)*. How transplantation will affect ongoing endogenous neurogenesis is unknown. Delaying transplantation for weeks, however, poses the disadvantage of allowing the formation of scar tissue, which might adversely affect implanted cells.

The choice of timing must also consider the natural course of recovery from stroke. Neurodegenerative disorders are inexorably progressive, and clinicians know patients will worsen over time. However, much less is known about stroke outcome, which can be quite variable. Impairments have different courses of improvement, depending on the type and severity *(7)*. In addition, individual brains are very differently wired. For example, some patients who become aphasic after a left caudate infarct regain some language function by using their intact cerebral hemisphere, although others do not. Many neurologists would, therefore, delay transplantation until deficits have plateaued. On the other hand, there is accumulating evidence that stroke recovery involves plasticity of connections, which occur early after a stroke but may disappear months or years later. The effects of transplantation might be enhanced from such plasticity and become maximally beneficial during this reorganization.

For these reasons and many others, some investigators have preferred to transplant at least a few months after a stroke. Indeed, the initial clinical trials on cell transplantation chose to study disabled patients at least 6 months after a stroke. Unfortunately, there are no corroborating animal models of chronic stroke to investigate transplantation several months after focal ischemia. Few outcome measures exist for animals with chronic stroke infarcts. Rodents recover relatively quickly after ischemic stroke. Furthermore, functional recovery in animals cannot be easily equated across studies or related to humans. Most behavioral tests focus only on motor deficits.

4. VASCULATURE

Transplantation is unlikely to succeed if there is a severe arterial occlusion without collateral circulation; inadequate blood supply would not support graft survival. The intimate role of the vasculature in stroke has been emphasized recently by the concept of the neurovascular unit. There is a dynamic interrelated process between brain cells in the parenchyma and the arterial vessel. In the acute and subacute stages of stroke, various factors are being released between neurons and endothelial cells within the neurovascular unit. It is unclear how cell transplants would affect the neurovascular unit. It is known that inflammatory cells travel from the vasculature into the ischemic region. Inflammation may therefore hinder implants from taking hold in infarcted areas. In contrast, transplantation efforts in progressive degenerative disorders are not necessarily concerned with arterial patency, the neurovascular unit, and inflammation.

5. SITE OF IMPLANT

Does the region of the brain that receives the transplanted cells influence different responses of the donor cells? From a mechanical standpoint, intracranial injection of cells into the fluid-filled cavity of a chronic infarct facilitates the migration of transplanted cells. Without a definable, cavitated area, intracranial transplantation requires more direct pressure to inject implants, risking damage to normal tissue. However, cavity fluid can dilute the concentration of donor cells.

Many studies directly inject cells into the core of an infarct, where it remains unclear whether new tissue can remain viable *(8)*. Specific neuropathological conditions may alter the balance of regional environmental signals by releasing, for example, proinflammatory and other modulatory cytokines, which, in turn, may adversely affect survival and differentiation of the implanted populations. Other studies suggest that the chronic ischemic region can support implanted tissue (see below).

In the acute setting, it may be more appropriate to inject cells in the salvageable penumbra, but grafts might still be exposed to the detrimental effects of spreading depression and excitatory neurotransmitters. Differences in graft behavior, depending on the injection site, were noted in a prior study *(9)*. Fetal cortical grafts to the ischemic rat brain have been shown to survive in the penumbra but not in the core lesion. However, in chronic infarcts, glial scarring might impede the delivery of cells to the penumbral areas.

Some posit that grafts could be more effective if the poorly vascularized, inflammatory environment of the ischemic region is avoided altogether and suggest the plausibility of transplantation to distant regions, even to the contralateral side *(10)*. A different approach is to introduce cells to the brain via the systemic circulation, and several studies using this approach are described in other chapters.

For some types of transplanted cells, there may be limited regions in the ischemic brain to support their growth. Conversely, certain areas of the brain may allow some types of grafts, particularly the more multipotential and proliferative types, to grow unchecked and form tumors in contrast to regions that promote implant differentiation *(11)*.

6. PATIENTS

The selection of stroke patients for transplantation trials depends upon a number of factors. Patients should have measurable deficits, impairments, and handicaps. The neuroanatomical relationship between the image-defined infarct and deficits should be well established. Basal ganglia strokes, for example, typically cause a hemiparesis that is easily quantifiable on neurological exam. The deficit should be sufficiently disabling to warrant such a procedure but not so severe that some dramatic effect would be necessary to produce measurable improvement. Practical issues, for example, comorbidities and the need for extensive follow-up, also play a strong role in determining which patients are good candidates for experimental therapies.

Transplantation studies in the acute stroke setting will also need to take into consideration whether to exclude patients who receive thrombolytic therapy. In addition, prior infarcts, hemorrhages, or other brain structural abnormalities might divert cells away from the fresh area of damage or impede the potential salutary effects of transplanted cells by other undefined mechanisms. The presence of shift, significant cerebral edema, or blood are also important factors in patient selection criteria.

7. DELIVERY

New safety trials are on the horizon testing direct intracerebral injections or systemic administration of cells. Both intravenous and intra-arterial approaches are being investigated. It will be important to determine which type of delivery is safest and most feasible.

REFERENCES

1. Lo EH, Dalkara T, Moskowitz MA. Mechanisms, challenges and opportunities in stroke. *Nat Rev Neurosci* 4:399–415, 2003.
2. Li Y, Chopp M, Jiang N, Yao F, Zaloga C. Temporal profile of in situ DNA fragmentation after transient middle cerebral artery occlusion in the rat. *J Cereb Blood Flow Metab* 15:389–397, 1995.

3. Ekdahl CT, Claasen JH, Bonde S, Kokaia Z, Lindvall O. Inflammation is detrimental for neurogenesis in adult brain. *Proc Natl Acad Sci USA* 100:13632–13637, 2003.

4. Li Y, Chen J, Chopp M. Cell proliferation and differentiation from ependymal, subependymal and choroid plexus cells in response to stroke in rats. *J Neurol Sci* 193:137–146, 2002.

5. Nakatomi H, Kuriu T, Okabe S et al. Regeneration of hippocampal pyramidal neurons after ischemic brain injury by recruitment of endogenous neural progenitors. *Cell* 110:429–441, 2002.

6. Arvidsson A, Collin T, Kirik D, Kokaia Z, Lindvall O. Neuronal replacement from endogenous precursors in the adult brain after stroke. *Nat Med* 8:963–970, 2002.

7. Hier DB, Mondlock J, Caplan LR. Recovery of behavioral abnormalities after right hemisphere stroke. *Neurology* 33:345–350, 1983.

8. Grabowski M, Johansson BB, Brundin P. Neocortical grafts placed in the infarcted brain of adult rats: few or no efferent fibers grow from transplant to host. *Exp Neurol* 134:273–276, 1995.

9. Hadani M, Freeman T, Munsiff A, Young W, Flamm E. Fetal cortical cells survive in focal cerebral infarct after permanent occlusion of the middle cerebral artery in adult rats. *J Neurotrauma* 9:107–112, 1992.

10. Veizovic T, Beech JS, Stroemer RP, Watson WP, Hodges H. Resolution of stroke deficits following contralateral grafts of conditionally immortal neuroepithelial stem cells. *Stroke* 32:1012–1019, 2001.

11. Miyazono M, Lee VM, Trojanowski JQ. Proliferation, cell death, and neuronal differentiation in transplanted human embryonal carcinoma (NTera2) cells depend on the graft site in nude and severe combined immunodeficient mice. *Lab Invest* 73:273–283, 1995

Index

Printed in the United States of America

EUROPEAN SOCIAL EVOLUTION

EUROPEAN
SOCIAL
EVOLUTION

ARCHÆOLOGICAL PERSPECTIVES

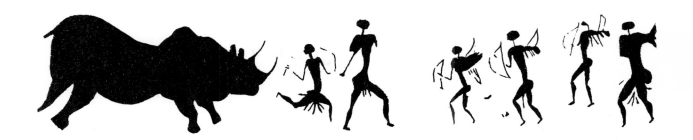

Edited by
JOHN BINTLIFF

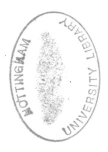

NOTTINGHAM UNIVERSITY LIBRARY

Production Editor: Shirley Johnson
Production Assistant: Susan Holland

600 **300086** X

ISBN 0 901945 52 8 (Hardback)
ISBN 0 901945 53 6 (Paperback)

cc

Published by the
University of Bradford
Bradford
West Yorkshire
England

Copyright: the authors 1984

Printed and bound in Great Britain by
Chanctonbury Press Ltd, West Chiltington, Sussex

This book is dedicated to
Colin Renfrew
for the selfless support and encouragement
he has given over the years,
both to myself and to innumerable scholars
of my generation.

CONTRIBUTORS

JOHN BINTLIFF is Lecturer in Archaeological Sciences, University of Bradford. Publications include Natural Environment and Human Settlement in Prehistoric Greece (1977), Mycenaean Geography (1977) and Palaeoclimates, Palaeoenvironments and Human Communities in the Eastern Mediterranean (1982; with W. van Zeist).

CLIFF SLAUGHTER is Senior Lecturer in Sociology, University of Bradford. Publications include Coal Is Our Life (1956; with N. Dennis and L.F. Henriques), Marxism, Ideology and Literature (1981) and State, Power and Bureaucracy (1982; with J.A. Dragstedt).

RAYMOND NEWELL is a Lecturer at the Biologisch-Archaeologisch Instituut, Groningen University, Holland. Publications include Automatic Artifact Registration: a Mesolithic Test Case (1972; with A.P.J. Vroomans) and The Skeletal Remains of Mesolithic Man in Western Europe (1979; with T.S. Constandse-Westermann and C. Meiklejohn).

ANDREW SHERRATT is Assistant Curator in the Ashmolean Museum, Oxford University. Publications include The Cambridge Encyclopedia of Archaeology (1980).

ANTHONY HARDING is Lecturer in Archaeology, University of Durham. Publications include The Bronze Age in Europe (1979; with J.M. Coles) and Climatic Change in Later Prehistory (1982).

MIKE ROWLANDS is Lecturer in Anthropology, University of London. Publications include The Evolution of Social Systems (1977; with J. Friedman).

ANTHONY SNODGRASS is Laurence Professor of Classical Archaeology, Cambridge University. Publications include Early Greek Armour and Weapons (1967), The Dark Age of Greece (1971) and Archaic Greece (1980).

TIM POTTER is Assistant Keeper in the Department of Greco-Roman Antiquities at the British Museum. Publications include A Faliscan Town in South Etruria (1976), The Changing Landscape of South Etruria (1979) and Roman Britain (1983).

RICK JONES is Lecturer in Archaeological Sciences, University of Bradford. His recently completed PhD thesis at London University (1982) is entitled Cemeteries and burial practices in the western provinces of the Roman Empire to AD 300.

TIMOTHY GREGORY is Professor of History, Ohio State University. Publications include numerous articles on Byzantine and Late Roman archaeology.

CHRIS ARNOLD is Lecturer in Archaeology, University College of Wales, Aberystwyth. Publications include Anglo-Saxon Cemeteries of the Isle of Wight (1982) and The Anglo-Saxon Kingdoms (1984).

KLAVS RANDSBORG is Senior Lecturer in Prehistory, University of Copenhagen. Publications include Chronological Studies of the Early Bronze Age of South Scandinavia (1968) and The Viking Age in Denmark (1980).

ILLUSTRATIONS

INTRODUCTION

John Bintliff

The evolution of human society would seem to be one of the most obvious themes for the historical archaeologist and prehistorian to tackle and, indeed, the general public might be forgiven for believing that this would be one aspect of the past that can stand to justify public support for 'the back-looking curiosity' (William Camden, quoted in Daniel 1967, p.35). And yet, paradoxically, the ability of the archaeologist to reconstruct the nature and transformational properties of past social systems continues to be one of the most controversial topics in the discipline, and only a few decades ago respected practitioners were resigned to confining their research to the more approachable economic and technological facets of Pre-Industrial communities.

It is the purpose of this introductory chapter, together with the social anthropological chapter of Cliff Slaughter, to examine the historical reasons for this rather unsatisfactory state of affairs. It is the purpose of this volume to present to the reader, period by period, what leading archaeologists consider to be the most significant processes and events that took European communities from Mesolithic hunter-gatherer bands to the emergent nation states of Medieval Europe. In each case, the contributor was asked to summarize the most important achievements of previous research in his period, as well as offering a progressive approach to current research problems. In a field that is widely agreed to be a methodological minefield, and given that serious attempts to establish a 'social archaeology' sub-discipline are less than 20 years old, it will be no surprise to learn that socially-oriented archaeologists differ amongst themselves both on matters of detailed theory and on specific social reconstructions. This is generally a feature of prehistoric and proto-historic research, because it is regrettably still the case (see further, below) that 'social archaeology' and even archaeology as an independent discipline have made but limited impact as yet upon historic archaeology in Europe. In recognition of the existence of contrasting models for social evolution in later prehistoric Europe, Andrew Sherratt and Mike Rowlands were invited to contribute chapters whose data base substantially overlaps with chapters by myself and Anthony Harding, in order to bring out the main positions in current debates.

The chapters themselves differ markedly in length, level of detail and analytical approach to the data. The one factor which is not relevant in accounting for this diversity is variance between the contributors on the way forward in social archaeology in terms of general method and theory. Since the pioneering revival of interest in social evolution amongst social anthropologists after the last War and amongst 'new archaeologists' since the 1960s, the questions to be asked, the issues to be investigated and the kinds of data and research programmes that offer the greatest potential, have become common ground for that sector of the archaeological community committed to making progress in this major research field.

In fact it is the relative amount of research conducted within each period on matters of social archaeology that provides the most crucial variable accounting for differences between contributions. In the Mesolithic period, as Raymond Newell points out, social evolutionary concerns have been made especially difficult, not just because of the exiguous traces of Mesolithic human communities but more importantly as a result of the dominance of eco-technic considerations on the theoretical plane. Newell's own continuing research demonstrates a strong element of pioneering into an uncharted research environment. At the other end of the period spectrum, post-Roman archaeology has proved highly resistant to the crusading inroads of 'new archaeology' and even more so to developments within post-War American social anthropology. Here again, Timothy Gregory, Chris Arnold and Klaus Randsborg represent a very small if vociferous minority of post-Roman archaeologists who both espouse the methodological advances of the 'new archaeology' and have an active research interest in social evolution. Whereas it is often the case in later prehistory that one can compare and contrast models and theories for the social system of a particular region and period, for these scholars of the post-Roman era there is all too little previous, archaeologically-based work to summarize. Much that is presented here, therefore, rests upon the contributors' personal efforts to assemble appropriate evidence from published work and their own research in order to create a provisional working model, or related set of insights, into the social evolution of their chosen societies. This factor is most evident in the virtually unparalleled essay on Byzantine archaeology by Timothy Gregory.

A second cause of difference of approach amongst contributors is due to the existence or otherwise of publications by a contributor that cover some of the same ground as his chapter in this volume, in which case the task of providing a comprehensive background and, frequently, detailed argumentation for particular points, has been omitted. Thus, Andrew Sherratt's and Mike Rowlands' chapters are the most recent in a series of seminal articles ranging widely over social issues in Neolithic to Iron Age Europe (cf. Sherratt 1976, 1980, 1981, 1982; Rowlands 1973, 1980, Frankenstein and Rowlands 1978). The chapters by Anthony Harding,

Anthony Snodgrass, Tim Potter and Klaus Randsborg represent succinct summary analyses of the state of play in social evolutionary research within the archaeology of their period, but which draw heavily upon major works of interpretation and synthesis they have published in the last few years (Coles and Harding 1979; Snodgrass 1980; Potter 1979; Randsborg 1980). Nonetheless, each of these contributors has created a totally up-dated and revised statement of his views and the current literature in preparing chapters for this volume. The chapters by Cliff Slaughter, Rick Jones, Chris Arnold and myself, in contrast, all represent our first (if carefully considered!) attempts to investigate the complexities of social evolution on such a scale, and therefore have generated a necessary proliferation of footnotes and packaged background information.

In the following section of this introduction, we shall take a detailed look at the historical development of an 'archaeology of social evolution'. We will thereby introduce the basic models and hypotheses that still dominate research in this area, within the context of the various transformations that the discipline of archaeology itself has undergone in the last 150 years.

Finally, I shall return to two central questions that are at the heart of current research endeavour in social evolutionary archaeology today:

(1) Does an attempt like the current volume to summarize developmental sequences for a particular region on a long time scale reveal fundamental regularities, basic repetitive processes at work, or coherent directional tendencies? Or is the generalizing, comparative and evolutionary approach forced to yield to an inevitable succession of highly particularistic studies, bounded narrowly by the interaction of circumstances both in themselves and in combination unique to specific chronological eras?

(2) If any such synthetic generalizations about social evolution as are posed by (1) appear possible with our current knowledge, what support do they offer to the more important theoretical schemes of social evolution current in the literature?

SOCIAL EVOLUTION AND ARCHAEOLOGY: AN HISTORICAL PERSPECTIVE[1]

Pre-nineteenth-century background

Archaeology had not yet cohered into a defined discipline and the collection and recording of antiquities was primarily conceived of as providing physical illustrations for the historical and biblical accounts of the past. Nascent social and political science had however begun to combine ancient and more recent historical sources with ethnographic accounts from colonial territories and original observations on contemporary society. Thus a number of important Enlightenment theorists discuss the cohesion and interdependence, rights and duties of the separate individuals, groups and classes in complex societies e.g. Hobbes, Locke, Rousseau. Several of the French 'philosophes' and Scottish Enlightenment thinkers indulged in 'theoretic or conjectural history': "This included the comparative study of living peoples, arranging them into logical developmental sequences, usually unilineal in nature, and projecting these sequences into prehistoric times. While most of their studies were based on ethnographic data, some of the Scottish Primitivists cited archaeological evidence in support of their theories" (Trigger 1978, p.59). Although their speculations on the nature of social development and society

itself have continued to be influential to this day, it is generally considered that their very limited data produced theorizing 'from a self-conceived past to a wished-for future' (cf. Service 1978). The emphasis was often on 'voluntaristic' theories, whereby complex society was seen as a necessary co-operation of individuals for their mutual benefit and protection (see Service, below). Another, older concept was that of 'conquest theory', which often took the form of a model of class origins based upon the permanent subjugation of a losing population in inter-community warfare (Ibn Khaldun, Jean Bodin and see Carneiro, below).

Nineteenth-century developments

Empirical analysis of political evolution only began on a major scale in the nineteenth century. A widespread confusion seems to exist in the literature about the interaction of social evolutionary concepts in archaeology or history and Darwinian evolution (Dunnell 1980). The idea of an 'evolution' of society existed by the mid-nineteenth century, before Darwin's discoveries, and was associated with a particular school of social philosophy led by Herbert Spencer. Darwinian biological evolution was influenced by this idealistic philosophical approach but concentrated on the material, empirical changes. Broadly speaking, therefore, scholars influenced by social-philosophical ideas of evolution, followers of Spencer and later Marx, have concentrated on generalizing schemes of stages of human evolution, in contrast to those developing Darwinian biological evolution who have concentrated on smaller scale processes of physical transformation. Dunnell (1980) has presented a strong case for arguing that these two approaches must be kept rigorously separate, stemming from very different premisses and practices. On this point I find his analysis convincing, but it does not seem to be the case, as he further suggests, that later nineteenth-century scholars and even mid-century pioneers of archaeo-anthropology did not make serious efforts to weave the two threads together into an evolutionary Social Darwinism. Thomsen (1836) and Worsaae in Denmark, even before Darwin, when establishing the Three-Age system that was revolutionizing the concept of time in human development (cf. Daniel 1967), clearly envisaged their successive, empirically verifiable, material stages of the human past in terms of levels of social and behavioural complexity, drawing on ethnographic parallels and ethno-historic records of 'savages', 'barbarian pastoralists' and so forth. More explicit syntheses of ethnography, ethno-history, 'modern' archaeology and the Spencer/Darwin sets of evolutionary concepts and theories typify major studies of man's past that dominate the later nineteenth century, chiefly from the pen of the 'evolutionist' school of Morgan, Lubbock, Tylor and Maine. "From biological evolution the idea of progress was extended to the history of human societies and culture; and two of the founders of anthropology, ... Tylor ... and ... Morgan ... saw in this principle of cultural evolution, and in the findings of archaeology with its Three-Age system and its demonstrated great antiquity of Man, the data from which to construct a model of the human social and cultural past" (Willey and Sabloff 1974, p.14).

Nonetheless, the **fundamental** stimulus behind these 'evolutionists', the related school of twentieth-century, official interpretations of Marx, and the important revivalist school of 'neo-evolutionists' of the post-World War II era (see below), does seem to reflect the philosophical, deductive position and the desire to establish models of human progress and social evolution on the grandest scale, which Spencer had developed from the Enlightenment progress models. "Archaeologists clearly had inherited the idea of cultural evolution from the speculative history of the eighteenth century and were working within an evolutionary framework that antedated the development of evolutionary frameworks in geology and biology" (Trigger 1978, p.62). The danger is continually present, therefore, that insufficient care is taken to validate such models against the complexities of the data; and at the worst, stage schemes or the emphasis on a particular general and world-wide 'process' behind human development are supported by reference to other theoretical work rather than constantly being tested against case studies. Understandably perhaps, Darwinian evolution has tended to concentrate upon the transformation of species through an endless succession of minor traits, shunning 'directional' inferences of a 'progressive' nature.

The 'developmentalist' or 'evolutionist' school has been particularly influential in providing a provocative conceptual framework for post-War social archaeology. These later nineteenth-century scholars sought to explicate modern ideas and institutions by tracing their connections to ancient society (from history) and 'contemporary survivals' i.e. considering less technologically and politically complex societies of their own age as 'the past in the present'. Once again, the Enlightenment was influential in providing the concept that human actions are comparable despite differences in time and space. Technology and economy were seen as major variables tied to social complexity. Change was generally gradual, with an overall tendency towards greater organizational complexity and more heterogeneous societies. The very title of Sir John Lubbock's classic volume (1865) Prehistoric Times as Illustrated by Ancient Remains and the Manners and Customs of Modern Savages says it all, although a succinct selection from the work of Edward Tylor is worth an additional citation: "In judging how mankind may have once lived, it is also a great help to observe how they are actually found living. Human life may be roughly classed into three great stages, Savage, Barbaric, Civilized, which may be defined as follows. The lowest or savage state is that in which man subsists on wild plants and animals, neither tilling the soil nor domesticating creatures for his food. Savages may dwell in tropical forests where the abundant fruit and game may allow small clans to live in one spot and find a living all the year round, while in barer and colder regions they have to lead a wandering life in quest of the wild food which they soon exhaust in any place. In making their rude implements, the materials used by savages are what they find ready to hand, such as wood, stone, and bone, but they cannot extract metal from the ore, and therefore belong to the Stone Age. Men may be considered to have risen into the next or barbaric state when they take to agriculture with the certain supply of food which can be stored until the next harvest, settled village and town life is established, with immense results in the improvement of arts, knowledge, manners and government. Pastoral tribes are to be reckoned in the barbaric stage, for although their life of shifting camp from pasture to pasture may prevent settled habitation and agriculture, they have from their herds a constant supply of milk and meat. Some barbaric nations have not come beyond using stone implements, but most have risen into the Metal Age. Lastly, civilized life may be taken as beginning with the art of writing, which, by recording history, law, knowledge and religion for the service of ages to come, binds together the past and the future in an unbroken chain of intellectual and moral progress ... So far as the evidence goes, it seems that civilisation has actually grown up in the world through these three stages" (1881, extracts prepared by G. Daniel 1967, pp.132-33).

However, despite the general features that the evolutionist school share in their writings, there are notable divergences in their detailed approaches that anticipate more recent developments. Morgan, for example, argued that there had occurred different developmental trajectories, contrasting in particular the Old and New World.

Morgan also laid emphasis on particular institutions which contained the potential for wider societal transformations, such as the 'gens' or clan which he considered to have paved the way from barbarism to civilization. His Ancient Society (1877) had a profound impact on later evolutionary thinking, particularly via Marx and Engels (see below) on Marxist theory up to the present day, with its dramatic contrast between primitive society: basically communistic, lacking commerce and entrepreneurs, private property, classes of rich and poor, and despots - and, civilized society: with private property, economic classes and the State. Great social changes, it was suggested, were due to major changes in the sources of subsistence.

Maine's especial contribution (Bock 1974) was the result of a doubt on his part as to whether the modern ethnographic spectrum of societies covered the range of past societies. He therefore operated a very extensive comparative method through historical and semi-historical sources (including Germanic, Roman and Slav history) to supplement contemporary observations on 'primitives' such as the peoples of India under British rule. His famous observation that societies tend to progress from relationships governed by status to those of contract echoes Enlightenment theory, but now was backed up by an impressive degree of cross-cultural observation.

Karl Marx developed his deep scholarly interest in social evolution in the reverse order to what one might expect. Firstly he set forth in his writings a critique of capitalism and a programme for social revolution; he then studied the peasant communities of Europe and Asia; and finally at the end of his life, he tackled primitive communities and the long-term evolution of human society (Krader 1976). As his timescale lengthened, Marx relied heavily on the research of the evolutionists, and the Ethnological Notebooks show lengthy quotes from them that were central to his own treatment of the past. Thus Marx, too, created a stage scheme. Like Morgan, however, he realized that different regions of the world had differing trajectories and rates of development, and he contrasted the more complex European sequence to that of Asia. But the most important emphasis in Marx's stage scheme was that each stage was characterized by the prevalent 'mode of production'. In Das Kapital, vol. 3, he describes this concept as "das innerste Geheimnis, die verborgne Grundlage der ganzen gesellschaftlichen Konstruktion". Simply put, Marx was here concerned to identify what he saw as the crucial relationship in considering any society: the social relations of production and, in particular, ownership of the means of production and control over labour.

In 1859 Marx conceived of a general law, a progression of mankind from the primitive to the historical stage. Four main periods were recognized, each with a dominant mode of production. The first and oldest was the 'Asiatic mode of production': here there was a relative freedom within communal village life, although these units were already obliged to offer a 'tax' to outside higher authorities, primarily in that most basic commodity, a corvée of surplus human labour. For Marx, this system lived on in Asia until the nineteenth century. Stages 2-4 were especially developed in Europe and consisted of the sequence 2: the production of Classical antiquity - especially dependent upon slave labour; 3: feudalism - serf/lord production; finally 4: capitalism -where the primacy of agriculture disappeared. Later, from Morgan, Marx developed the idea of the ancient 'gens' or clan as an alternative model for the communal village life of stage 1, from which develop the patron/client and master/slave relationships characteristic of his stages 2 and 3. The class exploitation emphasis of this overall model has had a profound effect on all subsequent discussions. Considerable interest has also been aroused by Marx's category of the Asiatic mode of production (India, China, Persia and Islamic lands). Marx and Engels argued that the exploitation of the producers living in village communities was not based on the existence of private ownership of land, but mostly on allegiance to a deified and despotic ruler who personified the state. Tribute was forthcoming for imagined/real protection of communities and/or trade, as well as for organizing water works (cf. Claessen and Skalnik 1978b). Archaeological and historical theorizing about Asian states has regularly concerned itself with these very issues (e.g. see below, Wittfogel).

Despite this acknowledged development in Marx of the contemporary work of the 'Evolutionists', it is generally pointed out that Marx was probably fully aware of the pitfalls of moving from particular historical types of precapitalist societies to general evolutionary stages (as may be observed from study of his Grundrisse, cf. Service 1978). Friedrich Engels is often considered to have been less critical in his historical speculations, though relying very much on Marx and Marx's sources. He produced two alternative models for the origins of the civilized State society. The first appears in his Anti-Dühring (1877/8); it is meant to be of more universal application (the Classical world being an exception) and stresses the shift from functional to exploitative power. Krader summarizes it thus (1975): "The servant of the community becomes the overlord; tribal chiefs, with the transformation of society from primitive to class society, become transformed into rulers. The oriental despotism is the crudest form of state" (which) "fulfils the peace-keeping function within the society, the war-making function without, and control of the water supply. The independence of social function as over against the society by these organs" of defence "was developed into dominance over the society" (p.275). Although war and conquest were significant for power concentration into the hands of managers (e.g. the old German State and its 'military democracy' under conquering war-lords) ultimately a more multi-causal explanation emerges: a number of 'functions useful for society' were operated by an elite stratum based on private land ownership or other wealth.

Engels's other major published contribution to evolutionism is his Origins of the Family, Private Property and the State (1884). Here the emphasis is closer to that of Marx, being that of the process of economic stratification. We begin with collectivist, communistic societies with common ownership of the means of production. With the growth of population and a diversification of the means of subsistence, encouraged by improvements in productive technology, overall productivity increases to produce a surplus which can be appropriated to cover the needs of non-primary producers. Surpluses are traded, middlemen arise and there is a shift from production for direct use to that of commodities; differences in private wealth consolidate to create economic classes. Key functions and capital become tied within particular families. The State arises to protect the vested interest of the rich as against those of the poor, as an instrument of repression and to maintain the stability of the status quo. Greek, Roman and German history were employed to show that some kind of stability in the resultant class conflict was indeed created by the state in favour of the elite. Although the merchant/entrepreneur group, skimming the cream off production, was given prominence, even more important was the recognition of private as opposed to public property (cf. the view that the 'Allod' or private property right of the Franks was the seed of feudalism). This 1884 model was primarily developed for Europe, passing through 'ancient', 'feudal' and 'bourgeois' stages.

In general, the Marx/Engels contribution was more penetrating than that of their fellow evolutionists, but differed little from them in its social-philosophical approach and often uncritical admixture of history, ethnography and 'Enlightenment theorizing'.[2]

Having set the stage for an explosion of fieldwork to test this body of evolutionary theory, circumstances combined to empty it of its company of actors, just when empirical observation was called for. For in the late nineteenth century and the early twentieth century, interest in evolutionary social science waned to insignificance, especially the caustic anti-bourgeois style of Marxism, in favour of down-to-earth fieldwork and a set of new ideas in anthropology based upon empiricism and the 'functionalism' of Durkheim (Harris 1968). Sociologists and anthropologists almost entirely abandoned the study of temporal process or social change, and scholarly effort returned to the identification and analysis of forms and functions (cf. Bock 1974).

The coming of age of social anthropology saw it cast itself loose of the constricting 'progress' and evolutionist models, to develop fresh analytical methods of understanding societies based upon their articulation at a given point in time, ignoring tendentious questions of directional advancement. The dubious nature of the stage schemes for the history of any particular region, in terms of the data available, led to a preference for localized minute descriptions of circumscribed societies over limited time-periods (Boas) and a gross suspicion of the comparative method of grouping societies remote in time and space. As Cliff Slaughter's chapter demonstrates, twentieth-century social anthropology in 'the West', at least until the post-War period (and longer in Europe), turned its back resolutely on social evolution (with prominent isolated exceptions), considering the period before modern observation as unworthy of serious analysis due to its poor data (unverifiable history or even worse -the speculations of the archaeologists from their refuse pit researches; see below, Leach).

However it is necessary to return to the archaeologists proper. The late nineteenth century witnessed evolutionary volumes that regularly utilized archaeological discoveries, but it is fair to say, bearing in mind the Spencerian/Darwinian dichotomy discussed earlier, that such field data were used to prop up a priori opinions about stages of the past, based in general upon the similarities between material remains and lifestyles of past cultures and those typifying contemporary Pre-Industrial societies. The evolutionists had indeed far more data about the past from the new science of archaeology and the great advances being made in ancient and medieval history, yet in many respects the underlying philosophical stance and questions being asked were not far removed from the work of the early nineteenth-century scholars, and even in certain respects from the social theorists of the preceding Enlightenment.

The early twentieth century

When social and political science began to part company with concepts of social evolution at the turn of the century, it is of considerable interest to ask what the reaction of the archaeological fraternity was to be. As scholars with diachronic developments to account for, the new synchronic approach of social anthropology was leaving archaeologists stranded in isolation, without theoretical support from wider developments in the social sciences. But that is not to say that synchronic analysis did not soon have a major effect on archaeological theory; the new mode of regional ethnographic mapping was to be closely linked to the identification of archaeological 'cultures' in the work of Childe (1925), Kossinna (1911) and others, allowing the supposed historical development of specific peoples to be traced. In fact two major responses can be recognized in the archaeological literature of the first half of the twentieth century.

Firstly, the unpopularity of general stage schemes and the popularity of regional material culture studies concentrated the archaeological focus on circumscribed peoples of the past. Material culture links between these 'cultures' and the reasons for the internal transformation of these cultures had now to be accounted for. Eschewing a priori processual models for parallel evolutionary trans-formations, there arose the 'diffusionist' model, whereby the radiation of innovatory adaptations and actual human colonization from historically-attested nuclear civiliza-tional zones (such as the Near East in the Old World), provided the constant motor for change around the globe. "The economic problems and growing class conflicts of the late nineteenth century eroded ... the idealism of the Enlightenment and began to produce serious doubts about the desirability of material progress ...". There arose "strong doubts that human behaviour was governed by regularities that could be discovered easily or expressed in comprehensive formulations ... This interest in the complexity of the archaeological record was part of a general concern with indeterminacy and unpredictability that was coming to dominate the study of man. It produced a growing preoccupation with the subjective and idiosyncratic and with the study of particular phenomena by inductive means ... Cultures were idealized as natural possessions suited to particular peoples. In keeping with this romantic outlook, human beings came to be viewed as conservative, resistant to change, and generally uninvent-ive ... Hence cultures tended to be viewed as static and cultural change was attributed to changes in population. This is exemplified in the work of W.M.F. Petrie ... who explained almost all cultural change in terms of migra-tions of whole peoples or transfers of small groups of artisans from one society to another" (Trigger 1978, pp.65-6). Effectively, the explanation of local change was in most cases totally bypassed by this 'deus ex machina' model. It must be said of course that in many ways this was an advance for archaeology (although familiarity with the archaeological realities had already led 'evolutionary' archaeologists such as De Mortillet to concede diffusion and migration as minor modifications to an over-riding parallel evolution model), because the new analysis of cultural assemblages and inter-cultural links has continu-ed to be a vital source of data for societal investigations, and diffusion versus autonomy is today as lively a debate as 60 years ago (see below, and the chapters by Rowlands, Sherratt, Harding, Bintliff, this volume). Nor was the diffusionist/migrationist approach (Elliot-Smith, Perry, Kossinna, Childe) quite devoid of social theory. The hyper-diffusionists "admitted that cultural evolution had taken place but ... each successive stage had evolved only once and accounted for present cultural complexity throughout the world by assuming cultural mixing and loss as this single sequence had diffused from its source" (Trigger 1978, p.66). And when, for example, the spread of an artifact type or complex suggested a conquering horde sweeping across indigenous communities, such as the infamous Battle-Axe and Bell-Beaker migrations (Gimbutas 1965; see Bintliff, this volume), then the long-established conquest theory re-emerged to account for subsequent visible signs of enhanced social hierarchy. Thus the democratic Neolithic villages of Europe, politi-cally isolated, were totally and rapidly altered by the migrations of such warrior folk in the Late Neolithic, leading to warrior social elites over subordinate indigenes, as were seen to characterize the subsequent Early Bronze Age with its chieftain burials. Such sweeping, continent-wide pulses at crucial points of change in the archaeo-

logical record, setting a trend of models of disjunction rather than evolution, had an unintentional ally in the constant search by archaeologists for more refined dating for their finds. Beyond the initially helpful, gross divisions of the ages of Stone, Copper, Bronze and Iron, the complex inter-digitation of the newly recognized cultures within each age created enormous difficulties of historical reconstruction, unless some universals could be established. The lead of Montelius, in tying together the burgeoning number of archaeological cultures in Europe via horizons of diffusion from the Eastern Mediterranean, seemed an ideal solution, since the origin point was taken to be closely dated from historical records. Although this framework was gradually eaten away by further dis-coveries, piecemeal, its public demolition was to await the coming of age of the absolute chronology of C14 dating in the 1960s (Renfrew 1973a). As Colin Renfrew has pointed out, the dates and ties were wrong, but more importantly, the whole theoretical framework of 'deus ex machina' explanation for local developmental sequences was largely false, leaving post-War archaeologists with the urgent task, sadly belated, of working out a new methodology for analyzing social change **within** specific cultures (see below, Renfrew).

The second major reaction, although this is hardly ever clearly stated or indeed acknowledged in the litera-ture today, was that most archaeologists seem to have dug their feet in over the major principles established by the theories and researches of the nineteenth-century evolutionists. In particular, they maintained the concept of fairly distinct successive periods in the world's past characterized by contrasting socio-economic modes, whose main lines could be paralleled by major varieties of primitive lifestyles still observable amongst contemporary or recent primitive peoples or recorded by the ancient authors. This is not to say that archaeologists clearly stated their allegiance to the discredited model and its associated deductive philosophy, with the exception of Sollas's (1911) Ancient Hunters and their Modern Rep-resentatives (where a classical evolutionary viewpoint was applied to the archaeological material, and an existing culture taken as representative of each stage of pre-history). But if one studies the numerous works of synthesis from the first half of this century, reading between the lines and assembling indirect comments, one can recognize that the evolutionist position still underlay the general models being used to interpret the past. Although the reasons for the transformation from stage to stage were now most frequently attributed to diffusion and migration, yet the very existence of stages and long-lived, world-wide modes of life continued to dominate the implicit but rarely explicit theorizing of archaeologists. When explicit evolutionism was revived in the United States after the last War, as neo-evolutionism (see below), it could hardly represent, as is usually portrayed, a total shift of emphasis **within** archaeology. Rather, one must view this conscious revival of the bold approach of the late nineteenth century as indicative of a desire for archaeology to reassert its right to elaborate its own theory and methodology, bringing out into the open what had always been there. The essential need for broad, generalizing models of the past that the more important synthesizers of archaeological discoveries demanded, had kept alive the stage scheme, but cryptically stated and unmodified, almost for fear of the wrath of the anthro-pological fraternity at this temerity of the archaeologists. An important additional stimulus to the survival of the nineteenth-century approach to social evolution was the unabashed prominence given to it in Soviet and East European archaeology and history. Though not given sufficient attention in the West because of its apparent dogmatic inflexibility, yet its parallel existence to the covert evolutionism of the West encouraged individual Western archaeologists towards more explicit evolutionary theorizing as the century developed (such as Childe, White; cf. Klejn 1974).

Since this covert evolutionism in European archaeology is not usually identified in the literature, it may be worthwhile to illustrate it from early to mid twentieth-century sources.[3] Miles Burkitt's (1926) Our Early Ancestors, appears to treat the development of Europe from Upper Palaeolithic to the Bronze Age in a 'culture historic' way, but always present is evidence for an implicit set of models about each stage (Burkitt uses the simile of a 'volume' of human history). We begin with 'primitive' hunter-gatherers in small groups, succeeded by a Neolithic peasantry, followed in turn by socially stratified, complex monument-building societies of the Copper and Bronze Age, whose wealth has accrued especially from trade. Into the last-named group impinge (notably in the Aegean) the ideas and behaviour of Near Eastern bureaucratic, commercial, civilized societies akin to today's. As is predictable for its era, ethnocentric and migrationist ideas are stressed by the author, but underlying such impulses is a stage concept where eco-technic forces and a priori social theories are important: "The change from the life of a small, sparse, hunting population to that of thickly populated villages introduces the necessity for a well-regulated community life ... Again the congregation into communities favours the growth of specialisation" (p.51). "Again, the possession of crops and herds, whether owned by the individual, by the family, or by the community, involves the necessity for protection which was far less pressing in Palaeolithic times. The conception of property, now introduced for the first time in human history on anything like a large scale, involves automatically the concept of war" (p.52). These extracts demonstrate a curious but typically nineteenth-century combination of empirical material culture study and general a priori theorizing along stage lines; the growing body of evidence collected and analyzed along cultural and cultural history lines has been slotted into an implicit stage model directly derived from the evolutionists. The two do not match very well, as the analytical techniques to test the general theoretical statements from the archaeological data have yet to be developed.

Grahame Clark's (1940) Prehistoric England offers a more contorted approach to questions of social evolution. The book is thematic, yet there is no major section on socio-political development. But once again, a whole series of references interspersed through the text and, characteristically, never explicitly linked into an overall theory, provides clear evidence for the underlying existence in the author's mind of a traditional stage model and the associated philosophical stance. We find unavoidable 'commonsense' observations regarding the gross contrasts over time in political organization and status indicators, the citation of ethnographic observations and some traditional social theorizing (e.g. on the effect of certain innovations on social change). Yet no 'social' chapter is risked.

For the Mesolithic we deal in 'bands' (p.4) and are told that a "food-gathering economy implies a low density of population and an organisation in small scattered groups" (p.26). After a direct parallel between the landscapes of Upper Palaeolithic Britain and north Canada, we learn that the richer Mesolithic environment must have led to 'tribal gatherings' at peak food productivity times, where 'natural leaders' from the congregation of a number of 'scattered bands' would have boasted of their prowess. Men hunted, women and children gathered plant food (p.16). By the Neolithic we have shifted organization to units of a 'people' and 'culture' (p.6ff). Initially and until the later Bronze Age these comunities are 'essentially pastoral nomads' with fortified camps such as Windmill Hill as the headquarters of 'pastoral tribes'

organized on a 'strictly patriarchal basis' (pp.13, 26). Population is rising and increasingly larger seasonal congregations occur. The great monuments imply complex social organization and "it is evident that people can only have been impelled to construct" these "... by persons vested either with prestige or royal authority" (p.115). Detailed discussion of the rise of these leaders is absent, although the inferred background is detectable in the statement "The conclusion that certain members of society exercised functions of a priestly character seems irresistible" (p.27). The rich graves of the Early Bronze Age in Wessex are linked to "the Breton incursion ... a few leaders endowed with special prestige through their control of trade in precious commodities" (p.10). Settled farming only arrives with the plough in the later Bronze Age.

In the Iron Age, despite the florescence of great monumental hillforts, it is assumed that village chiefs are little elevated above their peasant colleagues. Invaders from the continent find them easy to bully and rapidly reduce them to the status of "hewers of wood and drawers of water" (p.27). The late arrival of the Belgic tribes welds lowland England into large political units along continental lines and by introducing better agricultural techniques and strong commercial interactions with Rome, they shift the petty chiefs to the level of princes (pp.14, 89).

In all, the volume represents another uneasy compromise between 'acceptable' culture history and an underlying model of stages, the latter providing much of the basic social theorizing and period contrast at an a priori level. The author's works do after all include his book From Savagery to Civilisation (1946), with its direct reference to evolutionist terminology.

In Clark's Archaeology and Society (1947) we surely expect that the latter should be dealt with quite explicitly, and the author's views on the evolutionist position clarified. Yet unabashed, the subject of social structure and social change is given the barest treatment and no overall theory emerges. Clark admits how essential it is for archaeologists to study past social structure, yet confesses how extraordinarily difficult the task is (p.182). And yet, we can still approach it "by a cautious use of comparative material from still living societies", (more backtreading follows on the dangers); one example is given, a comparison of Mesolithic communities to recent aboriginal Tasmanians. Despite this bold stroke, Clark then retreats again for the Neolithic and Bronze Age, merely suggesting that 'tribes' were larger. Social structure is hard to clarify until the succeeding Iron Age proves the existence of princes from coins: "only with the minting of coins ... is it yet possible to say anything definite of the political organisation of southern Britain" (p.184). But indicative of the original thinking and pioneering spirit of this great scholar, is his use without further comment of a series of indicators considered crucial today for social inference in archaeology, such as grave wealth differential, house form differential and rank emblems, as well as his anticipation of recent research in pointing to the potential of the study of early field systems for identifying property and land rights. Yet possibly the constraints of this half century inhibited Clark's innovatory talents. Thus as late as his Prehistoric Europe: The Economic Basis (1952) the European Neolithic stone axe trade is conceived of in terms of merchants, and only in his pathfinding paper of 1966 on the same subject is the great potential of direct ethnographic comparison revealed, initiating the present-day widespread interest in prehistoric gift exchange systems.

A similar continuity with the nineteenth-century stadial concerns can be found underpinning the major contributions of European prehistorians such as Stuart Piggott and Maria Gimbutas, as in their respective magisterial general syntheses Ancient Europe (1965) and Bronze Age Cultures of East-Central Europe (1965). The intellectual and conceptual gulf that might sometimes seem to exist between such modern syntheses and more recent 'progressive' studies of the same data, such as Colin Renfrew's 'new archaeology' version of European prehistory - Before Civilisation (1973) and Coles and Harding's (1979) Bronze Age Europe, is far less striking when one bears in mind the underlying similarities of deductive stadial approach. In other words one is witnessing different (and doubtless with time, more sophisticated and better documented) routes to the same end. In 1966, with not a trace of irony, Glyn Daniel, in a volume to accompany a BBC series entitled Man Discovers His Past, could compose a chapter (and programme) headed 'Archaeology and the Discovery of the Ancient, Savage and Barbarian Societies'.

This discussion has hitherto been concentrated on the prehistoric picture and the archaeological data, for indeed it is the former sphere of operations that has always posed the main issue of the viability of an independent archaeological approach to social evolution, and this time span wherein it is considered most of the major transformations must have occurred prior to complex, literate, state societies becoming widespread. For historic societies both in the nineteenth and throughout the twentieth centuries, vigorous debate has naturally continued on socio-political issues, but this is a debate where archaeology has had very little to say until recently, and where an archaeologist is perhaps permitted to say that far too much reliance has been placed on squeezing every ambiguous drop out of largely biased and fragmentary sources (cf. Plumb 1969). Only tardily in ancient and medieval scholarship have archaeological data been included as a novel source of information, rather than as a mute source for the illustration of historically acceptable reconstructions (cf. below). Nonetheless, much relevant social theorizing of an evolutionary nature, relying primarily or exclusively on traditional philosophical speculation and historical sources, can be charted for the early twentieth century (e.g. Weber, Oppenheimer, Lowie, Thurnwald, Westerman, etc.).

For archaeology in its own right, therefore, it was more of a challenging voice crying in the wilderness when Brögger wrote in 1937: "For the time being social history offers archaeology its greatest possibilities" (cited in Hagen 1980). As late as the 1950s two oft-cited publications by prominent European archaeologists formally renounced any pretensions Old World archaeologists might continue to harbour regarding their role in contributing to social evolution (Hawkes 1954, Smith 1955). The theme here, that the distinctive material culture data of archaeology were best suited to technological and basic economic interpretations, was to be echoed in a characteristic shot across the bows given by the notable British social anthropologist Edmund Leach to an early 1970s conference of European proto-new archaeologists (full of the American dream of easy routes to social archaeology; Leach 1973).

And yet throughout all this period one figure pursued obstinately and, ultimately, very influentially, the search for generalizing explanations of a stadial character to fit the increasingly complex body of data for Old World cultural developments - V. Gordon Childe. In a continuous series of major archaeological syntheses from the 1920s to the late 1950s, Childe emerged increasingly from the limitations of an early allegiance to the diffusionist/migrationist model to revive and create major models for social evolution (cf. especially his Social Evolution, 1951). His authority on the raw data and skill

at weaving the minutiae of the record into a coherent narrative led to his works becoming standard textbooks, whose revised editions were eagerly awaited by the scholarly community. Thus his bold progression into a generalizing social prehistory and history, relying primarily on archaeology or giving it equal voice with history when both were available, could not be dismissed lightly, though virtually no one in the Old World dared follow him. "During his lifetime ... his explicitly theoretical work was largely ignored by his contemporaries" (McNairn 1980, p.3). A highly significant factor in this aspect of Childe's work was his sense of social commitment (Gathercole 1971). Childe felt that the results of archaeology should contribute to debates about burning contemporary issues in his own society; most especially, he was committed to social change, and much of his social theorizing adopts a materialistic socialist standpoint heavily influenced by Marxism. Such a stance, while providing an important point of connection whereby Western scholars could approach later and with less prejudice those major issues of social change and organization exhaustively and rather one-sidedly treated by Soviet archaeologists and historians throughout this century, does seem to have had a rather negative effect in the short-term on the further development of Childe's ideas by his contemporaries. As we have seen, the Old World establishment continued largely to underplay or even reject the theory of social evolution, and even in the United States, where by the 1950s the rise of the neo-evolutionist group of archaeo-anthropologists had produced an audience very receptive to Childe's approach, Childe's influence remained as a general example, and neo-evolutionism largely bypassed Marx and went back to a more Spencerian formulation (Dunnell 1980).

Nonetheless both at the time, and more particularly in subsequent decades, the transformational sequences and theories put forward by Childe formed an important contribution leading to the post-War revival of a dynamic, archaeologically-centred social evolution. Initially, most interest attached to Childe's emphasis on revolutionary changes: the Neolithic Revolution, where settled farmers produced a surplus that stimulated new needs and a differentiation of labour and role; the Bronze Revolution, where scarce consumer wealth created local nodes of power and capital, chiefs and merchant groups, yet at the same time the first class of international scientists and 'free thinkers'; the Urban Revolution, where hitherto unparalleled concentrations of labour and wealth were associated with the rise of the State. More recently, Childe's tendency to see these changes from a Marxist standpoint has been attracting most attention. In his mature works he argued that social organization and ideology reflect the underlying, dominant economic base of a particular kind of society, and that this economic base was to be studied from the viewpoint of control over the means of production (cf. Trigger 1978). The various cumulative revolutions in man's development produced ever larger surpluses of labour and foodstuffs which spawned ever more complex hierarchies and compartments of roles and elites, dependent on manipulation of the lower class 'primary producers'. The State legitimized the pyramid of dependence and acted repressively to protect the vested interests of the exploiters over the exploited (cf. Engels). Let us now investigate Childe's contribution in more detail.

After the central explanatory role given to diffusionism and migrationism in his The Dawn of European Civilisation (1925), The Aryans (1926) and The Most Ancient East (1928), during the 1930s Childe shifted radically towards economic interpretations, notably in The Bronze Age (1930) (where the contrast between Neolithic and Bronze Age socio-economy is emphasized). In his revised New Light on the Most Ancient East (1934) his earlier 'ex oriente lux' diffusionist approach to the European connection is combined with an economic and sociological analysis. In Man Makes Himself (1936) Childe gave an extended account of his new economic approach, indicating his debt to Marxism: "Marx insisted on the prime importance of economic conditions, of the social forces of production, and of the applications of science as factors in historical change. His realist conception of history is gaining acceptance in academic circles remote from the party passions inflamed by other aspects of Marxism" (p.7). And in his keynote Presidential Address (1935) 'Changing Methods and Aims in Prehistory', he said: "It is an old-fashioned sort of history that is made up entirely of kings and battles to the exclusion of scientific discoveries and social conditions. And so it would be an old-fashioned prehistory that regarded it as its sole function to trace migrations and to locate the cradles of peoples". The "materialist conception of history ... puts in the forefront changes in economic organisation and scientific discoveries" (pp.9-10). Commenting on this development in Childe's thought, McNairn writes: "here it should be noted that Man Makes Himself constituted a radical departure from the texts hitherto published. The Dawn, The Most Ancient East and The Danube in Prehistory were first and foremost archaeological textbooks comprising fairly detailed syntheses of archaeological data within the cultural diffusionist framework. Man Makes Himself, however, was essentially a history of man's social evolution from a hunting-gathering stage to civilization based on the archaeological patterns presented in the earlier texts" (1980, p. 29).

Nonetheless, the stimulus to internal socio-economic changes still seemed to be Near Eastern for European prehistory, even if the mechanisms were being given a new and more sophisticated treatment; to some extent Childe's oriental stress was a reaction to contemporary Fascist, nationalist and racist archaeology within Europe. So in the revised The Dawn of 1939, Marxist analysis of social change went hand in hand with a dependency model still looking outside of Europe for prime movers. Likewise in What Happened in History (1942) the orientalist position continues, contrasted to Soviet archaeology with its social evolution firmly unilineal and autonomous, despite the major role now given by Childe to class conflict. For the Bronze Age, for example, the armoured elite warriors are seen as controlling key resources by superior force, holding sway over a subordinate, exploited and poorly armed peasantry like the knights and their men-at-arms in later Feudal society. By the 1947 edition of The Dawn, and in Scotland Before the Scots (1946), Childe was sufficiently influenced by the Soviet local evolutionist position to cite such an interpretation as an alternative prime mover to the one he still favoured, that of Near Eastern stimulus to spark off internal socio-economic transformations. Prehistoric Migrations (1950) retains this view, but then a further major change in Childe's thought occurred in the last few years of his life, during the mid 1950s.

Although not surrendering his initial position on the eastern diffusion impetus, which he always opposed to the pure autonomy of the Soviets, he now considered that what the Europeans did with these stimuli was far more creative and progressive than anything the Near East was to achieve, thus laying the basis for the ultimate superiority of the European nations. Naturally he was at pains to discount any concessions to the racialist lobby, arguing instead that the structure of the two societies tended to favour this divergence: "the explanation must of course be sociological not biological. Science, like technology is the creation of societies not races" (The Prehistory of European Society, 1958, p.9). Taking up the nineteenth-century analysis of Asiatic despotism, Childe contended that the Near Eastern communities were over-central-

ized, 'closed' and despotic systems in which innovation of all kinds tended to stagnate; Europe, with its smaller political units gave far more freedom for social and professional mobility and all kinds of experimentation, an 'open society' anticipating his vision of the modern world.

A second vital influence upon Childe's adoption of an explicitly socio-economic approach to prehistory, which he was to combine with his Marxist models, was that of contemporary social anthropology. Childe considered archaeology and anthropology to be very closely related disciplines, and believed that the workings of past society should be investigated along similar functionalist lines to the approach dominant in contemporary ethnography, with the emphasis upon the articulation of all aspects of society into an interdependent, adaptive system (Grahame Clark, e.g. 1952, adopted the same model). This functional view of culture was likewise introduced in the 1935 Presidential Address, arguing for the archaeological culture to be tackled: "not as a dead group of fossils or curios but as a living functioning organism" (p.10). In contrast to the severe limitations other archaeologists felt to be inherent in archaeological evidence for attempting such an holistic view, Childe's materialist outlook removed the problems for him, since he argued that the major social issues and structures were so fundamentally tied to the mode and **means** of production that they could naturally be inferred even by a discipline where technology and material culture formed the vast majority of the evidence.

Childe's stated affinity with and borrowings from anthropology, his concern with socio-economic interpretations and directly Marxist approach, led his researches into a conscious reformulation and testing of the nineteenth-century evolutionist stage schemes. In his 1946 paper 'Archaeology and Anthropology' archaeology was assigned the special role "to test the schemes advanced by ethnographers on the basis of their synchronic analyses of contemporary cultures" (McNairn 1980, p.2). As with the late nineteenth-century evolutionist syntheses, Childe wished to integrate material culture stages, especially the Three Age scheme, with socio-economic stages. By the 1930s of course the original simplicity and all-encompassing fit of that model was no longer possible to support on the data, but Childe argued for the Ages that "I should like to believe they can be given a profound significance as indicating vital stages in human progress" (1935, p.7). As we have noted above, from the 1930s onwards, Childe's materialist position led him to argue that the typology of material culture should be a guide to social forms: "The archaeologist's divisions of the prehistoric period into Stone, Bronze and Iron Ages are not altogether arbitrary. They are based upon the materials used for cutting implements, especially axes, and such implements are among the most important tools of production. Realist history insists upon their significance in moulding and determining social systems and economic organisation" (1936, p.9). Each age was heralded by a major economic revolution and the body of characteristic technology indicated a specific form of economy and social structure. Thus in Social Evolution (1951) the Stone Age (Palaeolithic and Neolithic) is described as the era of self-sufficiency, and of independent, small communities with an economy of primitive communism and a kinship-centred organization. With the advent of metallurgy in the Bronze Age, communities became dependent one on another, and distinct intra- and inter-community castes arose, of elite entrepreneurs and warriors, of craft-specialists and merchants. The Iron Age, with easy access to that metal, broke this structure down, encouraging the development of broader based 'republican' polities.

McNairn comments: "throughout his career Childe ... frequently approached the past using a combination of Lewis Morgan's model of savagery, barbarism and civilisation and the three ages. In What Happened in History (1942) for example, he equated savages with the Palaeolithic as a descriptive label for the hunting-gathering stage of man's evolution, barbarism with the Neolithic for the subsequent food-producing stage, and the first two thousand years of civilisation with the Bronze Age" (in the Aegean and Near East) (1980, p.88). And Childe himself, in Social Evolution (1951, p.22), stated: "I have spent some twenty years trying to give some such value (i.e. economic and sociological) to the traditional 'Ages' and to make these archaeological stages coincide with what sociologists and comparative ethnographers recognised as main stages in cultural evolution". But importantly, Childe showed himself well aware of the local divergences in development that each region he studied was revealing, and continued to argue that parallel evolution was constantly interfered with or replaced by cross-cultural diffusion.

In Childe's mature and late works we see the prototype of the contemporary social archaeologist. He has the a priori social theories, the hypothetical schemes of the comparative ethnographic evolutionists. But he believes that archaeology can test these models from its own particular data base, since the functional interdependence of every sector of a past society's behaviour must allow inference from material culture back to social structure. But the importance of an explicit theory of archaeological practice, and a scientific aim of testing models against the changing patterns of new data, set Childe far ahead of his contemporaries. In all these aspects he strikingly anticipates the rediscovery of these principles in Binford's programme for the 1960s 'new archaeology' (1968). "Childe might be said to be the first archaeologist to employ both an explicit methodology and a clearly defined historical and social theory" (McNairn 1980, p.2). More remarkable still, is Childe's anticipation of the most current trend to reflect on the subjectivity that constantly perverts the rigorous process of model-testing. In his Retrospect (1958), he cast oblique comment on his final synthesis The Prehistory of European Society (1958). "While he was aware that his argument rested on insecure foundations, he was nevertheless enthusiastic about the whole approach" (McNairn 1980, p.43), since its message to modern Europe was important enough to seem to justify Childe's own life's work as an archaeologist.

The Neo-Evolutionary Revival in the Post-War Period

In the 1940s and 50s there developed in the United States a major school of anthropologists and archaeologists, who openly revived the concept of stages of human development and general theorizing about universal factors influencing societal transformation. The reasons for this are complex. It has recently been suggested, for example, that the great sophistication of many of the societies with which archaeologists were having to deal, involving settlement and personal hierarchies and interactions of great geographical scale, led archaeology away from a timid imitation of contemporary social anthropology and its largely synchronic structuro-functionalist approach, useful for small scale village societies, back to the nineteenth-century theorists and early twentieth-century scholars with equally large-scale models (the evolutionists, Marx, Weber, Durkheim), where major yet unperceived structures controlled the form of aggregate human behaviour (Cohn 1980). Certainly Childe's achievement with Old World data was also influential to members of the American neo-evolutionary school.

The overall character of the revival has recently been summarized as follows: "Evolution ... In American archaeology, the concept is equated with the idea that there is a relatively small number of socio-cultural types, such as bands, tribes, chiefdoms, and states (Service 1971), representatives of which share basically similar structural features. These types do not necessarily constitute a unilineal series and the similar features are not viewed as analogies but as structural regularities that are valuable for interpreting archaeological data"; "the forces which shape cultures are relatively constant and can be comprehended easily ... This faith in determinism constitutes the essence of American evolutionism" (Trigger 1978, pp.11-12).

Perhaps the greatest early influence within the movement was Julian Steward, who presented the first of a series of well-known neo-evolutionary paradigms (to be followed by those of Service and Fried, in particular). From careful analysis of the ethnographic and archaeological record, and a strong central desire to produce widely valid, explanatory models for socio-economic development, Steward aimed to identify the basic processes that could account for general similarities in independent sequences of cultural evolution. In particular he laid stress on ecological variables: groups with similar generalized patterns of resource exploitation had similar kinds of institutions and ideologies, and similar histories of adaptation. Furthermore, it was this insight into the interdependence of pre-industrial societies and their regional environments that led Steward, early on, to doubt the utility of the diffusionist concepts of 'pristine/primary' foci of civilization and state development, and 'secondary' nodes. One of the cornerstones of the new school was Steward's (1949) Cultural Causality and Law: for the first time a set of general hypotheses about the evolution of early civilizations was created from the integration of archaeology and anthropology. As in his other works, a cultural ecological approach accounted for social institutions in terms of adaptations to specific techno-environments. Special interactive formulations of subsistence, social and economic structures were proposed for individual environments, e.g. irrigation land, grassland, woodland. A model evolutionary sequence was argued, where the states investigated were all semi-arid or arid region examples, and hence where irrigation tended to dominate the course of development. This sequence ran as follows: (1) hunter-gatherers; (2) incipient agriculture; (3) formative (peasant communities being transformed towards the state); (4) regional florescence (of states); (5) initial (empire) conquests; (6) Dark Ages; (7) cyclical conquests.

The model evolution was of course but one variant, a particular one where high population densities arose from irrigation, encouraging co-ordination. But the general emphasis on local environmental relationships and the secondary role of conquest theory was a necessary first step to the freeing of social archaeology from 'deus ex machina' solutions to social change. Proceeding from the start with the premise that local ecological conditions were paramount for the regional evolutionary sequence, and that widely divergent adaptations could be recognized, Steward did not fall into the trap of trying to create a single or unilineal sequence valid for all societies; indeed even within major eco-adaptive cultural types it was obvious not only that variability occurred but could be predicted. Hence Steward coined the complementary concept of multi-lineal evolution, whereby he attempted to reconcile a number of simplified and idealized model evolutionary sequences for particular environments with a range of actual examples: "The methodology of evolutionism contains two vitally important assumptions. First, it postulates that genuine parallels of form and function develop in historically independent sequences or cultural traditions. Secondly, it explains these parallels by the independent operation of identical causality in each one". Multilineal evolution "is like unilineal evolution in dealing with developmental sequences, but it is distinctive in searching for parallels of limited occurrence instead of universals" (1963, pp.14-15).

Despite this sensitivity to the complexities of the data, Steward's approach was an affirmation of the deductive, philosophical generalizing stance, being tested against appropriate data, rather than one of genuine inductive, empirical research into the causes of specific social changes under discussion (cf. below).

From the late 1950s into the early 70s, Marshall Sahlins contributed major specific insights into social evolution theory, following the lead of Steward and in close agreement with another contemporary in the group, Elman Service. Sahlins and Service both promoted the classic neo-evolutionary taxonomy of increasing complexity of socio-political types (band, tribe, chiefdom, state) (cf. their joint 1960 volume) Sahlins' research was primarily directed at squeezing the ethnographic record to obtain generalising insights, particularly those linking economic behaviour and social structure. He laid great stress on the rise of community chiefs as nodes of redistribution, sharing out surpluses and connecting areas of differing productive potential. The contrast between traditional Melanesian 'big man' systems and the dominance of formal chieftain societies in Polynesia led to a further suggestion that the simpler, achieved status of the former might have preceded the latter. Observations were made linking island fertility to the size of potential food surpluses and hence degree of social complexity, though this was an early contribution (1958) that Sahlins later modified (cf. his Stone Age Economics, 1972) to allow for mutual feedback from hierarchical systems into total productivity. Indeed ethnography was demonstrating that surplus food and leisure was insufficient to promote social complexity, Sahlins himself coining the memorable phrase "the original affluent society" (1968, p.85) for the hunter-gatherer lifestyles as found amongst modern representatives such as the Kung Bushmen. The sheer boldness of Sahlins' confidence in evolutionary universals and his challenge to the orthodoxy of European social anthropology can be seen in the following remarkable passage, that in spirit and word is a direct revival of the grand stage schemes and comparative evolutionism of the later nineteenth century: "the native peoples of Pacific Islands ... present to anthropologists a generous scientific gift: an extended series of experiments in cultural adaptation and evolutionary development ... From the Australian Aborigines, whose hunting and gathering existence duplicates in outline the cultural life of the later Palaeolithic, to the great chiefdoms of Hawaii, where society approached the formative levels of the old Fertile Crescent civilisations, almost every phase in the progress of primitive culture is exemplified" (1963, p.285).

Closely associated with Sahlins, but also in many respects with another member of the school, Morton Fried, is Elman Service. All three theorists have developed models for social evolution on a generalizing basis, but mainly from comparative ethnographic research rather than by using a diachronic approach integrating archaeology and ethnography (though a recent exception is Service's (1975) Origins of the State and Civilisation). These scholars also tend towards unilineal evolutionary sequences, and continue the nineteenth-century and even eighteenth-century tradition of Spencerian deductive social reconstruction, linking description to typology and typology to hypothetical stages of socio-cultural evolution (cf. Sanders and Webster 1978). Also especially associated with this triad is the simple taxonomy very much in

vogue amongst social archaeologists of the last decade: band, tribe, chiefdom and state.

This succession, sometimes but not necessarily considered to be a real evolutionary sequence, begins at the level of least social and political complexity: egalitarian societies, which can be subdivided into 'bands' and 'tribes', the latter being essentially a larger population unit (a multi-community society integrated by theoretical descent affiliation, age sets or sodalities). Normally these societies are hunter-gatherers, they have low population density and overall size, status rests on personal achievement, age and sex. With chiefdoms: kinship lineages tend to be graded on a ladder of prestige and one typically provides the chief - rituals centre on him and his entourage, but there are too few persons in the elite set to create a genuine 'class'. The main power base of the chief is considered to be the redistribution of food and other surpluses to his 'court' and subjects. In general such societies are considered to be those of sedentary village agriculturalists. One of the major distinctions from this stage to that of the State is that in the latter a genuine elite class and non-farming specialist craft/trade/bureaucratic sectors arise and the statuses and obligations maintaining the structure of such societies are now reinforced by a legal apparatus of forceful repression.

Various features of this scheme require further comment. Most particularly there has developed a confusing debate about the significance of 'tribes'. Fried (1967) and, in his more recent writings (but inconsistently) Service, have considered the stage of tribes as devoid of evolutionary significance in terms of natural internal evolution, as they may represent a kind of social organization that evolved in response to pressures generated on bands by nearby state societies. However, although it is true that egalitarian units at a tribal level can seemingly be converted in this way into more effective units, as with the Iroquois Confederacy and European colonists, there are difficulties in converting bands into characteristic chiefdom societies if we deny the existence of a natural, autonomous tribal level. Service himself continues to use the type in recent social reconstructions as if it still had a potential evolutionary role; Sanders and Webster (1978) present a strong case for its retention, suggesting that there is no reason why internal inter-band interactions could not create tribal units.

A second problem has arisen with the prominence all three authors have given to the chiefdom stage (echoing nineteenth-century preoccupations). The vital role of redistribution has been critically weakened by recent study (Peebles and Kus 1977, Sanders and Webster 1978) and in its place there has been emphasized a more chief-centred high productivity maintaining elite power and influence.

This debate over economic structure brings us on to a notable variance between Service and Fried on the motivational elements and overall benefits of elites in chiefdom and state societies. Whereas Fried stresses class conflict and exploitation, Service's approach is very much a reversion to the 'contract theory' of the Enlightenment, emphasizing the benefits of social hierarchy to the governed (cf. Renfrew 1973a). Primitive leaders, becoming at some stage hereditary, try to perpetuate social dominance by organizing benefits to their followers. Centralized leadership developed in unusual contexts (competitive-selective and eventually environmentally and socially circumscribed, see Carneiro, below), leading to increasing benefits that are run by ever more complex central organizations; these are eventually transformed into the state apparatus. Service argues that a major role in this acceptance of elitism is played by the theocratic or priestly aura of the chief: "the power of religion is manifest. Its positive as well as its negative conditioning seems to be by far the most direct and pervasive cause of the 'consent of the governed'. And here, too, is the best context for that consent to be engineered" (1978, p.31). It is also worthy of note in this debate, that although both Service and Fried deny the existence of any underlying force or 'prime mover' to these changes of power and surplus, many scholars have detected an implicit acceptance of population pressure spurring societal elaboration (cf. Sanders and Webster 1978).

A final general point about these three authors is their demonstration that distinct types of socio-political form can be found with distinct forms of economic behaviour (especially dominant modes of exchange).

In Service's (1975) Origins of the State and Civilisation, there is a genuine attempt to harmonize archaeological discoveries and historical sources with the hypotheses derived from comparative ethnography and social theorizing. Settlement expansion into areas diverse in their productivity and range of goods and foodstuffs encourages inter-community exchange between nodal individuals, 'big men' (cf. Sahlins) and chiefs. Colonization completed, internal resource and population pressures reinforce the role of organizing redistributors of surpluses and imports. From such situations hereditary nodal chiefdoms arise, with a theocratic and benevolent aspect, until it becomes necessary for secular sanctions, backed by force, to regulate such a proto-welfare state (as these regional groups integrate and organizational/control problems become too great for charismatic leadership). Overall, there is a strong attempt to play down those factors of unequal access and deprivation/exploitation as are stressed by Fried, or other areas of conflict between different sectors of society (cf. Claessen and Skalnik 1978b; further detailed discussion of this debate can be found in Larsen 1979).

Despite the continual interest in, and reference to, archaeological discoveries, it remains true that all three scholars are essentially concerned with illustrating hypothetical developmental schemes (derived from a typology of comparative ethnographic origin) with the archaeological and ancient historical data, rather than with the careful analysis of the evidence for a particular series of processes by which a certain past society was transformed. Nonetheless, their combined hypotheses and insights have had a crucial effect upon subsequent archaeological research programmes and interpretations. These have frequently been designed to confirm the relevance of these models and identify further archaeological means to infer their operation (essentially amongst the 'new archaeology' fraternity of the Old and New World).

In Morton Fried's evolutionary taxonomy his suspicions of the 'tribe', and the importance of 'big men' are emphasized: (1) egalitarian (2) ranked (3) stratified (4) the state. The stratified or chiefdom society embodies a clear-cut group of leaders where communal ownership of the means of production has significantly shifted towards differential private ownership (cf. Engels). Fried's researches have been especially important on the transition towards elite societies or marked social differentiation. In his major work The Evolution of Political Society (1967) he suggested several pathways whereby such differentiation could arise, all of which might be seen as linked to population pressure: (a) daughter-parent settlement links in a process of land infill; (b) newcomers arrive in an old-established community for similar reasons; (c) inter-community subsistence exchanges; (d) trans-settlement sodalities to create peace between neighbouring communities. Furthermore, once more based on comparative ethnography, Fried has improved on the important stimulus that Childe had given by his functionalist models of class differentiation, in stressing the significance of kins-

hip patterns as a pre-adaptive basis for differentiation. Whereas Childe had thought of entrepreneurial castes as the basis of rich/poor contrasts, Fried developed the model of an 'egalitarian' kinship structure such as a conical clan, which under certain circumstances (e.g. those suggested above) could form a suitable structure for hierarchical role development and economic centralization. Particularly where there is competition for resources or the products of exchange systems, emergent managerial and redistribution figures, 'big men' and later chiefs provide an apparent solution to conflict and scarcity; yet by thus forming foci of control and economic power, self-interest amongst the elite grows dominant. Eventually we see "genuine socioeconomic classes associated with markedly contrasted standards of living, security, and even life expectancy" (1967, p.225). By this stage the distorted and abused kinship structure is unable to cope with the degree of social tension and the state develops as a non kin-based instrument of repression formally to protect stratification: "The state ... This formal organisation of power has as its central task the protection (and often extension) of the order of stratification" (Fried 1978, p.36).

Both in the origin and continued maintenance of social differentiation, Fried stresses unequal access to the basic productive necessities of life (though characteristically without invoking the close similarity to Marxist analyses): "It is not enough that the society should provide different or even grossly unequal levels of prestige for its members; it is essential that such differences of rank be intertwined with inequalities of economic access" (1978, p.36). The resources concerned are such as the basic subsistence capital: land and water; differential control of such resources gives status but also the opportunity to create patron-client systems.

To be associated with this important group of neo-evolutionary anthropologists are a number of other scholars who participated in the general opening-up of generalizing theory and analysis on questions of social evolution. In the main these scholars have been anthropologists or historical sociologists, though they have included anthropological archaeologists. What unites them is the new explicit boldness of speculation and a confidence that fundamental principles and processes can be elucidated from the traditional mine of comparative ethnography, history and, to lesser extent, field archaeology. Karl Polanyi (1957) and Robert Redfield (1953) contributed stimulating insights into economic history and prehistory, and historical sociology; Naroll (e.g. 1956) to questions of demography and organizational complexity. White (1943, 1949) stressed the irrelevance of particularistic and descriptive 'culture history' to which much archaeological interpretation had been reduced and, like Steward, tried to identify cross-cutting, large scale factors underlying developmental sequences, particularly the role of energy. Wittfogel revived earlier debates about irrigation societies and Asiatic despotic states in his much-quoted (1957) Oriental Despotism. Diakonov (1959, 1969) has investigated the rise of Mesopotamian civilization with a comparable class conflict model to that of Fried, but more explicitly relating to Marxist thought.

Carneiro, primarily from comparative ethnography and generalizing insights into the early civilizations, and to a far lesser extent making use of regional archaeological sequences, has produced an influential set of inter-related ideas concerning the rise of complex stratified societies, which have been widely quoted in recent archaeological discussion. Apart from cross-cultural analysis of the link between population size and organizational complexity (cf. Naroll), his most important contribution has been in a series of papers dealing with his theory of 'circumscription' (e.g. 1970, 1978). Following the underlying trend of Fried and others, Carneiro uses population

24

pressure as a major stimulus to societal elaboration, but has developed a more sophisticated environmental perspective recalling the work of Steward. As a population infills a given landscape, it comes up against natural barriers to expansion in terms of its economic and technological repertoire (environmental circumscription); or, it comes up against expanding colonists from adjacent nuclear settlement zones (social circumscription). In both cases the pressures over resources can lead to relationships of dominance and subordination arising. A further important elaboration of this model is the suggestion that even if no genuine wastelands or competitive neighbouring communities exist, the intense rivalry within a local population for control over the key natural resources within a region (irrigated land, terrace fields, etc.) can create similar pressures leading towards social hierarchy (cf. Gilman 1981). His adherence to the neo-evolutionist stage scheme meshes easily with this set of ideas (cf. Carneiro 1978): during the Palaeolithic, political organization is seen as that of a numberless succession of independent bands or villages. With the Neolithic, bringing agriculture and settled community life, perhaps some hundreds of thousands of independent village units are to be envisaged around the world. However, during this era, the fission of villages and the infill of the landscape set in motion the processes of circumscription. Aggregates of villages arise under the authority of a multi-community chief: "the most important single step ever taken in the course of political development ... Within a few millennia of" (this) "the first states emerged, and shortly thereafter the first empires" (1978, p.207). The continual swallowing up of each level of political unit into larger polities takes us finally to the present situation where political units within the world number some 150.

Dunnell (1980) finds the neo-evolutionists and associated social theorists guilty of a priori reasoning and trapped within a poorly-cognized tradition of 'stages' and 'progress': "The fundamental features of cultural evolution, whether one considers Morgan and Taylor or White, Sahlins and Service, preserve the transformational and typological approach to the study of variability that Darwin and his scientific successors had to reject flatly to move evolution into a scientific framework" (p.41). And this despite conscious attempts by Sahlins (1960) to reconcile 'general' and 'specific' evolution.

In the work of R. McAdams (1966), M. Coe (1961) and K. Flannery (eg. Coe and Flannery 1964), the urgent need to test this flurry of social theory against archaeological case studies began to find a serious response. Archaeologists of this generation have devoted particular attention to testing the now hefty body of social evolutionary theory against the archaeological data concerning the rise of the major ancient civilisations of the Old and New Worlds. Though initially the incompleteness and apparent muteness of the archaeological record often made them over-reliant on the hypotheses and models of the neo-evolutionists, the subsequent development of their researches has been towards the independence of the increasingly full archaeological data base, and to the use of the latter as the fragmentary master-mould against which all variety of putative casts (the competing theories of social evolution) have to be fitted. In this fundamental shift of analytical approach these authors have moved away from the core tradition of deductive social theorising that was both the controversial, generalising strength and scientific weakness of the Spencerian evolutionary position, and into a more volatile research area where new fieldwork can constantly create a serious re-orientation of interpretative models. Not surprisingly, therefore, many early ideas and insights have subsequently been rejected or drastically modified by the authors themselves. The empirical challenge that increasingly penetrates the important contribution of this group during

the 1960s and early 70s was to a major extent the creation of a new, wider methodological force in American archaeology - the 'new archaeology' that arose during this period to its maturity.

The New Archaeology and the current state of play

A post-War dissatisfaction with the limitation of archaeological aims and methods culminated in the rise during the 1960s of a highly influential pressure group, the so-called 'new archaeology'. The acknowledged leader or 'prophet' of the movement was Lewis Binford (1968), but it is generally recognized that the field for revolution had already been prepared by immediately preceding developments: firstly, the vigorous revival of generalizing theory about developmental trajectories and dominant universal processes represented by the anthropologists and historical sociologists of the neo-evolutionist school; secondly the undeniable challenge posed by the scholarly meticulous, yet boldly generalizing and evolutionist social archaeology of Gordon Childe (especially his late works); thirdly the example set and programmatic appeal launched by Gordon Willey. In Prehistoric Settlement Patterns in the Viru valley, Peru (1953) Willey demonstrated the untapped potential of research-orientated fieldwork for documenting societal change. For Willey, this shift towards asking far more from archaeological research went hand in hand with a commitment to the primacy of social archaeology. After the well-known, revolutionary dogma that opens Willey and Phillips' (1958) study of American archaeology: "American archaeology is anthropology or it is nothing" (p.2), the remainder of the volume, with its programme to mesh archaeological developmental sequences with socio-cultural stages, could be summarized as 'If archaeology is anything, it is evolutionary anthropology'. Willey and Phillips, however, still confined by the anti-evolutionist atmosphere of the period, shied away from any explicitly evolutionary interpretations, preferring to keep their 'historical-developmental' stages as 'descriptive' in nature.

These separate threads were spun together into the powerful new body of ideas and approaches associated with the 'new archaeology' of Binford. Not surprisingly, rather disparate elements found themselves in the same programme. Thus the early emphasis upon elucidating universals in human behaviour over time and space, 'the laws of cultural process' (Binford 1968), which is fully in the tradition of social-philosophical theory stemming from previous centuries, rapidly proved unrealistic and has been rejected (or 'postponed') in favour of tackling widely-valid issues that involve processes operative on a far smaller scale: Binford's 'middle range theory' (1977).

In fact it might now be considered that Binford's major contribution at this time was to stimulate archaeologists to drop their methodological inferiority complex and move to develop their discipline so as to tackle all the major aspects of human life covered by historians, anthropologists and sociologists. Binford not only argued for archaeology as a discipline that must concern itself, in its own data, with all such issues, but showed how it could be done in seminal papers designed to increase the interpretative potential of fieldwork programmes. His pioneer stress on field survey and sampling (1964) opened up vast field horizons for work that was to follow, in which the example of Steward and Willey could be applied and tested innumerable times. The apparent weakness and muteness of the archaeologist on questions of social status were tackled head-on in his studies of cross-cutting interpretative dimensions of artifactual patterns and mortuary behaviour (1962, 1971). The down-to-earth analytical approach to the study of socio-cultural phenomena at the core of this work, often combined with experiments with formal statistical techniques, challenged the material culture data to speak for themselves. Even Dunnell (1980) in his across-the-board criticism of the exponents of social archaeology, excepts this approach of Binford as most approximating to the scientific case-study methodology of Darwinian evolutionary tradition. Mortuary analysis has been vigorously pursued up to the present day as a central tool in social archaeology (cf. Tainter 1978). The proliferation of regional survey has been staggering (cf. for example, for the Mediterranean alone, Keller and Rupp 1983).

Despite the initial emphasis on methodological elaboration, the vast majority of studies that embrace the general philosophy and techniques of the 'new archaeology' have been dominated by a priori pressures to create or test generalizing explanations of the kind now familiar from the neo-evolutionist and evolutionist schools (i.e. within the philosophical tradition of Spencer and the Enlightenment). This apparent mismatch has hardly gone unnoticed within the 'new archaeology' fraternity, encouraging a lively and continual debate on the opposing hypothetico-deductive and empirico-inductive positions. The present writer is sufficiently a child of the first two decades of 'new archaeology' to prefer the former as more likely to justify the expense of archaeology to the public, and the expense of a lifetime to the individual archaeologist; to the scientific purist, he would recall Binford's citation from Hempel: "What determines the soundness of a hypothesis is not the way it is arrived at (it may have been suggested by a dream or a hallucination), but by the way it stands up when tested, i.e. when confronted with relevant observational data" (Hempel 1965, p.6, cited by Binford 1968). On the other hand, it is of course true, that an earnest desire to assemble archaeological data that are full enough and unambiguous enough to allow thorough exploration of major issues in social theory can, in the shortfall from such expectations, encourage unsupported 'leaps of faith' between field data and general models.

In the research climate of the last two decades of 'new archaeology', at least in the New World, a lengthy research programme without a theoretical aim seems obscurantist and anachronistic. The backwardness of Old World, 'establishment' reaction to these developments in the United States can be illustrated from the fact that in Britain only very recently did it become official policy to concentrate state funding into archaeological programmes with an explicit problem-orientation. Major progress **has** been made, if we superficially review the prolific outpourings of generalists directly or indirectly attached to the 'new archaeology'. Most recognize that however simple and a priori an explanatory model may be, (and regardless of whether it derives from comparative ethnography, historical analysis, imaginative social theorizing, or the apparent trends in empirical data), yet it is a totally valid exercise to go into the field with such a model and seek to test it against fresh data. The growth of competing teams of scholars focussing on the same culture or civilization, all armed with the same methodological approach but sporting very contrasting interpretative models, has meant that abuse of the data does not for long escape recognition. The research zone where this process is most highly developed is Mesoamerica. A regular series of symposia devoted to Mesoamerican civilizations and running battles in the academic journals bear witness to an ideal conjunction of traditional social theorizing, a commitment to generalizing social evolutionary reconstructions, and the essential scientific activity of competitive accumulation of new data and testing of rival theories (cf. for example Culbert 1973, Wolf 1976, Hammond 1977, Ashmore 1981 and contributions to American Antiquity over the last two decades). This overall approach is also very well represented in a single volume, Flannery's The Early Mesoamerican Village (1976). Yet

scholarly rivalry may also lead to the recognition that existing theories or existing data are obviously inadequate to provide the desired general explanatory reconstruction, as Wright's (1978) summary for Mesopotamia demonstrates with refreshing honesty.

The roll-call of archaeologists and archaeo-anthropologists involved in this recent surge of activity is too long to recite, but one might mention significant contributions in both New and Old World archaeology within this broader 'new archaeology' approach from American scholars such as McAdams, Flannery, Wright, Johnson, Chang, Redman, Sanders, Webster, Price, Peebles, Rathje, Wobst, Polgar, Goldman, Earle (and not forgetting of course the more recent works of the neo-evolutionists discussed earlier, where the archaeological 'renaissance' has had a visible effect).

Outside of America, not only 'new archaeology' but even the revival of social evolution has had but limited impact (cf. Zubrow 1980; Slaughter, this volume). Yet despite the negative approach to mortuary studies of Ucko (1969) and the scorn of most social anthropologists (Leach 1973), the two movements have gained a firm (if embattled) foothold in Europe, especially in Britain. It is probably true to say that the growth and eventual flourishing of both can be attributed to two individuals of almost equal charisma to Binford: Colin Renfrew and David Clarke. Whereas Clarke pioneered the methodological revolution (1968, 1972a), it was Renfrew above all who raised the banner not only of social archaeology (Inaugural Lecture, 1973b - the time lag to Willey and Phillips' equivalent gesture is noteworthy), but of social evolution (1973a). Elaborations of Binfordian and neo-evolutionary theory, particularly in the areas of spatial analysis and exchange networks (Renfrew 1973a, 1975, 1977) were applied to major interdisciplinary regional case studies with an impeccable attention to the raw data (Renfrew 1972, 1979, Renfrew and Wagstaff 1982). Disciples and 'clients' of these founding scholars soon scattered over the globe, though some stayed at home, to practise the new techniqes and to juggle the assorted social theories. The results of these activities can be seen in collected essays such as Clarke (1972a), Hodder et al. (1981), Renfrew and Shennan (1982).

Although the response to these innovations was generally much more restrained elsewhere in Western Europe, Scandinavia rapidly developed its own flourishing school of anthropological archaeology (cf. Kristiansen and Paludan-Müller 1978; Randsborg 1974, 1975, 1980). We will deal with the special case of Communist East European archaeology shortly.

Returning to our earlier discussion of 'covert evolutionism' amongst European archaeologists throughout the first half of this century, it will be recalled that the implicit need for a stage scheme, for generalized social models for specific areas, had never disappeared from their works of general synthesis (though expressed in guarded asides, to be read between the lines and from incautious slips of oblique reference). It is not surprising, therefore, that whereas the methodology of 'new archaeology' has met continued and powerful resistance amongst professional archaeologists in Europe, the neo-evolutionary models have been given a far wider and less critical acceptance. Anders Hagen (1980) from Norway complains that even amongst younger archaeologists in Scandinavia today, with evolutionary-processual views of the American 'new archaeology', the evolutionary model of Montelius for artifacts (earmarking cultures and also forms of society) has simply been grafted on to social archaeology, reaffirming Montelius' late nineteenth-century elaboration of the Three Age scheme of material-/cultural/social stages.

Another interesting development (cf. Chapman 1979) is the effortless introduction of explicit or implicit Marxist approaches into European social archaeology; though the right wing have now been alerted to this danger of creeping Socialism (Selkirk 1982-3). Yet it does not seem that Western scholars are directly inspired by recent or contemporary Eastern bloc archaeology or historical sociology. The East watches on, intrigued by the whole affair (Klejn 1977). Amongst factors that may be relevant are the example of Childe's later works, now the object of a revival of interest. Also contemporary trends in the socio-political and philosophical ethos of our age seem to be influential in a turning away from 'benefit theories', 'contract theories', towards class conflict models. Trigger has made the following observations concerning the development of a more pessimistic view of the past: "Into the 1960s, larger-scale societies generally were believed to cope more efficiently with their environments and to provide a richer, more secure and more leisured life for their members than did primitive ones. Soon after, however, American optimism was dampened by a series of political and economic crises that were accompanied by growing anxiety about industrial pollution, exhaustion of energy supplies and nuclear proliferation. Even the accelerating expansion of population which Childe had accepted as the key index of progress came to be viewed as a menace ... These conditions led many anthropologists to reconsider the concept of progress in a more sombre light". The 'leisured and noble savages' of the hunter-gatherer life were rediscovered (Lee and De Vore 1968) and Boserup (1965) argued that economic intensification was associated with loss of efficiency. Cultural progress was obviously neither inevitable nor necessarily desirable: "cultural development is attributed to ... pressures that compel men and women to work harder in order to survive in an increasingly complex social setting" (Trigger 1978, pp.71-2).

Yet throughout this century, Communist scholars have been relating Marx's and Engels's versions of evolutionism to the changing pattern of archaeological discoveries in Europe and further afield. In many respects therefore, Eastern bloc scholarship has a genuine advance upon Western archaeology, where even open discussion of evolutionary theory was for long an intellectually prohibited zone (Klejn 1974). On the negative side, strong pressure to treat the Marx/Engels canon as sacrosanct dogma has all too often stifled an otherwise natural development towards a constant modification of Soviet archaeologists' schemes in line with the accumulation of new evidence. At the extreme, the early Communist theorists are cited as if their models, based as they were on limited and often wildly inaccurate data, are in themselves solid facts. Both sides of the coin can be observed if we take a characteristic example of recent Communist treatment of social evolution - Beiträge zur Entstehung des Staates, edited by J. Herrmann and I. Sellnow (1976). The paper by Krüger on Old Germanic social structure makes impressive joint use of archaeology and the limited historical sources; independently of similar modern work in the West, he utilizes such aspects as burial form, settlement structure and patterns, craft specialization, hoards and trade networks, in his dynamic reconstruction of a simple yet stratified society growing gradually more complex. Herrmann's study of feudal origins stresses the social changes that ensued from productive transformations occasioned by the introduction of rye, metallurgy, the plough, soil fertilizers and water-mills. Yet in the same volume Sellnow reveals in his general study of state origins that to test early Marxist theory by appealing to early Marxist theory, decorating the argument on the way with unimpressive scraps of archaeo-historical data, takes us further away from making sense of the real message of the past than the position reached by nineteenth-century scholars who were at least trying to accommodate their

theories to the contemporary data base. Likewise, amongst studies of Neolithic Europe emanating from the Eastern bloc in the 1970s, some repeat the doctrinaire Marx/Engels stage schemes as if subsequent evidence and analysis is of no importance (cf. Taganyi 1977), whereas others suggest that their authors feel free to take every inherited dogma as open to revision or even rejection (e.g. Tabaczynski 1972).

Despite these constraints, it is frequently obvious that a Marxist perspective in its most general sense, i.e. the investigation of class conflict, is sadly lacking from much Western social theorizing (cf. for example Winzeler 1976, and the telling critique by Panoff that follows it).

Social archaeology in the Communist world (which is actually often emphasized there as the core of archaeology - cf. Otto and Brachmann 1975), makes no distinction in its approach to the remote prehistoric (Palaeolithic), later prehistoric (Iron Age,) Classical or Medieval epochs. But in Western Europe the barriers between those studying different eras continue to cripple attempts to create a general body of progressive theory, akin to American 'new archaeology', that could co-ordinate research workers towards the realization of common goals. More importantly, not only is it extremely difficult to compare research publications stemming from investigations of different periods, but it is basically only in prehistory that the discipline of archaeology is claimed to be self-sufficient as a provider of independent interpretations of past processes. By and large, Classical and Medieval archaeology continue to serve as subordinate illustrators to the mainstream activity of historical exegesis. It is a commonplace observation that this difference of attitude between America and Europe towards the role of archaeology as an investigative and interpretative discipline in its own right, reflects the far longer and more abundant historical record of the latter. Historians in Europe had begun to debate why and how societies changed and events occurred, in the fifth century BC and have never ceased doing so since that time. Archaeology, with its effective development of a mere 150 years, not surprisingly seems too immature for most historians to be prepared to give it an equal voice in debates about the past, wherever written sources exist to 'tell the whole story'.

It is perhaps ironical that the most lively controversies rage within historical circles about the social evolution of Classical or Feudal Europe, and the boldest general theories abound (cf. Postan 1975, Hopkins 1978, Finley 1973, for example), yet with a few notable exceptions, post-War Classical and Medieval archaeologists remain ignorant of social archaeology, and indeed of most of the entire package of methodological and theoretical advances contained within the 'new archaeology'. Even American Classical archaeology has generally insulated itself from the challenge of 'new archaeology', as Colin Renfrew has recently reminded its practitioners (1980). Anthony Snodgrass' Archaic Greece (1980), which for the first time asked the archaeology to speak for itself, to confirm or reject well-worn but untested historical models and interpretations for pre-Classical Greece, opened up an entirely new understanding of the period. For the Roman era, Britain has until recently been dominated by blind allegiance to (actually very inadequate) historical sources. The astonishing absence of genuine and independent archaeological interpretative theory in Frere's Britannia is a case in point (1978). This is still the standard archaeology textbook for the period, yet the treatment is pure culture history, and the few pages where 'society' is mentioned are glosses on historical sources. Rodwell (e.g. 1981) has recently pitched an advance base in the immediate pre-Roman Iron Age to repel the swarms of 'Renfrewsian' social archaeologists.

However there is evidence of a growing coherence of progressive scholarship crystallizing out within the Roman era in Britain and associated with linked research work by Hodder, Millett, Reece and Jones (cf. Jones, this volume). Even so, as the following anecdote reveals, Roman Britain has a long way to go to free its archaeology from being the uncritical handmaiden of history. A few weeks ago the writer was in a gathering where a prominent Roman archaeologist pronounced himself baffled at the interest aroused by Renfrew's Before Civilisation (1973); but, he continued, the section at the beginning explaining C14 **was** worth students' reading. In Italy, in contrast, partly for political reasons, but also from the growth of regional projects in which period interests have broken down to let general theory in (especially from prehistory), a Roman social archaeology and even social evolutionary archaeology is in vigorous health and indeed threatens to dominate the research scene (cf. Potter, this volume).

Over most of Western Europe, post-Roman archaeology is in a much worse state of immaturity. Archaeology as art-history and as an illustration of history remain paramount. The early twentieth-century goals for the discipline, concentrating on lifestyles, technology and economy, continue little changed into the 1980s. It is striking that scholars who attempt to break with this tradition by applying the techniques of the 'new archaeology' and an anthropological, evolutionary perspective as independent approaches to history, tend to have been trained, or be embedded, in research teams dominated by prehistorians (e.g. Hodges 1982; Arnold 1980, this volume), or even be marauding prehistorians themselves (Randsborg 1980, this volume). General textbooks, supposedly comprehensive, such as The Archaeology of Anglo-Saxon England (1976) edited by D.M. Wilson, show nothing achieved in response to the new questions and approaches emanating from the United States; the most progressive sector is that of spatial patterns, which actually represents something of an insular British specialization stemming from Fox and Crawford rather than cross fertilization from American archaeology. The book is arranged in chapters itemizing major facets of technology and economy, with settlements being discussed separately as 'urban', 'rural' and 'religious'. There is no chapter, or even extended treatment, on social and political evolution and its archaeological investigation. In his crusading paper of 1980, Chris Arnold states: "The archaeology of early Anglo-Saxon England is still primarily based on cemeteries and their contents and there is a continuing tendency to study the evidence in terms of art-history, cultural chronology and demography ... Even in the more optimistic climate of today where archaeologists are encouraged to ask more detailed and germane questions about the material, there remains a deep-rooted pessimism on the part of early medieval archaeologists" (p.81). And elsewhere he writes: "Anglo-Saxon politics ... are extremely complex, but while the particularism of the historians of the period has resulted in an understanding of much of the structure of institutions and the sequence of events, no attempt has been made to understand the causal processes" (p.84). A further anecdote illustrates the current situation in first-millennium AD post-Roman studies in Europe rather well: an eminent specialist on the period, reviewing Randsborg's The Viking Age in Denmark (1980), where Viking studies have been transformed almost overnight from text-orientation to archaeological, 'new' archaeological and anthropological archaeology perspectives, concentrated his dismissive critique on the absence of a chapter on art styles and some linguistic confusions. Americanist in author and approach, and 'transatlantic' in study area, is another exceptional study of Viking society (in Greenland) by McGovern (1981).

The historic archaeology of the Slav peoples in Central and Eastern Europe has long been the object of intensive study, with social and political evolution very much in the forefront, as can naturally by expected of Eastern bloc scholarship. Regrettably, much of this is little known in the West (though cf. Kidd 1980). It is indeed unfortunate that despite many enquires we were unable to secure the services of a specialist in Slav archaeology who would have provided the present volume with a further chapter.

Passing briefly to high Medieval archaeology, Professor Philip Rahtz, in his 1980 inaugural lecture (1981) and elsewhere (1983), has roundly challenged its practitioners to move their subject in a progressive direction, his 'New Medieval Archaeology', whilst he catalogues its current backwardness and theoretical poverty. Work by Professor Colin Platt shows exactly the right intentions and approach (e.g. his (1978) Medieval England: A Social History and Archaeology), yet characteristically Platt seems to have developed a progressive line in isolation and does not refer to parallel theoretical work in the United States or beyond his period. The same can be said for the very fine social archaeology of Ten Years Settlement Archaeology on the Island of Sylt (1974, Kossack et al.) which is an independent and anomalously progressive out-growth from German archaeology; as with Anglo-Saxon spatial archaeology in Britain, this excellent and forward looking work is the culmination of a long indigenous tradition of geographical archaeology. Promising developments elsewhere in Medieval archaeology such as Dixon's paper on Medieval border defence works and social structure (1979) must herald a change of attitude, although Dixon is another example of an archaeologist with equal professional interests in prehistoric archaeology. As for Byzantine civilization, there exists virtually no relationship between the innovative and theory-conscious school of historical research (social issues being well-treated) and the incredibly backward world of Byzantine archaeology (which has no pretensions beyond architectural and art-history). Timothy Gregory's paper (this volume) is eloquent enough, but his own attempts at a 'new Byzantine archaeology' on Americanist principles are hard to parallel elsewhere in current research on this neglected culture.

Nonetheless, there is absolutely no doubt that the unparalleled combination of an independent archaeological discipline and a rich documentation from historical sources will create an interpretative potential in many regions and periods of Europe that may well exceed anything widely available in America (excluding Colonial archaeology), and it does now seem not too far away when this potential will begin to be realized. At that point it is confidently hoped that European archaeology can begin to return the favour to America by exporting its own own elaborations of method and theory, together with a new depth of insight into the processes of social evolution.

SOCIAL ARCHAEOLOGY: TOOLS OF THE TRADE

The production of archaeologists trained in 'new archaeology' and anthropological archaeology is now a constant stream outpouring from the universities and institutes of America and Europe. Both the accumulated data base of some 150 years of archaeology and the unimaginable quantity of data that can be shown to be still available for new research projects in the field, provide intellectual food for this army, sufficient to fuel the academic warfare of rival theorists in social archaeology for centuries to come. With each year, new techniques and approaches emerge and are further refined. The following list represents no attempt to be complete, rather it is meant to illustrate some of the commonest analytical tools now in use by social archaeologists in Europe. For each approach one or two examples are given of applications on European data.

(a)   **Mortuary Studies:** for a useful recent overview see Chapman, Kinnes and Randsborg (Eds. 1981), with a full picture of the application of Binfordian (1971) inspired analyses of burial differentiation. Shennan (1975) was a pioneer application in Central Europe. Analysis is directed at such potentially socially-significant features as variability in the form of graves; burial rite; .nature, quality and quantity of gifts; clustering of graves. Recent work by Arnold and Jones (cf. this volume and Arnold 1980, Jones 1980) represents the extension of such an approach into historical archaeology. The pattern of burial monuments and cemeteries and its possible social implications has been discussed by Renfrew (1973a), Bintliff (1977b) and Frankenstein and Rowlands (1978).

(b)   **Palaeodemography, Palaeopathology:** the study of the population structure and health/diet aspects of past societies, primarily from burial remains, but in the former case, also from analyses of settlement patterns. Diet and disease studies have yet to become widespread in European social archaeology, and Shennan's review paper of the American literature (1980) was intended in part to stimulate greater interest. For cemetery population structure and its social implications cf. Arnold (1980 and this volume), Drewett (1979), and references discussed in my Neolithic chapter (this volume). Demographic aspects in broader terms, i.e. questions of population pressure and density, and the correlation with social change and social complexity, are standard research issues in Europe (cf. Kristiansen 1978; Welinder 1975; Bintliff 1982 and this volume, Neolithic and Iron Age chapters).

(c)   **Settlement Studies:** analyses of the internal structure of settlements can provide insights into social and professional differentiation and general features of communal organization; cf. Clarke (1972b), Raper (1977), Kossack et al. (1974), Gregory (this volume). Settlement systems on a regional basis can be studied for insights into organizational hierarchies, cf. Bintliff (1977a), and on an inter-regional basis cf. Renfrew (1975).

(d)   **Exchange Systems:** dominant modes of exchange in a society may indicate the operation of a particular kind of socio-economic structure, cf. Renfrew (1975, 1977), Sherratt (1976); tracing the precise circulation routes and circulation time of exchange goods may offer finer detail on social questions, cf. Frankenstein and Rowlands (1978), Kristiansen (1978), Ellison (1981).

(e)   **Symbolic Signalling in Material Culture:** symbols of rank and status, or role differentiation, have been widely studied, cf. Tabaczynski (1972), Randsborg (1974), Snodgrass (1980); the signalling of ethnic 'territories' is being investigated more analytically than in the traditional 'culture-people' model, cf. Gamble (1980), and Newell (this volume).

(f)   **Labour Input:** estimates of the man-hour requirements for large domestic structures, or monuments such as ceremonial centres and linear earthworks, have become a regular feature of studies aimed at demonstrating the degree of organizational complexity and central control prevalent in a particular society, cf.   Startin (1978), Renfrew (1973a), Muir (1980).

(g)   **Human Ecology, Land Use:** the mutual feedback between the exploitation of natural resources and the social organization of particular societies has been frequently explored (cf. Jochim 1976; Bintliff 1982; Gilman 1981; Kossack et al. 1974).   The evidence of field systems promises to be a major growth area for social insights (cf. Harding this volume).

(h)   Last, but not least, **Historical Sources:** now to be seen as but one source of evidence rather than the touchstone of confirmation for all the other lines of approach. The playing off against each other of textual evidence and field evidence is already becoming a very fruitful route to greater accuracy in following social developments for literate societies, cf. Potter (this volume), Jones (this volume).

SOCIAL EVOLUTION: THEORY OR FACT?

Scanning the publications of 'new archaeology', or edited collections of evolutionary papers such as Claessen and Skalnik (1978) The Early State, and Cohen and Service (1978) Origins of the State, one might gain the impression that the post-War revival of explicit evolutionism has swept all before it (excepting of course most of European historical archaeology).

In fact, apart from traditional archaeologists who find little of relevance in 'new archaeology' and anthropological archaeology, there is also a significant number of open-minded scholars who take issue with the assumptions, approaches and results of social evolution in archaeology. I have already cited more than once an important and thoughtful paper by Dunnell (1980), which correctly, to my mind, analyzed an obvious confusion concerning social evolution and Darwinian or biological evolution. Trigger (1978, pp.30-4) adopts a similar critique, and reminds archaeologists that biologists make no pretence at being able to predict past sequences of biological evolution, rather than post-dicting on the general processes that explain palaeontologically-attested small scale sequences of evolution. However I have voiced my opinion that 'hypothetico-deductive', problem-orientated research programmes are always to be preferred in archaeology, not least in social archaeology, provided they conform to two principles: (1) the models are genuinely tested and indeed testable against field data and (2) there exists a lively debate in which a number of scholars pit a range, or battery, of competing models against the same or a comparable data set. I have also stated my view that these conditions are regularly met with in Americanist archaeology, in Mesopotamian archaeology and increasingly in European archaeology (primarily prehistory).

But since it cannot yet be shown that any one major model, any particular unilineal or multilineal evolutionary scheme, has achieved a decisive advantage over alternatives in accounting for archaeologically-attested developmental tendencies in any major region of the world, it is not unreasonable that independent observers such as Trigger should remain sceptical of the priority given to such hypothesis testing: "I would agree with Murdock ... that the course of evolution, as distinguished from its processes, must be identified with what actually has happened in the past, not with highly abstract generalizations about what is believed to have taken place" (1978, p.xi).   Trigger's own attitude is nonetheless revealingly inconsistent (one might even comment 'Do as I say, not as I do').   On the one hand he takes a stance that seems to deny a serious role to social archaeology, reminiscent of traditionalists cited earlier: "The archaeologist who is interested primarily in formulating laws about sociocultural processes might better become a social anthropologist or an ethnologist and work with living or historically well-documented people rather than with the more refractory material of archaeology" (1978, p.34).   Then in the same volume of essays appears a chapter entitled 'Inequality and Communication in Early Civilisations' (pp.194-215), which uses an analytical structure of "differing levels of socio-cultural complexity" that is nothing less than a barely-modified neo-evolutionary stage scheme of bands, autonomous villages, tribes and state societies!

A second and rather more specialized critique stems from anthropologists who belong to the 'formalist' school (cf. Dalton 1981 for the terms of this debate). Whereas the opposing school of 'substantivists' (following the example of Weber and Polanyi, and with obvious connections to Marxist theory) argue for contrasting economic modes for distinct eras of the past, the formalists believe that certain fundamental principles of economic behaviour unite all eras, with the passage of time merely producing differences of scale in economy rather than differences in dominant mode. The relevance to social evolution in a broader sense is that the neo-evolutionist school and its archaeological followers have, like the substantivists, claimed to identify parallel sequences of social forms and economic forms from stage to stage of their sequences of development (cf. Reid 1979). An explicit or implicit formalist viewpoint can be found in the recent work of Rowlands and Sherratt (this volume); the substantivist viewpoint appears in other contributions (e.g. Bintliff, Harding), but it should be stressed that the debate over the existence of sequences of economic evolution must not be equated with that over the existence of social evolution.

For all the correctness of the criticism that social evolutionists are still at the stage of collecting (feverishly) new data and new archaeological techniques to try to discriminate between rival explanatory theories, it is surely absurd to deny that world societies have 'evolved' in a directional sense in the long term, whilst regional societies in the short term have, within that very simplified trend, undergone cycles of 'evolution' and 'devolution'. "Within limits, social evolution does go from less to more complexity, from less to more heterogeneity, from less to more efficiency ... Has not the modern state now taken over all previous forms of society?" (Cohen 1981, p.206; cf. Carneiro, 1978 in a similar vein, and Lenski 1976).

Turning to the results of the present volume, which we hope represents a desirable conjunction of theory and data, it is our belief that it demonstrates: (1) The reality of directional, evolutionary transformations in the development of European societies; (2) The utility of the models and processes, and indeed the evolutionary taxonomies, of the neo-evolutionist school; (3) The ability of archaeology as a discipline in its own right to recover and interpret from its own data, the material correlates of social structure and social change.

EUROPEAN SOCIAL EVOLUTION: ARCHAEOLOGICAL PERSPECTIVES - A PERSONAL COMMENTARY TO THE CONTRIBUTIONS

It is the aim of this final section of the Introduction to offer a personal view of what seem to be the main processes and trends in the development of European society over the immense time-period covered by this volume, based upon the individual contributions but incorporating my own (often divergent) critical opinions.

The Mesolithic

Raymond Newell suggests that ecological control was limited in the Palaeolithic, therefore social forms were narrowly defined and can be matched to the standard hunter-gatherer ethnographic analogues. The adaptive success of the early Mesolithic peoples, however, especially to Holocene changes in the landscape, was sufficient for the first time to free most communities to expand

their socio-political systems in more varied formats. In particular this allowed a very wide movement of marriage partners which was not inhibited by territorial behaviour (as was to arise in the later Mesolithic and subsequent millennia). However, gradual, uncontrolled over-expansion of population led to territoriality, social stress and perhaps the scope for decision makers ('rich burials', etc.) in the Late Mesolithic. As a **social** group the best model for the Mesolithic community is still that of the band.

Not surprisingly, Newell has difficulty in producing a clear resolution of the stimulus-response effects that link Holocene environmental changes and Mesolithic societal transformations. Although no emphasis is given to the potentially deterministic influence of ecology and population pressure, it might be suggested that the contrasts drawn between Early and Late Mesolithic, and between Palaeolithic and Mesolithic, are primarily expressions of relative population density to contemporary available resources under a novel technology. Finally, the overall treatment is not out of tune with recent versions of the nineteenth-century 'band-savagery' model for this 'stage', with shifts indicated towards 'tribal' configurations later on in the period (cf. 'lower barbarism').

The Neolithic to Iron Age

In his Neolithic and Iron Age chapters (which we shall examine as one unit here), within the context of the development of Europe from simple to complex farming communities at emergent state level, **John Bintliff** offers an extended treatment of the factors just identified i.e. the relative balance between population density, resource availability and extraction efficiency (cultigens, technical skills). It is suggested that imbalances lead to regular or cyclical 'crashes' of population and linked political superstructure; that dramatic rises in **absolute** population density produce cumulative increases in the surpluses of food, raw materials and manpower capable of supporting social hierarchies and complex division of labour; that high levels of **absolute** population density produce authoritarian potential and conflict-resolution needs that are met by the elaboration of leadership roles. Significant conflicts arise over rights over resources, especially if resources are increasingly fixed and intensively worked (cf. Gilman), or if the potential of further expansive colonization is reduced (cf. Carneiro). A further general point is the argument that the greater the concentration of population and resource surpluses, the more the emergent elites can be freed from local milieu constraints to indulge in inter-elite contacts, which can provide status-reinforcement (cf. the prestige-chains of Renfrew and Rowlands) and can stimulate the development of elite subcultures with a cross-cultural format (cf. the Hopewell Interaction Sphere and European parallels studied by Sherratt and Shennan). Such broader interactions have a potential, through subcultural alliances and intermarriage, to encourage a new spiral: of ever-increasing hierarchical development via regional chiefs/central places to paramount chiefs, then to princedoms. However there are important restraints on this development, imposed by practical communication factors and transport limitations, ecological and social overkill (the soil deteriorates, the people rise up, etc.). The result of these conflicting tendencies is that the European Neolithic-Bronze-Iron Age era, until the final stage of the Iron Age, seems to evidence a cyclical development of the elaboration and simplification of political systems, such that neither states nor coherent, long-lived, large scale polities of a lesser kind are achieved (except in the Aegean). This picture is contrasted to the longer cycles and greater stability of Egypt and Mesopotamia with their easier communications and annual renewal of fertility. Even with the latter examples, however, growth and decline cycles are detectable, though generally on a longer scale (cf. Butzer, McAdams). Further parallels of agrarian/political cycles are drawn from the Greco-Roman and Medieval Feudal worlds. Changes in land use and technology provide the potential for both quantitative and qualitative transformations in productivity and population, which have crucial effects in turn on the socio-political system. Although an elite structure may have positive, short term feedback on cultural take-off, in the long term it is suggested that more often than not a destructively negative feedback ensues on the original novel potential.

A major problem, however, in Bintliff's contributions is the essentially provisional nature of many of the case-study interpretations central to these arguments, since the relevant data base is still inadequate for definitive explanations to be proposed and alternative models cannot generally be ruled out. The overall sequence as presented is strongly comparable to the neo-evolutionist model of band/'big man'/tribe/chiefdom /early state module (cf. Renfrew)/state, but with one significant difference. It is suggested that conditions favourable to the development of a certain type of social structure could occur at virtually any point without even limitation on the mode of economy (cf. King), and conceivably in any order. However, it is argued that the set of causative conditions associated with each major type of social system tends to be prevalent and sustained only from certain points in time, as a result of which development 'stages' are nonetheless created, on the basis of the **characteristic** form of social organization for each region.

In his study of the Bronze Age, **Anthony Harding** adopts a similar emphasis on European developments as due to internal, and largely regional, evolution. The age is distinct from preceding eras in its far greater frequency of indications for people of high status, although the evidence is mainly from mortuary differentiation, which Harding handles with appropriate caution. Nonetheless it still seems reasonable to treat the largely positive evidence for a period of 'chiefdom' dominance as a basis for generalization, especially when exceptional cultural spheres such as the Lausitz, where status is rarely symbolized in burials, demonstrate alternative clues to complex hierarchical organization. The economic background to this phase of pre-state elites (the Aegean excepted) is sought primarily in unequal access to the most fertile land, rather than in trade and industry (although, significantly, the latter factors may affect the **expression** of status). In this Harding follows the Substantivist approach, as also in his suggestion that local elite groups administered trade instead of supposed guilds of international 'capitalist' merchants often favoured in the past. In general, the image of the age being presented is consonant with the neo-evolutionary model of stratified, chieftain societies intermediate between the preceding ranked and stratified societies of the first farmers, and the proto-state societies of the contemporary Aegean and subsequent European Iron Age.

The chapters by **Andrew Sherratt** on the Copper Age and **Mike Rowlands** on the Late Bronze to Early Iron Age deserve to be discussed together, as they adopt a significantly different approach from that of Bintliff and Harding. Both authors stress the interconnectedness of European later prehistoric societies, evidenced by exchange systems effective over great distances. These ties beyond the immediate district are seen as equally if not more effective in initiating social change than internal processes of social differentiation based on control over subsistence resources. Sherratt does not however abandon the notion of directional evolution, despite obvious reservations about 'stages' and the narrow dogma of unilinealism. The Copper Age is envisaged as a more complex society than the Neolithic and anticipates features of the Bronze Age, with notable emphasis being placed on wider communication, especially via exchange and prestige outlets, and greater diffusion of ideas - both symbolic and functional. This very process of widening horizons is argued to be in itself a most potent force for social evolution, particularly in the transformational stage between what are seen as agriculturally-centred, broadly 'egalitarian' societies of the Early Neolithic and the aggressive, elitist, trading-based societies of later prehistoric (Bronze to Iron Age) Europe. An invaluable insight is Sherratt's placing this phase in social development along a sliding timescale, broadly running from east to west. The gradual emergence (with temporary hiccups) of more elaborate social organization reflects in his analysis the continual expansion and intensification of regional and inter-regional exchange systems. Traditional, broadly egalitarian (with limited power assigned to kin-heads and 'big men') and internally-centred communities, experience disruption as they become plugged into elite-centred networks of trade goods of a practical or purely prestige kind.

It is important to note that despite the central role of a primitive 'international market' in exchange items, which has over-ridden and absorbed local value systems, Sherratt's analysis still argues for the later Neolithic and Copper Age as one where 'big men' form the key to social structure, and for perceptible differences in social complexity in comparison to the preceding early Neolithic (kin-based, egalitarian) and the subsequent early Bronze and Iron Ages (chiefdom, paramount-chiefdom to princedom) societies. It is in effect a modified stage scheme that retains the outline of the neo-evolutionist taxonomy. Secondly, as is argued in the chapters by Bintliff, it is equally valid to suggest that the progressive elaboration of inter-regional exchange, via elite nodal points, could reflect the local emergence of land- and herd-based elites with the leisure and wealth to participate in prestige exchanges. The east-west bow wave effect could solely be accounted for by emphasizing its similarity to the time-lag of the inception of settled farming across Europe (creating a consequent delay in internal evolution amongst the communities of most recent origin), an argument that Sherratt acknowledges but dilutes with his exchange-interaction model run in tandem.

Mike Rowlands' analysis of developments around the turn of the first millennium bc (Late Bronze/Early Iron Age), employs the same emphasis as Sherratt on the 'extra-regional' perspective to be adopted in the search for explanations of the move towards more complex forms of society: "changing sequences of political and economic forms in different sectors of ... Europe ... it is argued here, are responses to increasing elaboration and intensification of the exchange networks upon which they are based". But in contrast to Sherratt, Rowlands emphasizes that the main networks are normally keyed in to more powerful economic and political systems far beyond European borders. In particular, reviving older diffusionist ideas, transformations in European society are crucially tied in to historical events in the states of the literate Near East. For example, the third-millennium bc changes discussed by Sherratt in a European perspective, are here envisaged as bow wave responses to the Urban Revolution in the Near East. The rise of industrial and commercial powers in the Eastern Mediterranean led to trade-orientated elites in South East Europe, and from here the waves of exchange created an ever-widening circle of trade-based elites across Europe, culminating in the prestige burials of the English Wessex Culture and elsewhere by the early second millennium bc. In this model the influence of 'world system' theory (Wallerstein 1974) is visible, and some strongly Formalist assumptions. A second phase of major change is that of the European Late Bronze Age, when the Near Eastern palace societies are crumbling (together with their European limb, the Aegean civilization of the Mycenaeans); in their place merchant oligarchies and mercantile empires with more free enterprise arise, creating a renewed push of commerce towards Europe. As a result there is a notable elaboration of continental European prestige-exchange spheres and of networks of chiefdoms and princedoms dependent upon them. These tendencies are further reinforced with the Early Iron Age expansion of Greek and Etruscan colonies and traders on the fringes of the 'barbarian' communities of continental Europe. The associated commercial pressure transforms certain regions into major territorial 'princedoms', whose rise and fall is critically dependent on the stability of commercial exchanges to the Mediterranean literate civilizations.

Despite the broader canvas on which Rowlands traces causative processes, it is still possible to isolate a directional evolution in his analysis: from small-scale chiefdoms and 'big man' systems, to proto-state, territorial 'polities' under central and internally highly-stratified aristocratic groups. However, echoing the more recent doubts of Service, and those of Fried, the reasons for organizational transformation are here largely attributed to the impact of more highly developed societies beyond the study area. Secondly, I have already raised the issue of internal versus external economy in my critique of Sherratt's chapter, and the point is equally valid in this later context. The debate is entered into at greater length in my Iron Age chapter.

Greek Society

Anthony Snodgrass's chapter represents the first of several concerned with the rise of a literate, urban civilization in Europe with expansive tendencies. In discussing the author's interpretations we will incorporate aspects dealt with in much more detail in Snodgrass's Archaic Greece (1980).

On the question of the origins of Greek state societies, Snodgrass contrasts two models: (a) indigenous takeoff based on a population explosion, increased ranking and the rise of a settlement hierarchy, producing secondary transformations in trade and industry and the growth of urbanism; (b) a catalyzing effect of Near Eastern state and city-based trade (cf. the Orientalizing period), stimulating increased social and settlement hierarchies in Greece.

Overall, Snodgrass prefers model (a) as the more important causal chain, and in a similar Substantivist approach, in dealing with the subsequent spread of Greek colonies around the Mediterranean and Black Sea, places the emphasis firmly (with some exceptions) on a background in land and population pressure in the Greek homeland in contrast to a model of expanding commercial systems. This emphasis upon regional evolution, particularly the connection between social and political structure in early historic Greece and rights over arable land, provides an essentially internalized explanation for the rise of 'democracy', in terms of power-sharing amongst a class of militarily-powerful yeoman farmers. It is suggested that the failure of this nexus in post-Classical times drew with it a reversal towards early Archaic, oligarchic forms of government. The city, seen largely in terms of Finley's (1973) 'parasitic' model, the absence of genuine technological advances, and the dependence of the whole system upon the demography -land productivity relationship, focusses our attention on the new **social** arrangements that underlay the political evolution and devolution, in particular the role of agrarian slavery.

In summary, Greek society is seen as essentially a primary civilization. Archaeology has recently contribut-

ed dramatically to our understanding of evolutionary processes, for example in its demonstration of the population explosion and of the consolidation of elite claims to local eminence as elements preceding the rise of large central places (the city state centres). This sequence, seen in detail (cf. Snodgrass, 1980) tends to shift the emphasis away from the secondary elaboration of commerce and industry towards the primary changes in the relationships of production within regional land-based economies (cf. Bintliff 1982). These same issues are treated in a very different way in Tim Potter's study of a broadly similar cultural sequence in early historic Italy, but in a related way in Rick Jones' subsequent chapter on the rise of Roman society in the Western Provinces.

Iron Age and Roman Italy

With **Tim Potter's** chapter we move west to study again the creation of early state societies, combined with urbanism, a common grouping for traditional definitions of civilization. He emphasizes the new roles and specialist activities that typify urban civilization, often associated with political formalization in terms of territorially-defined rights for 'citizens'. This stress on the specific connotations of urban society is reflected in later chapters by Jones and Gregory, as a particularly significant aspect of early European civilization and its socio-political structure. For Archaic to Classical Greece, Snodgrass (1980, this volume), has likewise pointed to the importance of the urban focus, but despite obvious parallels between his Archaic state and those of early historic Italy, he adopts a broadly Substantivist approach notably distinct from Potter's broadly Formalist model developed in the Italy chapter. Potter argues that trade and industrial production were vital, progressive forces in the rise of Etruscan and sub-Etruscan (e.g. Roman) polities; a linked prestige-exchange model (interactions with the Greek world), with strong transformational properties catalyzing local communities, evokes obvious parallels with Mike Rowlands' (this volume) model for the continental Early Iron Age. Investment in land by dominant urban elites is seen (also in agreement with Rowlands on the Celts) to be a late development, with initial status emergence and elaboration being attributed largely to international trade. Subsequently, the creation of ever larger political units or state/empire systems - culminating in the mature Roman Empire, is seen in the context of trade/territorial competition.

But alongside these 'modernist' models there is, within his treatment of the development of the later Roman Republic in Italy, a contrasted emphasis upon the swallowing up of agricultural land into fewer and fewer private hands (cf. Hopkins 1978) and the rise of the slave economy to replace the cannon-fodder of the peasant army; merchants and industrialists are considered to be far less relevant to this sector and era of social evolution. Furthermore, in detailed comments on trends in the Imperial Roman period, overall decline is envisaged in terms of manpower shortage and related to the cessation of imperial expansion with its flow of slaves.

In general terms, therefore, Italian civilized/urban society is argued to have arisen as a secondary formation due to interactions with Greek colonies; subsequently the former expands by conquest over much of temperate and all of Mediterranean Europe. Typical features of the social structure include dominant landed aristocrat rule, but also a major private industrial and merchant sector which both broadens the source of elite support and increasingly penetrates the tradional elite circle itself, thus tending to enlarge the social catchment involved in administration of the system.

Current archaeological and historical research are clearly working in harness to clarify the relative explanatory value of the two basic models utilized in this chapter: the world systems, Formalist, free-market approach to social change, and the land-based, regionally-centred, Substantivist approach typified by Finley (1973). A further debate, already alluded to in our discussion of Sherratt's chapter, is the existence of an alternative model to account for the apparent 'chain-reaction' of early state and proto-state societies across Europe from Greece to Italy to the Celtic sphere. As a counterpoise to the 'core-periphery' approach of Rowlands and Potter, I have suggested (Iron Age chapter) that we may be witnessing slightly staggered, parallel evolutionary sequences for large areas of Iron Age Europe at this time, in which Greek, Italian and Celtic societies are independently approaching climax growth during the first millennium BC; population explosion and a takeoff in social superstructure lead to increasing interactions between these three cultural spheres and their eventual merging by conquest.

In general, allowing for the 'secondary civilization' factor, the area and period are treated by Potter in an analysis consistent with traditional views on the distinct nature of pre-industrial State society (post-'higher barbarism'/chiefdom society): urban centres, literacy, class differentiation, rural/urban contrasts, slave-dependent economy.

The Roman Western Provinces

Rick Jones follows the emphasis of Snodgrass and Potter on the characteristic urban core to Greco-Roman civilization and its associated dominant elite class. But in the Roman West we also have to deal with the assimilation of tribal and proto-state societies of the Celtic world. Consistent with traditional social evolutionary schemes, the major features of literacy, monumental architecture of a public nature, centralized government structure and population nodes/urban foci, are strikingly apparent and contrasted with preceding achievements. Yet at the same time, the ease of native assimilation reflects the incorporation, not elimination, of local elite groups, thereby bringing into play an already well-developed system of surplus accumulation in the hands of local aristocracies. Roman policy for these new provinces, as Jones points out, was a Do-It-Yourself affair, with only advice and some minor economic assistance given to indigenous populations in forming networks of local government infrastructure and towns: the desire to emulate the new power in every respect did the rest. In this remarkable process the long tradition of 'prestige spheres' in Europe reaches its climax in the Pax Romana.

Jones reminds us of central issues still under debate, such as the role of a 'market economy' in the Empire; or the concept, in contrast, of Finley's 'consumer city', the product of a very different socio-economic system to the model of widespread mercantile/industrial towns often associated with the 'market' lobby. Despite the evidence that can be presented for both viewpoints, it is undeniable that after the initial, highly disruptive phase of the early Roman conquest, there is a significant tendency for a distinct regionalization in the Western provinces of social and economic affairs. Imports are replaced by local industry, administration and responsibility devolve to a very considerable extent upon local notables who may generally have been native aristocrats, yet who strive to produce a plethora of miniature replica 'Romes' in each minor provincial town and its region.

On the other hand, there are clear changes in the archaeological record with the incorporation of Iron Age societies into the Empire - especially the evidence for a far higher population, not just the continuance of growth demonstrable from Late Bronze Age through to the Late (pre-Roman) Iron Age. This jump is clearly associated with the new colonial society and economy. It can be argued that the percentage of people to be supported 'internally' (i.e. by and in each province) rose sharply: administrators, craftsmen (new needs), businessmen and professional soldiers. This transformation was linked to far more effective 'towns' and garrison/defence measures, to more centralized and demand-stimulating manufacture and exchange. All this should imply a more productive economy at its base; yet since Celtic agricultural technology seems to have been in no way inferior to Roman, it must be postulated that actual as opposed to potential production rose to the colonial stimulus of greater demand. The rise of villas is often considered to indicate the openly commercial end of this farming intensification, producing for the new, more centralised and more widely-marketed consumer-trade of towns and garrison points. Are villa owners merely local nobles operating in the new economy?

Against such internal changes the role of long-distance trade, especially on an inter-province level, poses an as yet unresolved problem in its unclear effect on local social and economic processes. In many respects Jones seems to support a 'regional' viewpoint with the import/export flows being treated as only a minor sector in Western provincial socio-economic systematics. A far more extreme situation is nonetheless raised, in contrast, with the regional effects of very widespread factors such as the Empire-wide inflation-depression cycles relating to the Imperial coinage.

In any case, by the Late Empire a clear reversion is argued to a more 'embedded' and micro-regional socio-economy, with local landed magnates forming nodal points of authority across a landscape where the towns and their official superstructure are declining rapidly; possibly trade and commerce are also shifting towards rural, aristocratic estate foci. At least in Gaul and Germany there is a case to be made for a substantial degree of continuity of this estate-focussed society into early proto-feudal communities. Referring back to the very beginnings of Greco-Roman state societies in the Mediterranean, the process of political elaboration may now have come full circle, with incipient/shrunken town and rural, estate-based aristocrat/chieftain political structure (Snodgrass 1980, this volume; Bintliff, Iron Age chapter, this volume).

If we choose to prefer the regionally-centred model of Jones for the Western Provinces, relegating to a low level the proportion of the 'national product' leaving each region, one might envisage a model of provincial assimilation to Roman rule that achieved in the main a 'creaming-off' of regional products for extra-provincial purposes, coupled with the moving into the new provinces of people at all social levels who find an effective niche within a more productive, but largely still internalized, economy (cf. Fulford 1978). The leading area for research thus opened up is the process of transformation of the late Celtic patron-client network into that underpinning the new provincial leadership. In theory the Roman attitude, to consolidate then manipulate existing rights and obligations in all but the most brittle tribes, should have smoothed the transition. Yet as Jones makes quite clear, adoption of the new culture involved mobilization of far greater amounts of surplus food, raw materials and finished products than previously required or achieved. How were these produced without (as far as can be seen) direct Roman interference and funding?

The Byzantine World

Even more than in the previous chapters, the central role of urbanism, as an ideological and social phenomenon as much as a physical agglomeration, emerges from **Timothy Gregory's** analysis of social structure and social change in the Byzantine Balkans. Gregory's core argument is of the greatest importance: namely that the tradition of the early historic autonomous city-states of Greece, of innumerable district central places which formed distinct cultural and political foci, survived as a resilient regional structure in this area throughout the subsequent millennium of submergence within vast imperial systems. When the latter systems finally failed, in the Dark Ages of the seventh to ninth centuries AD for the Eastern Empire, but earlier, from the fourth to eighth centuries for the West, the inherent commitment of the elite class in the East to urban foci and lifestyle gave a greater survival strength there to the forms and traditions of the Greco-Roman world, than in the West. Both East and West suffered regular and major migrations by 'barbarians', and quite possibly the scale of population change was greater in the area of the Eastern Empire, yet the recovery of Mediterranean Classical civilization is only a reality in the East (even if tainted with the charge of 'fossilization', and despite the 'origin charter' posturing of Charlemagne). Ironically, this very strength of the small 'polis' unit had been achieved as an undisturbed characteristic largely as a result of the prolonged political irrelevance of Greece from Hellenistic through Roman Imperial times. The town and its integral hierarchy of local magnates existed across Greece as a vast series of petty rural societies with virtually no wider powers, yet with a formal pretence at sovereignty and government functions. With the breakdown in the much larger structures of real power, these city-state cocoons came into their own as bastions of complex society from which the mature Byzantine civilization was able to reconstitute itself.

The apparent paradox of scale, between effective imperial political structure and the anomalous persistence of regional and micro-regional socio-economic structures of pre-imperial origin, might be said to disappear if we opt for a 'creaming-off' model for ancient empires, as opposed to the Formalist position where each limb of the total system is essential to all the others in terms of market flows. If we follow the implications of the former, regionally-orientated model, we would characterize an ancient empire as a physical juxtaposition of regions that though formally dependent upon a central political focus and a central people, remained primarily internalized in the production and consumption of everyday foodstuffs and raw materials (excepting in particular certain categories of scarce commodities). The strength of an empire like Rome's lay, therefore, not in the flow of silver from the east nor in the latest artillery systems on the limes of the Danube frontier, but rather at the level of the health of its cumulative regional components in manpower and basic productivity. The phenomena of Roman decline in the West, as discussed by Potter and Jones, harmonise with such an interpretation. For the East, consequently, it should come as no surprise that the traditional 'polis' structure, an integrated unit developed from regional self-absorption, should prove to be a powerful adaptive module for a civilization under threat.

Post-Roman Western Europe

Chris Arnold's chapter takes up this analysis from the point of view of the former Western provinces of the Empire during the Dark Ages and beyond. Once more we seem to be on the threshold of the origins of the State and of civilized society, but over a thousand years after the processes that Snodgrass and Potter are concerned with in Greece and Italy. The usual debate of primary/secondary forces arises, and once again the early role of prestige exchange is discussed from the contrasted approaches of an externalist model (commercial catalyst) and an internalist model (subsistence changes lead to elite enhancement, which leads to wider inter-elite links). On balance, Arnold seems to favour the latter, with 'administered trade' of Polanyi (1957) type developing from emergent princedoms that have their roots in the regional 'privatization' and capital accumulation of land and local raw materials. (The recent study by Hodges (1982), however, gives greater emphasis to the externalist model for the same era). In the tertiary process of the cohesion of the Anglo-Saxon kingdoms, a role for territorial competition opens up links to the theories of Carneiro (1970). Only at the end of the development sequence does a semblance of 'market' economy arise.

In an intriguing parallel sequence for the first millennium **AD,** to what may be inferred concerning late prehistoric and early historic state origins in the first millennium **BC,** Arnold begins with small-scale, chieftain societies of the Migration Period, in many respects reminiscent of Neolithic-Bronze Age communities; from thence we proceed, via competing regional princedoms, to centralized kingdoms with the associated rise of a bureaucracy and town foci. A dramatic evolutionary pathway, yet compressed into the few centuries from the fifth to the ninth centuries AD. This short time scale for such a degree of social change might be explained by 'world systems' theorists as ruling out autonomous, internal evolution and demonstrating the role of complex societies in transforming more primitive neighbouring communities; however it could equally be argued that the accumulated agricultural and technological expertise achieved in much of Europe by the first millennium AD provided a hitherto unparalleled capacity (as the post-Dark Age population recovery bears witness), to nourish a remarkably rapid rerun of the process of local state formation.

However, unresolved problems such as the role of economic interactions with contemporary more complex societies (especially the Byzantine Empire), may still frustrate attempts to treat the 'rise of the West' as a 'primary' sequence to statehood. Yet if the apparent dominance of internal factors causing increasing social and economic differentiation is sustained in future research, it will serve to reinforce processual explanations offered elsewhere in this volume by Newell, Bintliff, Harding and Snodgrass.

Viking Society

Klaus Randsborg's chapter offers us a very clear, directional evolution for Denmark (taken as a microcosm for Scandinavian developments), running from egalitarian villages of the Iron Age (c.0 BC/AD) to the first Danish state in the tenth century AD. On the way we pass through chiefdom society, thus accomplishing yet another remarkable developmental cycle for a period of one millennium. In his analysis of the highly significant intermediate stage of chiefdoms, Randsborg attributes their power to the ability to attract and sustain a retinue via gift exchange and the organization of profitable raids. Crises in the flow of prestige wealth for maintaining the chiefdom structure stimulate the greatest frequency of external pillaging expeditions, but later in the millennium the energy of chiefs is absorbed into building up large landed estates as an alternative base of wealth and power. At this latter stage Danish society becomes prone to external attack itself. But until this later period, the overall explanatory emphasis of Randsborg is one of the rise and elaboration of a chieftain caste maintained by chains of prestige exchange, from one chief to another and from leader to support group; only limited scope is assigned to preferential access to land and labour within

Viking society. The element of a landed aristocracy, as with Rowlands and Potter on Celtic and early historic Italian societies, is seen as a secondary development.

Despite the emphasis on external factors (such as the supply of precious metal, interactions with neighbouring political systems), and a Formalist stress on social structure as dependent upon the Viking equivalent of portable symbolic capital, a notable attempt is made to relate these approaches to what may be inferred of regional subsistence economics (the role of climatic change, soil fertility and patterns of land ownership). Nonetheless, since Randsborg's conceptual emphasis aligns him with the chapters by Sherratt, Rowlands and Potter, and in order to take account of insights and models presented in other chapters of this volume, an alternative processual interpretation could perhaps be proposed for the same data. In particular, there does seem to be insufficient attention devoted to the articulation between the exchange of wealth items amongst the elite and the relationships of agricultural production and labour service between the elite and the subordinate majority of the population. Is it not conceivable to suggest that an initial degree of social differentiation, based upon private or traditional preferential land ownership, created circumstances in which the elite could obtain and circulate portable wealth?

The argument that our starting point in this chapter, Iron Age society in the Germanic-Teutonic area is generally one of egalitarian peasant families, is actually rather controversial. Princely burials of the 'Roman' Iron Age have been viewed as evidence for an atypical degree of social complexity nourished by 'prestige trade' relations with the Empire (cf. Hedeager 1980), yet contemporary settlements have evidenced what should be chieftains' establishments that seem to be well above the average family in terms of subsistence production. The analysis I have offered elsewhere (Iron Age chapter) of pre-Roman and Roman-era Iron Age society in both Celtic and Germanic spheres would seek to recognise the dominance of chieftain society from the first; I have further argued for its socio-economic structure being one in which preferential access to subsistence products, especially land, may have been central to elite maintenance.

If we turn to the celebrated Viking expansion overseas, Randsborg's emphasis on mobile capital accumulation underplays the settlement component, and the latter aim helps to explain the fact that much of the foreign loot failed to get back into the economy of the homeland. The very notable Scandinavian settlement of the English Danelaw, in Normandy, Iceland and Greenland, and colonization on a limited basis in America, require to be treated as an issue of central relevance to understanding conditions in the settlers' homelands. In the same vein, more weight ought to be given to the runic evidence for the importance of claims to aristocratic lands, one of the features taken by Randsborg as an indication of the emergent state (the comparison to Archaic Greek hero cults is illuminating in a closely parallel context, cf. Snodgrass 1980 and this volume). Land rights are admitted to be very relevant to the understanding of the final stage in the Danish sequence, state creation, but clearly their role in the earlier stages of the sequence towards statehood deserves greater consideration.

External pressures from the more developed Frankish society to the south are well attested (cf. the Danevirke walls, a co-ordinated response), yet despite the potential here for a 'secondary civilization' model, the emergence of the Danish Viking state is much later in time. The central argument on local state-formation revolves around processes integral to the pre-state, chiefdom societies of Randsborg's middle phase (although we

have suggested that a separation-off of his early stage on the grounds of it being **egalitarian** may not be supportable). For the middle phase, at one extreme, we might be led into a Formalist, world systems view where factors such as the flow of silver around the European subcontinent act as social catalysts. Or, to develop the alternative, regional model, one might conversely consider the increasing elaboration of local social hierarchies towards state level, as commencing with chieftains whose control over exotica (as power symbols and indicators of retinue allegiance) rests firmly on private control over surpluses of crops, herds and labour. If local resources become inadequate in this latter sense, rather than that of the first model, colonization of land abroad may be desirable if not essential. The Viking raids that were not made with the intention to settle would have provided plentiful status ornaments and personal prestige for an elite sector whose basic support base (for the chief and his immediate followers) was ensured by inequalities of land access in the homeland.

That debate, like that concerning all the other fundamental issues in this volume, continues. But it must be clear now, that the way forward, the direction in which the greatest potential is seen to lie for illuminating European, pre-industrial, social evolution, is along the pathway of social archaeology.

Bradford, June 1983

NOTES

Note 1
Sources that were particularly helpful in preparing this brief historical investigation were Cliff Slaughter's chapter in the present volume, Cohen and Service (1978), Trigger (1978), Claessen and Skalnik (1978), Dunnell (1980) and McNairn (1980). Cliff Slaughter also provided numerous comments and criticisms on the text which have been incorporated into this final version.

Note 2
We should in fact distinguish between (a) Marx's more empirically based analysis of the workings of capitalist society, which is more in tune with the 'processes' approach of Darwinian, biological evolution and (b) the more speculative reconstructions of Marx and Engels on the developmental stages and inner workings of pre-capitalist societies, akin in methodology to the social-philosophical tradition. It is the latter aspect of the Marxist heritage that is the object of critical comment here, since this body of theory has underlain the characteristic interpretations of social evolution to be found in Eastern bloc archaeology and history to the present day.

Note 3
Subsequent to my reaching this conclusion for European archaeology I discovered that a similar tendency was detected for American archaeology over the same period by Willey and Phillips (1958).

BIBLIOGRAPHY

ARNOLD, C.J. 1980 - "Wealth and social structure: a matter of life and death", pp.81-142 in P. Rahtz, T. Dickinson and L. Watts (Eds.) Anglo-Saxon Cemeteries 1979. British Archaeological Reports 82, Oxford.

ASHMORE, W. 1981 (Ed.) - Lowland Maya Settlement Patterns. University of New Mexico Press, Albuquerque.

BINFORD, L.R. 1962 - "Archaeology as anthropology", American Antiquity vol. 28, pp.217-25.

BINFORD, L.R. 1964 - "A consideration of archaeological research design", American Antiquity vol. 29, pp.425-41.

BINFORD, L.R. 1968 - "Archaeological perspectives", pp.5-32 in S.R. and L.R. Binford (Eds.) New Perspectives in Archaeology. Aldine Press, Chicago.

BINFORD, L.R. 1971 - "Mortuary practices: their study and their potential", pp.6-29 in Social Dimensions of Mortuary Practices, Memoir No. 25, Society for American Archaeology, (American Antiquity vol. 36).

BINFORD, L.R. 1977 - "General Introduction", pp.1-10 in L.R. Binford (Ed.) For Theory Building in Archaeology. Academic Press, New York.

BINTLIFF, J.L. 1977a - Natural Environment and Human Settlement in Prehistoric Greece. British Archaeological Reports, Suppl. Ser. 28, Oxford.

BINTLIFF, J.L. 1977b - "New approaches to human geography. Prehistoric Greece: a case-study", pp.59-114 in F.W. Carter (Ed.) An Historical Geography of the Balkans. Academic Press, London.

BINTLIFF, J.L. 1982 - "Settlement patterns, land tenure and social structure: a diachronic model", pp.106-11 in C. Renfrew and S. Shennan (Eds.) Ranking, Resource and Exchange. Cambridge University Press, Cambridge.

BOCK, K.E. 1974 - "Comparison of histories: the contribution of Henry Maine", Comp. Studies in Society and History vol. 16, pp.232-62.

BOSERUP, E. 1965 - The Conditions for Agricultural Growth. Allen and Unwin, London.

BURKITT, M.C. 1926 - Our Early Ancestors. Cambridge University Press, Cambridge.

CARNEIRO, R.L. 1970 - "A theory of the origin of the State", Science vol. 169, pp.733-38.

CARNEIRO, R.L. 1978 - "Political expansion as an expression of the principle of competitive exclusion", pp.205-23 in R. Cohen and E.R. Service (Eds.) Origins of the State.

CHAPMAN, R.W. 1979 - Comments to "The social anthropology of a Neolithic cemetery in the Netherlands", by P. van de Velde, Current Anthropology vol. 20, pp.37-58.

CHAPMAN, R.W., KINNES, I. and RANDSBORG, K. 1981 (Eds) - The Archaeology of Death. Cambridge University Press, Cambridge.

CHILDE, V.G. 1925 - The Dawn of European Civilisation. London.

CHILDE, V.G. 1926 - The Aryans. London.

CHILDE, V.G. 1928 - The Most Ancient East: the Oriental Prelude to European Prehistory. London.

CHILDE, V.G. 1930 - The Bronze Age. Cambridge.

CHILDE, V.G. 1934 - New Light on the Most Ancient East, the Oriental Prelude to European Prehistory. London.

CHILDE, V.G. 1935 - "Changing methods and aims in prehistory: presidential address for 1935", Procs. of the Prehistoric Society, vol. 1, pp.1-15.

CHILDE, V.G. 1936 - Man Makes Himself. London.

CHILDE, V.G. 1939 - The Dawn of European Civilisation (3rd Ed. revised). London.

CHILDE, V.G. 1942 - What Happened in History. Harmondsworth, London.

CHILDE, V.G. 1946a - "Archaeology and anthropology", Southwestern Journal of Anthropology, vol. 2, pp.243-51.

CHILDE, V.G. 1946b - Scotland Before the Scots. London.

CHILDE, V.G. 1947 - The Dawn of European Civilisation. (4th Ed. rev.).

CHILDE, V.G. 1950 - Prehistoric Migrations in Europe. London.

CHILDE, V.G. 1951 - Social Evolution. Watts and Co., London.

CHILDE, V.G. 1958a - "Retrospect", Antiquity vol. 32, pp.69-74.

CHILDE, V.G. 1958b - The Prehistory of European Society. Harmondsworth, London.

CLAESSEN, H.J.M. and SKALNIK, P. 1978a (Eds.) - The Early State. Mouton, The Hague.

CLAESSEN, H.J.M. and SKALNIK, P. 1978b - "The early state: theories and hypotheses", pp.3-29 in Claessen and Skalnik (Eds.) The Early State.

CLARK, J.G.D. 1940 - Prehistoric England. Batsford, London.

CLARK, J.G.D. 1946 - From Savagery to Civilisation. Cobbett Press, London.

CLARK, J.G.D. 1947 - Archaeology and Society (2nd Ed. Rev.). Methuen and Co., London.

CLARK, J.G.D. 1952 - Prehistoric Europe: the Economic Basis. Methuen and Co., London.

CLARK, J.G.D. 1966 - "Traffic in stone axe and adze blades", Economic History Review. pp.1-28.

CLARKE, D.L. 1968 - Analytical Archaeology. Methuen and Co. London.

CLARKE, D.L. 1972a (Ed.) - Models in Archaeology. Methuen and Co., London.

CLARKE, D.L. 1972b - "A provisional model of an Iron Age society and its settlement system", pp.801-69 in Clarke (Ed.) Models in Archaeology.

COE, M.D. 1961 - "Social typology and tropical forest civilisations", Comp. Studies in Society and History, vol. 4, pp. 65-?.

COE, M.D. and FLANNERY, K.V. 1964 - "Microenvironments and Mesoamerican prehistory", Science vol. 143, pp.650-54.

COHEN, R. 1981 - "Evolutionary epistemology and human values", Current Anthropology, vol. 22, pp.201-18.

COHEN, R. and SERVICE, E.R. 1978 (Eds.) - Origins of the State. Institute for the Study of Human Issues. Philadelphia.

COHN, B.S. 1980 - "History and anthropology: the state of play", Comp. Studies in Society and History, vol. 22, pp.198-221.

COLES, J.M. and HARDING, A.F. 1979 - The Bronze Age in Europe. Methuen and Co., London.

CULBERT, T.P. 1973 (Ed.) - The Classic Maya Collapse. University of New Mexico Press, Albuquerque.

DALTON, G. 1981 - "Anthropological models in archaeological perspective", pp.17-48 in Hodder, I., Isaac,G. and Hammond, N. (Eds.) Pattern of the Past.Studies in honour of David Clarke.

DANIEL. G. 1966 - Man Discovers His Past. BBC Publications, London.

DANIEL, G. 1967 - The Origins and Growth of Archaeology. Penguin Books, London.

DIAKONOV, I.M. 1959 - Social and Governmental Organisation of Ancient Mesopotamia. Nauka, Moscow.

DIAKONOV, I.M. 1969 (Ed.) - Ancient Mesopotamia. Nauka, Moscow.

DIXON, P. 1979 - "Towerhouses, Pelehouses and Border Society", Archaeological Journal, vol. 136, pp.240-52.

DREWETT, P. 1979 - "New evidence for the structure and function of Middle Bronze Age round houses in Sussex" Archaeological Journal, vol. 136, pp.3-11.

DUNNELL, R.C. 1980 - "Evolutionary theory and archaeology", pp.35-99 in M.B. Schiffer (Ed.) Advances in Archaeological Method and Theory, vol. 3. Academic Press, New York.

ELLISON, A. 1981 - "Towards a socioeconomic model for the Middle Bronze Age in southern England", pp.413-38 in I. Hodder, G. Isaac and N. Hammond (Eds.) Pattern of the Past. Studies in honour of David Clarke.

ENGELS, F. 1877/78 - Herrn Eugen Dührings Umwälzung der Wissenschaft .(Anti-Dühring). Marx-Engels Werke 20, pp.5-303.

ENGELS, F. 1884 - Der Ursprung der Familie, des Privateigentums und des Staats. Zürich.

FINLEY, M.I. 1973 - The Ancient Economy. Chatto and Windus, London.

FLANNERY, K.V. 1976 (Ed.) - The Early Mesoamerican Village. Academic Press, New York.

FRANKENSTEIN, S. and ROWLANDS, M.J. 1978 - "The internal structure and regional context of early iron age society in south-western Germany", Bull. of the Institute of Archaeology, University of London, vol. 15, pp.73-112.

FRERE, S. 1978 - Britannia. A History of Roman Britain. (Rev. ed.) Routledge and Kegan Paul, London.

FRIED, M.H. 1967 - The Evolution of Political Society. Random House, New York.

FRIED, M.H. 1978 - "The State, the chicken and the egg: or, what came first?", pp.35-47 in R. Cohen and E.R. Service (Eds.) Origins of the State.

FULFORD, M. 1978 - "The interpretation of Britain's late Roman trade: the scope of medieval historical and archaeological analogy", pp.59-69 in Roman Shipping and Trade, edited by J. du Plat Taylor and H. Cleere. CBA Res. Rep. 24.

GAMBLE, C. 1980 - "Information exchange in the Palaeolithic", Nature vol. 283, pp.522-23.

GATHERCOLE, P. 1971 - "Patterns in prehistory: an examination of the later thinking of V. Gordon Childe", World Archaeology vol. 3, pp.225-32.

GILMAN, A. 1981 - "The development of social stratification in Bronze Age Europe", Current Anthropology, vol.22, pp.1-23.

GIMBUTAS, M. 1965 - Bronze Age Cultures in Central and Eastern Europe. Mouton, the Hague.

HAGEN, A. 1980 - "Trends in Scandinavian archaeology at the transition to the 1980s", Norwegian Archaeological Review, vol. 13, pp.1-8.

HAMMOND, N. 1977 (Ed.) - Social Process in Maya Prehistory. Academic Press, New York.

HARRIS, M. 1968 - The Rise of Anthropological Theory. Crowell, New York.

HAWKES, C.F.C. 1954 - "Archaeological theory and method: some suggestions from the Old World", American Anthropologist vol. 56, pp.155-68.

HEDEAGER, L. 1980 - "Besiedlung, soziale Struktur und politische Organisation in der älteren und jüngeren römischen Kaiserzeit Ostdänemarks", Praehistorische Zeitschrift vol. 55, pp.38-109.

HEMPEL, C.G. 1965 - Aspects of Scientific Explanation. Free Press, New York.

HERRMANN, J. and SELLNOW, I. 1976 (Eds.) - Beiträge zur Enstehung des Staates. Akademie Verlag, Berlin.

HERRMANN, J. 1976 - "Allod und Feudum als Grundlagen des west- und mitteleuropäischen Feudalismus und der feudal Staatsbilding", pp.164-201 in Herrmann and Sellnow (Eds.)

HODDER, I. , ISAAC, G. and HAMMOND, N. 1981 (Eds) - Pattern of the Past. Studies in honour of David Clarke. Cambridge University Press, Cambridge.

HODGES, R. 1982 - Dark Age Economics. Duckworth, London.

HOPKINS, K. 1978 - Conquerors and Slaves. Cambridge University Press, Cambridge.

JOCHIM, M.A. 1976 - Hunter-gatherer Subsistence and Settlement: a Predictive Model. Academic Press, New York.

JONES, R.F. 1980 - "Computers and cemeteries: opportunities and limitations", pp.179-95 in P. Rahtz, T. Dickinson and L. Watts (Eds.) Anglo-Saxon Cemeteries 1979. British Archaeological Reports 82, Oxford.

KELLER, D.R. and RUPP, D.W. 1983 (Eds.) -Archaeological Survey in the Mediterranean Area, British Archaeological Reports, Int. Ser 155, Oxford.

KIDD, D. 1980 - "Barbarian Europe in the first millennium", pp.295-303 in A. Sherratt (Ed.) The Cambridge

Encyclopedia of Archaeology. Cambridge University Press, Cambridge.

KLEJN, L.S. 1974 - "Kossinna im Abstand von vierzig Jahren", Jahrb. Mitteldtsch. Vorgesch. vol. 58, pp.7-55.

KLEJN, L.S. 1977 - "A panorama of theoretical archaeology", Current Anthropology vol. 18, pp.1-42.

KOSSACK, G., HARCK, O. and REICHSTEIN, J. 1974 - "Zehn Jahre Siedlungsforschung in Archsum auf Sylt", Ber. der Römisch-Germanischen Kommission 55, pp.261-427.

KOSSINNA, G. 1911 - Die Herkunft der Germanen. Kurt Kabitzsch, Leipzig.

KRADER, L. 1975- The Asiatic Mode of Production. Van Gorcum, Assen.

KRADER, L. 1976 - "Social evolution and social revolution", Dialectical Anthropolgy vol. 1, pp.109-120.

KRISTIANSEN, K. and PALUDAN-MÜLLER, C. 1978 (Eds.) -New Directions in Scandinavian Archaeology. The National Museum of Denmark, Copenhagen.

KRISTIANSEN, K. 1978 - "The consumption of wealth in Bronze Age Denmark. A study in the dynamics of economic processes in tribal societies", pp.158-90 in K. Kristiansen and C. Paludan-Müller (Eds.) New Directions.

KRÜGER, B. 1976 - "Auflösungserscheinungen gentilgesellschaftlicher Produktionsverhältnisse bei den germanischen Stämmen in den Jahrhunderten um die Zeitwende", pp.147-163 in Herrmann and Sellnow (Eds.) Beiträge zur Enstehung

LARSEN, M.T. 1979 (Ed.) - Power and Propaganda. Akademisk Forlag, Copenhagen.

LEACH, E. 1973 - "Concluding Address", pp.761-71 in C. Renfrew (Ed.) The Explanation of Culture Change. Duckworth, London.

LEE, R.B. and DE VORE, I. 1968 (Eds.) - Man The Hunter. Aldine Press, Chicago.

LENSKI, G. 1976 - "History and social change", American Journal of Sociology vol. 82, pp.548-64.

LUBBOCK, J. 1865 - Prehistoric Times, as Illustrated by Ancient Remains and the Manners and Customs of Modern Savages. Williams and Norgate, London.

Mc C. ADAMS, R. 1966 - The Evolution of Urban Society: Early Mesopotamia and Prehispanic Mexico. Aldine Press, Chicago.

McGOVERN, T.H. 1981 - "The economics of extinction in Norse Greenland", pp.404-33 in T.M.L. Wigley et al. (Eds.) Climate and History. Cambridge University Press, Cambridge.

McNAIRN, B. 1980 - The Method and Theory of V. Gordon Childe. Edinburgh University Press, Edinburgh.

MARX, K. (1857-8) 1939 - Grundrisse der Kritik der politischen Ökonomie . Moscow.

MARX, K. (1867) 1970 - Capital. Translated from the 3rd German edition of 1883. Lawrence and Wishart, London.

MARX, K. 1972 - The Ethnological Notebooks of Karl Marx. Translated and edited by L. Krader. Van Gorcum. Assen.

MORGAN, L.H. 1877 - Ancient Society. World Publishing Company, Cleveland.

MUIR, R. 1980- "Cambridgeshire dykes retain their secrets", Geographical Magazine, December 1980, pp.198-204.

NAROLL, R. 1956 - "A preliminary index of social development", American Anthropologist vol. 58, pp.687-715.

OTTO, K.-H. and BRACHMANN, H.J. 1975 (Eds.) - Moderne Probleme der Archäologie. Akademie Verlag, Berlin.

PEEBLES, C.S. and KUS, S.M. 1977 - "Some archaeological correlates of ranked societies", American Antiquity vol. 42, pp.421-48.

PIGGOTT, S. 1965 - Ancient Europe: from the Beginnings of Agriculture to Classical Antiquity. Edinburgh University Press, Edinburgh.

PLATT, C. 1978 - Medieval England: A Social History and Archaeology from the Conquest to AD 1600. Routledge and Kegan Paul, London.

PLUMB, J.H. 1969 - The Death of the Past. Macmillan, London.

POLANYI, K., ARENSBERG, C.M. and PEARSON, H.W. 1957 (Eds.) - Trade and Market in the Early Empires. Free Press, New York.

POSTAN, M.M. 1975 - The Medieval Economy and Society. Penguin Books, London.

POTTER, T.W. 1979- The Changing Landscape of South Etruria. Elek, London.

RAHTZ, P. 1981 - The New Medieval Archaeology. Inaugural Lecture, University of York, 1980.

RAHTZ, P. 1983- "New approaches to Medieval Archaeology Part I", pp.12-23 in D.A. Hinton (Ed.) 25 Years of Medieval Archaeology. Dept. of Prehistory, Sheffield University.

RANDSBORG, K. 1974 - "Social stratification in Early Bronze Age Denmark: a study in the regulation of cultural systems", Praehistorische Zeitschrift, vol. 49, pp.38-61.

RANDSBORG, K. 1975 - "Social dimensions of Early Neolithic Denmark", Procs. of the Prehistoric Society. vol. 41, pp.105-18.

RANDSBORG, K. 1980 - The Viking Age in Denmark. Duckworth, London.

RAPER, R.A. 1977 -"The analysis of the urban structure of Pompeii: a sociological examination of land use (semimicro)", pp.189-221 in D.L. Clarke (Ed.) Spatial Archaeology. Academic Press, London.

REDFIELD, R. 1953 - The Primitive World and its Transformations. Cornell University Press, Ithaca, New York.

REID, P.E.W. 1979 - An Analysis of Trade Mechanisms in European Prehistory. University Microfilms. PhD thesis, University of New York (Buffalo).

RENFREW, C. 1972 - The Emergence of Civilisation: the Cyclades and the Aegean in the Third Millennium BC. Methuen and Co., London.

RENFREW, C. 1973a - Before Civilisation. Jonathan Cape, London.

38

RENFREW, C. 1973b - Social Archaeology. Inaugural lecture, University of Southampton.

RENFREW, C. 1975- "Trade as action at a distance: questions of integration and communication", pp.3-59 in J.A. Sabloff and C.C. Lamberg-Karlovsky (Eds.) Ancient Civilisation and Trade. University of New Mexico Press, Albuquerque.

RENFREW, C. 1977 - "Alternative models for exchange and spatial distribution", pp.71-90 in T.K. Earle and J.E. Ericson (Eds) Exchange Systems in Prehistory. Academic Press, New York.

RENFREW, C. 1979 - Investigations in Orkney. Thames and Hudson, London.

RENFREW, C. 1980 - "The Great Tradition versus the Great Divide: archaeology as anthropology?", American Journal of Archaeology vol. 84, pp.287-98.

RENFREW, C. and SHENNAN, S. 1982 (Eds.) - Ranking, Resource and Exchange. Cambridge University Press, Cambridge.

RENFREW, C. and WAGSTAFF, M. 1982 (Eds.) - An Island Polity. The Archaeology of exploitation in Melos. Cambridge University Press, Cambridge.

RODWELL, R. 1981 - "Iron Age coinage: a counter reply", p.56 in B. Cunliffe (Ed) Coinage and Society in Britain and Gaul. CBA Res. Rep. 38. London.

ROWLANDS, M.J. 1973 - "Modes of exchange and the incentives for trade, with reference to later European prehistory", pp.589-600 in C.Renfrew (Ed.) The Explanation of Culture Change. Duckworth, London.

ROWLANDS, M.J. 1980 - "Kinship, alliance and exchange in the European Bronze Age", pp.15-55 in J. Barrett and R. Bradley (Eds.) The British Later Bronze Age. British Archaeological Reports, 83, Oxford.

SAHLINS, M.D. 1958 - Social Stratification in Polynesia. University of Washington Press, Seattle.

SAHLINS, M.D. 1960 - "Evolution: specific and general", pp.12-44 in Sahlins and Service (Eds.) Evolution and Culture.

SAHLINS, M.D. 1963 - "Poor man, rich man, Big Man, chief: political types in Melanesia and Polynesia", Comp. Studies in Society and History vol. 5, pp.285-303.

SAHLINS, M.D. 1968 - "Notes on the original affluent society", Discussions, Pt. IIb, pp.85-89 in Lee, R.B. and De Vore, I. (Eds.) Man the Hunter.

SAHLINS, M.D. 1972 - Stone Age Economics. Aldine Press, Chicago.

SAHLINS, M.D. and SERVICE, E.R. 1960 (Eds.) - Evolution and Culture. University of Michigan Press, Ann Arbor.

SANDERS, W.T. and WEBSTER, D. 1978 - "Unilinealism, multilinealism, and the evolution of complex societies", pp.249-302 in C.L. Redman et al. (Eds.) Social Archaeology. Academic Press, New York.

SELKIRK, A. 1982-3 - Editorial comments and book reviews, Current Archaeology nos. 82-85.

SELLNOW, W. 1976 - "Marx, Engels und Lenin zu dem Problem der Staatsentstehung", pp.13-26 in J. Herrmann and I. Sellnow (Eds.) Beiträge zur Entstehung.

SERVICE, E.R. 1971 - Primitive Social Organisation: An Evolutionary Perspective. (2nd Ed.) Random House, New York.

SERVICE, E.R. 1975 - Origins of the State and Civilisation. Norton, New York.

SERVICE, E.R. 1978 - "Classical and modern theories of the origins of government", pp.21-34 in R. Cohen and E.R. Service (Eds.) Origins of the State.

SHENNAN, S. 1975 - "The social organisation at Branc", Antiquity vol. 49, pp.279-88.

SHENNAN, S.J. 1980 - "Osteology and prehistoric society", Nature vol. 283, pp.620-21.

SHERRATT, A.G. 1976 - "Resources, technology and trade", pp.557-81 in G. Sieveking et al. (Eds.) Problems in Economic and Social Archaeology. Duckworth, London.

SHERRATT, A.G. 1980 - "Early agricultural communities in Europe", pp.144-51 in A.G. Sherratt (Ed.) The Cambridge Encyclopedia of Archaeology. Cambridge University Press, Cambridge.

SHERRATT, A.G. 1981 - "Plough and pastoralism: aspects of the secondary products revolution", pp.261-305 in I. Hodder et al. (Eds.) Pattern of the Past. Studies in Honour of David Clarke.

SHERRATT, A.G. 1982 - "Mobile resources: settlement and exchange in early agricultural Europe", pp.13-26 in C. Renfrew and S. Shennan (Eds.) Ranking, Resource and Exchange.

SMITH, M.A. 1955 - "The limitations of inference in archaeology", Archaeological Newsletter no. 6, pp.3-7.

SNODGRASS, A. 1980 - Archaic Greece:The Age of Experiment. Dent, London.

SOLLAS, W.J. 1911 - Ancient Hunters and their Modern Representatives. Macmillan, London.

STARTIN, W. 1978 - "Linear Pottery Culture Houses: reconstruction and manpower", Procs. of the Prehistoric Society vol. 44, pp.143-59.

STEWARD, J. 1949 - "Cultural causality and law: a trial formulation of the development of early civilisations", American Anthropogist vol. 51, pp.1-27.

STEWARD, J. 1963 - Theory of Culture Change. University of Illinois Press, Urbana.

TABACZYNSKI, S. 1972 - "Gesellschaftsordnung und Güteraustausch im Neolithikum Mitteleuropas", Neolithische Studien I, pp.31-96.

TAGANYI, Z. 1977 - Comments, pp.224-26, to B.J. Price "Shifts in production and organisation: a Cluster-Interaction model", Current Anthropology vol. 18, pp.209-33.

TAINTER, J.A. 1978 - "Mortuary practices and the study of prehistoric social systems", pp.106-43 in M.B. Schiffer (Ed.) Advances in Archaeological Method and Theory, I. Academic Press, New York.

THOMSEN, C.J. 1836 - A Guide to Northern Antiquities. National Museum, Copenhagen.

TRIGGER, B. 1978 - Time and Traditions. Essays in Archaeological Interpretation. Edinburgh University

Press, Edinburgh.

TYLOR, E.B. 1881 - Anthropology. London.

UCKO. P.J. 1969 - "Ethnography and archaeological interpretation of funerary remains", World Archaeology vol. 1, pp.262-80.

WALLERSTEIN, I. 1974 - The Modern World System. Academic Press, London.

WELINDER, S. 1975 - Prehistoric Agriculture in Eastern Middle Sweden. Acta Archaeologica Lundensia series in 8º Minore No 4, Lund.

WHITE, L.A. 1943 - "Energy and the evolution of culture", American Anthropologist vol. 45, pp.335-56.

WHITE, L.A. 1949 - The Science of Culture. Grove Press, New York.

WILLEY, G.R. 1953 - Prehistoric Settlement Patterns in the Viru Valley. Bureau of American Ethnology, Bulletin 155, Washington.

WILLEY. G.R. and PHILLIPS, P. 1958 - Method and Theory in American Archaeology. University of Chicago Press, Chicago.

WILLEY, G.R. and SABLOFF, J.A. 1974 - A History of American Archaeology. Thames and Hudson, London.

WILSON, D.M. 1976 (Ed.) - The Archaeology of Anglo-Saxon England. Methuen and Co., London.

WINZELER, R.L. 1976 - "Ecology, culture, social organisation, and state formation in Southeast Asia", Current Anthropology vol. 17, pp.623-40.

WITTFOGEL, K.A. 1957 - Oriental Despotism. Yale University Press, New Haven.

WOLF, E.R. 1976 (Ed.) - The Valley of Mexico. University of New Mexico Press, Albuquerque.

WRIGHT, H.T. 1978 - "Toward an explanation of the origin of the state", pp.49-68 in R. Cohen and E.R. Service (Eds.) Origins of the State.

ZUBROW, E.B.W. 1980 - "International trends in theoretical archaeology", Norwegian Archaeological Review vol. 13, pp.14-23.

1

SOCIAL EVOLUTION:
SOME SOCIOLOGICAL ASPECTS

Cliff Slaughter

Prologue

For the general reader, I attach this note on some of the positions which have been taken in social theory with respect to the question of social evolution. After Vico (1725) I refer to the French Encyclopaedists, particularly the Physiocrats, and the political economists of the Scottish Enlightenment. In the nineteenth century, Comte and Saint-Simon continue the rationalist tradition. Spencer, independently of Darwin, it must be stressed, presented social evolution as a natural process. Maine was interested primarily in the 'jural' aspects of institutions. Bachofen, McLennan and Morgan are representative, in different ways, of those writers of the later nineteenth century who developed theories of the evolution of forms of the family and marriage. Morgan however incorporated this aspect of his theory into a more general scheme of social evolution. Marx and Engels considered his work to be an independent discovery of their own 'materialist conception of history'. Tylor's is a cultural evolution, the 'intellectualist' bias of which is characteristic also of Frazer's work.

With the coming of the twentieth century we find the development of modern sociology, which affects anthropology greatly, first through Durkheim and his school and then through the work of Max Weber. The consequence is a concern with function and equilibrium rather than social evolution, until the neo-evolutionist revival, in which the work of White, Steward, and of Service and Sahlins have been landmarks. Talcott Parsons attempts a paradigm of social evolution on structural-functionalist foundations.

I have omitted any reference to archaeological work on social evolution, especially as represented by American scholars (Adams, Flannery, Wright and others) influenced by Steward and 'cultural materialism'. Nor do I deal with the uses of systems theory, cybernetics and, more recently, catastrophe theory, in explaining social processes.

The yawning gaps in this outline will be filled, to a small extent, by the main text of my chapter, below. For a comprehensive outline the reader should consult Marvin Harris' The Rise of Anthropological Theory.

1 Vico, Giambattista, The New Science, 1725. Postulates three ages: the age of the gods, of the heroes, and of men. Although these are seen as characterized essentially by different relations between men and the supernatural, Vico nonetheless seeks to trace historical transformations in social institutions.

2 Turgot, A.R.J., Universal History, 1750, and Montesquieu, The Spirit of Laws, 1748. Turgot was a leading representative of the views of the 'Physiocrats', founders of political economy in France. He sees mankind as passing through three stages : hunting, pastoralism, and farming. Turgot and Montesquieu, like other writers of the Enlightenment, lay great stress on the effects of geographical environment in the development of civilization, and see the origins of social inequality and power in men's ability to produce a surplus over and above subsistence. Montesquieu differentiates between the stages of savagery, barbarism and civilization. In general it is considered that there are basic inadequacies in the eighteenth-century rationalists' view of social development, because of their inability to solve the riddle: 'man is the product of his environment', yet 'opinions govern the world'.

3 Ferguson, Adam, An Essay on the History of Civil Society, 1767. Ferguson connects the development of private property to increasing control of the means of subsistence, and draws conclusions from this about the origin of the state and changes in the family.

4 Millar, John, Observations Concerning the Distinction of Ranks in Society, 1771. Defines more sharply the connection between the growth of property and of the state, and especially the incompatibility between social orders based on kinship and descent, on the one hand, and the growth of division of labour and private property on the other.

5 Robertson, William, History of America, 1777. Again savagery-barbarism-civilization, this time advocating the use of archaeological as well as ethnological evidence.

6 Condorcet, Outline of the Intellectual Progress of Mankind, 1795. The rationalist exposition of historical evolution, par excellence: society's evolution is essentially a progressive enlightenment.

7 Comte, Auguste, Cours de Philosophie Positive, 1830-42. More important for his view of society as an organism (a view fundamental to the later functionalist sociology) than for his proposed three stages: theological, metaphysical, and scientific.

These stages are said to characterize all branches of knowledge. His notion of the source of such development is the rationalist-idealist one. Society develops as an organism, with its functions and its pathology. To a great extent, Comte took this concept from Saint-Simon.

8   **Spencer, Herbert,** Principles of Sociology and many other works, 1842 onwards. Considers society to be governed by a universal natural law of evolution, and fails to distinguish between biological and social evolution in important senses. Human nature has evolved, and genetic changes must be associated with social-historical changes.

9   **Maine, Sir Henry S.,** Ancient Law: its Connection with the Early History of Society and its Relation to Modern Ideas, 1861, and Lectures on the Early History of Institutions, 1875. Considers the patriarchal family to be the earliest form of social organization. The movement of all 'progressive societies', he says, has been 'from status to contract.'

10   **Bachofen, J.J.,** Mother-Right (Das Mutterrecht), 1861. Bachofen is the first to formulate the theory that matriarchy was the original form of family and society, giving way universally to patriarchy. His work is based not on ethnographical evidence, but on Greek classical literature and myth.

11   **McLennan, J.F.,** Primitive Marriage, 1865. Elaborates a scheme of stages of the development of marriage, in which social organization is not considered in relation to economic or property forms. The family is said to arise after earlier stages: tribe, then clan. The scheme is a speculative reconstruction of logical transitions between observed customs such as endogamy, exogamy, marriage by capture, etc.

12   **Tylor, E.B.,** Researches into the Early History of Mankind, 1865, and Primitive Culture, 1871. Thinks it the task of anthropology to fill out the origins and stages of development of human social institutions from the evidence of the customs of modern 'primitive' peoples. Fundamental is the common ability of human minds to solve problems by working always in basically similar ways. Lays great stress on the evolution of culture, rather than of social structure.

13   **Morgan, L.H.,** Systems of Consanguinity and Affinity in the Human Family, 1871 and Ancient Society, 1877. Social development is based primarily on 'enlargement of the sources of subsistence' through the sequence savagery-barbarism-civilization. To this Morgan relates sequences for the evolution of property, the family, and government. He surveys systematically contemporary ethnographic evidence in this framework. Thus, early societies had primitive communism, and private property developed only with civilization. The family evolved, after a hypothetical original promiscuity, from the 'consanguine' form through 'group marriage' to the 'pairing family' to monogamy. The classificatory system of kinship terminology evolved in a way which reflected this latter evolution, but always with delays, so that terminologies contained 'survivals' of earlier forms of marriage and the family. From a social organization by descent ('gentile society') societies evolved to territorial allegiance and the state. Morgan does not distinguish the materialist implications of his theory from his notion of the growth of 'the idea of government', 'the idea of property', and 'the idea of the family'.

14   **Marx, K.** Capital, 1867, and **Engels, F.,** Origin of the Family, Private Property and the State, 1884. Social evolution is essentially a necessary sequence of specific 'modes of production' and the social formations which are built on them. At points where the social relations of production become a fetter on the further development of men's productive forces, a social revolution is necessary and is fought out in the sphere of the class struggle. Through such historical crises, there has resulted a series of historical types of society: primitive communism, the slavery of the ancient world, feudalism, and capitalism. This is not to say that research may not demonstrate a different sequence in other parts of the world. Marx and Engels consider that Morgan independently discovered their own 'materialist conception of history', and embrace his views on the evolution of marriage and the family and of gentile society.

15   **Frazer, J.G.,** The Golden Bough, 1890, and many other works. Insofar as Frazer considers social evolution it is essentially as a manifestation of intellectual progress. The great stages of social development are magic, religion and science: a progressive shedding of ignorance and superstition through the intellectual labours of society's best minds in the light of experience.

16   **Durkheim, E.E.,** The Division of Labour in Society, 1893, and The Elementary Forms of the Religious Life, 1912. Society is above all a normative order, yet social facts can be studied 'as things'. Society develops, by means of increasing division of labour, from 'mechanical solidarity' of like parts, undifferentiated, to 'organic solidary' of differentiated unlike parts with functional interdependence. In Elementary Forms of the Religious Life Durkheim reaches the position that the religious consciousness is the basis of society, as shown in its earliest forms. Despite the 'evolutionary' implications of these works, it is generally considered that Durkheim's emphasis on functional explanation resulted in a mode of social analysis which neglected or could not conceptualize or explain social change.

17   **Weber, Max,** General Economic History, 1903, Theory of Social and Economic Organisation, 1947. Weber's stress is on the necessity of an 'interpretative' understanding (i.e., an explanation of social behaviour in terms of the orientations of actors). From this standpoint, research must consist of a series of studies of individual situations or characteristic orientations, selected for study according to stated value-choices and approached via 'ideal-type' heuristic concepts. Historical processes and situations are grasped as manifestations of types of meaningful action : 'end-rational', 'value-rational', 'traditional', or 'affective'; and in no sense as representative of 'stages'. Modern industrial societies are said to exhibit an overwhelming tendency to bureaucratic rationalization.

18   **Boas, F.,** The Limitations of the Comparative Method of Anthropology, 1896, The Mind of Primitive Man, 1911. Rejects evolutionist theorizing, first on the grounds that it is necessary instead to gather data on the actual historical sequences. However he soon developed the view that in fact there was nothing in the nature of social-historical reality to permit the assertion of uniformities of

process. For Boas, different parts of the total culture may influence and relate to one another in a number of ways. This leads him and some of his followers (e.g. Ruth Benedict) to lay the central emphasis on the unique patterning of particular cultures.

19 **Malinowski, B.** The Family among the Australian Aborigines, 1913; Crime and Custom in Savage Society,1926; article 'Culture' in Encyclopaedia Britannica, 1931. Institutions must be studied in terms of their functions in satisfying men's basic biological needs, and not historically, especially as we do not know the history of the primitive peoples studied by anthropology.

20 **Radcliffe-Brown, A.R.,** Structure and Function in Primitive Society (papers representative of the period 1914-1958). Characterizes the nineteenth-century social evolutionary theories, and especially Morgan's, as 'conjectural history' (a phrase borrowed from the early political economist Dugald Stewart), particularly because of the unfounded assumption that contemporary usages, such as kinship terminologies, may be interpreted as survivals of hypothetical earlier stages, instead of as functional components of the existing social order, contributing to the maintenance of its 'social structure'.

21 **Polanyi, K.,** The Great Transformation, 1944, and 'The Economy as Instituted Process' in Trade and Market in the Early Empires, K. Polanyi, C.W. Arensberg, and H.W. Pearson (Eds.) 1957. His stress on the social 'embeddedness' (in early societies) of the activities we call economic has been highly influential ('Substantivism'). Note also his conceptualization of the broad category of 'redistributive' societies, which in a sense stand midway between more primitive economic and later market systems.

22 **White, L.,** 'Energy and the Evolution of Culture', 1943 (see his The Science of Culture, 1949), and The Evolution of Culture, 1959. Influenced by Marxism, White tries to show that control of the environment, represented above all by the progress of production and control of energy, is the basis of cultural evolution.

23 **Steward, J.H.,** 'The Economic and Social Basis of Primitive Bands' 1936, and 'Cultural causality and law: a trial formulation of the development of early civilizations' 1947 (reprinted in The Theory of Culture Change: the Methodology of Multilinear Evolution, 1955). The fundamental component of any culture is the mode of its response to the given natural environment. The study of the 'form-functions' of the cultural-ecological and techno-environmental aspects of different cultures reveals parallel types of development sequence. Hence the multilinear evolution of the 'cultural materialists'. These parallel sequences are especially significant in the transition to civilization.

24 **Service, E.R.,** Primitive Social Organisation, 1962, Service and **Sahlins, M.D.,** (Eds.) Evolution and Culture, 1960; Sahlins, M.D., Tribesmen, 1968 and Stone-Age Economics, 1972. Sahlins and Service have been important in recent anthopological discussions of social evolution, especially through their postulated sequence of socio-cultural forms: band-tribe-chiefdom-state. It should be noted that this sequence of forms of social integration is not dependent on a theory of the priority of any one aspect of social life, say, the economic, and that

Service declared in a later publication that instead of band-tribe-chiefdom-state we should substitute another sequence: the egalitarian society, the hierarchical society, and in a few instances archaic civilization and classical empire.

25 **Parsons, Talcott,** Societies: Evolutionary and Comparative Perspectives, 1966. Arrives at the conclusion that "an increase in generalised adaptive capacity" of societies has produced "three very broad evolutionary levels ... primitive, intermediate, and modern." It is as 'normative structures' that societies evolve. Written language was the code of the essentially cultural change in the normative structure which transformed primitive societies into intermediate ones. In the transition from intermediate to modern, the fundamental change is "internal to the social structure, and centres in the legal system". The core processes behind these evolutionary transformations are said to be (a) 'differentiation' of roles and collectivities and of the functions attached to them, (b) consequent adaptive upgrading, by which the role or collectivities become more productive, and (c) integration of the system within which the differentiated roles and collectivities work. Finally, the 'value-system' of the society must undergo changes which adjust the orientations of the parts to the general or central value system. Parsons's later writings refer to the 'central value system' as the most crucial differentiating characteristic of social systems. 'Structural-functionalist' theorists take structural differentiation and integration to be the basic processes of the evolution of societies, but not all of them share Parsons's view of the relation between these processes and the value-system.

... ...

Asked to contribute an introductory paper on social-anthropological and sociological aspects of approaches to social evolution, one might reasonably have presented a descriptive account of the forms taken by social evolutionist ideas, together with the criticisms of these. Such an account is in fact easily available in Marvin Harris's The Rise of Anthropological Theory, and that book's open partiality is easily compensated for by reading any of the several outlines and histories of social anthropology. I have preferred, rightly or wrongly, to seek to indicate some of the general theoretical assumptions which predominate, often without any systematic elaboration or discussion, in interpretation of the 'social evolutionary' implications of archaeological findings, and to emphasize the need for a critical analysis of these. Nor have I thought it wise to confront directly the material presented recently in the volume The Evolution of Social Systems, edited by J. Friedman and M.J. Rowlands (Duckworth 1977). The latter contains contributions by the editors and others which explore the possibilities of discovering the structural-transformational properties of social systems as a key to the mechanism of social evolution. It is hoped that what follows here will be found to have some relevance to the question of the feasibility of such an approach.

THE USES OF ETHNOGRAPHY?

Archaeologists who take seriously the problems of development of the societies whose remains they study naturally find themselves referring to the ethnographic record of 'primitive' societies produced by the work of social anthropologists. Although there exists a considerable number of invaluable ethnographic works dating from the late nineteenth and early twentieth centuries,[1] the great majority of the field-studies consulted belong to the last 50 years. In any discussion of social evolution it should not be forgotten that such studies, especially those of British social anthropologists, were carried out almost entirely within the framework of one or another variety of functionalism, and with a quite explicit rejection of any concern with 'evolutionist' concepts or concerns. This emphasis predominates in the literature, notwithstanding the recent growing interest in social evolution among social anthropologists, which has been further stimulated by a renewed influence of neo-Marxist approaches, and which is paralleled in archaeology. Radcliffe-Brown, the dominant influence in social anthropology, characterized nineteenth-century evolutionism and interest in origins of institutions, and paticularly the work of Lewis Henry Morgan, as 'conjectural history',[2] and postponed the elaboration of any soundly-based theory of social evolution to the distant future, considering that in any case there was no way of knowing the history of the peoples studied by anthropologists - an opinion shared by Malinowski ("Primitive peoples have no History"). Nor, asserted Radcliffe-Brown, was there any reason whatsoever to suppose that the contemporary primitive societies should be considered as equivalents of earlier stages of our own. Franz Boas's historical particularism was the foundation of the education of a whole generation of American cultural anthropologists.[3] The highly influential work on kinship by Radcliffe-Brown, 'The Social Organisation of Australian Tribes'[4], carries no bibliographical reference to Morgan's works even though the weight of the monograph's argument is concentrated specifically against Morgan's own account of the significance of Australian kinship organization. Laufer, Boas's pupil, is famous (only) for his characterization of the concept of social evolution as "... the most inane, sterile and pernicious theory ever conceived in the history of science".[5] Alexander Goldenweiser announced at regular intervals in the 1930s the 'downfall of evolutionism'.[6] Evans-Pritchard wrote in 1951: "Modern social anthropology is essentially conservative in its approach. Its interests are more in what makes for integration and equilibrium in society than plotting scales and stages of progress".[7]

Criticism of the nineteenth century evolutionists has concentrated especially on their supposed unilinearism, i.e. the idea that a series of essentially uniform stages of development is common to the development of all societies. Later in this paper I discuss briefly the way in which the views such as those of Morgan on this matter have often been oversimplified. Like others, he made many allowances for 'exceptions' and divergent paths of development. More important than the question of unilinearism, now no longer disputed, is that of the nature of the causes of the development of societies. It would be true to say that, whatever the very considerable differences on this matter between nineteenth-century evolutionists, they did proceed on the assumption that it was through a demonstration of their historical interconnections and origins that institutions could be explained. Herbert Spencer considered that social systems had natural characteristics of organic-functional unity which were the key to their mode of evolution. (He furthermore considered that changes in the social organization were necessarily accompanied by changes in the human species).[8] Morgan considered "the progressive enlargement of the sources of subsistence" to be the source of historical development, but at no time did he see the need to consider the inconsistency between this and his idea of institutions developing in terms of the growth of major ideas (the idea of property, the idea of government, etc.).[9] Tylor did not have a materialist

starting point, but laid great stress on the uniformity of the human mind which lay behind culture and the differentiation of man from nature.[10] Within this perspective, he tended, as later did Frazer, to an 'intellectualist' intepretation of the origins and development of religion and other cultural phenomena.[11]

In the twentieth century, Radcliffe-Brown, from the standpoint of functionalism, and Boas, from that of 'culture-history', each stressed the detailed study of particular peoples, and rejected the concern with universal stages and the search for origins. But the dichotomy 'evolutionism/functionalism' (or evolutionism/particularist history) obscured the more fundamental matter of the causes and mechanisms of the development of societies.

It can safely be said that throughout the period when the structural-functionalism of Radcliffe-Brown reigned, such interest in social evolution as was shown in Britain found expression in the work of a minority of archaeologists rather than in social anthropology. V. Gordon Childe's works on the transition to civilization, influenced by Marxism, are well-known, and his mature view of social evolution[12] is summarized below. In the United States, Leslie White was something of an isolated figure from the early 1930s to the end of the 1950s. He worked quite independently of the prevailing functionalist anthropology; and, although his very early work reflected directly the Boasian 'culture-history' orthodoxy, he very soon, through his own Iroquois research, came to accept much of the approach of Morgan. Before the end of the 1920s he had visited Russia and become very interested in Marx's historical materialism. His subsequent work shows an attempt to assimilate Marxism to Kroeber's notion of the 'super-organic' character of culture.[13] For White, the progressive development of human society's command of energy resources was the objective basis and index of cultural evolution.[14] Alongside, and in the same period, there developed the work of Julian Steward, proceeding from the premise that each society's specific type of symbiosis with its natural environment shapes its cultural and social forms, from which it follows that social evolution will be 'multilinear'.[15] From the comparative study of the forms and functions of these multilinear evolutions Steward considered it possible to suggest parallels, particularly in the process of formation of civilizations. His work is related to that of Karl Wittfogel, who is best known for his 'hydraulic society' schema.[16] The large scale public works, the inevitable necessity of authority and co-ordination, and degree of separation of mental from manual labour, consequent upon the necessities of irrigation in great flood-valleys, were said by Wittfogel to give rise to a distinctive mode of social evolution and origin of the state, and he traced modern totalitarian regimes to these origins.

Despite the overwhelming anti-evolutionist influence, until very recently, of structural-functionalist theories in social anthropology, the meticulous field-work of the members of this school undoubtedly did provide material suggestive of certain conclusions which are very relevant to the understanding of social evolution, and these anticipate, to a certain extent, more recent discussions of 'cultural ecology' and of the inadequacy of any simple theory of economic surplus as efficient cause of the origin of civilization and the state. In 1947, Daryll Forde brought together the results of a considerable body of field-work to show that 'lineages' and 'clans', i.e. unilineal descent groups, are associated neither with the most elementary forms of relation to the environment (hunting and gathering), nor with those societies which have a developed division of labour, class divisions and centralized government (the state). Rather, the unilineal descent group is the dominant form of social organization in societies with an intermediate level of control of environment, technique, division of labour, population size and density, etc. At this intermediate level, there arises a need for definition of corporate rights in resources and regularized modes of co-operation and regulation of relations between groups, but not yet the necessity or possibility of distinct private property and private interest.[17] Forde did not advocate on this basis an evolutionary theory, and put forward no specific theory of the transition between the types of social organization to which he referred, but certain implications are clear. Meyer Fortes[18] was able to review virtually the whole of British social anthropological field-work since the 1930s within this framework and to demonstrate that the internal structural characteristics of unilineal descent groups were entirely consistent with Forde's approach.

When Peter Worsley[19] subjected to critical analysis the earlier study by Fortes of the Tallensi (in the northern part of what is now Ghana),[20] he showed that the abstract structural principles ('principle of the unity of the lineage group' etc.) adduced by Fortes and others of the Radcliffe-Brown school were not explanatory, and became quite superfluous when even the limited available knowledge of history and of the necessities flowing from the mode of agricultural production was brought to bear on Fortes' own material. Malinowski's findings on the people of the Trobriand Archipelago, and especially his account of the ceremonial exchange cycle called the kula,[21] are perhaps the best-known of all ethnographic works. The fact is, however, that his account has been shown to be vitiated by his one-sided and anti-historical approach. Marvin Harris's argument, that Malinowski virtually ignored the significance of economic aspects of the activities within which kula partnership operated, is incontrovertible, and is, from the point of view of theory, the most decisive of the criticisms of Malinowski which have been made. In this context, the papers by P. Lauer, 'Amphlett Islands pottery trade and the Kula',[22] and Edmund Leach, 'On the "Founding Fathers"',[23] are important. It must also be said that the work of Max Gluckman between 1941 and 1951 on the Lozi of Barotseland[24] anticipated by many years the discussion of surplus product and its role. Of the Lozi he wrote, "The cohesion of these systems of relations was not disturbed by economic cleavages, though struggles within them were set in economic terms; for the Lozi economy was primitive, possessing only primary foods and egalitarian standards of living. Chiefs and wealthy men used their riches only to attract dependants".[25]

Another 'structural-functionalist' who anticipated later theoretical issues was E.E. Evans-Pritchard. Polanyi's assertion of the 'embeddedness' of economics in other institutions, and the associated questioning of any application of Marx's concept of 'economic base',[26] have been central to 'economic anthropology' in the most recent period. Evans-Pritchard long ago made many statements in his work on the Nuer to the effect that: "One cannot treat Nuer economic relations by themselves, for they always form part of direct social relations of a general kind".[27] Insofar as Evans-Pritchard's emphasis here has a theoretical base rather than being only his conclusion from observation of the Nuer, that base is to be found in the work of Marcel Mauss. In his Essai sur le Don (1950),[28] Mauss suggested, among other things, that what appeared to be economic actions in primitive societies should be understood as 'total' social phenomena, expressive of social relations and cultural meanings of a 'non-economic' kind. This, as well as the general resort to 'gift-exchange' in explanation of transactions in primitive societies, has proved to be an important heritage in the models adopted by archaeologists and historians. Evans-Pritchard himself in later years became critical of his structural-functionalist colleagues, attacking particularly the project of Radcliffe-Brown for a 'natural science of

society' in which structural principles had virtually the status of scientific laws. Evans-Pritchard advocated instead an approach to ethnography which was historical.[29] However, he did not propose any actual theoretical framework for such an approach, and certainly did not revert to any sort of evolutionism.

SOME SOCIOLOGICAL INFLUENCES

In what follows, there is contained an outline of the views on social evolution put forward by thinkers like Sahlins and Service, which have in the past two decades become influential in shaping the general background of thought of archaeologists. I also make some reference to the issues which are raised by various attempts to analyze anew the implications of Marx's theories for the study of pre-capitalist societies. A less brief introduction than the present one would need full discussion of the theories of Durkheim and Weber as well as of Marx, in order to provide some framework for analysing the models and assumptions within which archaeologists and anthropologists proceed. Radcliffe-Brown's structural-functionalism was derived in the first place from Durkheim's view of 'society' as resting on systematically structured norms, external to the individual as such and exercising constraint on him,[30] and for Radcliffe-Brown, 'function' means, essentially, contribution to the permanence of this structure, the maintenance of its equilibrium. Insofar as Durkheim, in his earlier works particularly, had a theory of social evolution, it concerned changes in 'moral density', modes of integration, sentiments of solidarity, rather than any material basis of the social 'morphology' to which he pays lip-service. The most general of these changes was that from what he called mechanical to organic solidarity, i.e. from primitive, undifferentiated, simple social units consisting of like individual parts, to complex social organisms with units interdependent through division of labour.[31] It is possible to draw from The Division of Labour in Society the conclusion that Durkheim thought increase of population the primary cause of transition from mechanical to organic solidarity, but this thesis is not consistently stated or developed. But the transition is unexplained, and appears to be the result of some inherent property of social organization as such, a criticism which applies equally to late nineteenth-century theories of 'Gemeinschaft-Gesellschaft' polarity,[32] to Maine's "movement of progressive societies from status to contract",[33] and especially to Herbert Spencer's notion of evolution from simple to complex.[34] The influence of Durkheim's general approach has of course been effected, primarily, through the work of Radcliffe-Brown and the British school of social anthropology, but there is an important additional influence via the developments of structural-functionalism specifically into theories of social development, by Talcott Parsons and S.N. Eisenstadt (see below).

These sociological theorists have attempted a synthesis of the ideas of Durkheim and Max Weber (and to some extent, of Pareto and Alfred Marshall[35]). Weber is perhaps the strongest influence on recent and contemporary sociology. Whereas Durkheim's primary emphasis was on the legitimacy of studying 'social facts as things', having objective reality and thus amenable to scientific treatment,[36] Weber carried into sociology the distinction between Naturwissenschaften and Geisteswissenschaften, (roughly, natural and social-historical sciences) which dominated social and historical theory in the late nineteenth and early twentieth centuries in Germany. In the most general terms, Weber's approach results in a twofold impact on the comparative and historical study of societies. First, the insistence that sociological explanation must be adequate 'at the level of meaning' as well as 'causally adequate'.[37] This flows, according to Weber, from the particular nature of social reality: that human actors attach meaning to what they do; and so their social action is comprehended only insofar as the evaluations and orientations with which they endow their actions in relation to objects and to other actors are incorporated in the explanation. The method by which such interpretative understanding is to be gained, according to Weber, provides for a causal explanation, as against the intuitive approach of the adherents of Lebensphilosophie. It is a matter of constructing 'ideal types' of social action for the explanation of particular historical forms (say 'the spirit of capitalism', 'the Protestant Ethic', etc.). These ideal types are not averages or summaries, but projective meaningful wholes attributed (zugerechnet) to the orientations of actors of collectivities. They are heuristic devices for illuminating the historical reality. Weber furthermore eschews any notion of a 'prime mover' in history, and asks only for explicit statement of the researcher's value-orientation in selecting facets of the reality for study. For Weber, besides 'economic' man there is the man of religion, of aesthetic activities, of politics, of the family; and every historical situation is a 'mosaic' of the structured orientations and actions built up in each of these spheres of motivation. Any a priori notion of the primacy of one of these over the others must be rejected. The task of the scientific investigator is rather to define as clearly and scrupulously as possible the scope and limits of his own selected viewpoint. I leave aside the vexed question of whether Weber did not in fact, through his comparative sociology of religion, arrive at the conclusion that the decisive factor in the rise of capitalism was indeed a change in the religious sphere (viz. the 'this-worldly asceticism' and the notion of the 'calling' characteristic of Calvinism, phenomena which themselves are unexplained).[38]

One particular (rather than general) concept of Weber's, derived from this general approach, which has considerable influence on and implications for the study of the evolution of societies, is his theory of social stratification, in which status-position (Stand) is the dominant theme. In contrast to Marx's theory that class and class struggle were determined in the first place by position in the exploitation-relation in production, Weber saw class, economically defined, as one aspect of status divisions.[39] The implications of this emphasis are well brought out in the use of Weber's framework by M.I. Finley.[40] For him, ancient Greek society is characterized by a 'continuum' or 'spectrum' of statuses, rather than classes; and the social conflicts of classical Athens, for example, are struggles between different status groups over the division of rights and privileges. Clearly this approach will give rise to a very different emphasis, in studying the evolution of Greek society, from a Marxist approach[41] in which slaves and slave-owners constitute classes related by exploitation, a division which by no means coincides exactly with the slave-free division, and which a Marxist would seek to explain in relation both to other class divisions in the same society and to status divisions and the conflicts between status groups.

The different theoretical approaches to the nature of status and class and their interrelation are of importance not only in ancient Greece and Rome, in other civilizations, and in later complex class societies. Do the status differences in pre-class, pre-state societies have the same social, economic and political significance as do status differences in those societies where the transition to civilization, with a class structure and the state, has taken place? Is reference to a simple **accumulation** of status differences (in goods and in prestige) an explanation of that transition, or is it necessary to examine the relations of production (i.e. the class relations)? These problems reappear, in one form or another, in what follows here.

For the most part, it would be true to say that the influence of sociological and social-anthropological theory, in its non-Marxist forms, has been one based on an amalgam of the approaches of these major thinkers, or an eclectic combination of parts of their theories. Indeed, sociology itself could be so characterized. It has been noted more than once that through the many different approaches and detailed works available in the matter of social evolution the 'old' question of what constitutes the basic dynamic or 'prime mover' recurs just as insistently in our own day as it did for the nineteenth-century theorists. For example, it can hardly be contested that differentiation of functions is a characteristic of the development of societies. But does this **explain** anything? Why does it take place in some societies rather than others, under certain conditions, at a given time and not some other, at different tempos, etc.? Does it constitute, in and of itself, increasing adaptive powers, progress? Is it a natural property of systems as such? And so on.

If 'differentiation' is essentially the instrument of increased functional efficiency in responding to disturbances of the existing equilibrium between social system and external environment, and 'integration' is a response to the disturbance of the internal social equilibrium which has resulted from the differentiation, clearly integration is not an explanation of the change but only a description of the changed methods induced by other (unexplained) changes. These latter, in turn, are responses to some change or changes outside the social system. (I leave out the case of other societies as constituents of the environment in this argument, since that would only push the problem of **explanation** one step farther back). It appears, then, that the properties of **social systems as such,** in theories like those of Parsons and Eisenstadt, are equilibrium-promoting properties only. In these theories, the dynamic of historical change is **external,** even if its effects are mediated by certain properties of the social systems. The system itself, that is, has no dynamic and tends always to equilibrium through structural differentiation and integration (see below for Eisenstadt's attempted solution of this problem). For such an approach to arrive as a theory of social change, it becomes necessary to introduce notions of elites, enterpreneurs, etc., to infuse life into the structure. As an alternative, with different implications for the explanation of social evolution, one might begin by acknowledging that the relation between society and 'environment' (i.e. the rest of nature) is not an abstract one, nor is it one in which the social system receives 'information' from its environment, i.e. responding only to an external dynamic, nor is it a matter of how the social actors see the problems posed to them in the struggle for individual survival (including the survival of their cultural identity). The relation between society and its environment **is** production, the 'nature-imposed necessity' (Marx) of appropriating from nature sufficient energy to reproduce the human beings of which society consists. This necessity is not simply 'biological', but requires productive appropriation at a level of quantity and stability sufficient to reproduce the necessary organization and relations of production as well as the existent level of productive forces. On this basis, Marxists will locate the dynamic of social change ultimately in the **relation between** society and nature, the active and changing relation called production, which, through the labour process, must incorporate and transcend the necessities of the natural material on which it works. This dynamic is then neither simply internal to the social system (its properties qua system) nor external, but both at the same time. In the course of carrying out the necessary practice of transforming nature, men have also continuously created the conditions for changes in their relations of production.[42] The mode of production of the means of life in society is not only technique and its raw material, but a contradictory unity of forces of production and social relations of production which facilitate the development of these forces but do not develop in any planned way so as to adapt to every change in them, so that 'disequilibrium' from time to time requires that men become more or less conscious of the need to transform those relations, piecemeal or totally. Where, when and how such changes become necessary and are possible or not is a matter to be investigated empirically. Marx proposed that each type of mode of production and social formation built up on it would show its own characteristic 'law of motion' in this regard. I refer below to some of the issues involved in distinguishing this theoretical approach from the 'cultural materialism' of Harris and others, as well as to some of the problems which have emerged in recent attempts to develop the implications of Marxist theory in the analysis of pre-capitalist societies.[43] But first, it is necessary to return to a more general characterization of the problems involved.

SOCIAL EVOLUTION: DEFINING THE PROBLEMS

Given the development outlined above, it is not surprising that social anthropology, particularly in Britain, has made little explicit contribution to theories of social evolution. In the last two decades, there has been a growing recognition of the limitations of a functionalist, ahistorical (and even anti-historical) approach, but there has at the same time been a considerable growth in the influence of structuralism. In its most consistent form, structuralism explicitly separates its concerns and those of anthropology from those of history.[44] The cultural materialists following in the footsteps of Leslie White and Julian Steward have brought cultural anthropology and archaeology close together in the United States, especially in the study of New World history and prehistory, but also in the work of Adams and others on Near Eastern civilizations.[45] In Europe, however, this latter tradition has had immeasurably more influence on archaeology than on anthropology.

Social anthropologists have for the most part been very particularistic in their research concerns, reflecting the overwhelming emphasis on individual field-work monographs and functionalist analyses of societies as self-contained and self-perpetuating systems in equilibrium. If the explanation of any social or cultural phenomenon is to be sought in its functional contribution to the maintenance of the 'social structure' (however that may be defined), it is difficult to see the prospect of a theory of social change or social evolution.. Even the most careful selection of 'analogies' from a comprehensive range of ethnographic examples will surely suffer irreparably from the bias introduced into the anthropologist's findings by a functionalist approach.[46] This is indicative of the very general and basic nature of the theoretical questions - questions on which there is no consensus among sociologists and anthropologists - which still remain, even when one has rejected assertions such as that made by M.A. Smith in 1955: "Since historical events and essential social divisions of prehistoric people don't find an adequate expression in material remains, it cannot be right to try to arrive at a knowledge of them through archaeological interpretation."[47] Leach, more recently, has said that evolutionists have only made assertions, and have explained nothing.[48]

In the pursuit of a 'social archaeology', against these warnings, archaeologists have borrowed and developed the ideas of certain anthropologists and sociologists. In the nature of the case, they have found most congenial the writings of those anthropologists who have an 'evolutionist' approach and who concern themselves with ecological and economic matters more than have the functionalists in Britain. In the course of this development, there has

flourished recently an interest in Marxist theory. Such an interest is certainly part of a general tendency in the social sciences and humanities in the last two decades, but of course Gordon Childe and Leslie White were influenced by Marxism ever since the 1920s, and the most influential work of Sahlins, Stone Age Economics,[49] was written after his work in Paris and contact with the ideas of French 'structuralist Marxist' anthropologists. This latter influence, via the work of Godelier, Terray, Dupré and Rey, Bloch and others,[50] has also subsequently been a direct one in British anthropology and archaeology. As recently as the early 1950s, Marxism (or even 'evolution' for that matter) was virtually excluded from the literature and the teaching of anthropology in Britain. Now the academic atmosphere is greatly changed.

We may begin by noting that certain elementary considerations about social evolution are no longer controversial, or are much less open to challenge than they once were. Gordon Childe,[51] some 30 years ago, included a number of these points in his view on social evolution, which may be summarized as follows. Childe started from the fact that, in different geographical environments, a similar result had emerged from the histories of societies observed in temperate Europe, the Mediterranean area, the Nile valley and Mesopotamia. This end-result, civilization, meant, he maintained: "concentration of large populations in cities, class and occupational divisions therein (between producers and non-producers, between merchants, officials, rulers, priests, or various artisans and cultivators), a concentration of economic and political power, writing, and weights and measures, standardized. The starting-points for the development leading to this common result were also similar: the extension of agriculture to cultivation of cereals and domestication of certain animals."

But between starting-point and result there was "not even abstract parallelism". On the contrary, in rural economy, there was "not parallelism but divergence and convergence". Furthermore, no technological element as such could be shown to be necessary in all cases of the transition. In each case there are exceptions (plough, wheel, domestication of animals, stone-metal sequences). Trade "exhibits parallelism" but "is not very helpful"; it is not precisely measurable; and it is normally found as trade **with** civilized areas. In "social institutions" (e.g. state authority, war) there is "no closer parallelism".

All this, Childe thought, did not invalidate the concept of 'evolution'. But besides variation and differentiation we find **convergence** and **assimilation,** and not only by conquest, domination, or elimination of one society by another. Here the decisive importance of **diffusion** enters. Because culture is the specifically social mode of adaptation for survival, it is **diffusion** which "more than anything" distinguishes social from organic evolution. For an idea or technique to be diffused, the receiving society must have already evolved to a stage where adoption of the diffused item will be possible and "socially approved".

All this indicates a kind of explanation of the observed failure of the sequence Childe considered to exhibit parallelism of evolution. They were not sufficiently independent of one onother, free of mutual diffusion, to constitute "distinct instances" from which inductions could legitimately be drawn.

Despite the breakdown of the analogy between natural and cultural evolution, Childe considered that, "with modification", "variation, heredity, adaptation and selection" could be used more intelligibly for social than for organic evolution (I use 'cultural' and 'social' here exactly as did Childe). Accumulation is distinctive of

48

cultural evolution. In sum, Childe thought cultural evolution vindicated by his study, and more so by his having eliminated false analogies with organic evolution.

Ignoring for the moment the point at which one might object to these conclusions (e.g. the absence of consideration of cases when there **was** separation of the processes of development: Old World - New World, Greece - China) we might add one or two other general considerations.

It no longer seems sensible to dimiss ideas of social evolution because of the supposed uncritical faith in continuous progress of nineteenth-century thinkers. It is not true that they were all optimists in this regard. While Morgan, as the most important of them, did have a notion of progress, it was one which had contradictory development at its heart, and it is well known that he considered probable and desirable the historical demise of the modern social order based on private property. As much as anything else it was this historical criticism of a class society, where the product controlled the producer, that attracted the attention of Marx and Engels. Less often quoted is his conclusion on the family: "It is at least supposable that it (the monogamous family) is capable of still further improvement until the equality of the sexes is attained. Should the monogamian family in the distant future fail to answer the requirements of society, assuming the continued progress of civilization, it is impossible to predict the nature of its successor."[52]

It is hardly disputed in our day that no notion of moral progress is implied in the cumulative development of techniques of control of nature or the historical transformations of social relations. Evolutionists of the nineteenth century differed in their opinions of the mechanisms and motive forces of these developments, as we have seen. It is easy to demonstrate, however, that regardless of these differences and inconsistencies, these and many other evolutionists often stated explicitly that their idea of progress applied 'in general' to the course of humanity's history, and did not imply absence of historical stagnation and even regression.

Marx is often invoked in such discussion, especially because he and Engels embraced the conclusions of Morgan's Ancient Society,[53] but it is now more generally recognized that this latter aspect is secondary to the general implications for social evolution of the materialist conception of history. In the case of Marx, there is explicit recognition of, and attempt to account for, the fact that societies in certain circumstances do not progress. The Communist Manifesto contains the well-known assertion that the class struggle in any society may issue not in the victory of one or another class but in "the mutual ruin of the contending classes". In any discussion of Marx in relation to nineteenth-century social evolutionism, it must also be understood that all teleology was excluded from the historical materialist view of social development, and an explicit theory advanced of the relation between individuals' purposive activity, beginning in the labour process, and the structure and transformation of societies.[54]

Harris (The Rise of Anthropological Theory)[55] has shown also that it was an oversimplification to have thought that the most important evolutionist thinkers ignored the role of diffusion. It was 'diffusionism' itself, in the extreme form put forward by Eliot Smith, Perry and Lord Raglan, which reduced this question to an absurdity,[56] rather than one which must in each case be adjudged by concrete demonstration of the maturing of internal conditions which make possible the adoption of 'diffused' artifacts and behaviour-patterns. Actually involved in such demonstrations are theoretical questions of

a different order than 'independent invention v. diffusion': what meaning can be given to the concepts 'internal' and 'external' in particular cases? Does 'ability to accept' imply cultural values or stages of technological or social development, or a combination of some or all of these? And so on.

'Unilinearism' and the criticism of it figured for long as the villain of the piece in anthropology's dismissal of social evolution in the twentieth century, but is now generally recognized to be something of a red herring. There are good grounds for thinking that it was never anything else. Without doubt, citations may be taken from Morgan and others which suggest unilinearism, especially where these thinkers were held back by the failure to separate historical from biological evolution.[57]

But neither is there any doubt that Morgan, Tylor and others qualified their view of 'general' social evolution. Thus Morgan on the family: "I do not mean to imply that one form rises complete in a certain status of society, flourishes universally and exclusively wherever tribes of mankind are found in the same status, and then disappears in another, which is the next higher form ... Moreover, some tribes attained to a particular form earlier than other tribes more advanced ..."[58] At the most elementary level of discussion, we can say that Morgan and Tylor, as well as do anthropologists today, understood that great flexibility was necessary in considering the history of particular societies in the framework of social evolution, because of the influence, through war, trade, colonization, etc., of neighbouring, more advanced peoples and empires, and, to a varying extent, but in general increasingly as we go back in the historical record, because of geographical-environmental differences. It is doubtful if any 'evolutionist' today entertains the notion of a series of evolutionary stages immanent in social reality.

In their Evolution and Culture[59] Sahlins and Service have suggested that there is an 'easy reconciliation' of the problems of whether 'culture in general' evolves through 'grand stages' or only particular social systems evolve. Leslie White in his introduction says: "As Sahlins makes perfectly clear, evolution in its specific (phylogenetic) aspect is multilinear; evolution in its general aspect is unilinear". Sahlins and Service assert that 'general evolution' refers to 'advance' or 'overall progress', and 'specific evolution' to 'divergence', 'variation', effected through particular adaptations. The distinction is taken directly from biology. 'General evolution', it must be stressed, is considered to be not an abstract summary but to be objective and measurable in terms of "greater adaptability, greater dominance, greater complexity of organization".

Julian Steward's 'multilinear evolution'[60] illustrates the difficult theoretical problems in this area. Worsley has noted: "Steward's 'multilinear' evolutionism is little more than a simplistic environmental determinism which tells us that, given similar technological equipment, people respond to similar environments by producing parallel social forms. It is therefore a theory singularly restricted in scope and explanatory 'power', since many social and cultural forms appear unconnected with environment or technology in a close way; since they may be culturally communicated (borrowed, enforced, etc.) and not 'naturally' derived; and since technological innovation and social institutions and cultural forms became progressively less dependent on the determinations of Nature".[61]

Harris expressed one aspect of this criticism in a slightly different way, and one which has implications for the 'reconciliation' of Sahlins and Service, when he observed that adaptation to environment by particular societies produces convergence as well as divergence, and that 'phylogeny' is an unjustified importation from the concepts of biology: "Phylogeny implies speciation, and there is no concept less applicable to cultural evolution than that of biological 'species'. The adaptive significance of culture in the evolution of the biosphere is precisely its exploitation of a non-genetic feedback circuit which permits adaptation without speciation. All socio-cultural systems can exchange pasts with each other ..."[62] (clearly the last sentence is a gross over-simplification, but it is correct as against the 'phylogeny' analogy).

Readers may be forgiven for finding it difficult to find very much in this latter discussion which was not already in Childe's Social Evolution.

On the one hand, then, there has been a clarification of some of the cruder misunderstandings and distortions of what is implied by 'evolutionism', and thereby a clearer view of what are the substantive theoretical problems. Here, however, in these substantive problems of the sources and mechanisms of social evolutionary change, there is, perhaps understandably, a great divergence of views. Confronted by the considerable influence of 'cultural materialist' views of one sort or another, and the renewed interest in Marxist historical materialism, Service has asked: "**Where** is the locus of the evolutionary impulse? Does it lie in the mode of production, in technology, in the relations of production, in the class struggle, in the division of labor, in man's view of destiny; or is it a mystical force in the cosmos? It would seem that those who posited mode of production, class struggle, technology, or division of labor were much influenced by the industrial revolution, which has been, of course, a most striking evolutionary prime mover for the past century and a half and promises even more wondrous cultural transformations almost immediately. But has the material, technoeconomic aspect always been the prime mover? The change from primitive chiefdoms to early states and then to empires in Mesoamerica, Peru, and probably elsewhere seems to have been first in the political sector; even the important inventions of writing and mathematics could have originated in the occult mumbo jumbo of priests. The modern evolutionist accordingly wants to know more about particular instances of change and finds no need to insist that the initial loci must be always in the same sector of culture."[63]

One answer to this problem of 'prime mover' and causality has been the use by Renfrew and others of a 'systems' approach, which stresses the mode of inter-connection between different sectors or subsystems of society, rather than the causal priority of one section over another, as the key to understanding social change (see below).

In the same article (1967) Service concluded that 'philosophies' like those of Marx and Spencer, "... were too grand in scope and too schematic to be useful. They also became stultified dogmas as they were used by political parties and academic 'schools of thought'. A better fate may be expected of recent evolutionism, judging from the evidence of new empirical attitudes, particularly if its proponents remain guarded against unnecessary and untested preconceptions that can so easily impede a true evolutionary science of culture."[64]

It is perhaps remarkable that in the subsequent years, empiricism (which must, it goes without saying, be distinguished from the study of the empirical data) has come under heavy attack from many sides in the social sciences, and most work on social evolution and associated matters has been approached precisely within theoretical frameworks heavily dependent on 'philosophies' such as those of Spencer or of Marx (or claiming so to be).

Whether one thinks the use of such frameworks to be nothing but 'preconceptions' will depend on what explanatory force they are found to possess.

AN EXAMPLE: 'THE EMERGENCE OF CIVILIZATION'

In view of the central place (if that is the appropriate metaphor) occupied by Colin Renfrew in archaeologists' discussion of social evolution, it may be useful to refer to the way in which he has adapted some of the theories of social system, structural differentiation, and integration which have been dominant in sociology and may be traced in large part to Spencer.[65] In his best-known work[66] Renfrew proposes that "the key to change of structure ... in human cultural development ..." is to be found in "... the interconnectedness among the different activities of the individual in society, the interdependence of the subsystems of society ..." making possible "a new kind of positive feedback among innovations".[67] There appears to be a certain confusion here, between the level of individual actions, on the one hand, and "interdependence of subsystems of society" on the other; but Renfrew's general approach is that which can be found in most explicit and developed form in the works of S.N. Eisenstadt and Talcott Parsons and his collaborators.[68] Eisenstadt's proposed synthesis of social-structural causes and individual motives will readily be seen to approximate very closely to the emphasis placed by Renfrew on 'elites': "... It is this double aspect of social institutions - their organisational exigencies on the one hand, and their potential close relations to the realm of meaning on the other - which may provide us with clues as to how the ordinary and the charismatic are continuously interwoven in the process of institution building. New organisations and institutions are built up through the varied responses and interactions between people or groups who, in order to implement their varied goals, undertake processes of exchange with other people or groups. But the individuals or groups who engage in such exchange are not randomly distributed in any society. Such exchange takes place between people placed in structurally different positions, that is, in different cultural, political, family, or economic positions which in themselves may be outcomes of former processes of institutional exchange. Their very aspirations and goals are greatly influenced by their differential placement in the social structure and the power they can thereby exercise. The resources that are at their disposal - for instance, manpower, money, political support, or religious identification - are determined by these institutional positions and vary according to the specific characteristics of the different institutional spheres. These resources serve as means for the implementation of various individual goals, and they may in themselves become goals or objects of individual endeavors. Such resources always evince some tendency to become organised in specific, autonomous ways, according to the specific features of their different institutional spheres; this can be seen, for instance, in the fact that the exchange of economic resources is organized in any society in different ways than that of political or religious resources."

"The concrete institutional framework which emerges in any given situation is thus the outcome not only of some general appropriateness of a given solution proposed by such people to the groups acting in this situation but also of the relative success of different competing groups of such leaders and entrepreneurs who attempt to impose, though a mixture of coercive, manipulative, and persuasive techniques, their own particular solution on a given situation."[69]

According to Eisenstadt, earlier social evolutionism suffered not only from unilinearism but also from "... the failure to specify fully the systemic characteristics of

50

evolving societies or institutions or the mechanisms and processes of change through which the transitions from one 'stage' to another were effected ..." In Eisenstadt's rendering of modern sociological theory, concepts like specialization and complexity in the explanation of evolutionary change have been replaced by 'differentiation', which "describes the ways through which the main social functions or the major institutional spheres of society become dissociated from one another, attached to specialised collectivities and roles, etc." Thus "... different levels or stages of differentiation denote the degree to which major social and cultural activities as well as certain basic resources - such as manpower and economic resources -have been disembedded or freed from kinship, territorial, and other ascriptive units". From this differentiation there arise new problems, those of integration of the differentiated functions and roles, which are said to "... become more interdependent and potentially complementary in their functioning". This functionalist approach has of course been criticized for proceeding as if 'complementarity' and 'interdependence' **as such** are somehow forces of history, and thus obscuring from view the concrete mode by which this inter-penetration is actually effected, either 'spontaneously' or with an element of conscious response and initiative in face of perceived problems of integration.

It is evident that for Eisenstadt problems of social evolution are above all problems posed by the necessity of integration following 'new levels of differentiation'. At this point, we find once again the introduction of the factor of 'elites', in the same way that the role of elites, with initiative and authority, is so central to Renfrew's notion of social evolution. Thus Eisenstadt says: "... at any given level of differentiation, the crystallization of different institutional orders is shaped by the interaction between the broader structural features (sic) of the major institutional spheres, on the one hand, and, on the other, the development of elites or entrepreneurs in some of the institutional spheres of that society, in some of its enclaves, or even in other societies with which it is in some way connected."[70]

Such statements are so general that they may be interpreted and utilised in quite different ways, depending upon what other assumptions and/or theories are combined with them. Interestingly enough, the emphasis placed by Sahlins and some other commentators on the central role of relations of political dominance in determining the direction and tempo of social change, leads to very similar conclusions. Eisenstadt himself does not think it possible to draw conclusions about any general tendency or law in social evolution, and prefers this formulation: "The most that can be claimed at present is that the processes of differentiation in different societies exhibit similar formal and structural characteristics and that these create somewhat similar integrative problems."[71]

One wonders how **processes** might have **structural** characteristics; but the formal-sociological emphasis of this conclusion is clear enough. Because of this ultra-formalism (I mean to say that the problems are posed in terms of abstraction from any actual societies or their identifiable concrete-historical characteristics) the final link in the chain of Eisenstadt's argument proves to be a very fragile one. This is to be expected if, as is implied by Eisenstadt, some general but real force for differentiation and integration motivates social actors. Besides the problems which arise, he says, there must be a 'capacity to solve these problems'. It is of course a gigantic assumption, and one for which no argument is presented, that the resolution of society's problems, even if they can be defined as those of integration arising from differentiation, is tackled through some generalized capacity for dealing with such problems. Rather, one might argue,

men in their different activities set themselves certain particular purposes; they do so in the context of conditions and traditions which they find and which are not of their choosing: the interrelations between their activities, within one sphere (say, the political, or the economic, in certain societies) or between these spheres may assert themselves, go through transformations, and change the related spheres, determining or conditioning behaviour in hitherto unknown ways. Such sequences of unintended consequences have long been recognized in social and historical sciences. No one would deny the importance of an analysis of the role of individual and group initiative within and in relation to such changes, and the way in which that role differs under different conditions, but this is not what Eisenstadt proposes. For him, there are structural problems of integration, and there are capacities for dealing with them. "The crucial is the presence or absence, in one or more institutional spheres, of an active group of special 'entrepreneurs' - that is, an elite that is able to offer solutions to the new range of problems."[72]

He goes on to cite Max Weber's concepts of 'charismatic' groups and personalities as the anticipation of this theoretical discovery and notes the implications for social evolution. "The development of such 'charismatic' personalities or groups constitutes perhaps the closest social analogy to genetic mutation. It is the possibility of such mutations that explains why, at any level of differentiation, a given sphere contains not one but several, often competing, possible orientations and potentialities for development."[73]

This is not the place to argue whether or not the concept of 'structural differentiation' might be fruitfully employed independently of Eisenstadt's speculation about problem-solving elites. It is interesting, however, to see how Renfrew has left the door very wide open for such speculation by his advocacy of the 'multiplier effect' in explaining the transition to civilization. My aim in what follows is not of course to impugn Refrew's contribution to historical understanding of that transition by his work in the Aegean, but rather to point out what appear to me to be weaknesses and contradictions in the theoretical approach which he proposes. I shall argue that some of these result from loose and inconsistent definitions, while others repeat certain of the features to which I have drawn attention in Eisenstadt's schema.

Renfrew[74] is quite explicit in his intention, with the definition of the 'multiplier effect', to demonstrate the mechanism by which movement is possible in the system of interconnectedness, unity and equilibrium stressed by functionalist anthropology. "When the multiplier effect comes into operation, there is sustained and rapid growth, not merely in the scale of the systems of the culture but in their structure."[75]

It seems, then, that 'the culture' has systems, in the plural, and that these in turn each have properties of scale and of structure, both variable. At any rate, the first question is, precisely: when, and under what conditions, **does** the multiplier effect come into sustained operation? In the case of the emergence of civilization, says Renfrew, "... it seems that the crucial requirement is that there should exist the possibility for sustained growth (and for positive feedback) in **at least two** of the subsystems of the culture."[76]

One is led to assume here that 'subsystems of the culture' means what earlier were called 'systems of the culture'. The example of one of these 'subsystems', given in parentheses in Renfrew's sentence, is 'agricultural production'. In the next paragraph 'the "temple" culture' of Malta is named as a subsystem, and it is put alongside 'technological' and 'economic' subsystems.

In the previous chapter, in which 'interconnected-ness' is stressed at the expense of any 'prime mover' (see above), Renfrew had outlined five subsystems: the subsistence subsystem (composed of actions related to the distribution of food resources); the technological subsystem (composed of actions resulting in the production of material artifacts); the social subsystem (composed of actions which take place between men ... 'patterned inter-personal behaviour'), **including** what might in market societies be categorized separately as the economic subsystem; the projective or symbolic subsystems (giving formal expression to man's understanding of and reactions to the world); and the trade and communication subsystem (activities involving travel, of men or of artifacts).[77] Renfrew helpfully points out that "a given human action can exist in several dimensions at once."

In Malta, then, it was a matter of the religious subsystem developing but the technological and economic (social) subsystems failing to do so, having no freedom to move. No indication is given of under what conditions such 'freedom' does or does not occur. After a brief glance at the well-known argument that a surplus product is a necessary but not a sufficient condition for significant social and economic change, Renfrew says simply that the growth of civilization came about "through innovations in technique **coupled with** social and other development which at the same time made these subsistence improvements both possible and desirable". From this standpoint he criticizes Robert Adams's conclusion that "the transformation at the core of the Urban Revolution lay in the realm of social organisation."

Now Renfrew comes to formulating his idea 'as a testable proposition' for the case of the emergence of civilisation, and here it seems that **three** subsystems are involved: "... we shall not expect the archaeological record for the early development of a civilisation to show greatly improved production techniques (e.g. irrigation) and 'surplus' storage facilities arising prior to, or without evidence of social stratification (e.g. palaces) or religious specialisation (e.g. temples). Nor shall we, in the cases where the successful transition to civilisation was later accomplished, expect these social and religious advances to have developed markedly without development also in food production. On the contrary, the two were linked together by the multiplier effect."[78]

What can it mean to say 'linked together by the multiplier effect'? An **abstraction** from history, the **multiplier effect**, has become a **real** link, a cause. In reality, of course, Renfrew has not said any more than that increased food production, to the point of a significant surplus over and above the subsistence of the producers, is a necessary condition for the transition to civilization, and that history knows two paths by which this transition has been effected: through appropriation of the surplus by a newly emerging socio-economic class or classes, and through the domination over production and distribution by a religious bureaucracy. It will be noted that it is not **any** two of the three factors (subsystems) that may combine to produce the transition. Consequently the 'old' problems of the determining nature of 'the economic', or of the mode of production, cannot be so easily spirited away by incantating 'interconnectedness' and 'multiplier'.

For the Aegean civilization, Renfrew here mentions 'trade' (subsector five) and its need for 'strong (?) interaction with other sectors, such as social organization' as the elements of the multiplier effect. Assuming that 'sectors' here are 'subsystems' or 'systems' (or, later in the same passage, 'factors'), we are left with the same problem: acknowledging the 'interaction' of 'factors', nothing whatsoever is said to establish that all are of the

same real or potential significance. Renfrew does not go so far as Service, to say that any sector of social behaviour may be the determining one in any particular case, but he does assert that in general any **combination** of two (or three, in some definitions) elements may prove so to be. In the cases he cites, however, it is always a matter of how those activities concerned with production and distribution of the material means of life combine with certain other elements of social life. I would stress, of course, that the body of Renfrew's work is indeed a rich demonstration of the complex and many-sided processes making up the 'emergence of civilization', a demonstration which rises above (or, perhaps, wisely stays **below,** in a certain sense) the level of the theoretical apparatus outlined by the author.

If we follow Renfrew's theoretical introduction to its end, it is not because he finds ways of overcoming the difficulties pointed out here, but because he shows even more clearly, intentionally or unintentionally, that problems with a long history in sociology and anthropology are involved, problems with very broad implications. The archaeologist, no less than the sociologist and the anthropologist, needs to be aware of these implications, of the problems they have raised, and of the 'solutions' which have been proposed to them. It has become clear, from the years of revival of discussion of the uses of ethnographic analogy in archaeology, that in one sense the issue was wrongly posed. It is not a case of this or that suitable analogy, nor even the need for a wide knowledge of possible analogies because of the great variety of cultural response to similar environment and problems, as many have concluded. More to the point is that anthropology, sociology and history, in general theory and in their attempt to apply such theory in mastering empirical ('ethnographic') material, must be examined to discover the degree to which they have clarified the theoretical issues at stake in analyzing historical societies, the relations between their parts, the possible implications of material remains, and so on. Renfrew borrows and amalgamates various elements from current or past sociological theories, or from 'common-sense' assumptions about 'human nature' and motivation; and all these, whether we like it or not, have a history which it would be costly to ignore.

Following his outline of interacting subsystems, Renfrew asserts: "It is, of course, at the level of the individual in society that the multiplier effect actually operates" and "the various subsystems of the culture are linked at the level of the individual".[79] Actually, there is no 'of course' about it. Any truth in this resort to 'the individual' is exhausted by the truism that without individuals and their actions there would be no society. If 'interconnectedness' of subsystems is the 'key' to social change, as Renfrew has stated, and this inter connectednesss actually happens 'at the level of the individual', then it is difficult to avoid the conclusion that psychological rather than sociological explanations of social change are in order. Insofar as Renfrew stresses interacting subsystems, he is following the prescriptions of Binford and Clarke, and of other archaeologists like Flannery with his 'continually interacting factors'.[80] Into this he introduces a general concept from cybernetics (Maruyama's 'deviation-amplifying mutual causal process' and 'positive feedback'). Whatever may be one's criticism of this rejection of any notion of the primacy of the economic or some other element, the approach is, so far, capable of being made 'operational'. But is this consistent with the assertion that it is 'at the level of the individual' that the interconnections are established and work? Let us assume only that, say, the economic and the political subsystems (insofar as they can be defined and separated) mutually affect (cause) one another, and induce changes in each other. In what sense can this be deemed to be a process

52

'at the level of the individual'? If I say, for example, that a feudal economy is less likely to be associated with a parliamentary democracy than is a capitalist economy, or that early empires tended to outgrow their economic basis, in what possible way are the relations suggested by these 'hypotheses' testable 'at the level of individual behaviour'? It is no denial of the reality of individual choices to show that there are social-historical processes which have regularity and necessity at a level which cannot be reduced to the connections between **the individual's** (say) 'economic' and 'political' actions and thoughts. This is quite apart from the difficulties posed for **archaeology** if the vital connections are, after all, individual and psychological.[81] In case it should be thought that I exaggerate, I may point out that in the same work (The Emergence of Civilisation) we do indeed find social stability or equilibrium explained in terms of 'the working of habit and convention'. This 'habit' is, it seems, a property of individual behaviour which is necessary if the totality of individual actions is to constitute the **system** of culture, with the homeostatically-controlled equilibrium characteristic of systems as such. At no point does Renfrew explain (he only asserts) the relation between the individual and the social-system levels.[82] Renfrew then introduces as historical fact that instability is brought to 'the system' by external factors, their effects being controlled homeostatically, before proceeding to his 'multiplier' effect (see above) to explain change. Here culture is viewed as essentially a normative order, working through the conditioning of the individual's habits (Durkheim's "social facts ... external to and exercising constraint upon the individual"). This is indeed one of the solutions (not the same as Weber's) to the problem of the relation between individual and social reality. It is therefore in a sense quite correct for Renfrew to refer to functionalist anthropology as one of the bases of his approach. It leads however to the conclusion stated best, perhaps, by Radcliffe-Brown, with his "... the whole system of moral and religious sentiments on which the social order rests".[83] I would point out, furthermore, that Talcott Parsons, after his exhaustive work to establish a frame of reference bringing Durkheim's and Weber's ideas together[84], produced a series of systematic works which tried eventually to take full cognisance of systems theory and cybernetics, and emerged with the conclusion that in general, the distinguishing marks of cultures one from another will be found at the level of their 'central value systems'.[85] Renfrew himself does not discuss all these implications of his own assertions, but it is interesting to refer, in conclusion, to his remarks in a later publication. In his 'Space, Time and Polity' he says, "We have to ask ourselves what we mean by social organisation", and the core of his answer is, "The kind of social group we are speaking of here is relevant to the notion of identity, to the 'Who are You?' question. So that operative groups (e.g. 'middle income group' or group sharing a specific blood type) are not relevant. But for once we are not defeated by the evanescent, irrecoverable nature of past cognitive categories. For **it is precisely the recognition of the group that governs group behavior.** When we are dealing with social groups their cognitive existence, recognized by those included and those excluded, reinforces their operational existence or may indeed create it. And the distinctive group behaviour - the differential nature of interactions with members of the group in distinction to those outside it - reinforces its cognitive recognition. It is this feedback mechanism that gives social groups their distinctiveness - for the group does not count as such if you" (?) "cannot recognize it .... This being so, we ought to be able to recognize them in the archaeological record." (emphasis in original).[86]

This passage repeats, even more explicitly, the reductionist error of referring explanation of the reproduction and transformation of society to the level of consciously motivated behaviour (whether called 'group' or individual). It is quite explicit, also, in its subjectivist emphasis that for present purposes it is the meaning conferred upon groups and their behaviour by the actors that is significant. It is of course of great value for archaeologists to be able to use distinctive cultural features as marks of 'ethnicity',[87] but recognition of this relation is in the nature of a technical aid rather than a sociological or historical theory. Unless we know intimately the society concerned we cannot know **what** difference is implied by cultural distinctiveness, only that there is such distinctiveness - and this will be of great value at certain stages of research. (There is also the point that, even if only those groups are considered which are self-aware, not all of them will 'choose' to mark their self-awareness with material signs. The need or inclination to do so may vary between different kinds of groups and different types of societies). Renfrew does not take from here the road trodden by Levi-Strauss and the structuralists: to seek fundamental structures of the human mind which allow us to understand the patterning of these cultural meanings. Levi-Strauss: "History organises its data in relation to conscious expression of social life, while anthropology proceeds by examining its unconscious foundations."[88] Renfrew prefers to argue from group identity to the process of 'inhomogeneity' of social groups, their degree of differentiation and their 'hierarchy', which is introduced as the essential mechanism of control in differentiated organizations. The spatial correlates of these properties of systems are then offered as the meaningful data open to study by archaeologists. "For is not the most important feature of a chiefdom the existence of a central person, resident at a central place, whether this be periodic or permanent? And is not the distinguishing feature of the state generally accepted as the existence of a permanent hierarchical structure of administration and authority - a structure generally reflected in a hierarchy of central places, so that between the major centre (or state capital) and the minor residence unit (or village) there is at least one intermediate settlement and administrative unit, the regional centre?"[89] All Renfrew has done here is to list those characteristics of state systems which have 'spatial' reflection in the archaeological record, and show their 'fit' with his emphasis on formal structures of cybernetic control. **All** the questions about the origins and nature of the state are begged, in fact, and one is led to assume that this state is indeed only a response to the need, at a certain level of organizational complexity, for effective integration through hierarchical control. That such control is characteristic of states, no one disputes. That reference to it explains anything about the rise of states, or that the presence of such implies always the existence of a state, has simply not been argued. It is in this sense that I said (above) that Renfrew at least leaves open the door, in the explanation of culture changes, for the 'charismatic entrepreneur' explanation offered by Eisenstadt, just as his looseness of conceptual definition and argument leave him open to the conclusion that 'cognitive structures', or 'norms', or 'central values' are the essential content of social processes, even if we set out with the apparently 'neutral' assumption of mere 'interconnectedness'. Certainly Renfrew does not draw these threads together to adopt the specific conclusions of Durkheim or Eisenstadt or Parsons. Rather, he seems to assume the evidence of some ahistorical reservoir of human behaviour-patterns upon which systematic and structural changes work. Thus, "Regularities in response are dependent upon regularities in human behaviour"[90] and, in a formulation which, taken by itself, might lead us to revise our statement (above) that he does not share the view of Levi-Strauss: "The essential kernel of many of the interactions between activities and between subsystems, interactions which are the mainspring for economic growth, develops from the human inclination to give a social and symbolic significance to material goods."[91]

In line with this idea that the dynamics of social systems are 'developed from' some 'human inclination', we discover that market equivalents, just as much as gift-exchange equivalents, are 'constructs of the human mind'.[92] I have tried to indicate below some of the complexities involved in the relations between economic relations and ideology, insofar as they bear on questions of social evolution. For present purposes, this demonstration of a descent into an explicitly idealist interpretation of economic realities serves to complete our brief analysis of the questions raised by Colin Renfrew's view of the evolution of societies from the non-civilized to the civilized level.

'CULTURAL MATERIALISM' AND MARXISM

Against those sociologists and anthropologists who have emphasized the unique structure of meanings attached by a society's members to their actions, artifacts, institutions and behaviour, the point has often been made that, when this has been acknowledged, there remains the question of explaining under what conditions this given set of meanings arises, is capable of being sustained, and comes or may come to an end. The study of societies as adaptive systems in relation to their natural environment is said by the advocates of 'cultural materialism' to produce "... a theory which account(s) for cultural differences and similarities in terms of techno-economic and techno-environmental conditions".[93] It accounts for social evolution in terms of the same 'techno-economic and techno-environmental conditions', and Harris in 1968 welcomed, among American archaeologists, "a growing convergence towards the strategy of cultural materialism", reflected in serious collection of "data on population ... seasonal and climatic cycles; response of settlement pattern ...; food production techniques ...; techno-environmental effects; size of food-producing and non-food producing groups; incidence of warfare; contribution of disease vectors to mortality; nature of social organisation defined in terms of house groups, village or town units; and intercommunity organisation. These interests link archaeology to ethnology in a powerful new symbiosis, providing the two disciplines with a common set of assumptions emphasising etic events and a joint strategy which has already begun to yield a better understanding of evolutionary process".[94] It is not my intention here to outline the work to which Harris refers, since it is generally already familiar to archaeologists rather than to social anthropologists or sociologists. I confine myself simply to certain aspects of the relation between the view represented by Harris's work, on the one hand, and the recent growth of interest in Marxism in this field, on the other. 'Cultural materialists' and Marxists concur in giving priority in historical explanation to what Harris calls 'etic events'; that is to say, mental processes and products are viewed as secondary, derivative; and material, objective processes as primary, **not** derived from mental ones. Secondly, Marxists would not quarrel in any way about the need to work for accurate natural and techno-environmental information on the matters listed in our last quotation from Harris. Beyond this, the similarity ceases. It is not necessary to detail Harris's misconceptions about Marxism (typified by his outlandish notion that "Marx shared with Darwin and Spencer that curious nineteenth-century faith in the ability of violence and struggle to bring about unlimited social improvement"[95]), and it is enough to note that the difference between historical and 'cultural' materialism at the most general level concerns Marx's concepts of 'forces of production' and 'social relations of production'. Harris considers that the running controversy about "whether or not Marx and Engels intended to give the technological factors equal

weight with the 'relations' or organization of production", results from "ambiguity inherent in Marx's and Engels's definition of 'base'".[96] Harris thinks much confusion has resulted from Marx's and Engels's interpretation of the transition from feudalism to capitalism "as a result of the organisation of the craft and merchant guilds".[97] This is an unfortunate error on Harris's part. There is in Marx and Engels no worked-out theory of the transition, but there are many very definite indications that the most important sources of the transition must be found in the changes in the feudal mode of production rather than the intrusion of money economy and 'the craft guilds'. More immediately relevant here is the implication, in Harris's statement, that 'relations of production' means 'organization' of production. This was not Marx's view, and an 'evolutionist' theory which compounds the two, whatever virtues it may possess, will not be a Marxist one. Much of what is comprised by organization of production would be part of the forces of production, for Marx (or, as some Marxists argue, may be considered as necessary 'work-relations' not immediately relevant to the dialectical relation between forces and relations of production). The **social relations of production,** for Marx, means all those relations between men which are necessary to a given, specific, historical mode of effecting the coming together of means of production and labour, entailing, in class societies, the appropriation of the surplus product of one or more classes by one or more other classes, and normally having legal definition as property rights. Roughly speaking, they are all the social relations immediately essential to the structure of ownership and control of the means of production. For Marx, major socio-historical systems are characterized essentially by the specific mode by which the surplus product is 'pumped out of the direct producers'.[98] Furthermore, Marx asserts that the forms of social and political domination and the social struggles characteristic of a given social formation are structured by these relations of production.[99] The totality of the social relations of production constitutes what Marx and Engels called 'the economic structure' or 'base' upon which social relations and ideological superstructures are raised. Major social-historical changes, social revolutions, depend not upon the recognition of need for change and capacity for initiation of 'entrepreneurial elites' or on environmental changes alone. Each of these is strictly conditioned in its range of possibilities by an objective element: the transformation of the relation between development of productive forces and structure of social relations of production to a condition where they cease to be compatible; and this contradiction provokes class struggles on an intensified revolutionary scale, now having the content not merely of a conflict over the degree and conditions of exploitation within the given system, but of a struggle to break the power of the ruling class and bring a new class to power. The class struggle under capitalism, moreover, is the last of these struggles, because the forces of production have reached a level at which only a classless society corresponds to their effective use and development. The transition to the classless society is effected, according to Marx and Engels, by socialist revolution and the 'dictatorship of the proletariat'. One may consider Marx right or wrong, but it should be noted that he was quite explicit that without the elements here summarized, there was nothing distinctive about Marxism.[100] (I have of course dealt only with those distinctive elements which bear directly on the **general** question of social evolution).

It seems clear enough that Marx's theory gives an ontological priority to the development of humanity's growing control over nature (the development of the forces of production). He takes this symbiosis of men with the rest of nature to be a material necessity arising at a definable stage in the development of the material world. Social production is thus a ' nature-imposed necessity', and requires definite social relations of production. The struggle with nature presents itself afresh every day, and it consists of the labour process in its many forms, a series of actions not **directed** at the structuring or changing of social relations but, rather, at the maintenance or more effective production of the material means of life, while at the same time having consequences for the reproduction and transformation of social relations. It is the 'unity and conflict of opposites' constituted by the forces of production and the relations of production that is for Marx the most fundamental motive force of social evolution. It is through exploitation of labour that the reproduction of the social structure takes place, in class society. It is the class struggle inevitably consequent upon this exploitation that is the actual motion of society. From the Marxist standpoint, for example, the origin of the state could not be understood only as the centralized organization necessitated by a change in production like irrigation. That would imply a mere adaptive response of the social structure to the structure of production. Rather, a Marxist would seek to investigate the changing forms of exploitation connected with the practice of large-scale irrigation, the forms of social domination necessary to stabilize the conditions of that exploitation, the relations between the different classes involved, and the history of the creation of political institutions to control the exploited class or classes and to contain the competing interests among the exploiters. He would seek to trace in as much detail as possible the manner in which the previously existing social relations, say, the organization of a segmentary lineage and clan system with devolved rights in land, with self-acting corporate groups regulating disputes, came increasingly into conflict with the economic consequences of changes in the productive forces, or changes induced by the impact of other societies. He will be aware that it is not written into the nature of social formations that they each develop through contradiction to a point where they are inevitably displaced by a higher social form. The possibility of such a transformation must be discovered in the facts, by analysis, as Marx did for the origin and development of the capitalist mode of production (Marx's Capital). Strictly speaking, a Marxist account of the processes dealt with in the literature of 'social evolution' would dispense with vocabulary like 'societies' or 'cultures' and use only 'modes of production' and 'social formations' or 'socio-economic formations'. It should be stressed that Marx gave an extended analysis and account of only one such social formation, capitalism, and he did not complete his work on that. From the 'critique of political economy' he worked to an account of the 'law of motion' of capitalist economy. The historical record, for Marx, showed that several other types of social formation had existed, and these corresponded to levels of the development of men's control over nature, but it would be entirely against the spirit of Marx's theory to propose a theory of social-evolutionary stages, without having carried out analyses of the laws of motion of other modes of production and social formations than capitalism. This was not done by Marx or by any Marxist since his day. Furthermore, it is doubtful if the necessary materials exist for such an analysis. As Engels put it: "political economy in (its) wider sense has still to be brought into being".[101] This does not by any means exclude scientific work on pre-capitalist social formations in the light of Marx's historical materialist concepts; productive forces; social relations of production; exploitation; class; class struggle, etc. It is legitimate to regard Capital as a 'test' of the validity of the hypothesis on the nature of social development which Marx built out of these concepts.

Samir Amin, in his The Law of Value and Historical Materialism,[102] rejects the idea of 'political economy in its widest sense', preferring to restrict 'political economy' to the analysis of capitalism and regard 'historical materialism' as the theoretical framework for social formations in general. From one point of view, this is no more than a terminological dispute. Amin asserts that "... under the capitalist mode of production economic laws possess a theoretical status different from that which they possess under pre-capitalist modes; and even that, strictly speaking, economic laws are to be found only under the capitalist mode...".[103] It would be better to say, '... have only been discovered and defined for the capitalist mode'. Later he declares that in pre-capitalist societies, "... the relations between base and super-structure are not the same".[104] This could mean two totally different things: either that the way in which the base determines in general the superstructure differs and must be studied in detail in each case (which is surely not controversial among Marxists), or that the base does not determine the superstructure in pre-capitalist societies (which certainly is).

Evidently, the problems raised by attempting a Marxist analysis of pre-capitalist societies require a theoretical framework which is very different from that of 'cultural materialism' and any assimilation of one to the other must be rejected.[105] Given the emphasis above, on the distinctiveness of the economic and social structure of the one social formation analyzed by Marx, capitalism, does this mean then that his findings and method in political economy are irrelevant to the study of the evolution of earlier social formations? I shall try to show that, on the contrary, Marx's political economy has illuminating theoretical implications for the study of pre-capitalist economies.[106]

In the literature of what is called 'economic anthropology' there are many references to the relevance for pre-capitalist societies of economic categories proper to capitalism and economics. Meyer, Malinowski and many others attached considerable importance to what they thought to be the existence of something called 'capital' in early societies. The criticism of such attitudes and approaches should not be kept to the level of pointing out their ethnocentricism. If we can show that such use of economic categories is unhistorical, then clearly there will be significant implications for concepts of social evolution, of historical development. I do not mean to say that a 'Formalist' approach to pre-capitalist economics cannot have a theory of social evolution, but only that such a theory would have very definite characteristics and perhaps unforeseen implications for all manner of important questions.

THE EMERGENCE OF SOCIAL-ECONOMIC DISTINCTIONS: FORMALISM AND SUBSTANTIVISM

Polanyi answers the Formalists by stressing the social 'embeddedness' of economic activities, forms, institutions, relations, in pre-capitalist, in contrast to capitalist, societies, where they are 'disembedded'.[107] Godelier has long ago pointed out that this distinction "... is a questionable one, since the term 'disembedded' could suggest an absence of internal relation between the economic and the non-economic, whereas this relation exists in every society ... (capitalism's) rationality is that of competing individuals who may or may not be owners of the factors of production. It cannot be reduced to 'purely' economic significance, because it also means a particular way of functioning of the family, the state, etc., in these societies, and because its aim, the accumulation of wealth in money form, creates possibilities for the individual of playing a role in the political, cultural, etc., structures of his society. In other societies, at other moments of history, economic rationality would have a quite different context."[108]

It seems clear therefore that an uncritical use of the categories of economics in non-capitalist economies will not only result in a misunderstanding of the relations of production and distribution. The nature of other 'non-economic' social relations (or of other, non-economic, aspects of certain social relations) will also be mis-construed, because in each type of socio-economic forma-tion, each of them relates to the social totality and its economic structure in different specific ways, and not at all in the way (indicated in part by Godelier) that this interrelation is effected in capitalism. The totality of capitalist production-relations is continuously activated by the renewed acts of exchange between capital and labour and the consequent circulation of goods; this social relation appears as a 'mass of commodities', things. The social product takes the commodity form, universally, in capitalism, and so in Capital Marx starts with it, and moves by analysis to the actual relations of production and the class struggle, the history of capitalist society. In non-capitalist societies, the product is **not** commodity, the producers and the means of production do not come together **in this way,** and the actions and roles of individ-uals are not dependent on the relations of production **in this way** (i.e. as a consequence of their appropriation of 'value', an appropriation derived from the distribution of means of production between individuals). If we need an economic anthropology we need it first of all for the critical understanding of our own society, to demonstrate the social-historical 'embeddedness' of its 'rational' eco-nomic categories and imperatives. It is not that primitive economies should be patronizingly acknowledged as having 'their own' type of rationality. Rather, we shall not begin to ask the right questions until we question the notion that there is anything 'rational' about an economic system in which the relations between the different productive labours and between branches of the economy is decided by the blind play of 'market forces'. The rational motives of individuals in adapting sensibly to such a system do not make the system rational. There were rational place-seekers in Hitler's entourage to the last.

Now, in studying pre-capitalist economies, is the task one of comparing the 'behaviour and attitudes' of the individuals concerned with those of entrepreneurs and buyers and sellers under capitalism? Does anyone propose treating of social evolution, for example, as an evolution of such behaviours? I suggest that the discussion of economic rationality, and much of the discussion about motives in relation to surplus, as of 'dominance' and power, should be subjected to the same critical question-ing. We run the risk, not only of attributing to imaginary actors individual motives which are anachronistic, but also of reductivism, i.e. explanation of social-historical phenomena in terms of individual behaviour. It seems then that material goods, products of labour, in our own society, are mysterious things, bearers of social relations not only not visible to the naked eye but not discoverable or definable by orthodox economic or sociological treat-ment. Every product in capitalist economy contains within itself 'congealed labour time' which makes it automatically potentially representative of the value of every other commodity; and this quality, from the stand-point of the economic system, predominates over the palpable material qualities and uses of the commodity. Finally, the economic system is **not** the product or aggre-gate of meaningful acts informed by consciousness of these relations. On the contrary, the behaviour of actors is 'rational' only by asymptotic conformity to these char-acteristics of the commodity, the value-form and the resulting social relations. Men conform to these as to an external, natural necessity.

The archaeologist, confronted with the material products of extinct societies, is familiar with stern ad-monitions from anthropologists and sociologists, to the effect that things are not always what they seem, that they have been parts of a set of cultural meanings in which wealth or utility, as we understand them, are irrelevant. The 'cultural materialists' have taken from Marx the elementary proposition that nonetheless no society could exist for a week without a system of the production of the material means of life, and that there are necessary regularities of such a system, whatever motives and values surround it. Marvin Harris[109] has even shouted through the bars of the prison-window of anthropology, telling archaeologists that they should con-fidently get on with what they are doing, and be glad that they have been spared contamination by the 'emic', es-pecially in its virulent French form. The truth in this injunction is unfortunately very limited, and beyond its limits becomes an untruth. The cultural materialists themselves, that is to say, carry us into the opposite trap, where the economic is not distinguished from the techno-environmental. Instead of a dialectical relation between the two, we have a collapse of the former into the latter. It is as if the capitalist economy was to be understood simply as 'that set of social roles which corresponds to the predominance of large scale industrial production'. (This is indeed the view, I must say, of the vast majority of sociologists, who take their subject matter to be 'indust-rial society'. This is like interpreting Brecht's Arturo Ui as a warning against the men behind greengrocery busi-nesses). Again, there is a limited truth-content in such a proposition, but it turns into its opposite, becomes an untruth, precisely at the point where historical change, (the content of '**social** evolution'), comes into question. Degree of control over the natural environment includes techniques of production, and development of these tech-niques has implications for change in social systems, but without a knowledge of the historical context we **do not know** what these implications are. In general, for exam-ple, there develops a contradiction between private appropriation (through capital-ownership) and 'socializ-ation' of production, in capitalism, but the extent to which capitalism can contain this contradiction is not known in advance, is not at all a purely economic, let alone a purely 'technical' question, and depends on politi-cal and ideological developments, etc. Moreover, the system's degree of success in overcoming temporarily the contradictions produces new historical forms, unpredicted and unpredictable. In connection with the question of the relevance of Marxism for the study of pre-capitalist societies, I stress again that the foregoing propositions refer to the one society, capitalism, for which Marxism has ventured an analysis of the 'laws of motion'. One should not even begin to formulate the requisite analogous proposition for non-capitalist societies, on which the work has just not been done, and for which, in large part, the data simply do not exist for the same kind of analysis. There is no **general** answer to the question: is Marxism applicable to the study of the societies studied by archae-ologists? From the practice of Marx follows only the necessity of a detailed study of the history of each social formation, to discover if possible its law of motion.

Ignoring this 'discipline of the historical context' (E.P. Thompson) sociologists and anthropologists, cultural materialists among them, time and again impose the categories of the modern economic system on to earlier economies. R.F. Salisbury's work on the Siane of New Guinea[110] has understandably been one of the most influential ethnographic works of the recent period. It has provided unique and invaluable comparative data for the study of economic systems, just as did the work of Salisbury's teacher, S.F. Nadel.[111] Yet there is an important sense in which the author was separated from the implications of his own material. In his introduction we read: "The traditional Western economic concept potentially most applicable and useful in understanding the Siane material is that of 'capital' ".[112] On the

56

contrary. The "traditional Western economic concept, 'capital'" becomes 'applicable' to the Siane only when it is stripped of all historical-economic specificity and is used to refer to the elementary condition of **all** production in **all** societies, viz. that part of the product is set aside for future **productive** consumption. Insofar as Salisbury extends the meaning of 'capital' to Siane behaviour, it is no more than abstract comparison of selected aspects of Siane individual attitudes to wealth with those of individuals in capitalist societies. Such analogy becomes a substitute for independent analysis, and it is derived, once again, from an uncritical view of the economics of our own society. Thus, the "traditional Western economic concept" of 'capital', as Salisbury puts it, eliminates the specific social-historical relations of actual "traditional Western economy", capitalism. It "unthinkingly compounds the historically determined social forms of production with the material aspects of the real labour process".[113] I contend that we stand a better chance of making an objective appraisal of 'non-capitalist economy' and its evolution if we acknowledge, with Marx, the historical content and limits of the categories of political economy. Thus, for example, capital is value "which breeds surplus-value" (Marx) and not out of some inherently magical quality, but because it "rests on a particular historically determined relation - the relation of wage-labour" (Rosdolsky). This definition of capital in terms of the properties of the capitalist system should not be compounded with the form taken by capital in stages of its transformation in the processes of capitalist production and circulation: as a sum lent, as stockpiled goods, in which cases "it seems to be a mere thing, and to coincide entirely with the material in which it is present".[114]

At this point I indicate, though I cannot develop here, some of the general implications of this argument for studies of exchange and trade in pre-capitalist societies. It has been important to recognize that exchanges in these societies must not be interpreted on the model of sale and purchase, the equating of the value (price) of goods. Models of gift-exchange and reciprocity have in general been accepted as often more appropriate than a market model. (It is of course necessary to distinguish between these forms of exchange and the development of markets and merchant capital in pre-capitalist economies). Again, it has become a truism in archaeology that 'trade' is not important only as a medium of contact, of diffusion of culture, and evidence of it part of the proof thereof. Rather, one considers the actual effects of internal and long-distance trade on social **systems.** This has been part of the opening up of important and exceedingly difficult questions: the definition of the boundaries of economic and social systems, once we leave behind the old 'culture' and 'culture area'; the meaning of 'internal' and 'external'; the causal relations between external trade and internally generated need; and so on. Anthropology and archaeology most often deal with traditional social formations, in which only a **part** of the total social product takes the commodity form. Exchange does not concern "production in its totality but only superfluous production and superfluous products"[115] (no value-judgment is involved in the use of the term 'superfluous' here, it refers only to production over and above the needs of consumption and necessary means of future production in the given society). This is obvious enough, but perhaps we have not yet taken cognizance of the vast implications of the fact that in our own society **no** social relations of production are entered into without passing through the exchange of values (and above all of the exchange of the commodity labour-power for a portion of capital).

In capitalism, other social relations are built up on this economic foundation, including the political and ideo-

logical forms. The contradictions of capitalist societies, and the changes of which these contradictions are the motive force, are internal to the system of these social relations (or rather to the unity of them with the forces of production through which men confront nature). In the study of non-capitalist societies, however, there is need to pay attention to the contradiction **between** this sector in which exchange exists and the rest of production, which will no doubt be found to have its own internal contradictions in addition.[116] Which of these sets of contradictions will be predominant in the mechanism of social development should not be postulated in advance. That is a matter for research: to establish the developing relations between exchange-relations (and the production underlying them, and their social consequences) and that sector of production which is devoted to producing use-values (and its social relations). It is sufficient to refer to the rich discussion and associated research of the last three decades or so concerning the role of commerce and of change in social relations of production in the transition from feudalism to capitalism. Unfortunately, we do not have the same wealth of data for the periods studied by most archaeologists. It may well be that at this stage archaeological perspectives on European social and economic evolution are limited, on many questions, to defining the scope and limits of the evidence. Finley's many writings on the ancient economy, on the historical content of Homer, and on Aristotle's 'economics' have relied heavily on the analogy of gift-exchange systems in ethnography (in this way seeking to avoid ethnocentrism), in interpreting the available archaeological and literary evidence. It has already been suggested that Finley has over-generalized the ethnographic analogy here, and that there was, in classical Athens, besides the survival, in whatever proportion, of gift-exchanges and prestige-transactions, a growing commodity sector for which Aristotle recognized the necessity of a separate type of analysis, anticipating the theory of value in classical political economy.[117]

However specialists may decide what is at stake in this specific case of interpretation of the passages in the Politics and Ethics, it is I think clear that the whole area is only just opening up, and that knowledge of what are assumed to be analogous 'gift-exchange' ethnographic examples is by itself an extremely limited equipment. Of course Binford and many others made this point long ago: that the archaeology must itself provide the historical connections and systematic relations, i.e., analogy is no substitute for good archaeology. It must be said that functionalist bias in anthropology has produced a mass of material in ethnography which is of little use in this connection, having never asked the appropriate questions (above).

I return briefly to Salisbury's book on the Siane, since it bears on many of the problems involved in discussion of the relation of archaeology to anthropology and is invaluable in spite of the infelicity to which I have referred. In every lineage of the Siane there are several 'big men', i.e. men who are listened to more than others, accumulate more consumption-goods and prestige items, and have a wider range of contacts, who are also partners in gift-exchange. However, it should be noted that the existence of a number of 'big men' of this type has no significance for production. There is no 'economic' division between them and other men. Such a situation is not uncommon in simple economies. If an archaeologist were to excavate Siane graves he might well find differentiation in the quantity of burial goods. He certainly could not legitimately infer anything about social stratification or (what I consider to be a different question) social relations of production. Clearly, no way exists of analyzing a piece of funeral paraphernalia which will determine its economic function, or whether it relates to class or to status difference (where 'status' might be decided by all sorts of criteria). Among the Siane, accumulation of goods is in order to consume more in a certain way so as to extend one's social contacts. That, and not the accumulation of wealth to put a man in a position to exploit the labour of others, is the sole aim of appropriation. At death, in accordance with the outlook prevalent in such a society, much or even all of a man's personal property will be given away at the funeral. For this and other, perhaps chance, reasons, some burials contain no grave goods, and whether they do or not is not dependent to any detectably significant degree on wealth at time of death. In some societies, wealth in graves reliably indicates wealth at death. In others, it seems, death is something of a leveller, and not only in the moral sense. Of course, even if graves did give us an accurate picture of differences in personal property, we would have to adjudge the significance of these differences in a case like the Siane (who are not exceptional in this respect) where personal property is rigidly separated off from property in means of production (primarily of course the land). The latter cannot be owned privately. It is one of a category of things, rights over which involve account-ability and responsibility of the possessor to the community and to the ancestors. With land, in this category, are included sacred objects such as flutes used in ritual, and the lore of ritual. All are inalienable, and are assimilated in Siane culture to the rights of a man over his children. In the opposite category are personal items of dress, implements, and objects such as trees and pigs which depend upon personal labour and use. A complex set of rules establishes the priority of the collective and sacred category, in which personal rights are not separated from the overriding rights of the collective, past, present and unborn. Land tenure itself need not concern us here: it is on the familiar pattern of localized and segmented lineage-group rights. These segmentarily-organized rights would be highly unlikely to show in any archaeological record. There are no boundary ditches, fences or hedges, only a particular species of plant used as boundary markers at certain points. Let us note, in any case, that 'material' goods are to be found on both sides of the property-classification, as are goods of 'economic' significance. It is not possible to anticipate or interpret the classification (and whatever implications it may have for the disposition of material remains in some archaeological find) on the basis of any a priori criteria. The 'fit' between what status-stratification there is and this pattern of ownership and control of means of pro-duction is not one which could be seen in even the most ingenious analysis of material remains. We are all familiar with the literature on the way in which distinct-ions of rank and status in tribal societies can become the forms through which a quite new economic content develops, but we cannot but note that such differences exist over a vast span of space and time - the whole period of what used to be called barbarism and the transition from barbarism to civilization (and probably in some sense and in some cases in conditions of 'savagery' also) - and without considerable additional data we just do not know how to interpret their significance for social evolution in particular cases. In cases like the Siane, there seems little doubt that the cultural meanings[118] attached to property-forms would have been a consider-able historical obstacle to the evolution of new economic forms in response to changes in division of labour and forces of production. This is of course a bigger question than that raised by the albeit interesting material presented in Salisbury's book on the impact of colonial rule, steel implements and the rest, since first contact was made with the Siane in the early 1930s.

I have not meant to say that the uniqueness of cultural form in each such society makes impossible any comparative or historical study which would contribute to a theory of social evolution. Rather, I suggest that in each case we need to analyze the relation between what Marx called 'phenomena' and 'their hidden substratum'. "The former appear directly and spontaneously as current modes of thought; the latter must first be discovered by science".[119] We do not, I repeat, know anything about these necessary relations by way of deductions from something called historical materialism, or by analogy with Capital, any more than we do by 'applying' orthodox economic concepts, or by proceeding with a supposedly neutral common sense, or by application of an a priori scheme of social evolutionary stages.[120]

THEORIES OF SOCIAL EVOLUTION WHICH TAKE AUTHORITY OR DOMINATION TO BE PRIMARY. SAHLINS AND SERVICE.

Marshall Sahlins and Elman Service have perhaps been the most influential anthropologists in the revival of evolu-tionist thinking. Despite the fact that Leslie White wrote an approving introduction to the volume edited by Sahlins and Service in 1962, Evolution and Culture[121] and despite Sahlins' liberal use of phrases such as 'mode of pro-duction', it should be noted that both Sahlins and Service present social evolution in frameworks which are not consistent with that of White and flatly contradict Marxism. Their works are readily available, and I deal with certain crucial theoretical issues rather than giving a thorough critical presentation of their theories. Service's classification of levels of cultural development (band, tribe, chiefdom, state) has tended to become a common-place wherever archaeologists discuss social evolution. It is in point of fact little more than a general descriptive summary in loose terms relating primarily to the type of socio-political integration observable.[122] This is of course an implicit theory of social evolution, and one must assume that it is meant to be broadly related to what Service and Sahlins call 'the law of cultural dominance', i.e. the growing capacity of men to control their environ-ment.

Service, as we have seen, considers that the impetus to major social change may come from any sector or subsystem of society or culture. Let us take his view of the transition to civilization and the state. Interestingly, as the following quotation shows, Service ends up with an emphasis on organizational complexity, the initiative of elites, and the inherent power of leadership, which is reminiscent of the explanations put forward by Renfrew and by Eisenstadt (above): "essentially, the road to civiliz-ation was the developmental route taken by a few simple bureaucracies formed by hereditary (institutionalized) leaders and their relatives. Under rather unusual environ-mental conditions (competitive-selective and eventually circumscribed) this development fulfilled the tremendous potentialities that lay in centralized leadership. Redistri-bution (and especially trade), military organization, and public works were all basic in the classical civilizations, but all must have had small beginnings in the simple attempts of primitive leaders to perpetuate their social dominance by organizing such benefits for their followers. These organizational benefits, growing ever more complex, more useful, and finally necessary to the society, assured the continued maintenance and defence of the society - and the continued growth in power of the bureaucratic organization itself."[123]

Service considers this sweeping conclusion valid because, he says, all early states and civilizations are marked by the emergence of a distinction between those with and those without power, "and this power was so absolute that it needed no buttress such as economic advantage". Consequently "... the question thus turns on the origin of this political power ... the nature of the power structure itself ...".[124]

58

This is not the place to consider the wealth of evidence which contradicts Service's contention. Few would agree with Service that the powerful in the early state enjoyed no economic advantage, or that the state did not enforce a 'law and order' within which a newly-arisen economic exploitation (i.e. extraction of surplus product) could take place under stable conditions. It would be difficult to cite an example where this was not the case. However, Service poses the question of the origin of political power itself, and clearly asserts that changing "rather unusual environmental conditions" permitted the expression of "the tremendous potentialities that lay in centralised leadership". This is a new 'immanentism', putting in a very secondary place the necessities through which human choices had to battle in order to advance from one condition to another. One can only account Service's case here to be an explanation if one is prepared to accept as natural the drive of (some?) men for dominance. Thus, the enormous historical processes involved in 'redistribution (and especially trade), military organization, and public works' are reduced to the small change of individual motivation: "... all must have had small beginnings in the simple attempts of primitive leaders to perpetuate their social dominance".

Even if one considers it an unassailable truth of 'human nature' that men seek to perpetuate their 'social dominance' (a dominance whose origin is itself unexplained), one still could hardly call Service's argument an explanation. Consider an 'explanation' of war by the statement: 'it must have had small beginnings in the aggressive actions of men ...'; or of the history of the institution of marriage: 'it must have had small beginnings in the sexual instinct ...'.

Definite types of authority are born and prove necessary to definite modes of social production and social organization. 'Necessary' needs definition. Authority is a matter not only of a required division of labour at a given level of development of the means of production, but also of the imposition of a definite level of exploitation of the direct producers. This latter is a factor determined in a struggle between classes, and not one flowing directly from technical necessities. It is evident that the relation of authority necessitated by division of labour to the power exerted over the producers in order to ensure their exploitation is not a static one, even within the historical limits of the same mode of production and its economic formation. In the first place, it is of course permanently more or less subject to modification by the changing relationship of class forces. But secondly (a point analytically but not empirically distinct from the first) the given social relations of production and accompanying authority structures may be historically 'necessary' at one stage of the development of productive forces, but may then become barriers to their further development. The relation between these two aspects (i.e. between class struggle within a given mode of production, on the one hand, and the historical tendency of that mode of production, on the other) is one of mutual interaction, interpenetration, transition, and transformation; and it is not the same for every mode of production and type of society. Within this broad analytical framework, the concept of 'necessity' or 'function' of a given 'elite' and its authority becomes definably problematical and amenable to scientific investigation. Such a framework might well provide a way out of the impasse evident in recent discussions about the inadequacies of functionalist explanations in the study of the origins of social stratification (e.g. Current Anthropology, 22, 1, February 1981). In his stimulating paper 'The Development of Social Stratification in Bronze Age Europe', Antonio Gilman points to the exploitative and oppressive nature of some 'elites' or 'ruling classes', and his critics in discussion point out that this aspect and that of functional necessity

are not mutually exclusive. This correction is justified, but leaves the matter at a formal and ahistorical level.

At any rate it is clear that there are different, competing or complementary frameworks for such analysis. Service tends to abstract and reify the factor of 'the tremendous potentialities of centralized leadership' from the social-economic relations which produce and sustain authority. At crucial points this can be decisive, and raises questions for which entirely new hypotheses must be introduced. For example, if we assume that the 'absolute power' referred to by Service is essentially a growth from 'small beginnings' in primitive society, the natural fulfilment of the 'enormous potential of centralized leadership', we are hardly disposed to ask the question: is there a point at which authority was no longer based on belief in its legitimacy or sacredness but needed to be sustained (at least in part) by organized coercion? Morton Fried,[125] as well as many others, has noted that it is the monopoly of force which characterizes the state, echoing at least in part the central importance given by Marx and Engels to 'bodies of armed men' as the core of the definition of the state machine.[126] For Service, on the contrary, the division between governors and governed concerns "aspects of the division of labour" and "there apparently was no class conflict resulting in forceful repression".

We have referred above to Marx's criticism of those who confused economic categories like capital with the particular material forms in which they function, a procedure which obscures their historical content. Marx comments on a similar distinction necessary in the study of the state power: "Just as in the despotic states, supervision and all-round interference by the government involves both the performance of common activities arising from the nature of all communities, and the specific functions arising from the antithesis between the government and the mass of the people".[127]

Sahlins confronts more directly the relation between economic and political development. He writes a great deal about the 'big men' in tribal societies,[128] who later figure so prominently in Renfrew's theories, and it is clear from his account that the basis of their status is not in opposition to reciprocity and egalitarianism but actually works through it. The 'big-man' phenomenon is the form taken by individuality in a tribal society. It does not mean appropriation of wealth to exploit others and to create a permanently differentiated class but, on the contrary, it means distribution of wealth by the 'big man' to preserve and enhance his prestige. Under changed economic circumstances (the impact of colonialism, or presumably, of a change in the mode of production making possible a new division of labour, diversifying of production, a surplus product sufficient to sustain non-producers, the possibility of individuals surviving economically if they break from their descent groups, the break-up of such groups as their solidarities came into conflict with a new and more effective mode of exploiting resources etc.) then certain social characteristics of the 'big men' became important for rapid social development. The 'big man', say, in Melanesia, may have already, in pursuit of contacts and gift-exchange partners, created a network of relations transcending his own settlement. He may have sown the seeds of rivalries and factions based on interests other than distance of kin by his selection and building up of a body of followers or clients. Sahlins is able to show that in Polynesia there is a long record of revolt and threat of revolts against tendencies to inequality. Such revolt can be avoided only by expenditure on ceremonial display, potlatch, or a relaxation of the demands made on followers. As for chiefs, they are in a more formalized position of prominence. Here "The accumulation of funds of power and their redistribution was the underpinning of Polynesian politics".[129] Chiefs here were much richer than the Melanesian 'big men', and could use wealth for more elaborate purposes, but it is clear from Sahlins's account that the difference is one of degree. "Like Melanesian big-man systems, the development of Polynesian chiefdoms was eventually short-circuited by an overload on the relation of chief to people", though "the cut-off point was high ... The limits of chieftainship are the limits of primitive society itself. Where kinship is king, the king is in the last analysis only kinsman, and something less than royal".[130] Whatever significance we attach to the redistributive mechanisms developed in 'chiefdoms' we should remember that, speaking of the chiefdom as a temporal phase of development, the kinship base of social organization still serves as the defining system for production relations, and this social-economic framework must be broken before classes, exploitation, private property in means of production, and the state, can emerge.

Such an argument seems consistent with the data presented by Sahlins, but it would appear that other interpretations could also fit, since Sahlins himself adopts a different standpoint on social evolution here: "Quite apart from technological improvements, political transformation can play the decisive role in economic development".[131] This has since become a common view. It is one which should be tested against long-term development rather than single events or short sequences of events. If not, then we cannot distinguish the degree of historical importance of those cases in which politics are the direct cause of economic developments and those in which the opposite seems true. It is not a question of counting the one series against the other. May it not be, for example, that, within the evolution of one social formation, the capacity of political events and decisions to make significant economic change varies greatly? The words 'decisive role' and 'economic development' here are too general and indefinite.

In his Stone Age Economics, however, Sahlins is much more explicit, stating clearly his view of how societies evolved towards civilization. Thus: "Everything depends on the political negation of the centrifugal tendency to which the Domestic Mode of Production is naturally inclined". To this role of politics, population is secondary and land-use is tertiary, he says: "... and political organisation harbours a coefficient of population density, thus in conjunction with the ecological givens, a determinate density of land use".[132] What the source of the political 'given' is, we are not told. As Cook[133] has pointed out, Sahlins here combines a 'Hobbesian' view of the anarchic tendency of society in its immediate relation with nature (that relation is production) with an essentially idealist notion of how social integration is achieved, i.e. from the realm of what Marx called the political superstructure. Here we are emphasizing the essential difference between historical materialism and the general theory put forward by Sahlins. A more detailed development of the Marxist theory would lay greater stress (as Marx, Engels and other Marxists did on many occasions, and always when analyzing particular historical processes) on the interaction of politics and economics.[134]

ECONOMY AND POLITY IN SOCIAL EVOLUTION: THE STATE, PRODUCTION AND EXCHANGE.

Marxism does not hold that only economic causes are to be found in historical development. Furthermore, it would be necessary to consider much more seriously than has so far been the case in the work of Marxists, the significance of the element of compulsion in the economic process of exploitation itself in pre-capitalist societies.[135] Marx notes that capitalism is distinguished from other societies by its being able to dispense with the 'extra-economic coercion' which characterizes pre-capitalist forms, with their unfree labour. Anthropologists have often discussed the question of the conditions under which the ability to produce a surplus in excess of subsistence results in the formation of class society and the state. One might pose the question, then, as: what is the evidence in each case for a stable system of extra-economic coercion being established, able to ensure the regular exploitation of the direct producers, i.e. the appropriation of the surplus by another class? Such a method of procedure would anchor the discussion of origin and early forms of the state in the whole complex of socio-economic relations, and take it beyond a discussion simply in terms of complexity, efficiency, forms of hierarchy and co-ordination, and so on. In this context, one might arrive at a definition of the crucial importance of 'politics' which would have a great deal more content than has the assertion of Sahlins.

The emergence of centralized control which is noted by all writers on the early state is, moreover, not simply a matter of a functional response to complexity 'on behalf' of society at large, but in a Marxist framework would be considered as necessitated as much by the need to regulate those private interests which became differentiated from group or societal interests at a certain level of economic development. Insofar as such differentiation is absent from primitive society, sanctions and social control are 'diffuse and generalised'[136] but such sanctions are inadequate for the coercive maintenance of exploitation relations and the regulation of conflicting private interests, as well as for the increasing number of social functions which transcend the capacity of descent groups and kinship networks, as adaptation to the environment becomes less localized. The interests to which we refer imply class relations, in that opposed economic interests in relation to the exploitation relationship are the basis of class and class struggle. Differences of rank and status are to be found in pre-class, pre-state societies as well as in civilized, class, state societies. Rank and status have been shown to be compatible with a social organization based on descent and kinship groups, class is not. This distinction is of course directly relevant to the interpretation of archaeological evidence of status difference and the use of such interpretation in argument about social evolution. Here, recent work on the Near East[137] is of exceptional importance. Mario Liverani, discussing in a recent paper the breakdown of the Syrian regional system of trade at the end of the Bronze Age, noted: "The Syrian system of the Late Bronze Age is based on a convergence of interests by the king and the class of high functionaries (maryannu, scribes and administrative personnel, merchants, etc.) with a particularly crude exploitation of the village communities".[138] The historical crisis and collapse of this state arrived when the level of exploitation provoked desertion from the villages and abandonment of basic tasks of village production, and the formation by the runaways of semi-nomadic groups which then attracted other villagers, processes which combined with the weakening of the military links between aristocracy and palace, and the desertion of palace administrative and other specialists. So weakened was the state system, that several attacks from the outside on the Syrian coast at the end of the Bronze Age produced collapse. Liverani also points out that "the particular concentration of all the element of organisation, transportation, exchange, etc., - a concentration which seems to reach its maximum in the Late Bronze Age - has the effect of enlarging the physical collapse of the Palace into a general disaster for the entire kingdom".[139]

The precise mechanism of the decline is not clear here, but the summary suggests that an internal economic-political crisis, concerning the exploitative as well as administrative role of the state, and its place in the conflict of classes,[140] is, in this case at least, central to an understanding of why blows from the outside could bring about collapse. Many European parallels suggest themselves.

One might also add that, although direct evidence of the development of class structure and exploitation, and thus of the law of motion of past societies, may not be available, it will be of great value to be able to ascertain the degree to which it was possible in particular areas to establish stability over time in the production of a surplus and a corresponding set of relations between centre, regions and local social groups.

The ethnographic and the historical evidence suggest that the elements necessary for the formation of the state (which is always a necessary component of the transition from economically undifferentiated to class society, from 'barbarism to civilisation') are developed and come together in processes which are long drawn-out and contradictory,[141] involving innumerable regressions and 'false starts' (which moreover have a different pattern and outcome according to the historical circumstances and the possibilities offered by particular environments). Development of efficiency of food production and the first social division of labour provide the potential of a contradiction between productive forces and the primitive descent-solidarity basis of social organization. Though individual interests begin to emerge, they may be restricted in scope for development by the paucity of external contact and possibility of exchange and accumulation; by the relative slowness or stagnation of further development of division of labour and technique; by cessation of supplies of raw materials; and especially by the members of the society resorting to their systems of rights and obligations, redistributive mechanisms and so on, to prevent the break-up of the existing order. The establishment of any degree of permanence or stability of a distinct social group able to appropriate the surplus product, the consolidation of rights of possession into private-property right, transformation perhaps of traditional gifts to tribute, the coming together of particular individuals of separate lineages, clans or tribes (or, in some cases of individuals from villages which do not have kinship or descent definition) into new types of group with common interests is a long evolution, and requires always not merely the emergence of an elite (above) able to resolve increasingly complex problems, but a struggle to reduce the communities to the permanent condition of a subject, exploited class, to give fixed social form to the loss of freedom. In the historical record, we find that among the direct producers themselves, in village communities, community forms of life remain, often for centuries; and the imposition of large scale tax and/or rent mechanisms does not necessarily destroy them. In every case, then, attention should be paid to the way in which individual interest emerges to go beyond the status-difference recognized in tribal societies and become consolidated into a class interest. Along with this one must ask: how did hitherto undifferentiated relationship to the land, of men in communities organized on the principles of descent, become transformed into a relation of labour bound to the means of production, the land, as an exploited class, forced by extra-economic coercion, backed crucially by the state, to yield up the surplus?[142]

When Sahlins does discuss economy, even in terms of 'domestic mode of production', it will be found that he deals with relations of distribution and exchange (in Polanyi's case it is forms of integration) and not social relations of production. That is of course an entirely legitimate concern, though it is also pertinent to indicate that theories like those of Sahlins and Polanyi do not offer any systematic analysis of the relation between exchange

/distribution and production relations. Since the work of these economic anthropologists is often discussed in connection with the criticism of Marxism, and particularly of any analytical separation of the economic realm from other social relations in pre-capitalist societies, it should be noted that Marx and some Marxists have in fact done a considerable amount of work on the interaction between relations of production and distribution.[143] The most general and fundamental sense in which the ideas of Sahlins oppose Marx's historical materialism is in his rejection of the notion of the economic structure as the 'base' of the social formation, and this must of course have momentous implications for any concept of social evolution. In Stone Age Economics, we find: "But then, even to speak of 'the economy' of a primitive society is an exercise in unreality. Structurally, 'the economy' does not exist. Rather than a distinct and specialised organization, 'economy' is something that generalised groups and relations, notably kinship groups and relations **do.** Economy is rather a function of the society than a structure, for the armature of the economic process is provided by groups classically conceived as 'non-economic' ". The essential content of this passage is that economy is 'a function of society rather than a structure'.[144] Claiming to follow Marx here, Sahlins seems to have in mind the remark in Critique of Political Economy: "The communal system on which this mode of production is based ... causes individual labour to appear rather as the direct function of a member of the group organisation".[145]

It is not clear why the common ownership of means of production by families, joint families and/or lineages and clans should not be characterized as social relations of production which take the specific form of descent-relations, obligations and rights. That these relations are in themselves not characterized by conflict, and in this sense relate both to the productive forces and to the political and ideological superstructure in different ways than do the production relations of primitive society, is surely no surprise, and can hardly in itself justify abandoning the general concept of 'economic structure'. Indeed, there is good reason for assuming that accumulating contradictions between this economic structure of common ownership and the development of new productive forces and division of labour are as central to the development process here as are analogous contradictions at later stages of history.[146] Contrast the 'band-tribe-chiefdom-state' sequence of political-social forms, which, insofar as it has any reference to economic development, is a classification in terms of a sequence of mechanisms of exchange, rather than of modes of production.[147] In any case one would like to see Sahlins explaining in what sense the "coefficient of population density," and "thus, in conjunction with the ecological givens, a determinate density of land use" supposedly proper to each political organization can be abstracted from and determined independently of the productive forces themselves and the corresponding relations of production. Clearly Sahlins's 'economy as function, not structure', is closely related to Renfrew's view of the economic as a social subsystem, an idea derived from structural-functionalism and its reification of 'the social'. In Sahlins's scheme, social groups and modes of activity are explained as having the function of maintaining the social system (which, again, is undefined except as consisting of the relations or interconnections between subsystems). This simple functionalism is the solution awaiting all those approaches which lay the main emphasis on the impossibility of separating in any way the economic from other social relations. Some of the best-known Marxists writing in anthropology take the same path, in my opinion mistakenly. Godelier[148] for example: "We need in fact to analyse more closely kinship relations, for if they determine the places occupied by individuals in production, their rights to land and goods, their obligations in respect to work and gifts, etc., then they **function** as production-relations, just as they function as political, religious, etc. relations. Kinship is thus here both infrastructure and superstructure ..."

If this argument was taken to its logical conclusion, it is difficult to know what would remain of Marxism. Let us agree that 'kinship determines the place occupied by individuals in production, their rights to land and goods, etc ...'. Is not the same true, at least in part, of the inheritance laws, or the educational system, or the structure of class and racialist prejudice in some cases, in capitalist societies? Would it therefore be necessary to say that these legal and ideological factors 'function as relations of production'? I contend that there is a structure of necessary production relations in primitive as in other societies and that the allocation of individuals to roles and positions in these relations does not constitute the structure but supplies it and in that sense expresses it.[149] The degree of freedom of movement of the relations of production is systematically related to the nature of the environment and the level of development of productive forces. If we conclude, with Godelier, Althusser and others, that the economic relations are constituted largely by other domains, and these domains in turn are in no way definable as non-economic,[150] it is difficult to see how we can avoid the conclusion produced (and referred to above) in the theory of Eisenstadt or of Sahlins, that 'any factor' may provide the principal impetus to social evolution.

Dupré and Rey[151] have indicated that the approach of Polanyi, emphasizing the 'embeddedness' or 'submergence in social relations' of the economy in pre-market societies, proceeds always in terms of **exchange-mechanisms** as the defining characteristic of economies, and that this emphasis is just as ethnocentric as is the Formalist approach. When Polanyi insists that his classification of modes of social integration (reciprocity, redistribution, exchange) is not an evolutionary sequence, this is, as Dupré and Rey argue, perfectly accurate. Reciprocity, redistribution and exchange do appear to correspond to a factual sequence in time, but the classification contains no theory of the transition from one to another type of integration. Here it is useful to revert to an earlier argument about the need for the cultural anthropology of our own market (capitalist) society before we can usefully analyze earlier ones. For example, Polanyi attempts an explanation of the observed phenomenon of a difference between the fixed equivalent of redistributive systems and the haggling of the market system, directing us to the 'psychosociological' attributes connected with each, attributes proper to solidarity on the one hand and individualism and the pursuit of gain on the other. What is missed here is again the fact that the phenomenal form of market exchange and the 'law of supply and demand', reflect and give form to social relations of production. The fluctuations of price, 'haggling' included, are **oscillations around** value, the labour-content of the commodities, and this is an expression precisely of social relations of production. Failure to consider this content (in production relations) of 'market relations' may well play a part in blinding us to the role of (different) production relations in earlier societies in the course of their evolution.

A section 'Conclusion', would not be appropriate to these introductory remarks. In the papers which follow will be found a wealth of data on the development of social formations in pre-historical and early historical Europe. The authors do not by any means subscribe to a common theory or group of theories. The only purpose of this first paper has been to refer to a number of the theoretical issues which are at stake in the understanding of the material produced by archaeology, ethnography and historiography.

NOTES

Note 1
Among the most important Morgan, L.H. League of the Ho-do-no-sau-nee, or Iroquois, Rochester, Sage and Broa, 1851; Junod, H. The Life of a South African Tribe, Neuchâtel: Imprimerie Attinger Frères, 2 vols. 1913; Malinowski, B. Argonauts of the Western Pacific, London, Routledge 1922; The Sexual Life of Savages in Northwestern Melanesia, London, Routledge 1929; Coral Gardens and their Magic 2 vols. London, Allen and Unwin 1935; Spencer, B. and Gillen, F.J. The Native Tribes of Central Australia, 1899, London; The Arunta: a Study of a Stone-Age People, 1927, London.

Note 2
Radcliffe-Brown, A.R. Stucture and Function in Primitive Society, Cohen and West, London 1952.

Note 3
Boas, F. The Mind of Primitive Man, Macmillan, N.Y., 1911; Boas, F. General Anthropology Health. N.Y. 1938; Boas, F. Race, Language, and Culture, Macmillan, N.Y. 1942; and cf. Harris, M. The Rise of Anthropological Theory, Crowell, N.Y. 1968, ch. 9.

Note 4
Radcliffe-Brown, A.R. 'The Social Organisation of Australian Tribes', Oceania, I, 1932.

Note 5
Laufer, B., Review of Lowie's Culture and Ethnology, in American Anthropologist vol. 20 (1918), pp.87-91.

Note 6
e.g. Goldenweiser, A. History, Psychology and Culture, N.Y. Knopf, 1933.

Note 7
Evans-Pritchard, E.E. Social Anthropology 1951, Routledge and Kegan Paul, p.41.

Note 8
Spencer, H. Principles of Sociology, London and New York, 1872-96.; The Evolution of Society (Selected from 'Principles') University of Chicago Press 1967.

Note 9
Morgan, L.H. Ancient Society 1877, World Publishing, New York, ch. I.

Note 10
Tylor, E.B. Primitive Culture, Murray, London 1871.

Note 11
Frazer, J.G. The Golden Bough, Macmillan, London 1890.

Note 12
Childe, V.G. Social Evolution, Watts, London 1951.

Note 13
This does not of course mean that Kroeber himself was an advocate of theories of social or cultural evolution or that he shared White's views. Kroeber's anthropological-geographical approach contained no theory of social change.

Kroeber, A.L. "The Superorganic" in American Anthropologist vol. 19, 1917, pp.163-213; Kroeber, A.L. Anthropology, Harcourt, Brace, New York 1948.; Kroeber, A.L. The Nature of Culture, Chicago University Press, 1952.

Note 14
White, L.H. The Science of Culture: a Study of Man and

62

Civilisation, 1949, Grove Press, New York.; The Evolution of Culture, 1959, McGraw-Hill.

Note 15
Steward, J.H. Theory of Culture Change: the Methodology
of Multilinear Evolution, University of Illinois Press,
Chicago, 1955.

Note 16
Wittfogel, K. Oriental Despotism, Yale University Press,
New Haven and London 1957.

Note 17
Forde, C.D. 'The Anthropological Approach in Social
Science', Address to Section H of the British Association
for the Advancement of Science, 1947.

Note 18
Fortes, M. 'The Structure of Unilineal Descent Groups' in
American Anthropologist vol. 55, 1954, pp.17-41.

Note 19
Worsley, P.M. "The Kinship System of the Tallensi: a Reevaluation," JRAI 1956, vol. 86, part I, pp.37-75.

Note 20
Fortes, M. The Dynamics of Clanship Among the Tallensi,
OUP, London 1945; The Web of Kinship among the
Tallensi, OUP, London 1948.

Note 21
Malinowski, B. op. cit.

Note 22
Mankind, vol. 7, pp.165-76.

Note 23
Current Anthropology, vol. 7, pp.560-76.

Note 24
Gluckman, M. Economy of the Central Barotse Plain,
Rhodes-Livingstone Institute, Paper no. 7, 1941.;
Gluckman, M. Essays on Lozi Land and Royal Property,
ditto, no. 10, 1943.; Gluckman, M. "The Lozi of Barotse-
land in North-Western Rhodesia", in E. Colson and M.
Gluckman (Eds.) Seven Tribes of British Central Africa,
1951, Manchester University Press.

Note 25
Gluckman, M. op.cit. (1951) p.87.

Note 26
Polanyi, K. The Great Transformation, 1944, New York,
Holt Rinehart Winston Inc.

Note 27
Evans-Pritchard, E.E. The Nuer, Oxford, Clarendon Press,
1940, p.90.

Note 28
Mauss, M. English translation: The Gift: Forms and
Functions of Exchange in Archaic Societies, Cohen and
West, London 1970.

Note 29
Evans-Pritchard, E.E. op.cit. 1951.

Note 30
The Rules of Sociological Method, Free Press, New York,
1938.

Note 31
Durkheim, E. The Division of Labour in Society, 1933,
Macmillan, New York.

Note 32
Tönnies, F. Community and Society, Harper, New York
1957.

Note 33
Maine, H.S. Ancient Law, Murray, London, 1861.

Note 34
Spencer, H. op.cit.

Note 35
Parsons, T. The Structure of Social Action, McGraw Hill,
N.Y. 1937.

Note 36
Space does not permit here a discussion of the issue of
whether Durkheim's 'scientism' was at the same time not
materialistic in character.

Note 37
Weber, M. The Theory of Social and Economic Organisation, The Free Press, Glencoe 1947.

Note 38
The Protestant Ethic and the Spirit of Capitalism,
Scribner, New York, 1958.

Note 39
Weber, M. Economy and Society. An Outline of Interpret-
ive Sociology, 3. vols. Ed. S. Roth and C. Wittich. From
Max Weber: Essays in Sociology, ed. H. Gerth and C.W.
Mills, Routledge, 1946.

Note 40
Finley, M.I. The Ancient Economy, Chatto and Windus,
London, 1973, for example.

Note 41
G.E.M. de Ste-Croix, The Class Struggle in the Ancient
Greek World, 1981, Duckworth, London.

Note 42
Lukacs, clarifying Marx's remarks in Grundrisse (Pelican,
1973) pp.711-12; "Economic practice is carried on by
men, in their decisions between alternatives, but its
totality forms an objectively dynamic complex whose laws
run beyond the will of any individual man, confronting him
as an objective social reality with all the stubbornness
that characterises reality. Yet in the objective dialectic
of this process, these laws produce and reproduce social
man at an ever higher level, or to put it more precisely,
they produce and reproduce both those relations that
make possible man's higher development, and those capabilities in man himself that transform these possibilities
in reality". Lukacs, G. The Ontology of Social Being, 3,
Labour, Merlin, London, 1980, p.85.

Note 43
An alternative framework for the understanding of those
properties of social systems which affect historical evolution is to be found in J.Friedman and M.J. Rowlands,
'Notes towards an epigenetic model of the evolution of
'civilisation' ', in J. Friedman and M.J. Rowlands (Eds.)
The Evolution of Social Systems, Duckworth, London,
1977, pp.201-76.

Note 44
Levi-Strauss, C. Structural Anthropology, I, 1968,
Penguin, London, pp.1-25 and 277-315.

Note 45
e.g. Adams, R.M. The Evolution of Urban Society: Early
Mesopotamia and Prehistoric Mexico, Aldine, Chicago,
1966.

Note 46
Elman Service has gone so far as to assert: "... for evolutionary purposes of the comparative method, travellers' and missionaries' accounts are still useful, whereas our modern dissertations by trained anthropologists are not, except for such rare cases as Chagnon's study of the savage Yanomamo ..." 'War and our Contemporary Ancestors' in War: the Anthropology of Armed Conflict and Aggression, 1967 Ed. M. Fried, M. Harris and R. Murphy, Garden City, New York, Natural History Press, p.166.)

Note 47
Smith, M.A. 'The Limitations of Inference in Archaeology', Archaeological Newsletter, no. 6, 1955, p.6.

Note 48
Leach, E.R., 'Concluding address'', in Renfrew, C. (Ed.) The Explanation of Culture Change: Models in Prehistory, London 1973.

Note 49
Sahlins, M.D. Stone-Age Economics, 1974, Tavistock, London.

Note 50
Dupré and Rey (see note 151); Godelier, M., Papers collected in Perspectives in Marxist Anthropology, Cambridge, 1977; Terray, E. Marxism and 'Primitive' Societies, London, Monthly Review Press, 1972; Bloch, M. (Ed.) Marxist Analyses and Social Anthropology, New York, Wiley, 1974.

Note 51
Childe, V. Gordon, Social Evolution, 1951, Watts, London.

Note 52
Ancient Society, Part III, Ch.V.

Note 53
I suspect, also, that modern commentators have too easily assumed that the ideas of social evolution and progress met with an enthusiastic reception from nineteenth-century 'public opinion'. For the most part, the 'educated' public probably were no more appreciative of the proposition that their forefathers were some sort of communists than that they were some sort of monkeys.

Note 54
See note 42, above.

Note 55
Harris, M. The Rise of Anthropological Theory, 1968, Crowell, New York.

Note 56
cf. Lord Raglan's famous aphorism: "... savages never invent or discover anything". Raglan, How Came Civilisation?, 1939, Methuen, London.

Note 57
e.g. Morgan, in letter to The Nation: "... how could (the Indians) any more than our own remote barbarous ancestors, jump ethnical periods? They have the skulls and brains of barbarians, and must grow towards civilisation as all mankind have done who attained to it by a progressive experience".

Those who derive amusement from such statements might do well to ask it they are not caught in a crude anachronism. In the state of knowledge in the nineteenth century, and given Darwin's demonstration of biogical evolution, it was not unreasonable to fail to define the discontinuity between biological and social development. Similarly, until science itself clarified the matter, it was not 'racism' to suppose that there might be racial differences in brain capacity. Engels was among those who wrote that change to a meat and fish diet implied a development of the brain. Such errors were the consequence of an attempt to consider human social development as part of a scientific world outlook, and the errors which flowed from the limitations of the prevailing level of knowledge should be judged with a proper sense of the historical context.

Note 58
Morgan, Ancient Society, Part III, Ch. IV; for other, similar, passages in Morgan and Tylor, see Harris, op.cit.

Note 59
Sahlins, M.D. and Service, E.R. Evolution and Culture, 1960, Ann Arbor. University of Michigan Press.

Note 60
Steward, op.cit.

Note 61
Worsley, P. 'The Origin of the Family revisited' in Marxist vol. 4, no. 1, 1965.

Note 62
Harris, op.cit. p.652.

Note 63
'Evolution: Cultural Evolution' in International Encyclopaedia of the Social Sciences, 1967.

Note 64
Ibid p.227.

Note 65
The concept of structural differentiation is also made use of by Sally Humphreys (Anthropology and the Greeks, London, 1978, ch. 10, 'Evolution and history: approaches to the study of structural differentiation', reprinted from Friedman and Rowlands, 1977, op. cit. and passim) though for the most part in a more specialist sense, as explanatory of the emergence of 'intellectuals' as a social stratum, the division between public and private lives, and the beginnings of abstract thought. Use of the concept in another context may be found in Keith Hopkins, Conquerors and Slaves: Sociological Studies in Roman History, vol. I, Cambridge University Press, Cambridge, 1978.

Note 66
Renfrew, C. The Emergence of Civilisation: the Cyclades and the Aegean in the Third Millennium B.C., Methuen, London, 1972.

Note 67
Ibid.

Note 68
cf, Eisenstadt, S.N. 'Evolution: Social Evolution' in International Encyclopaedia of the Social Sciences, 1973, and Max Weber on Charisma and Institution Building, Chicago, 1968; and Parsons, T., Societies: Evolutionary and Comparative Perspectives, 1966, Eaglewood Cliffs, New Jersey, Prentice-Hall.

Note 69
Eisenstadt, op.cit., 1973.

Note 70
Ibid.

Note 71
Ibid.

Note 72
Ibid.

Note 73
Ibid.

Note 74
Renfrew, op.cit., chs. II and III.

Note 75
Ibid., p.38.

Note 76
Ibid., p.39.

Note 77
Ibid., pp.22-3.

Note 78
Ibid., p.40.

Note 79
Ibid., p.41.

Note 80
Flannery, K.V., 'Culture history v. culture process: a debate in American archaeology', Scientific American vol. 217 (1967), pp.119-22.

Note 81
I leave aside for the moment the 'social action' framework put forward as a solution by Max Weber to these questions. Weber sees the distinctiveness of the social as inhering in the fact that subjective meaning is attached by the actors to their actions and the actions of others. Some archaeologists, who give their main emphasis to the cognitive mapping of the cultural and natural environment, have begun to follow through the implications of Weber's sociology. I intend to deal with this elsewhere, showing that it does not escape the problems which I have suggested remain in Renfrew's work.

Note 82
His citation of a passage from Hawkes is interesting -"The human activity which (archaeology) can apprehend conforms to a series of norms, which can be aggregated under the name of culture ... The notion of norms in man's activity ... is an anthropological generalisation based on the extensive degree of conservatism shown by primitive man in his technological traditions ... without this the whole subject would crumple up."

Note 83
Radcliffe-Brown, A.R. African Systems of Kinship and Marriage, OUP, London 1950, p.72.

Note 84
Parsons, T. The Structure of Social Action, 1937.

Note 85
Parsons, T. Evolutionary and Comparative Perspectives, 1966

Note 86
Renfrew, C. 'Space, Time and Polity' in The Evolution of Social Systems, Ed. J. Friedman and M.J. Rowlands, Duckworth, 1977, p.97.

Note 87
See Newell's paper in this volume.

Note 88
Levi-Strauss, C. Structural Anthropology, vol. I, p.18.

Note 89
Renfrew op.cit. 1977, p.101.

Note 90
The Emergence of Civilisation, p.495.

Note 91
Ibid., p.497.

Note 92
Ibid., p.498.

Note 93
Harris, op.cit. p.25.

Note 94
Ibid., p.685.

Note 95
Ibid. p.222.

Note 96
Ibid., p.232.

Note 97
Ibid., p.233.

Note 98
Marx, K., Capital, vol. III, Lawrence Wishart, London 1972, ch. xlvii, section 2, p.791.

Note 99
Ibid.

Note 100
Marx, letter to Weydemeyer, September 11, 1851, in all editions of Marx-Engels selected Correspondence.

Note 101
Engels, F. Anti-Dühring, Lawrence and Wishart, London 1934, p.171.

Note 102
Amin, S. The Law of Value and Historical Materialism, 1979, Monthly Review Press.

Note 103
Ibid, p.2.

Note 104
Ibid. p.110.

Note 105
For a similar conclusion, though with rather different arguments, cf. Dominique Legros, 'Change, Necessity and Mode of Production: a Marxist critique of cultural Evolution', American Anthropologist, 1977, pp.26-41.

Note 106
Marx's historical materialism and political economy do **not** consist only of a theory of capitalism, and the question of Marxism's uses in the study of pre-capitalist societies is not the same as the question of applicability of 'formal' economics in those societies. Orthodox economics is not 'historically critical' of capitalism. That is to say, it tends to regard the laws or principles of operation of capitalist economics as laws of economy as such, not recognizing that their applicability is historically limited to a particular stage in the development of social production. Adam Smith's assumption that to exchange and barter was human nature is a fundamental matter for economics. ("This division of labour ... is the necessary, though very slow and gradual consequence of a certain property in human nature which has in view no such extensive utility; the propensity to truck, barter, and exchange one thing for another." The Wealth of Nations (1776), Penguin Books, 1970, p.117). At the 'other end' historically, so to speak, the self-negation of capitalism by the operation of its own 'law of motion', effected in the struggle of classes necessary to capitalism's functioning, is excluded by economics. This is the meaning of Marx's assertion that bourgeois political economy was

scientific, through the development of the labour theory of value and even to the anatomy of the social classes, but only up to the point where the class struggle in its specifically capitalist form (i.e. the replacement of sporadic conflict of workers and capitalists by confront-ations of the classes as such) appeared in history. (Preface to Second Edition of Capital, 1873). Henceforth, he thought, bourgeois economics became apologetics, 'vulgar economics'. From a Marxist standpoint, there is no need to suppose that sociology would be any less 'vulgar', i.e. unhistorical, uncritical. (cf. Slaughter, C., Marxism and the Class Struggle, London, New Park, 1975).

Marx means that in 'vulgar economics' as in everyday thinking, the forms in which products and persons appear in experience are taken to be their natural forms, and their properties to be properties natural to them as products and persons, while in reality these **forms of appearance** conceal their own essential content. This content is, that they are the end-results (historical ex-pressions and bearers) of a definite historical (not 'natural') process. Historical here means: having a given historical origin (transition from other social forms), a given development according to its own law of motion (to be determined by historical analysis, cf. Capital) and a given historical end (transition to another social form). Marx, as we have seen, developed a materialist theory of the source of transitions, evolutions and revolutions, ultimately in the developing contradictory relation between the forces of production developed by man in response to a 'nature-imposed necessity', on the one hand, and the economic structure or totality of social relations of production, on the other.

Now, returning to the economic concepts with which anthropologists and economists approach other societies, we find ourselves in complications. According to Marx, the concepts of economists have only a very limited validity even for capitalist economy, and these concepts are essentially nothing more than the consistent and systematic working out of the forms of thought (ideology) current in capitalist society generally. So soon as it is a matter of considering capitalism's law of motion, its contradictions, and not only its functioning, there is collapse, because of the fundamentally unhistorical nature of the concepts. Here we can begin after all to get closer to the problems of studying non-capitalist economies and their evolution. Men and women in capitalist society find in their everyday experience that money incarnates value, and, in some definite quantity, represents the essential social characteristic (the value) of every other thing, as if by nature. These other things - products, and even other people - 'behave' in the world, are related to one another, and to us, by means of a property, price (the phenomenal form of value), which they possess 'objectively', i.e. not according to one's subjective estimation. That we should relate our own private labour (through its products and the money for which they are exchanged) to the total collective labour of society, in **this** way is unquestioned, and taken for granted. Yet, of course, this 'absurd form' of relation of individual to society, where money becomes the only community, is the product of a long historical development. That individuals enter into mutual relations as 'free' individuals disposing of their marketable com-modities is not 'natural' but is the product of historical processes, and in particular, of the 'freeing' of the produc-ers from the means of production. That all labours and products can be equated in this way, stripped of their particular qualities, is a result which can only come from the highest concrete development of particular divisions of labour in the technical sense. The market, where isolated individuals seek only their self-interest in produc-ing and appropriating goods, is at the same time the regulator of the social division of labour. The money form and the market conceal this social character and at

the same time are its only form of objectification, the only visible social relation (or series of social relations) between men.

Classical political economy could explain certain regular-ities of the functioning of capitalist economics within definite historical limits. For this order of (functional) explanation, the outlook of 'the isolated individual in civil society' was appropriate. (It was even liberatory, for a definite period, as part of the ideology of individual liberty against the remnants of feudal order). "They are forms of thought expressing with social validity the conditions and relations of a definite, historically deter-mined mode of production, viz. the production of com-modities." (Marx, Capital, vol. I, ch. I, section 4). It is the next sentence which summarizes the implications of Marx's 'critique of political economy' for anthropology and historiography: "The whole mystery of commodities, all the magic and necromancy that surrounds the products of labour as long as they take the form of the commodities, vanishes therefore, so soon as we come to other forms of production. What follows in Marx's text is familiar ground. Let me extract only those short passages which bring out most clearly the necessity of breaking from bourgeois economic categories which is basic to any use of Marxist method in analysis of pre-capitalist societies: in the European Middle Ages, "... instead of the independent man, we find everyone dependent, serfs and lords, vassals and suzerains, laymen and clergy. Personal dependence here characterises the social relations of production just as much as it does the other spheres of life organised on the basis of that production. But for the very reason that personal dependence forms the groundwork of society, there is no necessity for labour and its products to assume a fantastic form different from their reality. They take the shape, in the transactions of society, of services in kind and payments in kind. **Here the particular and natural form of labour, and not, as in a society based on production of commodities, its general abstract form is the immediate social form of labour ...   The social relations between individuals in the performance of their labour,** appear at all events as **their own mutual personal relations,** and are **not disguised under the shape of social relations between the products of labour.**" (my emphasis, C.S.)

In the peasant family, "... **The different kinds of labour,** such as tillage, cattle tending, spinning, weaving and making cloths, which result in the various products, **are** in themselves, and such as they are, **direct social functions,** because functions of the family, which, just as much as a society on the production of commodities, possesses a spontaneously developed system of division of labour. The distribution of work within the family, and the regulation of the labour-time of the several members, depends as well upon differences of age and sex as upon natural conditions varying with the seasons ... The labour-power of each individual, by its very nature, operates ... merely as a definite portion of the whole labour-power of the family, and therefore, the measure of the expenditure of individual labour-power by its duration, appears here by its very nature as social character of their labour." Finally, Marx asks us to picture "... a community of free individuals, carrying on their work with the means of production common, in which the labour-power of all the different individuals is consciously applied as the com-bined labour-power of the community... The total product of our community is a social product. One portion serves as fresh means of production and remains social. But another portion is consumed by the members as means of subsistence... We will assume, but merely for the sake of a parallel with the production of commodities, that the share of each individual producer in the means of subsist-ence is determined by his labour-time. Labour-time would, in that case, play a double part. Its apportionment in accordance with a definite social plan maintains the proper proportion between the different kinds of work to be done and the various wants of the community. On the other hand, it also serves as a measure of the portion of the common labour borne by each individual, and of his share in the part of the total product defined for individual consumption. **The social relations of the individual producers, with regard both to their labour and to its products, are in this case perfectly simple and intelligible, and that with regard not only to production but also to distribution."** (my emphasis, C.S.)

It seems perfectly clear that for the understanding of this latter (socialist) society neither classical political economy, nor the 'vulgar economy' which succeeded it, nor Marx's critique of political economy, will be necessary, since 'the life-process of society' will 'strip off its mystical veil' and be 'treated as production by freely associated men, consciously regulated by them in accordance with a settled plan'. This contrasts with commodity-producing society, 'in which the process of production has the mastery over man, instead of being controlled by him'. To the men and women of such a society, the representation of labour by the value of its product and of labour-time by the amount of that value appears '... as much a self-evident necessity imposed by nature as productive labour itself'. I contend therefore that while it may be useful to criticize as un-historical this or that characterization of some item of particular ancient or primitive economies in terms of its empirical correspondence to a concept like 'capital', the import of Marx's critique of political economy is much more general and radical. It shows that for most 'economic anthropology' and sociology, societies where 'the particular and natural form of labour is the immediate social form of labour' are viewed through the uncritically accepted categories of our own society, where 'the general abstract form' of labour is its immediate social form. Marx's analysis of commodity fetishism is thus not just an example of the development of his theory of ideology, here in the specific case of capitalism. It is central to the critique of all social and economic theory developed in capitalist societies including sociology and anthropology. This takes us directly into the endless debate about formalism and substantivism in economic anthropogy. If Marx is right, that the social relations between men necessarily take on, in capitalism, the appearance-form of the property of a thing, namely value as an objective property of commodities, and that this value has laws of movement in the market which can be given expression, and quantification, then the social relation between producers which is its real substratum is systematically obscured, not explained, by the categories which describe these movements of commodities. If the same economic categories - supply and demand, maximization of profit, etc. - are then transferred to study of a society where goods are not produced as commodities, for exchange, at all (or where the commodity sector concerns only one part of the total product), then the 'error' (if that is the right word) is compounded, to the point of a complete nonsense. The fact that in all societies men are carrying out productive labour, and that part of the product is set aside as future means of production (only in capitalist society is it transformed into capital) is the only reason for even a semblance of relation to the facts.

Note 107 Polanyi, op.cit. p.144, 1957.

Note 108
Godelier, M. Rationality and Irrationality in Economics, New Left Books, London 1972 p.268.

Note 109
Harris, op.cit.

Note 110
Salisbury, R.F., From Stone to Steel, 1962, Cambridge

Note 111
Nadel, S.F., A Black Byzantium, 1942, Oxford

Note 112
Salisbury, op.cit. p.4.

Note 113
Rodolsky, R. The Making of Marx's 'Capital'. Pluto Press, London, 1974, p.29.

Note 114
Marx, K. Grundrisse (Foundations of the Critique of Political Economy - Rough Draft) Pelican, Harmondsworth 1973, p.513.

Note 115
Ibid. p.406.

Note 116
This distinction has force despite the fact that of course capitalist production and exchange, where dominant, do not exist in pure form but are articulated with elements of earlier modes of production.

Note 117
See Scott Meikle, "Aristotle and the Political Economy of the Polis" in Journal of Hellenic Studies vol. XCIX 1979, pp.57-73, G.E.M. de Ste. Croix, op. cit., and, with a different emphasis, Dupré and Rey, 1969, op. cit.

Note 118
I hesitate to say 'ideological' meanings because of the technical problems of interpretation of that concept, which I prefer to leave for treatment elsewhere.

Note 119
Marx, K. Capital vol. I, p.507.

Note 120
The relation between phenomena and their underlying structure(s) is not of the same type in all societies. We have already noted Marx's distinction between the 'direct' or transparent nature of economic relations in non-capitalist societies and the 'commodity fetishism' of capitalism. However, this should not be allowed to obsure the fact that the necessary interconnections of the mode of production in these non-capitalist societies are by no means coincident with the repetitious surface forms of existence, let alone the way in which these are conceived by the social actors.

Note 121
See note 59, above.

Note 122
Cf. Service. "First, we find societies at widely varying levels of cultural and social complexity. Some are lowly hunters and gatherers with a simple **band** type of social organisation. Others are hunters in a rich environment, or horticulturalists and pastoralists with a larger society compounded of several segments, forming a **tribe**. A few societies reached a productivity which permitted large populations and a hierarchical form of centralized leadership or **chiefdom**. Out of chiefdoms in some areas a more complex state organization developed. Finally, some are peasant or folk communities, local subcultures within contemporary national states. The primary consideration, then, has been to select societies that illustrate these five levels or stages of complexity". (Preface to Service, E. Profiles in Ethnology, Harper and Row, New York, Second

Edition, 1971). This formulation appears as late as the 1971 edition, though Service himself had rejected it. Thus: "... the stages, Band, Tribe, Chiefdom, and Primitive State are not true to the aboriginal state of affairs. They may be useful for a classification of modern ethnography but not useful if they are to be used in extrapolating from extant stages to extinct stages. Morton Fried (1966) recently criticised my formulation of the band tribe dichotomy by arguing against the concept Tribe. I accept that but go further and also abolish Band ... the true egalitarian, acephalous, stage of society was probably somewhere between these two poles - varying, to be sure, but not nearly so greatly before the enormous disturbance caused by European expansion. I think, therefore, that the safest way is to abolish both Tribe and Band in favour of the single type, the Egalitarian Society. Similarly, the distinction between Chiefdom and Primitive State is worrisome ... The only safe way, until further documentary research suggests something more plausible, is to think of only three aboriginal types which might represent evolutionary stages: (1) the Egalitarian Society, out of which grew (2) the Hierarchical Society, which became replaced in only a few instance in the world by the empire-state that led to the next stage (3) the Archaic Civilisation or classical empire." (in War: the Anthropology of Conflict and Aggression, See note 46, above).

Note 123
Service, E.R. "Classical and Modern Theories of the Origins of Government", in Origins of the State, Ed. R. Cohen and E.R. Service, Philadelphia 1978, p.32.

Note 124
Ibid.

Note 125
Fried M.H. The Evolution of Political Society : An Essay in Political Anthropology, 1967, Random House, New York.

Note 126
And cf. Malcolm C. Webb. 'The Flag Follows Trade' in J.A. Sabloff and C.C. Lamberg-Karlovsky, Ancient Civil-isation and Trade, Albuquerque, University of New Mexico Press, 1975.

Note 127
Marx, K., Capital vol. III p.384.

Note 128
See especially Sahlins, M.D. Tribesmen, 1968, Prentice-Hall, Eaglewood Cliffs, New Jersey.

Note 129
Ibid. p.91.

Note 130
Ibid. p.93.

Note 131
Ibid. p.79.

Note 132
Sahlins M. Stone Age Economics. p.131

Note 133
'Structural Substantivism: a Critical Review of Marshall Sahlins' Stone Age Economies', in Comparative Studies in Society and History 1974, pp.355-79.

Note 134
For example, Marx: "This does not prevent the same economic basis - the same as far as its main conditions are concerned - owing to innumerable different empirical circumstances, natural environment, racial peculiarities, external historical influences etc., from manifesting infinite variations and gradations of aspect which can be grasped only by analysis of the empirically given circumstances" (Capital III, pp.791-2) and Trotsky: "While Marxism teaches that class relations arise in the process of production and that these relations correspond to a certain level of productive forces; while Marxism further teaches that all forms of ideology and first and foremost, politics, correspond to class relations, this does not mean at all that between politics, class groupings and production there exist simple mechanical relations, calculable by the four rules of arithmetic. On the contrary, the reciprocal relations are extremely complex. It is possible to interpret dialectically the course of a country's development, including its revolutionary development, only by proceeding from the action, reaction and interaction of all the material and superstructural factors, national and world-wide alike, and not through superficial juxtapositions, nor through formal analogies. ('Thoughts on the Progress of the Proletarian Revolution: En Route,' in Izvestia, 29 April 1919).

Note 135
Marx, on surplus product and feudal rent: "It is not this possibility (of surplus) which creates the rent, but rather compulsion which turns this possibility into reality" Capital vol. III, p.792.

Note 136
Krader, L., Dialectic of Civil Society, Assen, van Gorcum, 1976

Note 137
Some of the Mesopotamian evidence against the traditionalist view of the state, which plays down class conflict and repression, is summarized by Fried in The Early State, edited by J.M. Claessen and P.S. Skalnik, the Hague, Mouton, 1978

Note 138
Liverani, M. "Collapse of the Near Eastern Regional System at the End of the Bronze Age", paper read at a conference at Aarhus, Denmark, August 1980.

Note 139
Ibid.

Note 140
Brinkman, for example, notes "... a novel Assyrian stress on the importance of the intelligence system, and on quick responses by small local forces in order to retain control over a seething countryside" in (Power and Propaganda, ed. M.T. Larsen, Copenhagen, 1979)

Note 141
"...the transformation was not an abrupt mechanical one, but, on the contrary, was an extremely lengthy process" (Claessen and Skalnik p.211). Also, the historical unevenness resulting from the interplay of many different factors should always be borne in mind, as, for example, in this example from Northern Nigeria: "In Borno, and Fombina, the state emerged out of the relations between immigrant pastoral or semi-pastoral peoples and local agriculturists. In Biu, a people - the Bura - with a common sociopolitical and cultural background have differentiated into state and non-state factions" (Cohen, R.& E.R. Service, (Eds.) Origins of the State: the Anthropology of Political Evolutions, Philadelphia Institute for the Study of Human Issues. 1978.

Note 142
It is beyond the scope of this article to consider the question of the 'Asiatic Mode of Production'; a matter of whether there is a relationship between surplus, interaction and state formation distinctive to certain Eastern

68

social formations, in that specialization of function within the framework of the primitive community rather than the emergence of private property and private interest lies at the origin of state and class. For two opposed views of the place of the concept in Marxism, see Perry Anderson Lineages of the Absolutist State, New Left Books, 1974 and Lawrence Krader The Asiatic Mode of Production Assen, van Gorcum, 1975 and Dialectic of Civil Society (see note 136 above).

Note 143
Besides Marx, Capital vols. I, II & III cf. Marx, "Introduction" to Contribution to the Critique of Political Economy (published also in Nicolaus' translation of Grundrisse), Rosa Luxemburg Cours d'Introduction de l'Economie Politique; R. Rosdolsky, The Making of Marx's Capital; and , directly criticising theories like Polanyi's Dupré and Rey (cf. note 151, below).

Note 144
Stone Age Economics, p.66.

Note 145
Critique of Political Economy, p.34.

Note 146
A similar point is made in another context by Samir Amin: "Marshall Sahlins and others who have followed him have tried ... to substitute the domestic mode of production for analysis of the precapitalist modes of production, thereby erasing the modus operandi of the specific exploitation which imperialism imposes on the dominated peasants of the periphery". Amin refers to Sahlins' 'domestic mode of production' as 'transhistorical' (Amin, op.cit, p.121 and cf. Amin and Gunder Frank, Accumulation, dépendence et sous-développment, (Paris 1977).

Note 147
This has been pointed out by Cook, op.cit. 1974.

Note 148
Godelier, op.cit. 1972.

Note 149
cf. Meillassoux, C. : "Kinship expressses the social relations which form the basis of social cohesion but it is not basic itself," (in 'Essai d'interpretation du phénomène économique dans les sociétés traditionnelles d'autosubsistence', Cahiers d'études Africaines, vol. 4, 1960, pp.38-67.

Note 150
cf. D.E. Goodfriend "Plus ça change plus c'est la même chose: The Dilemma of the French Structuralist Marxists", in Diamond S. (Ed.) Toward a Marxist Anthropology, p.96.

Note 151
"Reflections on the Pertinence of a theory of the history of exchange", reprinted in Wolpe H. (Ed.) The Articulation of Modes of Production. London 1980.

2

ON THE MESOLITHIC CONTRIBUTION
TO THE SOCIAL EVOLUTION
OF WESTERN EUROPEAN SOCIETY

Raymond Newell

Social Evolution: A Working Definition

From the myriad of definitions of social evolution which can be found in the literature, it is difficult to find one which suits the problem at hand, the available data base, or the particular direction which seems to characterize the Mesolithic period. Instead of trying to force the data to conform to a specific definition, it would seem more constructive to think in terms of a working definition. For the purposes of this paper, social evolution may be broadly defined as directional culture change, i.e. culture change which was sufficiently successful as to be experienced by some societies to be adaptive and which served as the basis for their further change(s). Proceeding from that definition, the study of social evolution may be conducted in three levels, i.e. (1) The unbiased observation of the empirical data in order to identify the direction of culture change, (2) the interpretation of those data in order to explain the relevant process(es) and reason(s) for that change, and (3) implicit in the foregoing is the hope that if we are successful in attaining levels 1 and 2, we should be able to predict further and future change. The study of Mesolithic social evolution must, of needs, concentrate on level 1 and conclude with some hypotheses by which level 2 may be approached in future. In an attempt to operationalize the above working definition, we will start with an abridged history of research into Mesolithic social change.

Early Approaches to Mesolithic Social Evolution

In any discussion of social evolution in the Mesolithic period it must be realized that it is the most recently recognized and accepted period or stage in European prehistory. Therefore, by comparison with other periods, very little work has been done. The hiatus theory was dispelled in 1867 and the period which seemed to fill the gap between the Palaeolithic and the Neolithic received its name only a little over 100 years ago, i.e. in 1874 from Torrel, a Swedish archaeologist. Following that late and painful birth, research proceeded in fits and starts, but never on the scale enjoyed by earlier or later periods. Nevertheless, processes and mechanisms of culture change were recognized and cited by earlier authors, e.g. local invention or adaptation in response to environmental change (Clark 1939 pp.xiii, 131, 215; Schwantes 1934), difference in origin (Vignard 1929; Clark 1936 pp.xiii, 131, 214-15; Barrière 1956 p.333), diffusion (Clark 1936, pp.xiii, 131, 214-15), ethnic movement (= migration) (Vignard 1929; Mendez-Correa 1933; Clark 1936 pp.156, 214-15), and acculturation (Clark 1936 pp.xv, 214). Also, ethnic homogeneity was the implicit point of departure in the earlier works. Against this background, the above

mechanisms were seen to operate, e.g. Clark (1936 p.215). Finally, most authors proceeded on an implicit dependence on the band model of social organization: usually without any cognizance of its implications and operation. Only Barrière (1954 p.229) used a different term, i.e. 'tribus' to describe his 'Post-Tardenoisian' of the Paris Basin.

Together with the foregoing exceptions, most researchers have conducted their field-work and analytical efforts on the safer and more mundane work of establishing the basic building blocks from which the foundation of future work could be built, e.g. describing material culture and defining types, e.g. Breuil (1912), Déchelette (1924), defining time and space units and describing the relationship of the Mesolithic inhabitants to their natural world. Such work has been aptly categorized by Harp (1976 p.119) in the context of Arctic archaeology: "In reviewing past investigation of Arctic prehistory, I have been struck by our substantive preoccupation with material culture, mainly with artifacts. That is quite natural because our powers of interpretation and reconstruction are circumscribed in well-known ways by the paucity of our data, particularly so as we are dealing with the culture of Arctic hunter-gatherers. Therefore, we should be forgiven a natural tendency to submerge in the warm realities of artifacts and the comforting procedure of mensuration and taxonomy. These are legitimate scientific concerns, and they may lead us toward useful statistical formulations, definitions of cultural parameters and complexes, and so on. However, to the extent that we think solely in such statistical and materialistic terms, the fundamental human nature of our quest may be diminished, if not lost altogether".

Unfortunately, what started as a means to an end, tended to become an end in itself (Newell 1971a, 1973). Despite the awareness of some of the many possible sources and mechanisms of culture change, little use was made of them for the observation of social evolution. At best, broad comparative statements regarding the foregoing Palaeolithic (Clark 1936 pp.9-10) or the succeeding Neolithic (Childe 1927 p.20; Clark 1936 pp.6-7; Schwantes 1934) were made. For a perpetuation of these ideas or the re-invention of sliced bread vide Kozłowski (1973) and Fortea Perez (1976 p.122). Clearly, something better was needed.

The Pioneering Work of J.G.D. Clark

The only investigator consistently to attempt to break through and escape from the above constraints and to expand the frontiers of knowledge on Mesolithic social dynamics was J.G.D. Clark. His pioneering work brought Mesolithic fieldwork, and our approach to same, far enough for the study of social evolution to become possible. As such, that work merits special mention. In succession, he recognized and strove to define: the social consequences of the economic basis and Mesolithic land-use system (Clark 1932 p.10; 1972), the seasonal movement of Mesolithic social and economic groups, which varied in size (Clark 1932 pp.92, 127; 1954, p.10; 1972 pp.21-23; 1975 p.13), social territories (Clark 1975 pp.5, 12, 13), social organization (Clark 1975 p.21), and the interrelationship of all of the foregoing elements (Clark 1972 p.18; pp.4-5). While I would not insist that Clark was correct in every respect, I will say that due to his work alone, we are now in the position to start to relate our Mesolithic data and ideas to the fruiful input provided by cultural anthropology, more recent ethnographic research, and the fledgling sub-discipline of ethno-archaeology (Binford 1962). Without such careful and judicious applications of ethnographic analogy, an understanding of Mesolithic social systems and social evolution will remain in the sphere of speculation. As I shall attempt to demonstrate below, the combination of Clark's pioneer work and the above sources of input has proved to be a fruitful catalyst for the most current research. But before going on to that current research, it is perhaps just as well to take stock of the state of the art or the current position to which Clark's work has brought us.

The Current Position on Mesolithic Culture Dynamics

Despite great advances in the quality and intensity of fieldwork and the pioneering endeavours of J.G.D. Clark, little real progress in the recognition and definition of social systems has been made in the more than one hundred years of Mesolithic research. To date, most work has been aimed at the improvement of data resolution and analysis for the definition of settlements, as analytical units, in order to serve the time and space paradigm and what Chang (1968) would call settlement patterns (Newell and Dekin 1978). Very little has been done to reconstruct community patterns. Making use of the few notable exceptions, it is useful to try to formulate a position statement, from which we can evaluate current and future work. The basic premises are eight in number and will be annotated below:

1   A greater or lesser/implicit or explicit reliance upon the carrying-capacity model or Liebig's Law, e.g. Jacobi 1973 p.246; Jochim 1976; Larsson 1978 p.201; Meiklejohn 1978 pp.72-76; Woodman 1978 p.367.

2   Small and/or exogamous social groups, e.g. Clark 1936 pp.92, 127; 1954 pp.10-12; 1972 p.20; Barrière 1956 pp.230, 332, 335; Jacobi 1973 p.243; Larsson 1978 p.203; Gräslund 1974; Newell 1973 p.405.

3   Reliance upon a static model of the band level of social organization, e.g. Clark 1972, 1975; Gräslund 1974; Meiklejohn 1978; Rozoy 1976 p.32; 1978 pp.1110-14; Odell 1980 pp.414-16.

4   Ecologically based group-size, e.g. Clark 1936 p.127; Gräslund 1974; Mellars 1976 pp.382-84 citing Birdsell 1968 p.234; Meiklejohn 1978 pp.68-69.

5   Low population densities, e.g. Clark 1932 p.10; Larsson 1978 p.201; Gräslund 1974.

6   Non-permanent site occupation and cyclic seasonal economic/settlement patterns, e.g. Clark 1936 pp.92, 127; 1972 pp.13, 21; Newell and Vroomans 1972 p.57; Newell 1972 pp.405-6; Rozoy 1973 p.511;

Gräslund 1974; Jochim 1976; Meiklejohn 1978 pp.68, 72; Jacobi 1978 pp.301, 307; Larsson 1978 pp.201, 203; Mellars 1978 p.383; Odell 1980 pp.414-24; Woodman 1978 pp.364-5; Newell 1980.

7   Intensification of the food quest, including range of species exploited and/or range of subsistence equipment and/or techniques employed, e.g. Clark 1948, 1968; Bandi 1963; Newell and Vroomans 1972 p.57; Andersen 1973; Newell 1973 pp.414-18; Newell and Andersen (in prep.).

8   A biological (physical anthropological) population which:

a   demonstrates a continuous transition from the Palaeolithic through the Mesolithic, e.g. Vallois 1930; Boule and Vallois 1937, 1952; Barrière 1956 pp.314-24; Ferembach 1974; Vallois and de Félice 1977;

b   demonstrates a continuous transition from the Mesolithic to the Neolithic, e.g. Scheidt 1923; Barrière 1956 pp.314-24; Ferembach 1974;

c   can be divided into various races or 'types', e.g. 'type de Ofnet', 'type de Téviec', 'type de Muge', etc., which display continuities with present 'racial' types in Europe, e.g. Vallois 1930; Boule and Vallois 1952; Ferembach 1974; Valois and De Félice 1977;

d   Implicit in the above three arguments is the existence, or formation, of demes, in the sense of Murdoch 1960 pp.62-63, although Barrière 1956 p.332 denies any linear relation between 'race' and 'industry'.

Generally speaking, all the foregoing position statements or premises are very static, being merely a list of disarticulated parts which have not been put together or formulated into a mutually compatible and consistent system. Furthermore, it lacks the dynamism or the motor which makes it work. There has been too great a reliance upon unproven models and the methodology to date has been aimed at the acceptance of fixed positions and the forcing of the data into conformation to those models and positions. There has been insufficient understanding of the concept of range of variation and too much effort directed toward the search for **an** explanation or **the** explanation of the observed phenomena. Part of the blame lies in an insufficient knowledge of the range of relevant analogues. In some cases, the above negative criticism may seem unjustified because many potential data sources appear to be lacking. However, as J.G.D. Clark has demonstrated, the data are extant, but (1) we have not looked for them and/or (2) we have not looked in the right way and/or (3) we have not geared our surveys and fieldwork toward the generation of the requisite data (Newell and Dekin 1978). Only when we face these problems squarely will we be in a position to build upon the firm foundation laid by Clark and the first generation workers. But before going into the attempts of the current research to fill these lacunae, it is perhaps useful to look at the Mesolithic period in a broader chronological framework, i.e. compared to the foregoing Palaeolithic and the following periods.

Continuity and Contrast: Mesolithic Social Evolution Compared to the Palaeolithic

At present, comparisons between the Mesolithic and the Palaeolithic are made in what I would call the 'big picture' mode, whereby the whole of the Mesolithic en bloc is compared to the Palaeolithic, in toto. They are also made on a qualitative and relative scale, and, in most cases, without satisfactory measurement of the attributes being discussed. Such comparisons are all too often biased by one or more of the research-historical legacies, i.e. the 'poor starving savages' syndrome (Waterbolk 1964 pp.232-34; 1968), the 'paradise lost' syndrome (Fortea Perez 1976 p.122), and the ghost of the hiatus, either at the Palaeolithic/Mesolithic transition or, more currently, at the Mesolithic/Neolithic transition (Waterbolk 1964; 1968).

In the comparative mode, the Palaeolithic/Mesolithic transition can be seen as a study in continuities and discontinuities. The continuous elements consist of the following: (1) the biological population; (2) much of the flint, bone, and antler technologies; (3) most house or hut types and materials; (4) some aspects of the subsistence base and procurement strategies; (5) some decorative ornaments; (6) some art forms and stylistic motives; (7) some mortuary rituals. The discontinuities (= innovations) consist of the following: (1) some new flint techniques; (2) some expansions of final Palaeolithic types; (3) new flint, bone and antler types; (4) possibly new wood types; (5) most of the Mesolithic decorative ornaments; (6) some new elements of the subsistence base: a, plant exploitation, b, greater accent upon fishing, c, whales; (7) expanded range of subsistence equipment; (8) expanded marine navigation; (9) the domestic dog; (10) some new mortuary rituals. However, and in addition to this unabashed trait-listing, it is our contention that the Palaeolithic/Mesolithic transition is more than just a list of comparable or contrasting traits. Of greater importance is the way in which Mesolithic man articulated and mobilized these elements to provide himself with a qualitatively better adaptation than that available to his Palaeolithic predecessors. This better adaptation was made possible by a wider range and more even distribution of subsistence resources (Schwabedissen 1964; Rozoy 1976; 1978 pp.1029-78; Clark 1972; 1975 pp.85-98; Meiklejohn 1978 pp.65-8), improved transportation facilities, such as boats, skis, (and possibly the dog as a pack animal?) (Steward 1955 p.41; J.G. Taylor 1974 p.4), and a progressive reduction or release from the break-up/freeze-up regime and concomitant dispersion/aggregation settlement patterns. These factors permitted or promoted the following observable differences between the Palaeolithic adaptation and that of the Mesolithic period:

1   a more uniform distribution of the population over the landscape, e.g. Clark 1932; Brinch Petersen 1971, p.96; Newell 1970a; 1973 pp.405-6; Rozoy 1976 p.32; 1978 pp.1105-6; Meiklejohn 1978 p.71 citing Wilmsen 1973;

2   greater number of sites per land area, e.g. see above and Andersen 1973; Jacobi 1973 pp.246-7; Gräslund 1974; Cullberg 1975a, b; Welinder 1973; and Odell 1980 pp.405-8;

3   larger settlements (= greater areas and greater artifact densities), e.g. Newell 1970a; 1973 pp.404-9; 1980; Newell and Vroomans 1972 p.57; Andersen 1973-4; Rozoy 1978 pp.1105-6; Mellars 1976; Odell 1980;

4   more regular land-use/settlement systems, e.g. Andersen 1973; Newell 1973 pp.404-9; Broadbent 1978 p.194; Bonsall 1980; Newell et al. (in prep.);

5   more permanent house structures, e.g. Newell 1980;

6   intensification of the food-quest, e.g. Clark 1968, 1972, 1975; Bandi 1963; Newell 1970a, c; 1973 pp.414-18; Newell and Vroomans 1972 p.57; Andersen 1973; Meiklejohn 1978 pp.66-7; Newell and Andersen (in prep.).

All the foregoing observations lead to one conclusion, that in comparison with the Palaeolithic, the Mesolithic is marked by less mobility and a trend toward more permanent settlement, based upon a more secure subsistence base, and expanded range of subsistence equipment and means of transportation, as well as the personnel to articulate efficiently the one with the other. Whether the social system was sufficiently developed and adaptive enough to effect the maximal integration and provide a maximal yield and/or buffer surplus will be discussed below.

Proceeding from the foregoing, the observed increase in population and therefore population density, e.g. Newell 1970a, b; 1973 p.409; Andersen 1973; Brinch Petersen 1973 pp.103-27; Gräslund 1974; Cullberg 1975a, b; Rozoy 1976; 1978 p.658; Welinder 1973; Indrelid (1978), indicates that these changes allowed Mesolithic societies to break through the short-term and long-term cyclic fluctuations in population, documented for the Palaeolithic (David 1973). The consequence of the resulting increase in Mesolithic regionalization will be dealt with below. For the moment, it is sufficient to state that the Mesolithic period is the chronicle of the adaptation of the late glacial population of Western Europe to the rapid ecological change which marked the Pleistocene/Holocene border. It is my thesis that their attempt to achieve a harmonious articulation with their changing environment was not only successful but allowed them to break out of the cyclic constraints of their former Palaeolithic adaptation and to develop in a direction which would not, of itself, have led to the development or acceptance of food production. In terms of the theme of this volume, one can do no better than to quote Leacock (1969 p.3): "From an evolutionary point of view, social development does not simply involve a series of accumulative changes. Instead, there is the point at which a real transformation is effected, and something qualitatively different has developed".

In order to understand more fully the nature and the magnitude of the difference, we must first look at the other end of the problem: the Mesolithic/Neolithic transition.

Social Evolution at the Mesolithic/Neolithic Border

Assessments of the Mesolithic/Neolithic continuities and discontinuities have proceeded from a wider range of premisses or positions. These have clearly coloured the way in which the data have been viewed and in varying measures predetermined or biased the resulting interpretation(s). Perhaps the strongest position is that of total discontinuity over large areas of Western Europe. This is the environmentally determined calamity/hiatus theory proposed by Waterbolk (1962, 1968) on the basis of extrapolations from Troels-Smith (1953, 1957, 1960, 1967) and negative evidence due to skewed field sampling. This position is contra such contemporaries as Bandi 1963; Barrière 1956, 1973-74; Escalon de Fonton 1956, 1966, 1967a, b, 1968, 1971; Schwabedissen 1957-58, 1960, 1962, 1967, 1968; Taute 1967a, b, 1971 and Wyss 1968, who were working from original data. The continuity hypotheses are more complex, but may be roughly divided into six basic ideas. In practice, and as most authors have recognized, there will be innumerable shades of combinations and permutations, according to local and/or chronological circumstances. The six basic hypotheses are as follows:

1   Invasion/migration followed by:
     a   ecologically conditioned mutual exclusion of the Mesolithic and Neolithic populations due to a presumed absence of competition for the same resources, e.g. Clark 1932 pp.89-91;

72

1936 p.216; Newell 1970a p.32; 1971 p.9; Taute
1967, 1971, 1973-74, 1977; Escalon de Fonton
1971; and Andersen 1973. Such a suggested
Mesolithic 'survival' can be either short-term
or long-term, the process is the same;

   b   culture contact, which can proceed in two
dimensions, time and space, i.e. short-
term/long-term absorption of the Mesolithic
population, e.g. Escalon de Fonton 1967a, b,
1971; long distance/short distance acculturation, e.g. Clark 1932 pp.89-91; 1938 p.216;
Schindler 1961; Van der Heide 1966; Lomborg
1963; and the acculturation process can effectively go both ways, i.e. Neolithic traits to
the indigenous Mesolithic population and/or
Mesolithic traits to the emigrant Neolithic
societies, e.g. Newell 1970a, b, c. 1971b,
1973.

2   Symbiotic relationships, e.g. Newell 1970c pp.32-6;
1971b.

3   Indigenous adoption of food production due to:
   a   ecological motivation such as climatic change,
e.g. Iversen 1967, but vide 1973; and Troels-
Smith op. cit., and/or significant reductions in
critical resources, e.g. Troels-Smith op. cit.,
and Waterbolk op. cit.; Andersen 1973; Bailey
1978; Mellars 1978;
   b   demographic pressure, e.g. Binford 1968;
Andersen 1973; Newell 1973.

4   Independent, local invention of food production, e.g.
Schwabedissen 1968; Ducos 1958; Escalon de Fonton
1967a, b.

Some of the above ideas can be laid to rest, while
others still have to be tested adequately. Since Waterbolk
has changed his position on the question of the Mesolithic
occupation of Western Europe in the Atlantic period
(Waterbolk and Van der Waals 1976; Waterbolk 1977), it is
now being followed by his collaborators, e.g. Whallon and
Price 1976; Lanting and Mook 1977; De Roever 1976,
1979; Van der Waals 1976; and Harsema 1978. Furthermore, other dimensions of the problem have not been
taken into account, e.g. social structure, level of integration in the respective societies, levels of organization
of resource technologies (= extractive efficiency), etc.
Only when this is done in combination with the proper
scale of analysis, will we be in a position to assess the
complexities of the transition.

Moreover, it is beyond the scope of this paper to go
into the strengths and weaknesses of all of the foregoing
continuity hypotheses. This is further discussed in the
following contribution by J. Bintliff. Instead, I would
merely call the reader's attention to the fact that all or
nearly all of the possible combinations of elements have
been proposed already. At the same time, I would
emphasize that in the past, the choice of interpretation
has invariably proceeded in an 'either/or' paradigm. I
would plead for an 'and/or-and/and-or/or' paradigm which
is to be applied at the strictly local level so that regional
variations on the main themes may achieve greater
resolution.

It is in any case clear that the carrying-capacity
model, which relies on Liebig's Law (Odum 1971) and the
Law of the Optimum Yield (Dansereau 1957), and which
was first espoused by Linton (1936 p.211), Kroeber (1939)
and White (1959 p.65), is no longer adequate. Contrary to
Clark (1975 p.4), no foraging society achieves a perfect
adjustment to and maximum yield from its environment
(Washburn 1968; Thompson 1966; Casteel 1972; Sahlins

1972; J.G. Taylor 1974; Bailey 1978 p.49). Instead, the
level of extractive efficiency must be proven and not
assumed (Rostlund 1952 pp.85-6; Dunning 1959 p.25;
Washburn 1965; C. Martin 1978; Schalk 1977). In a wider
context, it has been noted that hunter-fisher-gatherer
populations never attain the maximum utilization of their
potential resources nor grow to the point of demographic
saturation (Hayden 1972; Constandse-Westermann and
Newell 1984). Instead, it has been observed that they are
maintained surprisingly far below 'capacity' (Steward
1955; Casteel 1972; Divale 1972; Yellen and Harpending
1972). Rather than looking toward the carrying capacity
model as providing the best vehicle by which to explain
the Mesolithic/Neolithic transition, it is perhaps better to
amend its relevance to a position whereby the relative
abundance of food resources and the society's ability to
harvest those resources will both have a bearing on that
society's social structure. That the level of social integration and cohesion is equally as, if not more important
than the resource potential, has been convincingly demonstrated by Rostlund (1952), Damas (1963, 1969), Nelson
(1969, 1973), Sahlins (1972) and J.G. Taylor (1974).

It is my contention that later Mesolithic societies
achieved what Caldwell (1958) has called 'forest efficiency', in the sense that the subsistence quest no longer
formed a significant problem of the societies concerned.
The early Holocene autochthonous inhabitants of Western
Europe were no longer constrained by the temporal and
spatial cyclic fluctuations of their resource bases. Nor
were they demographically constrained in its exploitation.
To my mind, the best indication of this success is the fact
that after the original Bandkeramik incursion in the fifth
millennium BC, it took an additional 1,200 years for
various combinations of elements of the food-producing
economy to spread throughout the rest of Europe. Bintliff
has made the same observation, but deals only with the
colonization process (Bintliff this volume). He does not
address the question of the lack of acceptance of food
production techniques by the local, indigenous societies.
If the Neolithic were the great salvation for the poor
starving savages, as Kozłowski (1973 p.333) would have us
believe, the transition would have been effected more
quickly and more permanently. Instead, the rapid disintegration and fragmentation of the Bandkeramik culture
in the fourth millennium BC forces one to wonder whether
that social and economic adaptation was as successful as
some would have us believe. When looking for mutual
influences, a stronger case can be made for Mesolithic
foraging elements in the Bandkeramik than vice versa, e.g.
Lautereck (Taute 1967a), Stuttgart-Bad Cannstatt (Taute
1967b), Mannlefésen (Thevenin and Sainty 1972, 1974),
Reichstatt (Thévenin 1976), Burghöhle von Dietfurt
(Dämmer et al. 1974), see also Gersbach (1956), Niquet
(1963), Taute (1977) and Wyss (1980). Instead of clinging
to old models, we would do better to think in terms of a
different direction of development - of a polythetic
approach to Mesolithic social and economic adaptations,
in the way proposed by King (1978; Fig. 1) for some
prehistoric and proto-historic Indian cultures in
California. When that has been done, I think that we shall
find ourselves in agreement with Constandse-Westermann
and Newell (1984) when they write: "The pattern which
emerges for the population of the later Mesolithic is far
closer to that of the Neolithic than has often been
perceived. The site sizes, population densities and growth
rates of the two are apparently not that different. The
growth rates suggested here are similar to rates posited
for the Neolithic elsewhere. Population growth is not an
exclusively Neolithic pattern, marked by its previous
absence. It is clear that the Mesolithic population has
already become part of the initial major transformation in
demographic parameters which Deevey (1960) attributed
to the Neolithic 'revolution'. We are, in some senses at
least, dealing with a continuum".

Improving the Resolution of Mesolithic Social Evolution

While the foregoing are the large scale trends in social evolution which we observe during the Mesolithic period (our level I of analysis), the following is an outline of ongoing work which is designed to substantiate and/or more precisely define those and additional trends. The current co-operative research can best be described as an inter-related two-pronged or 'pincer' attack upon our present ignorance. It consists of a biological (physical anthropological) project and a project in Mesolithic ethnicity. The biological project is being conducted in collaboration with Dr. Trinette Constandse-Westermann of the Instituut voor Antropobiologie of the University of Utrecht and consists of the integration of the following elements and goals:

I   Skeletal analysis for the establishment of the variability in the Mesolithic skeletal population in order to approach: a, the population-genetic structure and population dynamic processes of the Mesolithic inhabitants of Western Europe; b, sex ratios; c, birth rates; d, growth rates; e, age at death and life expectancy; f, pathology and trauma for the assessment of cause of death and level of inter-personal/inter-social violence; and g, diet and nutritional stress.

2   The contact or immediate post-contact demographies of 261 pedestrian hunter-fisher-gatherer Native Indian societies in North America. This explicitly analogue part of the project is aimed at providing data resolution at the band, tribe, and language-area-network levels of organization.

3   The social context in which the biological and demographic mechanisms are operating.

The main thrust of the biological investigation is to provide a satisfactory answer to the question of the existence of closed marriage networks or demes, in the sense of Murdoch (1960 pp.62-3) and as they might co-incide with our recognizable archaeological time and space units. Preliminary analysis of the greater part of the skeletal population (Constandse-Westermann and Newell in prep.) has indicated that genetically based demes cannot be recognized in the sample used. Since the formulation of a more complete and more critically assessed data base (Newell et al. 1979), this investigation is being continued so that the final analysis can be based upon a uniform and mutually comparable set of 50 metric and non-metric attributes. In lieu of that final study, it is possible to reject the original Valloisian 'type' approach and its alleged results. If the final analysis confirms our preliminary result, the absence of demes has significant social implications. It would appear that the Mesolithic breeding population was significantly larger than its constituent social populations (daily face-to-face contact) and/or constituent ethnic groups. This implies an exogamous marriage structure in the sense of Adams and Kasakoff (1975). They, Boyce et al. (1967, 1970) Harrison and Boyce (1972), Hiorns et al. (1969), Fix (1964) and Swedlund (1972) have defined some of the operative parameters of such a system, whereby the 80% endogamous group (= breeding population) tends to have an upper demographic limit of 10,000 souls. In a broader context, Adams and Kasakoff have observed that the 80% endogamous group may vary in its composition and level of ethnic identity. In a hunting-fishing-gathering situation, the breeding population is generally considerably larger than a social population or a single ethnic group. Like Carneiro (1967), they cite population density as being the critical variable. They have also observed that the social group (the band) is seen to articulate over an area having a radius of c.7kms. and to be one of a number of

equivalent groups which make up the ethnic group (=dialectic tribe). They go on to state, and our own demographic analysis has confirmed that the named ethnic group has a maximum size of c.10,000 people, in a hunting-fishing-gathering context. At the other end of the scale, in peasant villages, they observed the existence of demes within the same range of a 7kms. radius, while the size of the 80% endogamous group remained more or less constant, i.e. c.10,000 souls, and the size of the ethnic group (nationality) had risen. These observations suggest a transformation model something like Fig. 2.

From the foregoing observation and the transformation model, it would appear that one could expect a deme to be established only after the point at which the breeding population becomes equivalent to, or smaller than, the ethnic group, i.e. when the two sets of transformation lines cross. This is also the point at which band level societies have achieved the tribal level of organization (Steward 1955, Owen 1965, Service 1971). Because the breeding population and social population area parameters remain constant, it follows that only time and the size of the ethnic group are variable. Having broken through the cyclic nature of population growth and crash, Mesolithic population growth became cumulative. Therefore, time will be a non-linear function and produces the following modified transformation model, vide Fig. 3.

For our purposes, the critical question is how far along this sliding scale Mesolithic society came. The inquiry into the level of social organization proceeds from a reliance on ethnographic analogy and cultural anthropological theory, so as to satisfy the full range of multivariate constraints, e.g. biology, social ideas and norms, communication and transport, population dynamics and demography, environment, and level of technology. From that analogous base, there are three alternatives open to us, i.e. the band level, the tribal level, and the chiefdom or ranked society level. After weighing the definitions and attributes of each level, Newell et al. (in prep.) have argued for the acceptance of the band level of social organization. However, an 'identification' based upon best-fit inference is not good enough, it is too static. Nevertheless it does give us a point of departure from which developments during the early Holocene can be understood. It also entails the acceptance of certain implications and consequences. These are to be sought in the very essence of societies: their ethnicity.

This half of the attack is being conducted in conjunction with Dr. Constandse-Westermann and graduate students of the Biologisch Archaeologisch Instituut , i.e. Annelou van Gijn, D. Kielman and W. van der Sanden and incorporates the input of the anthropological colleagues mentioned above. The first problem we addressed is the problem of recognition of the scale or proper units or level of abstraction for the measurement of social change and therefore, social evolution. It has been argued that the optimal resolution of ethnicity is to be found at the level of the dialectic tribe. Defined by Henshaw and Swanton (1907), it is most aptly described by Brown (1918 p.222). "A collection of persons who speak what the natives themselves regard as one language, the name of the language and the name of the tribe being generally one and the same".

Implicit in this level of social resolution is a clear reliance upon the Sapir-Whorf hypothesis, which is best expressed by the latter as follows: "We dissect nature along lines laid down by native languages. The categories and types that we isolate from the world of phenomena we do not find there because they stare every observer in the face; on the contrary, the world is presented in a kaleidoscopic flux of impression which has to be organized by our minds - and this means largely by the linguistic systems in our minds. We cut nature up, organize it into concepts, and ascribe significances as we do, largely because we are parties to an agreement to organize it in this way - an agreement that holds throughout our speech community and is codified in the patterns of our language. The agreement is, of course, an implicit and unstated one, but its terms are absolutely obligatory; we cannot talk at all except by subscribing to the organization and classification of data which the agreement decrees" (Whorf 1940 p.231).

Our study then consists of the search for a material manifestation which is the functional equivalent of language and which embodies the material expression of codified ethnic information in a non-subsistence-related field, i.e. a material equivalence to Steward's 'Secondary Cultural Features' (Steward 1955 p.37). The following two quotations portray this line of thought: "First, I regard language as a means of conveying, amongst other things, a set of traditional, regionally oriented, adaptive symbols. The total matrix of the language is a device whereby one generation passes to another the knowledge, values, attitudes, and techniques necessary to cope with the total environment wherein it has been traditionally located. Second, I regard 'culture', or better 'a culture', as a complex of traditionally derived adaptive symbols -including, of course, both material and non-material. Thus, the old adage 'every language is sufficient to the needs of the speakers' takes on a specific, evolutionary meaning: **the** language is a device whereby regionally appropriated knowledge and understanding are transmitted to later generations" (Owen 1965 p.77).

And from E. Leach: "all the various non-verbal dimensions of culture, such as styles in clothing, village layout, architecture, furniture, food, cooking, music, physical gestures, postural attitudes and so on are organized in patterned sets so as to incorporate coded information in a manner analogous to the sounds and words and sentences in a natural language. I assume therefore it is just as meaningful to talk about the grammatical rules which govern the wearing of clothes as it is to talk about the grammatical rules which govern speech utterances" (Leach 1976 p.10).

The project in Mesolithic ethnicity commences with an assessment of Mesolithic personal decorative ornaments as signs and symbol systems of multiple levels of ethnic identity, e.g. inter-society, intra-society, long-range (language area) networks in the sense of Hill (1978). The same ethnicity of ornaments has been observed and reported by Fortes and Evans Pritchard. "The Aboriginal Africans feel their unity and perceive their common interest in symbols, and it is their attachment to these symbols which more than anything else gives their society cohesion and persistence" (Fortes and Evans Pritchard 1941 p.17).

Proceeding from the foregoing, we can thus look at the Mesolithic ornaments as insignia of group membership and as the signs of the internal ordering and structure of Mesolithic societies. As such, these signs may be seen to function as reliable indicators of ethnic identity (Barth 1969, Langer 1953, Mahr 1945). Therefore, by analyzing the distributions of these signs in time and space, we may be able to discover the ethnic boundaries of the societies which made, used, and ascribed cultural significance to them. In a broader sense, this study is also an attempt to utilize some aspects of material culture as a valid approach to the discovery of the non-material dynamics of culture and of the indigenous attributions of meaning and signifcance by the respective societies themselves. In that work, we have discussed some of the most critical cultural processes and phenomena whereby ethnicity is expressed and perceived in living hunter-fisher-gatherer

societies (Newell, et al. in prep.). An attempt has been made to present them in the form of related variables, which may be expected to bear on the formation and identification of ethnic groups. When attempting to test the archaeological resolution of ethnic groups, it is desirable that it be done in such a form that all the relevant variables, and the patterning of their data are, or can be, accounted for.

Clearly what is needed is a model based upon empirical and/or ethnographic data, which can be applied to the problem at hand. Both the model and its operational algorithm must proceed from and account for the following processes and phenomena:

1 the observed structure of the Mesolithic Mendelian population;
2 the epi-centres or aggregates of habitation and interaction (= home bases);
3 territorial behaviour and the seasonal availability of resources;
4 functional communication networks;
5 population density;
6 spatial and border maintenance behaviour;
7 fluid group membership (= fission and fusion of PSUs = Primary Subsistence Units and bands);
8 a measure of cultural and linguistic heterogeneity of the bands, at their respective levels of social integration,
9 clinal variation in level of social integration;
10 emic relevance (i.e. relevant to and in their own society).

Also, the same three levels of ethnic resolution (e.g. band, tribe, language-area network) are being investigated by means of an analysis of the mortuary rituals of Mesolithic societies. Through the variation in the mortuary ritual, the final elements of the ethnicity study, i.e. status and role, are being successfully approached.

While we feel that the dialectic tribe is the proper unit of measure for the study of social evolution, we would concur with Hodder's warning about too great a measure of optimism: "The archaeologist cannot hope to identify all the tribes or ethnic groups that existed in the past, but he can identify ethnicity if by this is meant (A. Cohen 1974) the mechanism by which interest groups use culture to symbolize their within-group organization in opposition to and in competition with other groups" (1979 p.452).

Conclusion

With the research still in progress, the emerging tendencies and conclusions can only be regarded as tentative. Nevertheless there are some results which have bearing on the central theme of this volume and which can be reported in their preliminary form. The increase in population and the intensification of the food quest, as well as a trend toward increased sedentism have been mentioned above. Concomitant with these trends is an increased regionalization, e.g. Newell 1973 p.427; Indrelid 1978 p.172; Jacobi 1978 p.317; Rozoy 1978; Newell et al. (in prep.). This increased regionalization expresses itself in reduced territory size and increased border maintenance behaviour. This may be due to the increased population, real or imaginary competition for resources (Lewis 1966) and/or a response to the contraction of available land area (Clark 1948, 1950, 1968; Newell 1970a, b,c, 1973; Jacobi 1973 p.247; Cullberg 1975a, b).

Whatever combination of the above elements is most germane, the fact remains that increased levels of border maintenance are reflected in the Mesolithic skeletal population and the decorative ornaments. From the skeletons showing signs of violence and/or trauma, such as lesions, contusions, embedded bone points and microliths (or fragments thereof), a statistically significant proportion is male. Secondly, the proportion of injured skeletons is equally significantly skewed toward the later part of the Mesolithic period. Finally, we have been able to demonstrate an increase in the variety and total number of decorative ornaments toward the end of the period. Also, those ornaments which are characteristic of the latter half of the Mesolithic tend to display a greater measure of spatial discretion and mutual exclusion.

All of these factors indicate the increased need for greater social organization and control in order to keep the various Mesolithic societies intact (Carneiro 1967; Meiklejohn 1978 p.68; Constandse-Westermann and Newell 1984; Newell et al. in prep.). From both the ornaments and the mortuary practices, we can discern a movement toward such an increased level of social organization. From an original base of age and sex, there are indications of a change from earned to both earned and ascribed statuses, e.g. Péquart et al. (1937), Péquart and Péquart (1954); Barrière (1956 pp.335, 355); and Taborin (1974). In contrast to Clark (1975 p.21), at least some societies do not appear to be entirely egalitarian. Bintliff (this volume) would argue that this measure of social differentiation did not become general until the Neolithic. Such hierarchical structures as the cemeteries at Téviec and Hoëdic may be indicative of a trend toward an increase in the strength of leadership and the emergence of a headman. However, and despite these indications, or incipient trends, Constandse-Westermann and Newell (1984) and Newell et al. (in prep.) would emphasize that the level of tribal society was not achieved. Deme formation has not been observed in the Mesolithic population or societies. Centralized village structures, such as we find in certain western Eskimo, Northwest Coast, and California Indian societies are lacking. Also, all signs of a centralized ceremonial, dance, or 'men's house' are absent.

The foregoing recalls the question begged earlier on. Perhaps the reason that food production was not readily accepted in North Western Europe lies not in the economic sphere, but rather that the delay had social causes. As Peebles and Kus (1979) have suggested, perhaps Mesolithic society first needed to develop a functional tribal level of organization before the labour-intensive work of food-production could be successful on the long term. If the Mesolithic social and economic adaptation were as successful as they appear, the Meso-lithic inhabitants of Western Europe may have opted for the retention of their 'original affluent society' (Sahlins 1972) until operated upon by compelling outside influences, e.g. environmental change (Andersen 1973) and/or social and/or demographic pressures (Binford 1968, Peebles and Kus 1979) from the immigrating Neolithic societies.

BIBLIOGRAPHY

ADAMS, J.W. and A.B. KASAKOFF, 1975 - 'Factors underlying endogamous group size'. In: M. Nag (Ed.), Population and Social Organization (World Anthropology Series). Paris, Mouton Publishers, pp.147-74.

ANDERSEN, S.H. 1973 - 'Overgangen fra aeldre til yngre stenalder i sydskandinavien set fra en mesolitisk syns-vinkel'. In: P. Simonsen and G.S. Munch (Eds.), Bonde-Veidemann Bofast-Ikke Bofast I. Nordisk-Forhistorie. Tromsø, Universitetsforlaget, pp.26-44.

ANDERSEN, S.H. 1973-74 - 'Ringkloster, en Jysk indland-boplads med Ertebøllekultur', Kuml, pp.10-108.

ANDERSEN, S.H. 1979 - 'Pelsjaegere,' Skalk, pp.2-8.

BAILEY, G.N. 1978 - 'Shell middens as indicators of postglacial economics: a territorial perspective'. In P. Mellars (Ed.), The Early Postglacial Settlement of North-ern Europe. London, Duckworth, pp.37-63.

BANDI, H.G. 1963 - Birsmatten-Basisgrotte. Eine Mittel-steinzeitliche Fundstelle im Unteren Birstal (Acta Bernensia I) Bern.

BARRIERE, C. 1956 - Les Civilisations Tardenoisiennes en Europe Occidentale. Paris, Bière.

BARRIERE, C. 1973-74 - 'Rouffignac, l'archéologie'. Travaux de l'Institut d'Art Préhistorique de l' Université de Toulouse -le Mirail vols. 15 and 16.

BARTH, F. 1969 - Ethnic Groups and Boundaries. Boston, Little, Brown and Company.

BINFORD. L.R. 1962 - 'Archaeology as anthropology', American Antiquity vol. 28, pp.217-25.

BINFORD, L.R. 1968 - 'Post Pleistocene adaptations'. In: S.R. Binford and L.R. Binford (Eds.), New Perspectives in Archaeology. Chicago, Aldine, pp.313-42.

BIRDSELL, J.R. 1968 - 'Some predictions for the Pleisto-cene based on equilibrium systems among recent hunter-gatherers'. In: R.E. Lee and I. DeVore (Eds.), Man the Hunter. Chicago, Aldine, pp.229-40.

BONSALL, C. 1980 - 'The coastal factor in the Mesolithic settlement of North-West England', Veröffentlichungen des Museums für Ur- und Frühgeschichte Potsdam vols. 14/15, pp.451-74.

BOULE, M. and VALLOIS, H.-V. 1937 - 'Anthropologie'. In: M. and St. J. Péquart, M. Boule and H-V. Vallois Téviec: Station-Nécropole Mésolithique du Morbihan. Archives de l'Institut de Paléontologie Humaine, Mémoire 18, pp.111-223.

BOULE, M. and VALLOIS, H.-V. 1952 - Les Hommes Fossiles. Paris, Masson.

BOYCE, A.J., KUCHEMANN, C.F. and HARRISON, G.A. 1967 - 'Neighbourhood knowledge and the distribution of marriage distances', Annals of Human Genetics vol. 30, pp.335-38.

BOYCE, A.J., KUCHEMANN, C.F. and HARRISON, G.A. 1971 -'Population structure and movement patterns'. In: W. Brass (Ed.), Biological Aspects of Demography. New York, Barnes and Noble, pp.1-9.

76

BREUIL, H. 1912 - 'Les subdivisions du Paléolithique supérieur et leur signification'. XIVe Congrès International d'Anthropologie et Archéologie Préhistorique, Genève, pp.165-238.

BRINCH PETERSEN, E. 1971 - 'Le Bromméen et le cycle de Lyngby', Quartär vol. 21, pp.93-5.

BRINCH PETERSEN, E. 1973 - 'A survey of the Late Palaeolithic and Mesolithic of Denmark'. In: S.K. Kozłowski (Ed.), The Mesolithic in Europe. Warsaw, University of Warsaw Press, pp.77-128.

BROADBENT, N. 1978 - 'Prehistoric settlement in Northern Sweden: a brief survey and case study'. In: P. Mellars (Ed.), The Early Postglacial Settlement of Northern Europe. London, Duckworth, pp.177-204.

BROWN, A.R. 1918 - 'Notes on the social organization of Australian tribes', Journal of the Royal Anthropological Institute of Great Britain and Ireland vol. 48, pp.222-53.

CALDWELL, J. 1958 - Trend and Tradition in the Prehistory of the Eastern United States (=American Anthropological Association Memoir 88). Springfield.

CARNEIRO, R.L. 1967 - 'On the relationship between size of population and the complexity of social organization', Southwestern Journal of Anthropology vol. 23, pp.234-43.

CASTEEL, R. 1972 - 'Two static minimum population density models for hunter-gatherers', World Archaeology vol. 4, pp.19-39.

CHANG, K.-C. 1968 - Settlement Archaeology. Palo Alto, National Press Books.

CHILDE, V.G. 1927 - The Dawn of European Civilization. London, Kegan Paul.

CLARK, J.G.D. 1932 - The Mesolithic Age in Britain. Cambridge, Cambridge Univ. Press.

CLARK, J.G.D. 1948 - 'The development of fishing in prehistoric Europe', Antiquaries Journal vol. 28, pp.44-85.

CLARK, J.G.D. 1950 - 'The earliest settlements of the West Baltic Area in the light of recent research', Proceedings of the Prehistoric Society vol. 16, pp.87-100.

CLARK, J.G.D. 1954 - Excavations at Star Carr. Cambridge, Cambridge Univ. Press.

CLARK, J.G.D. 1968 - 'The economic impact of the change from Late-Glacial to Post-Glacial conditions in Northern Europe'. VIIIth Congress of Anthropological and Ethnological Sciences, Tokyo, pp.241-44.

CLARK, J.G.D. 1972 - Starr Carr: a Case Study in Bioarchaeology (= A McCaleb Module in Anthropology from the series Addison-Wesley Modular Publications, Module 10). Reading, Mass.

CLARK, J.G.D. 1975 - The Earlier Stone Age Settlement of Scandinavia. Cambridge, Cambridge Univ. Press.

COHEN, A. 1974 - Two-Dimensional Man. London, Routledge and Kegan Paul.

CONSTANDSE-WESTERMANN, T.S. and NEWELL, R.R. 1984 - 'Human Biological Background of Population Dynamics in the Western European Mesolithic', Proceedings of the Koninklijke Nederlandse Akademie van Wetenschappen, series B, vol. 87, pp.139-223.

CONSTANDSE-WESTERMANN, T.S. and NEWELL, R.R. in prep. - 'The biological Aspects of Mesolithic Population Structure Studied by means of a Metrical Analysis of the Skeletons'.

CULLBERG, C. 1975a - 'Prospecting the West Swedish Mesolithic', Norwegian Archaeological Review vol. 8, pp.36-54.

CULLBERG, C. 1975b - 'Forntiden i Göteborg del I,' Fynd Meddelanden vol. 15, pp.1-47.

DAMAS, D. 1963 - 'Iglugigmiut kinship and local groupings: a structural approach' National Museum of Canada Bulletin 196, 216 pp.

DAMAS, D. 1969 - 'Characteristics of Central Eskimo band structure'. In: D. Damas (Ed.), Proceedings of the Conference on Band Organization. National Museum of Canada Bulletin 228, pp.116-38.

DAMMER, H.-W., H. REIM & W. TAUTE 1974 - 'Probegrabungen in der Burghöhle von Dietfurt im Oberen Donautal', Fundberichte aus Baden-Württemberg vol. 1, pp.1-25.

DANSEREAU, P.M. 1957 - Biogeography: An Ecological Perspective. New York, Ronald Press.

DAVID, N. 1973 - 'On Upper Palaeolithic society, ecology, and technological change'. in: C. Renfrew (Ed.), The Explanation of Culture Change. London, Duckworth, pp.277-303.

DECHELETTE, J. 1924 - Manuel d'Archéologie Préhistorique Celtique et Gallo Romaine. Paris.

DIVALE, W. 1972 - 'Systematic population control in the Middle and Upper Paleolithic: inference based on contemporary hunters and gatherers', World Archaeology vol. 4, pp.222-43.

DUCOS, P. 1958 - 'Le gisement de Châteauneuf les Martigues. Les Mammifères et les problèmes de domestication', Bulletin du Musée d'Anthropologie Préhistorique de Monaco vol. 4, pp.119-33.

DUCOS, P. 1976 - 'Quelques documents sur les débuts de la domestication en France'. in: J. Guilaine (Ed.), La Préhistoire Française II. Paris, C.N.R.S., pp.165-67.

DUNNING, R.W. 1959 - Social and Economic Change Among the Northern Ojibwa. Toronto, Univ. of Toronto Press.

ESCALON de FONTON, M. 1956 - 'Campagne de fouilles 1956, 3. La Baume de Montclus (Gard)', Cahiers Ligures Préhist. Archéol. vol. 6, pp.211-14.

ESCALON de FONTON, M. 1966 - 'Du Paléolithique supérieur au Mésolithique dans le Midi Méditerranéen', Bulletin de la Société Préhistorique Française vol. 63, pp.66-180.

ESCALON de FONTON, M. 1967a - 'Origine et développement des civilisations Néolithiques méditerranéennes en Europe occidentale,' Palaeohistoria vol. 12, pp.209-48.

ESCALON de FONTON, M. 1967 - 'Recherches sur la Préhistoire dans le midi de la France,' Cahiers Ligures de Préhistoire et d'Archéologie 16, pp.175-170.

ESCALON DE FONTON, M. 1968 - Préhistoire de la

Basse-Provence Occidentale. Syndicat d'Initiative Office du Tourisme de la Région de Martigues.

FEREMBACH, D. 1974 - 'Les hommes de l'Epipaléolithique et du Mésolithique de la France et du nord-ouest du Bassin Méditerranéen,' Bulletins et Mémoires de la Société d'Anthropologie de Paris vol. I, pp.201-36.

FIX, A.G. 1974 - 'Neighbourhood knowledge and marriage distance: the Semai case,' Annals of Human Genetics vol. 37,pp.327-32.

FORTEA PEREZ, J. 1976 - 'El arte parietal epipaleolitico del 6º al 5º milenio y su sustitución por el arte levantino'. In: S.K. Kozłowski (lir.), Les Civilisations du 8e au 5e Millénaire Avant Notre Ere en Europe (=Colloque XIX; U.I.S.P.P. IXe Congrès, Nice 13-18 Septembre 1976). Nice, pp.121-33.

FORTES, M. and E.E. EVANS PRITCHARD (Eds.) 1941 - African Political Systems. London, Oxford Univ. Press.

GERSBACH, E. 1956 - 'Ein Harpunenbrucstück aus einer Grube der Jungeren Linearbandkeramik,' Germania vol. 34, pp.266-270.

GRASLUND, B. 1974 - 'Befolking-bosattning-miljo', Fornvännen vol. 69, pp.1-13.

HARP, E. 1976 - 'Dorset settlement patterns in Newfoundland and Southeastern Hudson Bay'. In: M.S. Maxwell (Ed.), Eastern Arctic Prehistory: Paleoeskimo Problems. Memoirs of the Society for American Archaeology mem. 31, pp.119-38.

HARRISON, G.A. and A.J. BOYCE 1972 - 'Migrations, exchange and the genetic structure of populations'. In: G.A. Harrison & A.J. Boyce (Eds.), The Structure of Human Populations. Oxford, Clarendon Press, pp.128-145.

HARSEMA, O.H. 1978 - 'Mesolithische vuurstenen bijlen in Drenthe,' Nieuwe Drentse Volksalmanak vol. 95, pp.5-30.

HAYDEN, B. 1972 - 'Population control among hunter/gatherers', World Archaeology vol. 4, pp.205-221.

HEIDE, G.D. van der 1966 - 'Enkele aantekeningen betreffende prehistorisch bewoning van het oostelijk deel van het Suiderzeegebied', Kampener Almanak, pp.200-14.

HENSHAW, H.W. and J.R. SWANTON 1907 - 'Eskimo'. In: F.W. Hodge (Ed.), Handbook of American Indians. Bureau of American Ethnology Bulletin vol. 30 pp.433-36.

HILL, J.H. 1978 - 'Language contact systems and human adaptations', Journal of Anthropological Research vol. 34, pp.1-26.

HIORNS, R.W., G.A. HARRISON, A.J. BOYCE and C.F. KUCHEMANN 1969 - 'A mathematical analysis of the effects of movement on the relations between populations', Annals of Human Genetics vol. 32, pp.237-50.

HODDER, I. 1979 - 'Economic and social stress and material culture patterning', American Antiquity vol. 44, pp.446-54.

INDRELID, S. 1978 - 'Mesolithic economy and settlement patterns in Norway'. In: P. Mellars (Ed.), The Early Postglacial Settlement of Northern Europe. London, Duckworth, pp.147-76.

IVERSEN, J. 1967 - 'Naturens udvikling siden sidste istid. Forskere og methoder'. In: Norrevang & Meyer (Eds.), Danmarks Natur I. Copenhagen, pp.343-445.

IVERSEN, J. 1973 - The Development of Denmark's Nature Since the Last Glacial (=Denmarks Geologiske Undersøgelse V. raekke 7-c). Kobenhaven, Reitzel.

JACOBI, R.M. 1973 - 'Aspects of the 'Mesolithic Age' in Great Britain'. In: S.K. Kozlowski (Ed.), the Mesolithic in Europe. Warsaw, Warsaw Univ. Press, pp.237-265.

JACOBI, ·R.M. 1978 - 'Northern England in the eighth millennium BC: an essay'. In: P. Mellars (Ed.), The Early Postglacial Settlement of Northern Europe. London, Duckworth, pp.295-332,

JOCHIM, M. 1976 - Hunter-Gatherer Subsistence-Settlement Systems: A Predictive Model. New York, Academic Press.

KING, T.F. 1978 - 'Don't that beat the band? Non-egalitarian political organization in prehistoric central California'. In: C.L. Redman, M.J. Berman, E.V. Curtin, W.T. Langhorne, N.W. Versaggi and J.C. Wasner (Eds.), Social Archeology Beyond Subsistence and Dating. New York, Academic Press, pp.225-48.

KOZŁOWSKI, S.K. 1973 - 'Introduction to the history of Europe in Early Holocene'. In: S.K. Kozłowski (Ed.), The Mesolithic in Europe. Warsaw, Warsaw Univ. Press, pp.331-66.

KROEBER, A.L. 1939 - Cultural and Natural Areas of Native North America (=University of California Publications in American Archaeology and Ethnology vol. 38).

LANGER, S. 1953 - Feeling and Form. New York, Charles Scribner's Sons.

LANTING, J.N. and W.G. MOOK 1977 - The Pre-and Protohistory of the Netherlands in Terms of Radiocarbon Dates. Groningen.

LARSSON, L. 1978 - Agerød I: B - Agerød I: D. A Study of Early Atlantic Settlement in Scania. (= Acta Archaeologica Lundensia vol. 4, no. 12). Lund.

LEACH, E. 1976 - Culture and Communication. Cambridge, Cambridge Univ. Press.

LEACOCK, E. 1969 - 'The Montagnais-Naskapi Band'. In: D. Damas (Ed.), Proceedings of the Conference on Band Organization. National Museum of Canada Bulletin 228, pp.1.-17.

LEWIS, O. 1966 - 'The culture of poverty', Scientific American vol. 215, pp.19-25.

LINTON, R. 1936 - The Study of Man. New York, Appleton-Century.

LOMBORG, E. 1963 - 'Zur Frage der bandkeramischen Einflüsse in Südskandinavien', Acta Archaeologica vol. 33, pp.1-38.

MAHR, A.C. 1945 - 'Origin and significance of Pennsylvanian Dutch barn symbols', The Ohio Archaeological and Historical Quarterly vol. 54, pp.1-32.

MARTIN, C. 1978 - Keepers of the Game. Indian-Animal Relationships and the Fur Trade. Berkeley, Univ. of California Press.

MEIKLEJOHN, C. 1978 - 'Ecological aspects of population size and growth in Late-Glacial and Early Postglacial North-Western Europe'. In: P. Mellars (Ed.), The Early

78

Postglacial Settlement of Northern Europe. London, Duckworth, pp.65-80.

MELLARS, P. 1976 - 'Settlement patterns and industrial variability in the British Mesolithic'. In: I.H. Longworth and G. Sieveking (Eds.), Problems in Social and Economic Archaeology. Cambridge, Cambridge Univ. Press, pp.375-99.

MELLARS, P. (Ed.) 1978 - Early Postglacial Settlement of Northern Europe, London, Duckworth.

MENDES-CORREA, A.A. 1933 - 'Les migrations préhistoriques. Le témoignage spécial de la Péninsule Ibérique', Revue Anthropologique, pp.267-92.

MURDOCK, G.P. 1960 - Social Structure. New York, Macmillan.

NELSON, R.G. 1969 - Hunters of the Northern Ice. Chicago, Chicago Univ. Press.

NELSON, R.G. 1973 - Hunters of the Northern Forest. Chicago, Chicago Univ. Press.

NEWELL, R.R. 1970a - The Mesolithic Affinities and Typological Relations of the Dutch Bandkeramik Flint Industry. Ph.D. Diss., Univ. of London.

NEWELL, R.R. 1970b - 'Een afslagbijl uit Anderen, gem. Anloo en zijn relatie tot het Atlantisch Mesolithicum,' Nieuwe Drentse Volksalmanak 1970, pp.177-84.

NEWELL, R.R. 1970c - 'The Flint industry of the Dutch Linearbandkeramik', Analecta Leidensia vol. 3, pp.2-41.

NEWELL, R.R. 1971a - 'Comptes rendus J.-G. Rozoy, Typologie de l'Epipaléolithique (Mésolithique) Franco-Belge,' Helinium vol. 11, pp.174-75.

NEWELL, R.R. 1971b - 'The Mesolithic affinities and typological relations of the Dutch Bandkeramik flint industry,' Alba Regia Annales Museum Stephani Regis vol. 12, pp.9-38.

NEWELL, R.R. 1973 - 'The post-glacial adaptations of the indigenous population of the Northwest European Plain'. In: S.K. Kozłowski (Ed.), The Mesolithic in Europe. Warsaw, Univ. of Warsaw Press, pp.399-440.

NEWELL, R.R. 1980 - 'Mesolithic dwelling structures: fact and fantasy'. Veröffentlichungen des Museums für Ur- und Frühgeschichte. Potsdam, vol. 14/15. pp.235-284.

NEWELL, R.R. and S.H. ANDERSEN (n.d.) - 'A Mesolithic Fish-Story'. Manuscript in prep.

NEWELL, R.R., T.S. CONSTANDSE-WESTERMANN and C. MEIKLEJOHN 1979 - 'The skeletal remains of Mesolithic man in Western Europe: an evaluative catalogue,' Journal of Human Evolution vol. 8, pp.1-228.

NEWELL, R.R. and A.A. DEKIN jr. 1978 - 'An integrative strategy for the definition of behaviorally meaningful archaeological units,' Palaeohistoria vol. 20, pp.7-38.

NEWELL, R.R., A.L. VAN GIJN, D. KIELMAN and W. VAN DER SANDEN (in prep.) - 'An Inquiry Into the Ethnic Resolution of Mesolithic Regional Groups: A Study of Their Decorative Ornaments in Time and Space'.

NEWELL, R.R. and A.P.J. VROOMANS 1972 - Automatic Artifact Registration and Systems for Archaeological Analysis with the Philips P1100 Computer: A Mesolithic Test-Case. Oosterhout, Anthropological Publications.

NIQUET, F. 1963 - 'Die Probegrabungen auf der frühbandkeramischen Siedlung bei Eitzum, Kreis Wolfenbüttel,' Neue Ausgrabungen und Forschungen in Niedersachsen vol. 1, pp.44-74.

ODELL, G.H. 1977 - The Application of Micro-Wear Analysis to the Lithic Component of an Entire Prehistoric Settlement: Methods, Problems and Functional Reconstructions. Ph.D. Thesis Cambridge, Mass., Harvard Univ.

ODELL, G.H. 1978 - 'Préliminaires d'une analyse fonctionnelle des pointes microlithiques de Bergumermeer, Pays Bas," Bulletin de la Société Préhistorique Française vol. 75, pp.37-49.

ODELL, G.H. 1980 - 'Toward a more behavioral approach to archaeological lithic concentrations', American Antiquity vol. 45, pp.404-31.

ODUM, E.P. 1971 - Fundamentals of Ecology. Philadelphia, W.B. Saunders.

OWEN, R.C. 1965 - 'The patrilocal band: a linguistically and culturally hybrid social unit,' American Anthropologist vol. 67, pp.679-90.

PEEBLES, C.S. and S.M. KUS 1979 - 'Some archaeological correlates of ranked society,' American Antiquity vol. 42, pp.421-48.

PEQUART, M., and ST.-J., M. BOULE and H.-V. VALLOIS 1937 - Téviec: Station-Nécropole Mésolithique du Morbihan (=Archiv d. l'Inst. d. Paléont. Humaine. Mem. 18). Paris.

PEQUART, M. and ST.-J. PEQUART 1945 - Hoëdic, Deuxième Station-Nécropole du Mésolithique Côtier Armoricain. Antwerp, De Sikkel.

ROEVER, J.P. de 1976 - 'Excavations at the river dune sites S21-22. Swifterbant contribution 4,' Helinium vol. 16, pp.209-21.

ROEVER, J.P. de. 1979 - 'The pottery from Swifterbant - Dutch Ertebølle? Swifterbant contribution 11,' Helinium vol. 19, pp.13-36.

ROSTLUND, E. 1952 - Freshwater Fish and Fishing in Native North America (=University of California Publications in Geography 9).

ROZOY, J.-G. 1973 - 'The Franco-Belgian Epipaleolithic'. In: S.K. Kozłowski (Ed.), The Mesolithic in Europe. Warsaw, Warsaw Univ. Press, pp.503-30.

ROZOY, J.-G. 1976 - 'Evolution des groupes humains en France et en Belgique de 6500 à 5000 avant J. C.' In : S.K. Kozłowski (lir.), Les Civilisations du 8e au 5e Millénaire Avant Notre Ere en Europe (= Colloque XIX; U.I.S.P.P. IXe Congrès, Nice 13-18 Septembre 1976). Nice, pp.32-51.

ROZOY, J.-G. 1978 - Les Derniers Chasseurs de L'Epipaléolithique en France et en Belgique. Privately published.

SAHLINS, M. 1972- Stone Age Economics. Chicago, Aldine.

SCHALK, R.F. 1977 - 'The structure of an anadromous fish resource'. In: L.R. Binford (Ed.), For Theory Building in Archaeology. New York, Academic Press, pp.207-249.

SCHEIDT, W. 1923 - Die Eiszeitlichen Schädelfunde aus der Grossen Ofnet-Höhle und vom Kaufertsberg bei Nördlingen. München, J.S Lehmanns Verlag.

SCHINDLER, R. 1961 - 'Rössener Elemente im Frühneolithikum von Boberg,' Hammaburg vol. 13, pp.9-29.

SCHWABEDISSEN, H. 1957-58 - 'Die Ausgrabungen im Satruper Moor,' Offa vol. 16, pp.5-28.

SCHWABEDISSEN, H. 1960 - 'Die Ausgrabungen im Satruper Moor,' Zur Frage nach Ursprung und Frühester Entwicklung des Nordischen Neolithikums vol. 16, pp.5-28.

SCHWABEDISSEN H. 1962 - 'Northern Continental Europe.' In: R. Braidwood & G. Willey (Eds.), Courses Toward Urban Life. Chicago, Aldine, pp.254-66.

SCHWABEDISSEN, H. 1964 - 'Sinngehalt und Abgrenzung des Mesolithikums nach den Forschungsergebnissen im nordlichen Teil des europäischen Kontinents,' Report of the VIth International Congress on Quaternary. Warsaw 1961, pp.383-404.

SCHWABEDISSEN H. 1967 - 'Ein horizontierter 'Breitkeil' aus Satrup und die mannigfachen Kulturverbindungen des beginnenden Neolithikums im Norden und Nordwesten,' Palaeohistoria vol. 12, pp.409-68.

SCHWABEDISSEN, H. 1968 - 'Der Ubergang vom Mesolithikum zum Neolithikum in Schleswig-Holstein.' In: Führer zu Vor -und Frühgeschichtlichen Denkmalern ol. 8, Schleswig-Haithabu-Sylt. Mainz am Rhein, Philipp von Zabern, pp.9-26.

SCHWANTES, G. 1934 - Vorgeschichte von Schleswig-Holstein. Neumünster.

SERVICE, E. 1971 - Primitive Social Organization. An Evolutionary Perspective. 2nd ed. New York, Random House.

STEWARD, J.H. 1955 - Theory of Culture Change. Urbana, Univ. of Illinois Press.

SWEDLUND, A.C. 1972 - 'Observations on the concept of neighbourhood knowledge and the distribution of marriage distance,' Annals of Human Genetics vol. 35, pp.327-30.

TABORIN, Y. 1974 - 'La Parure en coquillage de l'epipaléolithique au bronze ancien en France,' Gallia Préhistoire vol. 17, pp.307-414.

TAUTE, W. 1967 - 'Grabungen zur mittleren Steinzeit in höhlen und unter Felsdächern der Schwäbischen Alb, 1961 bis 1965,' Fundberichte aus Schwaben vol. 18, pp.14-21.

TAUTE, W. 1967a - 'Das Felsdach Lautereck, eine mesolithisch-neolithisch-bronze-zeitliche Stratigraphie an der Oberen Donau,' Palaeohistoria vol. 12, pp.483-504.

TAUTE, W. 1967b - 'Neolithische Fundschicht mit Harpunen-fragmenten im Travertin von Stuttgart-Bad Cannstatt', Fundberichte aus Schwaben vol. 18, pp.43-60.

TAUTE, W. 1971 - Untersuchungen zum Mesolithikum und zum Spätpalolithikum im Südlichen Mitteleuropa. BD. 1. Habilitationsschrift d. Fachbereiches Erdwissenschaften d. Eberhard-Karls-Universität zu Tübingen.

TAUTE, W. 1973-74 - 'Neolithische Mikrolithen und andere neolithische Silexartefakte aus Süddeutschland und Österreich,' Archäologische Informationen vols. 2-3, pp.71-125.

TAUTE, W. 1977 - 'Zur Problematik von Mesolithikum und Frühneolithikum am Bodensee'. In: H. Berner (Ed.), Bodman -Dorf Kaiserpfalz Adel. Sigmaringen, Jan Thorbecke Verlag, pp.11-32.

TAYLOR, J.G. 1974 - Labrador Eskimo Settlements of the Early Contact Period (=National Museum of Man Publications in Ethnology no.3). Ottawa.

THEVENIN, A. 1976 - 'Paleo-histoire de l'Est de la France du 7º au 6º millénaire avant J.C.'. In: S.K. Kozłowski (dir.), Les Civilisations du 8e au 5e Millénaire Avant Notre Ere en Europe (=Colloque XIX; U.I.S.P.P. IXe Congrès, Nice 13-18 Septembre 1976). Nice, pp.71-92.

THEVENIN, A. and J. SAINTY 1972 - 'Une Nouvelle stratigraphie du Post-Glaciaire: l'abri du Mannlefelsen I a Oberlarg (Haut-Rhin)', Bulletin de la Société Préhistorique Française vol. 69, pp.6-7.

THEVENIN, A. and J. SAINTY 1974 - 'Achenheim, Oberlarg, 600,000 ans de préhistoire', Archéologia vol. 75, pp.49-61.

THOMPSON, H.P. 1966 - 'A technique using anthropological and biological data', Current Anthropology vol. 7, pp.417-24.

TROELS-SMITH, J. 1953 - 'Ertebøllekultur-Bondekultur. Resultater af de sidste 10 ars undersøgelser i Aamosen, Vestsjaelland', Aarbøger, pp.5-62.

TROELS-SMITH, J. 1957 - 'Maglemosetidens jaegere of fiskere,' Fra Nationalmuseets Arbejdsmark, pp.101-33.

TROELS-SMITH, J. 1960 - 'Ertebølletidens fangstfolk og bonder', Fra Nationalmuseets Arbrejdsmark, pp.95-119.

TROELS-SMITH, J. 1966 (1967) - 'The Ertebølle culture and its background', Palaeohistoria vol. 12, pp.505-29.

VALLOIS, H.-V. 1930 - 'Recherches sur les ossements Mésolithiques de Mugem', L'Anthropologie vol. 40, pp.337-89.

VALLOIS, H.-V. and S. DE FELICE 1977 - Les Mésolithiques de France (=Archives d. l'Institut de Paléontologie Humaine. Mémoire 37). Paris, Masson.

VIGNARD, E. 1928 - "Une nouvelle industrie lithique: le Sébilien," Bulletin de la Société Préhistorique Française, pp.200-20.

WAALS, J.D. VAN DER 1976 - 'Een tand met een beestje uit Swifterbant', Festoen, Feestbundel Prof. Dr. A.N. Zadoks-Josephus Jitta. Bussuem, pp.611-22.

WAALS, J.D. VAN DER and H.T. WATERBOLK 1976 - 'Excavation at Swifterbant - discovery, progress, aims and methods', Helinium vol. 16, pp.3-14.

WASHBURN, S.L. 1968 - 'The Central Eskimo: a marginal case?' In: R.B. Lee & I. DeVore (Eds.), Man the Hunter. Chicago, Aldine, pp.83-5.

WATERBOLK, H.T. 1962 - 'The lower Rhine basin'. In: R. Braidwood & G. Willey (Eds.), Courses Toward Urban Life. Chicago, Aldine, pp.227-53.

WATERBOLK, H.T. 1968 - 'Food production in prehistoric Europe', Science vol. 162, pp.1093-1102.

WATERBOLK, H.T. 1977 - 'De prehistorie' In: Winkler Prins Geschiedenis der Nederlanden DI. I. Amsterdam, Elsevier, pp.11-46.

WELINDER, S. 1973 - 'The chronology of the Mesolithic Stone Age on the Swedish west coast'. Studies in North European Archaeology vol. 9, pp.1-28.

WHALLON, R. and T.D. PRICE 1976 - 'Excavations at the river dune sites S11-13. Swifterbant contribution 5'. Helinium vol. 16, pp.222-29.

WHITE, L.A. 1959 - The Evolution of Culture. New York, McGraw-Hill.

WHORF, B. 1940 - 'Science and linguistics', The Technology Review vol. 42, pp.229-31, 247-48.

WILMSEN, E. 1973 - 'Interaction, spacing behaviour, and the organization of hunting bands', Journal of Anthropological Research vol. 29, pp.1-31.

WOODMAN, P. 1978 - 'The chronology and economy of the Irish Mesolithic: some working hypotheses.' In: P. Mellars (Ed.), The Early Postglacial Settlement of Northern Europe. London, Duckworth, pp.333-70.

WYSS, R. 1968 - 'Das Mesolithikum'. In: W. Drack (Red.), Ur-und Frühgeschichtliche Archäologie der Schweiz I. Basel, Verlag Schweizerische Gesellsch. f. Ur- und Frühgesch., pp.123-44.

WYSS, R. 1980 - 'Mesolithische Traditionen im neolithischen Kulturgut der Schweiz'. Veröffentlichungen des Museums für Ur- und Frühgeschichte Potsdam vol. 14/15, pp 91-104.

YELLEN, J. and H. HARPENDING 1972 - 'Hunter-gatherer population and archaeological inference', World Archaeology vol. 4, pp.244-53.

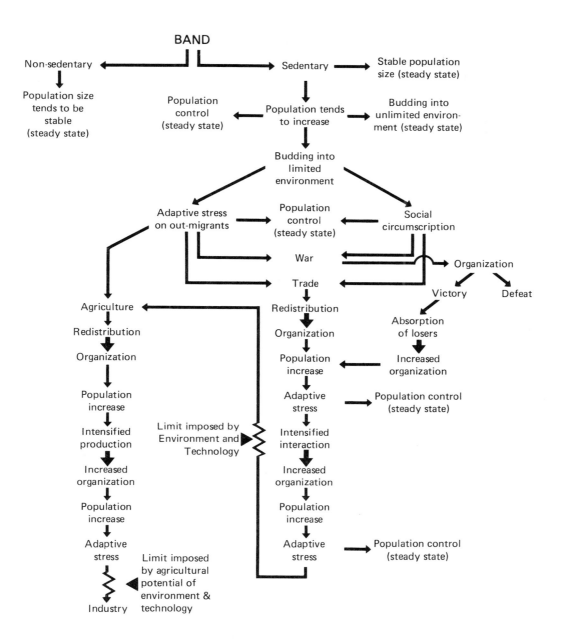

Fig 1
Organizational trajectories of hunter-gatherers (after King 1978).
Thickened lines indicate tendency toward increased political differentiation.

82

Model A   LINEAR TIME SCALE

OBSERVATION:

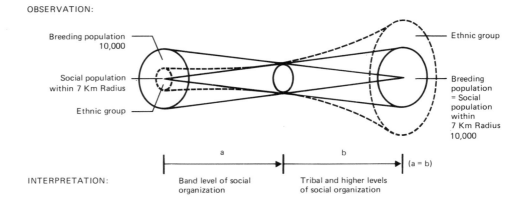

Breeding population
10,000

Social population
within 7 Km Radius

Ethnic group

Ethnic group

Breeding
population
= Social
population
within
7 Km Radius
10,000

INTERPRETATION:

a

b

(a = b)

Band level of social
organization

Tribal and higher levels
of social organization

Fig 2

Model B   NON-LINEAR TIME SCALE

OBSERVATION:

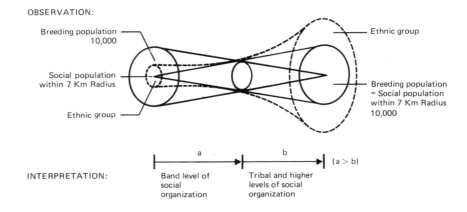

Breeding population
10,000

Social population
within 7 Km Radius

Ethnic group

Ethnic group

Breeding population
= Social population
within 7 Km Radius
10,000

INTERPRETATION:

a

b

(a > b)

Band level of
social
organization

Tribal and higher
levels of social
organization

Fig 3

3

THE NEOLITHIC IN EUROPE AND SOCIAL EVOLUTION

John Bintliff

Introduction

The most significant change inaugurating the Neolithic or New Stone Age in Europe is the arrival and diffusion over the subcontinent of a farming and herding economy. Beginning around 6000 bc in Greece we can trace the gradual changeover to a generally more productive economy in a series of waves across Europe, identified with specific archaeological cultures, or human groups characterized by recurrent sets of artifact types and settlement patterns. The far north of Europe, up to the limits of cultivation, and the British Isles, see the new economy some 2000 years later at the end of the pioneer process, after 4000 bc. The spread of mixed farming appears to be a combination of colonization from early agricultural communities of the Near East, and adoption by indigenous Mesolithic hunter-gatherer groups within Europe, and there are notable time lags from region to region due to adaptations to new environmental conditions, the relative necessity or advantages for local groups to change, and the phase of regional population build-up in the case of colonizing farmers before an adjacent region is opened up for colonization.[1] A combination of these factors seems to account for the remarkable delay in the general adoption of farming in the western Mediterranean region, of some 2-3000 years from the first contacts with the new lifestyle.[2]

Subsequent to the earliest establishment of farming communities in each region of Europe, one can trace an overall trend over several millennia towards increasingly dense populations, often directly linked to further innovations such as the plough, traction animals, as well as to successful local adaptations to the particular potential of each district in terms of crop preferences or the role and variety of the stock component.[3] In some regions, these concentrated populations supported a degree of craft specialization, some of the products of which were widely exchanged. Less commonly, we can observe the equivalent of a number of villages, or even all the population of a region, being organized to construct monuments or defensive earthworks. Associated with these trends in demography, occupational structure and communal activity, are signs in the archaeological record, in cemeteries and settlements, of significant social or status distinctions between members of the same community.[4] The frequently inferred picture of denser populations that become internally specialized as time progresses into farmers, herders, craftsmen and organizers (chieftains, headmen), - can be seen as a natural trend that is merely accentuated in the following Copper, Bronze and Iron Ages: one of concentrated populations crystallizing into proto-urban settlements, and district craft classes deriving their sustenance from farmer clients, or more frequently, the chief or prince of each area (and with the latter class identifiable by abnormally rich burials in cemeteries).

There is, then, broad agreement that European populations seem to get denser from the early to the late Neolithic, and it is arguable that in certain areas high densities are somehow closely linked to social change (cf. Phillips 1980, p.187). It has also been claimed that the general shift in economy away from the conditions of hunter-gatherer exploitation, was matched by a shift from 'bands' to 'tribal societies' (Service, 1962), involving less emphasis on the family ties and more on larger kin units (cf. the Marxist Gentile Society). This general viewpoint is based on long established ethnographic observations concerning the more complex nature of farming groups' social organization and the generally larger scale on which it operates. The 'tribe' is seen as a grouping comparable to a number of bands, and described further as a higher population unit, with greater socialization and wider range of co-ordinated activities. On the ground, for example, Sahlins (1968) sees it as a cluster of villages linked together by kinship, clanship and 'sodalities' (non-kin associations such as warrior castes, secret societies, age sets). Yet the larger unit would characteristically lack centralized control in socio-economy, or a permanent hierarchy - each village would be autonomous. Status in such a society is expected to be based on age, sex and talent - with an absence of inherited status or individuals monopolizing the use of force. Key resources would be under communal or corporate (especially kin-group) control. However, based on work in Melanesia, Sahlins also indicates the possible importance of so-called 'big men' on the economy and village decisions: individuals more successful than the average on their own achieved efforts.[5]

There is clearly a nineteenth-century inheritance here, where the size of the social group is directly correlated with its complexity, or better the **density** of the group. As an empirical generalization this seems broadly predictive, but falls short of being an explanation. Likewise the same ethno-historic generalization process that informs us that there exist numerous 'egalitarian' farming societies as a natural 'intermediate' stage to stratified farming societies from egalitarian band communities - is also short on explanatory power. Again, it is the nineteenth-century inheritance that provides us still with current major theories about the rise of leadership structures in such communities (cf. Introduction), especially the implicit or explicit role of ideas such as those of Engels (1877/8, 1884) on the shift from common ownership to private ownership. To Engels and others this key change was linked to increasing division of labour and the rise of 'useful' leaders (e.g. war-leaders) who then grew despotic via unequal control of land or other private wealth. In a related way, traditional theories about regular tribal movements across prehistoric Europe (e.g. Corded Ware, Unětíce, Lausitz), borrow the concept of Conquest States with the assertion that conqueror/conquered statuses provided a natural inequality over rights to key resources (Gimbutas 1965, Piggott 1965). A more recent set of ideas on leadership, associated with Sahlins (1974) and Renfrew (1973a) argues that competition between 'big men' and chiefs, for prestige and status, involving the use of luxury exotica, monumental constructions and communal redistribution, offers a key catalyst for increased social complexity and moves towards the State. In a neo-diffusionist elaboration of this competitive elite model (applied to the European Bronze and Iron Ages), Frankenstein and Rowlands (1978) and subsequent followers (e.g. Haselgrove 1982) have developed a widely applicable model of economic dependency for European developments on the aggressive external economies of the established states in the Mediterranean and Near East. Local European elites form the key nodes for such interaction and in the process, they and their societies are radically transformed into higher level chiefdoms, kingdoms and states.

PALAEOLITHIC - MESOLITHIC BACKGROUND:

Despite the rather hypothetical nature of recent generalizations on Palaeo-Mesolithic societies, it is of importance for models of Neolithic and later social systems that:

1   A large number of families coming together as a social group, on a seasonal or permanent basis, appears to be a basic, perhaps essential, feature of human societies - thus offering potential for group activities and indeed group control, well above the level of the family - the 'band' of Steward (1969) and Service (1962), (cf. Wobst, 1974).

2   Already from the end of the last glacial era, inadequate population control, or merely the fluctuations of natural subsistence resources, favoured larger cultural groupings on a regional basis (cf. Gramsch's (1973) Mesolithic cultural territories in northern Europe), whose function was perhaps to identify traditional communities in each area with their localized resource base.[6]

3   Much wider cultural linkages, comparable to Clarke's technocomplexes (1968), show the readiness of these small communities to assimilate new functional adaptations beyond their regional culture.

4   The more stable and localized that high quality resources become, the more there is opportunity (especially if population is relatively dense and a wide economic approach less flexible - cf. Newell and other authors on late Mesolithic Europe)[7], for development of more permanent settlements - in which that resource dependence encourages corporate ownership and symbolic group-awareness, reflected in territorial markers such as formal cemeteries (cf. the important paper by Chapman, 1981a).[8] The possibility that these unusual contexts may encourage elementary ranking of individuals receives some ethnographic support, but is ambiguously documented in variability in observed archaeological burial practice for the periods concerned. More plausible are inferences relating to corporate

residential groups with an emphasis on roles open to all, for example adult male status, female childbirth status, etc. (Pavuk 1972; Phillips 1980, 141 ff; Chapman 1981a).

Cases of particular relevance to this last point are such as the 'formal' burials in late Mesolithic Brittany, the shell midden cemeteries at Téviec and Hoëdic, with the former exhibiting multiple graves often under stone structures and associated with ritual hearths and food gifts (Péquart et al. 1937, 1954). Also, and even more striking, Mesolithic communities such as that at Lepenski Vir (Srejovic 1972) on the Yugoslav Danube shore: around 20 houses per phase built on a modular plan, also a central larger house considered a community focus. The houses are divided into a living space and a ritual space, and in the latter occur successively-interred, extended burials - but only a minority of the population and with an age range remarkably concentrating in the 40-80 year bracket. A site that was contemporary to the earliest Neolithic groups in the area but now being convincingly interpreted as the culmination of millennia of successful adaptation to the rich environment of the Danube Gorge. John Nandris sees a parallel and interactive development between the evolution of the Holocene climax vegetation and fauna here and the climax of human groups adapted to them with a hunter-gatherer strategy, as behind such elaborate communities and their unusual burial and artistic tradition.[9]

GENERAL DEVELOPMENT OF THE NEOLITHIC

As we have seen, and appropriately relating directly to the last point just made concerning Mesolithic 'climax development', a plausible theory in social evolution research at present is one of density-dependency, whereby dense populations allow of more occupational specialization, and may demand social complexity to control their cohesion - both factors encouraging the circulation of special prestige products (to reinforce social controls and the authority of controllers). (By 'prestige' are meant the rare and/or time-consuming artifacts in terms of manufacture, that may be seen to single out status and inter-group differences).[10] It must be borne in mind that the arrival of 'surplus' and 'leisure' to allow of division of labour in two such basic directions, is clearly no creation of the farming economy, and was probably available to most hunter-gatherer groups far back into the past. Study by anthropologists and demographers of both hunter-gatherer and semi-autonomous farming societies demonstrates that they tend to maintain carrying-capacities well below regional potential, often at 20-30% or less, to allow a safety margin (Polgar 1975, Brumfiel 1976, Hassan 1978, R.E. Adams 1978), and therefore there is generally a latent potential for much greater productivity, and often a significant surplus actually produced beyond basic needs. As for leisure-time, possibly this decreased with the change to farming, but overall population density clearly increased vastly, and because of the locally-intensive nature and high productivity of mixed farming, led to what had been a rare and localized phenomenon in the Mesolithic - relatively permanent pockets of dense population often in a village or cluster of inter-visible discrete homes - becoming increasingly the norm over large areas of Europe.

One particularly significant change would now be the much greater number of people available at close distance for the supply of a specialist's craft - thus crossing an hypothetical threshold to encourage personal investment in such labour. Likewise the dense sedentary or semi-sedentary populations offered greater potential for aspiring leaders to organize them in regional activities, and a greater necessity for the role of mediators in the increasingly disruptive conflicts over localized resources. Finally, the accumulated surplus within easy access of potential part-time producers, such as craftsmen and leaders, or for redistribution for communal work (whether building monuments, war parties or religious festivals), was also far greater in potential than that easily culled from lower density and more mobile and 'open' societies of pre-agricultural time. The development of specialist leaders, priests and craftsmen and the deployment of surpluses for group leadership purposes (including wasteful display) in unusual hunter-gatherer societies such as the Pacific Coast Indians and in California, might seem to support this interpretation, from consideration of the broad similarity in ecological and economic factors involved, which compare to those underlying more complex sedentary farming communities.

If the degree of concentration of population and surplus is significant, we can note two things: firstly that the 'catchment' or surrounding territory (Vita-Finzi and Higgs 1970) of a site may already determine from local fertility the existence of larger settlements and longer-lived communities.[11] Secondly, the addition over time, to the economy and technology, of features such as simple ard ploughs, animal traction, a more developed use of animal products (as Andrew Sherratt (1981) has shown), new cultigens and more intensive cropping systems (shorter fallow rotations) (cf. Boserup 1965, Fowler 1978, Welinder 1975, Bintliff 1982), will tend to raise the overall human density in Europe in terms of the parameters of crop and herd yields per district over time. This is borne out by the overall rise in population throughout the Neolithic, and the increasing numbers of larger, more stable tell communities.

THE EARLY NEOLITHIC

In the early expansion of the new economy across Europe, we might expect that initially there would be little problem of resource abundance, with either low numbers of colonizers (option A), or Mesolithic populations now able to reduce possible density-tension by adopting the more intensive mode of economy (option B), or combinations of the two (most probable : option C). In this view, a clear period of development relative to the timing of the initial economic change in each area and to the regional potential for continuous increased productivity, would ensue, before the detectable traces of density-dependent phenomena such as leadership structures or group territorial markers (arising from internal disputes over resources, or from the threat of adjacent groups). But if we prefer to emphasize not strife, but merely the potential for more public co-operation, such as might become more available to aspiring leaders of a secular or religious kind in denser localized populations, we might expect from the first a greater degree of specialization and evidence for higher achievement in communal activities (monument construction, etc.).

In both the Early Balkan Neolithic (FTN) (Nandris 1970, 1976b, 1977) and the Early Central European Neolithic (LBK) there is now widespread evidence for long-term stability of settlement in chosen niches of mixed farming exploitation. The more concentrated rich soils may explain the more nucleated villages of the Balkan tells (cf. the mosaic of large village territories studied by Dennell and Webley (1975) in the Karanovo region), contrasted to the hamlet scatters of the LBK, although much of the FTN has also a more dispersed and less permanent settlement pattern (Chapman 1976). But it is clear, looking at the packing of villages and their long life in many regions of the Balkans, or at the highly fertile plateau on which Neolithic Knossos in Crete lies, that the potential is there for sustained dense population and the support of craftsmen and other roles in society. Perhaps

significantly, in view of the theory (Chapman, 1981a) that population stress on fixed resources, such as land, is often met by the erection of group ownership monuments (the 'corporate group') such as communal cemeteries or monumental tombs (e.g. megaliths), to stress inheritance and the rights to resources, there is no tradition of formal communal burial in the FTN.[12] However communal cemeteries do exist in the LBK, and not only late on; this could reflect a new and growing importance of rights to land, especially appropriate now that we have moved from the popular shifting-cultivation model for the LBK (Soudsky 1962, Piggott 1965) to one of fairly fixed settlement.[13]

Very significant for general theories about the role of trade in social change, is the recognition that much of the FTN and nearly all of the LBK settlement areas, as Andrew Sherratt (1976) has reminded us, were poor in fine quality stone sources for tools of various sorts; yet scientific documentation evidences major and long-distance flows of such raw materials across Europe from the sources. There is no notable evidence to show that this led to the rise of leadership structures to control and foster such important supplies of everyday material, although it does seem clear that basic status differences, based primarily on age and sex, can be highlighted with it; for example in the LBK cemeteries the spondylus shells used for ornaments and exchanged from the Aegean Sea as far as Holland, are especially associated with older adult males in the community. All this contrasts to Gordon Childe's (1951) view of the dichotomy between the local self-sufficiency of the Early Neolithic compared to the wide exchange systems of the metal ages.[14]

Often associated in the literature with the earlier Neolithic is a predominance of matrilineal inheritance, or even 'matriarchy'. The origin of this concern seems to be Bachofen (1861), who in the nineteenth century sought an elusive primeval society, where women dominated, from the Classical sources and under the influence of legends of the Amazons. Morgan (1877) developed the theory with the addition of ethnographic parallels such as the Iroquois (who are actually matrilineal, the males controlling decision making). The general, but rarely closely-examined, assumption is that simple hoe agriculture is primarily a female role, thus stressing female descent in principles of inheritance, whereas the arrival of ploughs and oxen demand a primarily male role, as do intensive herding and the associated protection of flocks from predators and robbers. We must dismiss immediately, from sober research in ethnohistory, any claims for past societies where authority is normally invested in females, and the patrilineal/matrilineal association is far from clearcut in documented societies with the appropriate balance of labour. Nonetheless, authorities such as Otto (1960) and many other Eastern European scholars (cf. Behrens 1976/7), begin a priori with the belief that the Late Neolithic shift to greater herding activity and the use of the plough, together with increased signs of endemic warfare, would naturally correlate with supposed archaeological evidence for status changes from an emphasis on the female to one on the male.[15]

The Early Balkan Neolithic (FTN)

Houses in villages or hamlets seem, in general, to reflect nuclear or extended families, sometimes with internal storage facilities and ovens. In the early, long-settled plains of central Greece (Theocharis 1973, Halstead 1977), over many centuries, we can observe the continual increase in the number and size of villages (e.g. increases by a factor of five from Early to Middle Neolithic), some of the largest of which, by the fifth millennium bc seem to be organized on a central plan. Sesklo is the best known, 20-25 acres and a population believed to be over

86

3000, with defences, an 'acropolis' and lower town, and in the elevated part of the community an internal enclosure with a large central building and courtyard. A chieftain's residence? There is no confirmatory evidence from burials to support such distinctions (until the Late and Final Neolithic cf. Schachermeyr, 1976), but the domestic features of the central enclosure make it less likely to be a shrine or clubhouse. It is also possible that the site was producing fine pottery for its region. Significantly paralleling population rise and increasing signs of hierarchy are continual advances in the range of cultigens and types of land in use (Renfrew J. 1979, Renfrew C. 1972, Halstead 1977). For parallel later developments in the North Balkans see below.

The Early Neolithic in Central Europe (LBK)

It is now considered that LBK communities were small and dense in preferred niches of loessic river valleys,[16] linked by networks of raw material exchange and intermarriage, and by co-operation in building the typical wooden longhouses - but not apparently involved in a larger scale of co-operation (Van de Velde 1979). Startin, for example, has shown that some of the construction work on the houses would have required the help of what must have been, in many areas, a number of adjacent hamlets.[17]

In favoured areas the evidence is good enough to suggest many centuries or even as much as 1000 years of continuous or discontinuous habitation in the general area of each hamlet, coupled with continual population increase. Our best known area study is the Aldenhoven Plateau near Cologne; here a density is revealed, along the Merzbach valley, of five contemporary hamlets and several more temporary sites over a distance of about 1.5kms. With each hamlet possessing two to six houses, this would seem to reflect a population of 60-150 down the valley (something like a quarter of the nineteenth-century density for the same area).[18]

Despite the view that variable LBK house sizes reflect multiple family units (Soudsky and Pavlu 1971), in general the house 'core' is an extended family module (rather comparable to the FTN), with variable additional space for animal and food storage (Modderman 1970, 1975). Also there exists the larger 'clubhouse', possibly only one per larger site or district per phase, sometimes seen as a chief's house or communal cattle shed. This has more elaborate wooden stalls and is often of greater dimensions than the normal longhouse (often even as much as 80m. long) and has the same internal features as the domestic longhouse. There is growing agreement on the 'module' nature of LBK houses,[19] and the occurrence in later houses, of similar type, of several hearths need not be seen as indicating family multiples as opposed to differential heating and cooking requirements. The relative representation of the longhouse with storage facilities, and its central living area on its own - the 'dwelling', in contemporary phases at particular sites, has been plausibly seen as reflecting the fission of families and the creation of new households on a generation by generation basis. The linking of these household units into a larger community is now seen as of a different nature from the traditional 'village' picture, with the application of horizontal stratigraphy and more refined chronology. Hamlets or even single dwellings seem to be the more normal pattern. But the clear interactions between such communities to obtain stone, for mating networks and longhouse construction, would argue strongly for regular social gatherings. Given the small size of each settlement, is it possible perhaps, that the greathouses (if not also the residence of a leading family) served for such district gatherings?[20] Nonetheless the individual settlements of the LBK are generally considered to be autonomous units in terms of decision-making.

Scope for recognizing social statuses in these sites is made more difficult by the loss of living floors from erosion of the loess, although current research is trying to separate out cultural debris belonging to each house from adjacent pit debris.[21] At present it seems most plausible to suggest that the variability in longhouse versus small-house numbers relates to age seniority and the larger 'establishment' of heads of extended families.

It is reasonable to assume that hamlets within walking distance of each other in the favoured loess environment of the culture, the apparent absence of defences and prominent weapons, and the limited scale of leadership roles inferred from the settlement and burial evidence, argue jointly for an absence of territorial aggression for most of the long lifespan of the LBK. Considerable interest has therefore been aroused, (already in the work of Childe - cf. Tabaczynski 1972), by the development in late LBK times of quite striking defence works, such as the final great ditch at Köln-Lindenthal, or the Aldenhoven ringwork defences; but the pattern is very general.[22] At the same time the LBK population rise is abruptly reversed, large areas of the loess depopulated and a new expansion occurs into a whole new range of previously unoccupied or neglected environments (see below). Given the evidence for progressive erosion and podsolization of the loess soil, held due to cumulative early human misuse, it has been argued (Kuper et al. 1975, Kuper and Lüning 1975) that the prolonged intensive exploitation of the landscape by the LBK, under increasing population, led to its deterioration and the necessary disruption of the settlement pattern. The beginnings of land scarcity at the end of the LBK are seen then to be marked by more aggressive inter-community relations.

If we are correct in seeing a minimal level of LBK social ranking ('big man', lineage elder on the scale of several related hamlets?), we may consider whether the apparent lack of resource shortages or warfare, at least until the later phase of the culture, accounts for the absence of distinct stratified elites in the society concerned. That exchange was important to each community is clear, yet as noted, even the long distance 'prestigious' spondylus exchange served apparently merely to enhance the most basic statuses of adult male, 'elder' or 'big man' in the community.

Given this vagueness over LBK 'ranking', not surprisingly careful study has been devoted to the burial data. The existence for the LBK, in contrast to the FTN, of formal cemeteries, would be seen in the Chapman model as indicative of greater corporate identification, linked to lineage land rights, and we have suggested that this might not have applied equally to the larger and more stable FTN villages, if one were to argue that the LBK had a more localized and intensive cultivation.[23] The classic study of the Nitra LBK cemetery by Pavuk (1972), and his comparisons to other cemeteries, showed that in general males ranked higher than females and both ranked higher than children, in terms of the number of gifts and the presence of imports. Adult males were especially associated with fine stone axes and spondylus, and sometimes fineware pottery. However variability is apparent and sometimes the 'richest' graves are those of children, whilst female burials can also contain, at times, spondylus and even at some sites, numerous axes. There seems to be no exclusive and definitive status kit, uniform for the wide spread of the LBK culture, or even within a particular cemetery, except for a consistent trend for higher emphasis on adult male status. In addition to these observations, there also seem to be clusters of graves within cemeteries that seem to represent individual kin plots.

Having made these points, there are however further problems in detail. There are large numbers of graves with no gifts or just pottery, and if we look carefully at the 'rich' graves we seem to see that a certain proportion of adult males do not receive adequate status objects - at Nitra, for example, about half lack the axe and other equipment. This is technically a 'ranked' society, and we cannot reasonably argue, as some have, that the males buried with axes must have 'lent' theirs to other males during their lifetime; for the axes are working tools, as wear studies have shown, and fundamental to everyday tasks of mature males. In other words, the differential presence is more likely to be symbolic rather than identifying minority ownership.[24]

The most thorough recent attack on these problems is Van de Velde's (1979) study of the Elsloo cemetery. Perhaps 10-15 families formed the community burying here over a century or so. The number of 'wealthy' burials, argued to be mainly but not predominantly adult males, is at first sight perhaps only a quarter of that of total adult males; but if we then make allowance for numerous children being buried in the cemetery (the human remains have unfortunately not survived and all inferences are made on gift combinations), wealthy males would rise to just under half of all adult male burials. However, the author suggests that female burials are also assigned axes, though a different variety from the male symbol. Some of the especially 'rich' burials are interpreted as possible 'big men' of the community. Detailed study of pottery designs was rather inconclusive in detecting clusterings that could reflect exogamous kin groups, though it is stated that similar work from the associated settlement site argues for patrilocal residence. Here again, the potential 'ranking' (as opposed to 'stratification') within the adult male class, one might suggest, could relate to the distinction between the great house, the longhouse and the nuclear house in settlements (cf. Modderman 1970, 1975).[25]

The Early Neolithic in the West Mediterranean (Impressed Ware)

As with the Balkans and the LBK across the centre of Europe, we can see from the first development of a full farming economy in a few favoured areas of the Western Mediterranean, c. 5000 bc, a continuous development of denser populations. In Iberia these will grow into the early Copper Age cultures with proto-urban centres, from the early third millennium bc onwards.[26] But we can observe once more in southern Italy that cycle of expansion, then settlement retraction and disjunction, that punctuates the record of prehistoric Europe and continually seems to destroy a promising cultural florescence: in the Tavoliere Plain hundreds of large ditched villages are known in an arid but potentially fertile environment, but after a millennium or so there is a severe depopulation that may reflect both soil exhaustion and the highly variable and marginal rainfall in the area.[27]

THE MATURE NEOLITHIC (Danubian 2 of Childe, primarily the fourth millennium bc)

The infill of the FTN and LBK econiches or zones of preferred soils and locations leads to overflow into adjacent, more varied resources, possibly aided by overuse of the core settled areas. We can demonstrate a vigorous human expansion, both within these old settled zones and out of them in entirely new regions, into new niches - upland, lake and other lowland habitats, with associated shifts in the balance of the economy between wild and domestic components and between stock and crops. As a result we have the Neolithic expansion into France, Switzerland, the British Isles, southern Scandinavia and north east Europe to the Ukraine.[28]

Yet equally important must have been the adoption of the new economy by local Mesolithic groups, that especially in north and north-west Europe are argued to be highly populous, and perhaps requiring a more intensive economy to reduce population stress.[29]

By the end of the fourth millennium bc agricultural communities are established in virtually every region suitable for pre-plough farming in Europe. If we are to predict that this process will lead, by continued infill, to a need for greater organization and will stimulate communal activity, then it is notable that a 'climax' of East European high culture is reached c. 3500 bc, from a continuous local development beginning c. 5500 bc; in Iberia, the 'climax' proto-urban high cultures of Portugal and Spanish Almeria have arisen by c. 2500 bc from the first significant proliferation of farming in the fifth millennium bc[26]; whilst in north western Europe - to judge from the regional co-operation manifested in monument building, it is reached by c. 2500 bc, from a local inception of agriculture in the Atlantic coastlands c. 4000 bc.[30]

In Eastern Europe, the broadening of the areas of settlement and the exploitation of the total wild and domestic resource base, that characterizes the fourth-millennium Copper Age 'climax' society, is seen by Nandris (1976a, 1978) as the culmination of a trend throughout the local Neolithic from a generalized, adaptively unsophisticated, Early Neolithic 'pioneer' economy to one of a very broad and intense combination of locally feasible specialist modes of exploitation, associated with a peak of population, and of social and technological complexity, - a revival to him of the Lepenski Vir 'climax' phenomenon.[31] In some instances there are even hints of leadership superstructures beyond that of headman, or clan-head level, for example the Varna cemetery, or from consideration of prestigious artifacts. At the same time it is of interest to note that as all available land is taken in, and there is some evidence for long-term environmental decline during the Neolithic from both human overuse and perhaps climate (Dennell and Webley, 1975), we have the first general appearance in Eastern Europe of formal cemeteries, with their implication of enhanced stress on corporate rights in each district.[32]

There is a reasonable archaeological case to be made in various parts of Europe, that with the expansion of groups into new regions, and into new niches in old regions, conditions favoured the rise of community leaders or even elites. At present there are numerous theories (cf. earlier discussion) to explain their origin - e.g. the land scarcity/warleader model, or one of increased pastoralism leading to 'pastoral capitalism' with war leaders again. Indeed a lively debate exists from this period into the Iron Age as to the source of the power and wealth of elites in prehistoric Europe, as believed made manifest in wealthy graves. The Service-Sahlins view favoured by Renfrew (1973a) and others, emphasizes the initial advantage of a clan head or 'big man' in accumulating status, with a large household, associated craftsmen, and access to imported goods; communal surpluses as well as the household surplus, together with the imports, are then redistributed to those giving formal and informal allegiance to the person concerned. Randsborg, however, has pointed out (1982) that an alternative system might exist (here he cites Old German society), in which local leaders offer services to the community such as guidance in government, in war parties, as well as providing the products of craftsmen kept at their own expense; kinship here need not be of significance, but rather the continued support of the 'big man's' own achieved resources. Yet, any stability of authority would nonetheless seem to rest on inheritance of such resources, and therefore of such a 'role', hence the interest shown in many studies in the exact timing of the inception of private as opposed to group/corporate ownership of resources; and sometimes such a transformation is seen as manifest when we have rich child burials or of adults with a feeble physical appearance (!)[33]

Settlement evidence: The large numbers known for Europe show, in general, a continuance of the village-hamlet pattern through the fourth millennium bc, with increasing densities especially in Eastern Europe where the larger communities also seem more planned and perhaps more centrally controlled.[34] But houses are still normally of nuclear to extended family size.[35] Yet occasionally within the settlement can be seen one house larger than the others or given a special siting, and discussed variously as a shrine, a male clubhouse, a chieftain's residence, - with very rarely any supportive evidence to assist such an identification being adduced or preserved (as with the range of theories advanced for the curious settlement pattern of the Kolomischina site).[36] Overall, burial evidence (see below) provides little confirmation for a distinct aristocracy over most of Europe, as opposed to the widespread ranking already probably in existence during the LBK period, but there are some strikingly exceptional regions to this generalization, especially to the north and west. On the other hand, the late LBK trend to fortifications becomes a general characteristic of the fourth millennium in both older settled, and newly settled, farming zones (cf. the TRB site of Dölauer Heide). Yet possible ritual features at some of these, for example Sarup on Fünen, and the postulated greater need to protect the larger pastoral component of this period, have to be taken into account. Moreover, English causewayed camps seem to show the likelihood that communal defence, communal ritual and the protection of large herds, can all be catered for in the more complex earthwork systems of the developed Neolithic. And there are some clear cases of defended villages, for example the Goldberg (Schröter 1975) or Büdelsdorf.[37]

Burial: In general, a pattern comparable to the LBK emerges from cemetery studies, with gift variety and quantity broadly relating to age and sex, and with adult males especially notable in such richness as well as being associated with axes; some exceptionally furnished male burials are seen as community headmen or those of a special clan, or might be considered as local 'big men'.[38]

However, this pattern characterizing much of Central and Eastern Europe, (with some rare hints of a higher degree of ranking or even formal stratification, as at Varna), is contrasted to that to be found in many of the newly settled regions of the North and West, where burial data seem regularly to indicate more complex divisions within society. This is more surprising since the rare settlement evidence is comparable to the former areas, with family structures exhibiting no obvious distinctions in domestic accommodation.

The first group we shall look at is the TRB (Funnel Beaker Culture) in Northern Europe. The majority of burials here were probably simple earth or stone packed graves, but a minority stand out. In Poland and Czechoslovakia, for example, we have stately grave chambers under prominent tumuli, and most notably in the Kujavian Barrows where the monuments can be 100m. long, consist of 100 tons of earth and boulders overlying a carefully constructed chamber of stone and organic structure, but containing usually but a single burial. In Denmark, Klavs Randsborg (1975) has compared the relative distribution of early megalithic complex tombs of this period, and the simpler earth graves, showing their relationship to the density and spacing of population; he suggests there is selection from the community of important individuals for the more complex monuments and wealthier graves, in order to provide an integrative focus for district populations.[39]

Similar evidence comes from contemporary Neolithic Britain (see below). In the developed Neolithic in France (Chassey Culture) there are examples of increasingly large 'activity areas' or 'villages', such as St. Michel du Touch, a 50 acre site with traces of several hundred structures, ditches and palisades, and associated with elaborate pits, one with relatively rich offerings and two human burials.[40]

Exchange: There continues to exist very vigorous exchange, especially for axes and cores of hardstone and flint, but still not easily linked to the creation of status via control of such systems - even for the communities believed to be mining the raw material and feeding it into what is assumed to be village-to-village exchange (though we should expect some subsistence support from adjacent villages to the mining group).[41] And yet calculations on the possible scale of production of such mines suggest that tens of thousands of people, possibly far more, over a very wide radius, could have been provided with a large part of their yearly artifact needs from a single such source - although at the same time this requirement might have been fulfilled in no more than half a dozen exchanges between adjacent communities in the chain.[42] The same specialization and type of organization seem arguable for instances of Neolithic pottery exchange, such as English Hembury Ware (Peacock 1969).

Neolithic Britain The total archaeological and environmental evidence suggests an overall trend of population rise and settlement expansion over the Neolithic period from c.4000 -2000 bc. In the early third millennium the scale of this process seems already to have led to localized soil degeneration and a phase of abandonment of cleared land and retraction of settlement, or shift from arable to pasture.[43] This is followed by a renewed attack on the landscape, probably assisted by the arrival of plough traction. Now seen to be contemporary with, or not long after the inception of, the first farming, we begin to see two notable features in the landscape (regrettably settlements are poorly known apart from isolated houses) - both of which are considered to reflect a new stress on land rights, territoriality, and corporate group enhancement activities with land territory associations.

Firstly we have a very wide distribution of communal burial monuments, earthen long barrows and megalithic tombs. Renfrew (1973a, b) has argued that the dispersal pattern of these monuments reflects their role as territorial markers for a society of autonomous hamlet or sub-clan groups.[44] In this view the early tombs, such as the early Orkney series, vary in size merely because of insignificant local group size variations, and calculations suggest that c. 5000 man hours were required in such constructions - a task for the suggested small group of families to encompass in a season or two of pre-harvest labour. Supporting this view is the fact that anthropological study of tomb burials has several times confirmed that they represent a closely-related kin group (e.g. West Kennet, and further examples from the Severn-Cotswold tombs). As Chapman (1981a) notes, this major feature of the British Neolithic landscape could indeed plausibly be linked to rights to land, but is there sufficient evidence to suggest population pressure? It must be borne in mind that informed estimates of the British Late Mesolithic population are surprisingly high (some consider hundreds of thousands - R. Jacobi, pers. comm.), and it is clear that these people, whose cultural debris diminishes almost to extinction with the Neolithic period, 'became' a major (possibly **the** major) component of the Neolithic population together with hypothesized fully Neolithic colonizers from Holland and perhaps France (Case 1976). Here there might rapidly have developed the appropriate response (or, better, its adoption) of formal territorial symbolism.[45]

In Renfrew's study, these Early Neolithic egalitarian hamlet/sub-clan groups, at least in central and southern England, were co-operating to construct our secondary feature, earthwork complexes called causewayed-camps, generally interpreted as ceremonial centres for each region (Renfrew 1973b). Clusters of 20-30 long-barrows in the Wessex Chalklands were used to suggest the size of such co-operating groups, 400-2000 people, and this scale of population was seen as neatly of the right order to construct the camps in several seasons of off-peak agricultural labour. Territories of this larger social group were plotted hypothetically and for each camp territory a local leadership or smallscale proto-chieftain society was proposed.

However, this neat fit of data to model, where egalitarian hamlets (of the LBK type) in the circumstances of increasing density of population and surplus, are co-ordinated by ambitious 'big men' or chiefs to construct group-enhancing monuments, suffers from two serious flaws. Firstly, as Atkinson (1968) pointed out many years ago, earthen and megalithic tombs in Britain seem to have been built and used over a period of at least a thousand years, but contain remarkably few bodies - 30 or more is a rarity. The total number of known monuments is also relatively small. In this calculation we are reminded of the other basic flaw in Renfrew's model, for the summing up of group totals for 20-30 long-barrows in each causewayed camp territory takes no account of the fact that these monument clusters represent **cumulative** construction activity of such monuments, at irregular intervals over this period of up to 1000 years in each area. Without a doubt only a tiny proportion of the total population was destined to be buried in these prestigious structures. Whether these selected few were truly a 'privileged elite' or any other category up to and including social outcasts, is hitherto unclarified, though the family factor suggest that at least in some cases the special group was inheriting the right or role.[46] Further insight has been achieved from the recent excavation of the causewayed camp at Hambledon Hill (Mercer 1980). It is now clear here that a vast interrelated complex had been constructed by the third millennium bc (but the camp **type** now dates back to the mid fourth millennium bc),[47] consisting of perhaps three or more fortified domestic settlements of hamlet-village character, large enclosures for hundreds of head of cattle, and a great enclosure where it is arguable that almost the total dead of these communities were exposed for excarnation. Of the probable thousands thus exposed, a small proportion had their bones (generally skulls) deliberately collected and placed in the fill of the numerous ditch segments. Two long barrows are also part of the complex, and would probably have contained a half dozen or so bodies at the most. The earthworks of the whole complex now represent about half to three quarters of a million man hours of work, and the population involved is considered by Roger Mercer to be the villages themselves and probably numerous surrounding communities. If we take merely a 500 year period, some tens of thousands of dead bodies would have almost all rotted away in the open, with a mere 1% or so reinterred in the ditch silt 'ritual' deposits and in the local and district long-barrows contained in the putative causewayed camp territory.[48]

The picture that now seems to be emerging is one of individual districts participating, from dispersed and nucleated communities (some defended), in considerable co-ordinated efforts on ritual monuments and settlement and stock defences. The minority receiving special burial **could** be a co-ordinating class, - chiefs or priests and/or war leaders. And indeed Hambledon Hill and other similar sites such as Crickley Hill show clear traces of attack, destruction and slaughter.[49] In general, current thinking sees a more highly structured society, if not a stratified one, for the earlier Neolithic in Britain, than until recently envisaged, but comparable in such hints to the inferences being drawn from burial data in contemporary Scandinavia and Poland.

THE LATE NEOLITHIC AND CHALCOLITHIC (primarily the third millennium bc)

The continual push of population into less favourable soils and topography (cf. Jarman 1977, Figs. 3 and 4) was only partly compensated for by adaptation towards herding, hunting, and mining for exchange, and could be seen as frequently the result of declining yields in older cultivated areas. One can see this for example, in Kruk's (1980) sequence for Poland over the span of the Neolithic and Copper-Age, as sites move increasingly into the dry and poorer-soiled interfluve area.[50] In the third millennium bc, however, the general diffusion of more intensive agriculture utilizing the ard plough and animal traction, would have enabled greater productivity to be obtained even in the more marginal zones, at least for a time, as would the greater use of domestic herd products discussed recently by Andrew Sherratt (1981).[51] It may be significant that this possible revitalization of the European economy is associated with the rise of vast 'spheres of interaction', probably of a cult-prestige nature, such as the Corded Ware/Bell Beaker phenomena (see below); in some areas, with larger scale expenditure of effort and skill on monument construction e.g. Britain and Brittany; in other areas with the rise of putative primitive settlement hierarchies (Milisauskas 1978, p.202, and see below). At the same time the takeoff of olive production in the Mediterranean, as emphasized by Renfrew (1972), was a major additional boost to productivity at the basis of the flourishing Early Bronze Age high cultures of Greece and, possibly, of the proto-urban high cultures of Copper Age Iberia (Gilman 1976, 1981).

That all these changes were nonetheless those of intensification in ecologies that were perhaps unable to take the strain, seems demonstrable from the rise of heathland and poor acid soils in early cultivated areas such as Denmark (Kristiansen 1980) and the conversion of arable in parts of England to less intensive pastoral use (and see further possible examples below).[52] One might argue in many regions of Europe for the densest populations yet achieved, but this would seem to be the result of a very full use (cf. Nandris's (1976a, 1978) concept of 'climax') of a variety of soils and locations and economic strategies, often by the same cultural group. One can give little support to any idea that this is intimately linked to the spread of copper metallurgy from the fourth millennium bc, since it is now seen to be a material of little value for everyday agriculture and craft work and, with gold, was primarily used for decoration and display. Increased production of subsistence products has been seen as stimulated by the requirements of exchange for these prestigious materials, but as Sherratt (1976) has shown, the relevant exchange networks seem comparable in scale to earlier ones for obsidian and hardstone.[53]

One feature observable in the third millennium bc is the build-up of efficient adaptation and population growth in the newly settled areas such as the Polish late TRB culture, supporting by now a simple settlement hierarchy. The site of Bronocice, for example, of this time, is a giant site over 50ha., including tens of thousands of pits, and defence works, associated with a number of smaller settlements and perhaps acting as some kind of regional focus in its valley.[54]

Expansion of southern French populations over the 1000 years or so from the main fourth-millennium agricultural takeoff in this region, leads by the third millennium to colonization of the tough limestone country, and here, rapidly, competition for scarce arable and grazing land may have encouraged the rash of megalithic tombs and be linked to the appearance of some defended village sites, perhaps even the beginnings of some kind of regional authority in the latter (cf. Lébous, Boussargues).[55]

In Iberia the same process of population infill in various favourable regions for early farming, associated with the erection of megalithic tombs (markers for corporate group territories?), develops into a complex higher culture, the Copper Age, by the later third millennium bc (see again, note 30). This is characterized by a settlement hierarchy with major defended centres and associated cemeteries containing evidence of elite groups (on variety and degree of exoticness of tomb contents, as well as tomb placing), and with these centres also distinguished by an assemblage of special, often prestige artifacts rarely found on presumed 'satellite' rural sites (Chapman 1975, 1977, 1981b). The old view of external conquest or colonization of Iberia from the Eastern Mediterranean (Blance 1961), in order to account for these elites and the defended foci, has been effectively disproved on both chronological and typological grounds and supplanted by a model emphasizing internal differentiation (Renfrew 1967, Chapman 1975, Gilman 1976). In order to explain further the basis of such local elite emergence, several theories have been proposed. A rather doubtful case for artificial control over prime irrigated land has been made (Gilman 1981, Chapman 1978), but it might be more plausible to consider a more basic land control, by a minority, over prime dry-farmed land (both high water-table valley bottom fields, and moisture-retaining Neogen soils of the lower hill-lands).[56] Contemporary with these developments, in the Aegean, the fruitful olive-cereal culture of southern Greece was giving rise to dense populations and associated social developments - chieftains' mansions (?) (Renfrew 1972, 1973a) and burials indicating social stratification (Branigan 1975, Renfrew 1972).

By the third millennium bc, the continual push of population, and related movement into new and often more marginal land, leads inevitably in many areas to crisis, as seems to have occurred for instance at the climax of the long rise of Copper Age civilization in the north Balkans, and with the contemporary later Neolithic in north Greece. The subsequent changes in settlement pattern are radical, and are linked to a much greater emphasis on defence and an apparent widespread population decline. This development is plausibly interpreted by Renfrew (1972; n.d.) and others as reflecting agricultural over-exploitation. Such a truncation of cultural stability, and collapse of the support base for the highly elaborate life of these tell communities, reinforces Tringham's (1978) view of the constraining effect of the environment in a context of uncontrolled agricultural expansion and a primitive technology.[57]

A remarkable laboratory for social development is the Maltese archipelago, colonized c. 4000 bc as part of the expansion of early farming groups that had become established in strength in southern Italy c. 5000 bc. Its virtually isolated development is typified (in a microcosm for many regions of Europe) by population growth in a very fertile environment (comparable to Knossos on Crete) and the development of increasingly elaborate rock-cut tombs, from which arose above-ground temples (Evans 1971a, Trump 1976, 1980, 1981, Guilaine 1981). Renfrew has plausibly suggested that spatially discrete clusters of temples over the islands reflect local territorial groups (1973a). The considerable population suggested by these works and the high degree of organization inferrable by the third millennium bc, has been taken by Evans (1973) and Renfrew to denote a ruling elite, of priests or charismatic chieftains (with explicit parallels to the social evolution of recent island communities in the Pacific). Evans further points to details of the temples that imply the activities of a minority of 'specialists' and participants, and to the physical anthropology of burials in a complex chamber tomb that suggests a population group unfamiliar with manual labour (!). At a late stage, the amalgamation of temples into a connected complex at Tarxien may even suggest an elite 'palace'. Finally the great Hypogeum temple/mausoleum with its many thousands of bodies interred over perhaps 1000 years or so may also represent a small and perhaps privileged minority of the total population. This complex and innovative, highly organized and internally-absorbed high culture declines rapidly and apparently catastrophically, and although the succeeding Tarxien Cemetery culture is sometimes seen as a destructive incursive group from Italy, ecological overkill by a large population in a small archipelago has also been suggested as a viable alternative (there seems to be a simultaneous abandonment of temple sites and a perceptible interval before the arrival of the totally alien culture) (Trump 1976, 1981).

To see what might have happened had population increase been effectively matched by increased productivity and maintenance of soil fertility, we can turn to the great Neolithic settlement of Knossos on Crete. John Evans (1971b) has shown how this community developed gradually in size over the 3000 years or so of its existence before effective metallurgy, already betraying by the latter part of this period traces of a more integrated building plan compared to the small, individual family structures typical for the rest of Europe. By the threshold of the Bronze Age the population is estimated to be several thousand strong, and there is a natural development into the well-planned building complexes of the Cretan Early Bronze Age, which some already see as perhaps representing simple 'mansions', offices and stores of a growing managerial elite for large communities, (or at least highly organized, planned villages). From this point it is also considered no great step to the first great integrated palace structures on the Knossos site and elsewhere on Crete c. 2000 bc. Associated with this overall settlement transformation are clear signs of enhanced craft specialization and external exchange (cf. also Warren, 1975).

The minimal role of the continuing extensive flows of exchanged raw materials and finished artifacts over Europe, in creating, as opposed to emphasizing pre-existing, status distinctions, appears to apply equally well to fourth- and third-millennium bc societies in Europe as a whole (see again, notes 14, 32, 33, 42, 53). However, the contacts created by movements of hardstone for axes, and flint and obsidian for cutting tools, and many other items, including less practical but more display pieces such as metal, associated with indications of privileged access to these items for adult males and, perhaps, a special status group within that class (clan/family heads, 'big men', chieftains), could of course lay the basis for a network of a more enhanced prestige nature. This may already be anticipated in the earlier rare and often carefully status-linked burial of exotic spondylus ornaments. In the Late Neolithic/Copper Age era (in West, Central and North European terms), c. 2500 -2000 bc and beyond, much of Europe, both north of the Alps and in the central to west Mediterranean, betrays the existence of at least one or two very large networks, in which certain members of each district community are buried with a well-made beaker pot and a special set of warrior equipment (with the 'Corded Ware/Battle Axe Culture' a battle axe, with the 'Bell-Beaker Culture' often archery equipment and knives). Shennan (1980, 1982) has effectively demonstrated the appropriateness of a model of 'Spheres of Interaction' linking innumerable local communities, for these phenomena, in contrast to traditional ideas of migrating warrior peoples who established local aristocracies by right of conquest. That a cult aspect is part of this interactive package is very plausible, and it is suggested that local notables (the usual vagueness interposes itself here in terms of clan head/family head/'big man'/chief), would be those involved in this prestigious participation in an international (in our geography) belief and status system. In the absence of a network of major population or cult centres associated with these specific cult/ritual networks (with the possible exception of Late Neolithic Britain), it still seems as if the long-established inter-village flow of raw materials and ideas was acting as a pre-set circuit for such a reinforcement of already existing status in each community.[58]

Later Neolithic to Earlier Bronze Age Britain

After the possible over-expansion of the fourth millennium bc, and the conversion of much arable to pasture and woodland, a revival of land intake occurs, associated inevitably with renewed population rise, and probably fundamentally linked to the adoption of the traction plough. The success of this adaptation can be seen in notable community co-operation in the erection of special classes of giant or elaborate megalithic tombs, or megalithic and wooden sanctuaries such as the henges, stone alignments and cursus earthwork monuments, over large areas of Britain (Burl 1976, Renfrew 1979). Despite this visible demonstration of the size of concentrated surplus labour and food supplies, the Bronze Age that follows seems to show a progressive shift of population and the centres of craft production and status to new zones of the landscape, and a decline or collapse of major activity at nearly all the earlier ceremonial centres and burial sites (Bradley 1978, Barrett and Bradley 1980). It might be argued that the adaptations of the Later Neolithic were inadequate for resolving a continued strain between what are clearly, from the man hour calculations on monuments, very sizeable regional populations, and available local resources. With the shift of population comes the decline of the traditional signs of leadership and regional control - the monuments and the burials of elite groups.[59]

But during the climax of Late Neolithic centralized labour co-operation, as Renfrew has shown, the scale of monumental construction was far greater overall than in earlier Neolithic times. A small number of very large and impressive tombs are built, involving large numbers of people but for the interment of relatively few bodies - such as the great Maes Howe passage-grave in Orkney and the giant Boyne Valley tombs in Ireland (Renfrew 1973a,b, 1979). Parallel to this later concentration of effort at Maes Howe is the erection nearby of two stone circles in the centre of the Orkneys, representing to Renfrew a group of prestigious monuments constructed by the total regional population at the behest of an Orkney 'paramount' chief. In contemporary Wessex he considers the building of the henge monuments and particularly the giant 'cathedral' henges, such as Avebury and Durrington Walls, as reflecting an exercise in authority of a few leading chieftains who controlled similar territories as were previously focussed on the causewayed camps. Finally, in Wessex, a paramount chief unites these smaller chiefdoms into a large regional 'polity' marked by the

construction of the earthen mound of Silbury Hill, estimated at 18 million man hours of work.

The general scenario of increasing integration and co-operation under some kind of effective leadership is highly plausible. We may note that the already hypothesized elite nature of earlier Neolithic tombs is further developed here in the later period into what may be intra-elite stratification; within the minority burial structures the top of the pyramid is reasonably recognizable in the giant passage graves.[60] A curious physical (and possibly sociological) parallel to the Silbury Hill mound is the creation of a large mound by the 'egalitarian' Nuer of the Sudan, under the influence of a catalyzing regional prophet and war leader (Evans-Pritchard 1940, cf. plate 25). However, this does bring us to a further serious flaw in the Renfrew thesis: his emphasis on chiefdom societies as arising from economic and status competition between 'big men', chiefs and paramount chiefs. What is neglected is the detailed ideology that may have legitimized the elite and enabled regional corvées to construct these ceremonial monuments. The wide parallels throughout the European Atlantic world in types of megalithic tomb, and within Britain in ritual monument forms, seem to suggest contacts and similar belief structures over large areas, possibly linked to widespread participation in a religious system. Ironically, Renfrew (1979) compares his central Orkney cluster of Maes Howe and the two stone circles, to the similarly located Medieval cathedral of the Orkneys, St. Magnus, without recognizing that this latter was after all a cult centre for an international religion.[61] There is plenty of scope for priestly roles for the elite, as research into the mathematical and astronomical skills demonstrated by the layout and alignment of both burial and ritual sites has shown, although it now appears that these skills have been rather exaggerated (Burl 1976, Ruggles and White 1981). It is of particular interest that Brittany, also with early evidence for 'territorial' burial monuments, participates in this later Neolithic investment of effort in stone alignments and great standing stones.[62]

If the Boyne and Maes Howe passage graves are reasonable signs of personal elite status, the henges and other ritual monuments such as the cursus (which can be several miles in length), are seen as more public achievements, though the product likewise of chieftain co-ordination (Renfrew's (1974) 'group-orientated' versus 'individualizing' chieftain monuments). We are left to fill in the complexities of a more rounded, and I think acceptable reconstruction, with the addition of an overarching ideology (cf. Drennan 1976; Bintliff 1977a, pt.I, ch.7) that masks the simple exercise of power and charisma by community leaders. A further insight into these phenomena may also be obtained by relating them to the 'interaction spheres' of Shennan[58] belonging to the latter part of this same period, networks of common belief structures articulated by contacts and shared ideologies between district elites.

Conclusion

If initially the **average** European Neolithic community was larger than its Mesolithic predecessor, so also local resource variations should have conditioned the existence amongst the former of larger, more complex villages. By later Neolithic times these larger communities of several hundred people are increasingly common, reflecting a continual adaptation to local ecological opportunities and the accumulation of new technology.

The overall dominant impression given by the data available on the European Neolithic, and one that we would suggest will faithfully characterize, also, the succeeding Bronze Age, is one of an almost continuous distribution of village-hamlet communities across the cultivable zones of Europe. Within this, individual sites or districts stand out with larger communities and/or denser populations, and with associated incipient 'central-place' functions in some instances.[63] Such centralization is inferred in terms of craft production, exchange control, and organization of labour and surpluses, and is primarily to be related to a local basis of unusually rich and renewable soils or grazing land, or much more rarely in the Metal Ages, on the surpluses that can be drained from surrounding farming communities by a group with control over localized sources of copper or tin, gold or salt.[64] A very broad generalization seems to distinguish Eastern and South-Eastern Europe with a higher frequency of larger sites from the rest of temperate Europe, with smaller and less long-lived communities - a dichotomy that will continue into the Bronze Age and even beyond. At present it is possible to suggest that this difference rests at least in part on the greater degree of adaptation to local resources, linked to a longer development of mixed farming exploitation (and its technology), and differential availability of high quality and renewable farming and grazing land.

Despite the apparent development, over time, of more stratified society in Europe from the Early Neolithic to the Early Bronze Age, this is possibly too superficial a judgement. Admitting that in very localized and rare contexts, regional leadership and striking stratification may have arisen, (but indeed only for a limited period), the overwhelming picture for Europe as a whole exhibits merely small-scale distinctions, reconcilable with communities autonomous on a village/hamlet level, and in which status generally accrued with age, according to sex, and to those prominent in community leadership (headman, 'big men', clan elders, war-party leaders, small-scale chiefs). Occasional instances of higher status female burials may indicate inherited or ascribed rank and reflect a greater degree of social complexity. The total set of archaeological indicators for inegalitarian ranking does indeed exhibit variable expression over time and space, but this may be widely accounted for in terms of the density and stability of population and fluctuating success in achieving highly productive subsistence farming and ecological adaptation. The fluctuations in exchange networks for prestige or functional items seem at present to be less valuable in accounting for (as opposed to symbolizing) such status distinctions. Looking forward, from the Neolithic, the overall development of European society in the Copper Age and Bronze Age appears to be merely a continuation of the trends isolated in the Neolithic (and even perhaps incipient in the Palaeolithic-Mesolithic). The predominance of autonomous local groups, small in size,[65] with ranking and small scale stratification, though

now general and more emphasized than the Neolithic, probably reflects similar factors of demography and subsistence adaptation, and the continued limited significance of inter-community exchange to status-creation.

Again, sporadic in time and place, but more common than in Neolithic times, are signs of more developed stratification, almost entirely on the inferences obtained from burial differentiation. However, the regional scale of the latter statuses is not generally greater than similar phenomena of the Neolithic, and generally represents an evanescent florescence.[66] A unique exception to this recurrent picture in Europe is formed by the rise of palace civilization in Minoan and Mycenaean Greece.[67]

The sporadic differentiation of corporate groups, becomes general, as we move from Mesolithic to Neolithic times, as a partial result of the greater identification with more high yielding and localized resources, and the role of personal leadership and individual status emerges increasingly in density-dependent disputes, warfare and more peaceful communal group-enhancing activities.[68] In the Metal Ages the rare appearance in the Neolithic of marked stratification, also becomes more general yet far from customary or universal, but lower-level ranking and stratification now become commonplace. If any overall limiting factor is major here in inhibiting civilizational or state-society takeoff, it may perhaps be sought in the inadequately controlled growth of regional populations and recurrent failure to conserve subsistence resources. This instability hindered settlement continuity. It also hindered the emergence and long-term maintenance of dense nucleations of population and long-lived regional centres of leadership, servicing and general administration, and may be responsible for the overwhelming predominance of village-hamlet settlement and the implied relative or absolute autonomy of such small units from the Neolithic until Iron Age times. It is also possible that the associated stress favoured a greater emphasis on the rank of headman, clan elder, or temporary 'big-man': such a person might successfully steer the community economy, encourage and safeguard the flow of raw materials and socially valuable imports from considerable distances via neighbouring and potentially hostile communities, and engage supernatural forces in mutually-benefitting interactions for the safeguarding and advancement of public welfare. From the mature period of the Neolithic, defended refuge sites and settlement fortifications became a regular feature of the archaeological record, occasionally revealing evidence for attack and fatalities. Competition for limited and fluctuating resources is probably the source of this recurrent phenonomen.

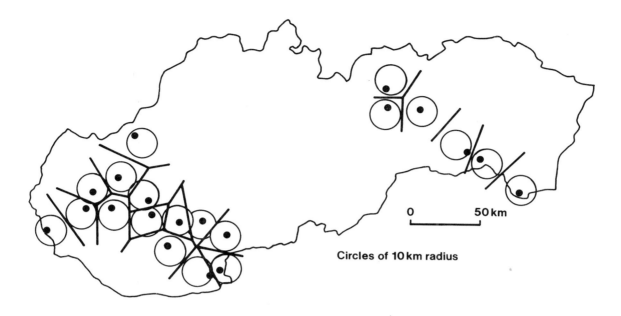

Fig. 1

Territorial analysis of 'central places' in the Early Bronze Age of Slovakia. Fortified centres of the MADAROVCE (west group) and OTOMANI (east group) cultures. After Vladar 1973 (Slov. Arch. 21)

NOTES

Note 1
For a discussion of these processes and interactions, see Ammerman and Cavalli-Sforza (1973), Modderman (1976), Chapman (1976) and Alexander (1978). N.B. In this paper, dates 'bc' are uncalibrated C14 years, 'BC' are calendar years.

Note 2
As recently argued by Lewthwaite (1981) and Phillips and Moore (1981).

Note 3
The overall trend to increasingly denser population from settlement, cemetery and other activity traces has been supported by a wide series of regional and inter-regional studies. Typical for different levels of investigation are Lies (1974), Modderman (1976), and Pavuk (1976). While indicating a higher overall population for Neolithic Britain in the later as opposed to the earlier Neolithic, Whittle has made a convincing case for superimposed major peaks and troughs on such a 'smoothed' trend, an important observation to which we shall return (Whittle, 1978).

Note 4
The relative dominance of funerary evidence over settlement data in European prehistory places an uncomfortable burden on 'social archaeology', namely the necessary defence of the proposition that variations in mortuary behaviour will reflect the complexity of the social structure (especially status distinctions) existing in the associated living community. The arguments in this debate have been frequently rehearsed (cf. Ucko 1969, Binford 1971, Saxe 1970, Tainter 1978, Van de Velde 1979; Chapman, Kinnes and Randsborg 1981), both from ethnography and archaeological case-studies. Present evidence suggests that the proposition is indeed a reasonable assumption or working hypothesis, but although more

likely to be true than not, it is certainly not infallible. In particular, whilst a culture with an elaboration of mortuary variability offers practical scope for confirmatory analysis of the significance of such behaviour, those cultures with undifferentiated mortuary symbolism or even a cultural prohibition on permanent mortuary signalling can include both relatively undifferentiated and highly differentiated societies (cf. Harding, this volume, and the writer's paper on the Iron Age, this volume). The contributors to this present volume, apart perhaps from a traditionally sceptical anthropologist, share this viewpoint.

Note 5
For the ethnographic background to these generalized expectations for Neolithic societies, see Sahlins (1963, 1968), Lewis (1968), and Service (1971). A distinction proposed by Fried (1967) will be found useful in this chapter, that between 'ranked' and 'stratified' societies. In the former case, society is basically egalitarian; certain individuals may be entitled to limited authority due to seniority in years and in the kinship network, or in terms of a specialized role (due to personal talent in war or religion). In addition, individuals may achieve higher status in their lifetimes due to personal economic or social success ('big men', cf. Sahlins) - it is assumed that this is not normally an inherited (ascribed) status. In **stratified** societies, however, there is an institutionalized hierarchy of elite/commoner type, where status accrues to those belonging to particular familial networks on an ascribed basis e.g. chiefs. Although achievement in economic production, community leadership, war and social success (e.g. marriage ties) may be important to the real authority and effectiveness of power of this elite group, membership of this class need not rest on such aspects but rather on the inheritance of status and privilege. In the light of the ambiguous nature of

Service's apostasy concerning 'tribes' and 'chiefdoms' (cf. Cliff Slaughter, this volume, and Introduction) we shall continue to credit him with interest in such socio-political arrangements as potential developmental stages.

Although the denser Neolithic populations in more confined areas seem to call for a social model distinct from the hunter-gatherer band, the degree of interaction between Neolithic settlement units is highly variable over time and space. It would not be difficult to conceive of tribe-like configurations for the European Neolithic if we were able to accept Childe's definition of the archaeological 'culture' (1950 p.2): "A culture is defined as an assemblage of artefacts that recur repeatedly associated together in dwellings of the same kind and with burials by the same rite. The arbitrary peculiarities of implements, ornaments, houses, burial rites and ritual objects are assumed to be the concrete expressions of the common social tradition that binds together a people". Indeed we do still treat the era in terms of Childean 'golf-balls', but the degree and kinds of social interaction that can have existed, say, within the giant Linear Pottery Culture were clearly quite distinct from those conceivable for the distinctive Breton Early Neolithic. Such taxonomic confusions were decisively exposed in Clarke's Analytical Archaeology (1968), which showed convincingly that once the different levels of human interaction within prehistoric Europe were clearly categorized, regional concentrations of internalized interaction could be discerned, offering real potential for comparison with ethnographic 'tribes'. Regrettably since the premature death of this great scholar, little progress has been made in applying his techniques of taxonomic differentiation, although most prehistorians continue to work with implicit or explicit 'tribal' groupings for the Neolithic on the basis of selected cultural norms (cf. for example the discussion by Milisauskas of this issue, 1978 p.42 ff).

The apparent neglect of 'tribes' in recent social archaeology in Europe relates partly to the real taxonomic abuses exposed by Clarke, partly to a general critique of the 'normative' culture model adopted by Clarke (cf. Norwegian Archaeological Review, 1970), but more importantly to the great emphasis placed instead upon role differentiation within regional societies ('big men', chiefs) as opposed to the question of the socio-political implications of 'ethnicity' on a tribal scale. Raymond Newell's modelling of social boundary evolution (this volume) from Mesolithic into Neolithic times provides a major new initiative to advance our understanding of the problem. In a recent paper, Braun and Plog (1982) have revived the 'tribal' concept, introducing a model in which demographic pressure and/or declining ecological resources could stimulate such a social formation as an organizational reaction to inter-group competition.

Note 6
For the beginnings of such a development during the latter part of the last glacial in Europe, cf. Gamble (1980).

Note 7
For increasingly dense Mesolithic populations over time throughout Europe, especially by the Late Mesolithic period, cf. Newell (1973; this volume), Clarke (1976), Meiklejohn (1978), Jacobi (1978), Whittle (1980), Bradley (1978), Barrett et al. (1981), Lewthwaite (1981) and Nemeskeri (1976). The trend in research on the typical Late Mesolithic coastal shell-middens, towards evaluating them as population-stress food rather than a healthy broad-spectrum staple (Bailey 1978), is significant in this respect. Others, however (Zvelebil, pers. comm.) see the Late Mesolithic emphasis on fish and shellfish as providing secure sustenance for the otherwise lean months of the year, and thereby allowing populations to expand to new heights by lakes and coasts (with concomitant stimulus to socio-political differentiation).

Note 8
Chapman develops his theory of formal cemeteries from the ethnographic observations of Meillassoux (1972). The latter contrasts the generally open group membership and flexible territorial relationships of hunter-gatherers, with the fixed residential groups and territorial obsessiveness (based on localized labour investment) of fixed-plot agriculturalists. The role of descent and of ancestor cults becomes a key one and is manifested in increasing concern for formal burial points as signals and reinforcements of the rights of the corporate group over confined and thereby defined localized resources (Saxe 1970). Hayden and Cannon (1982) have recently provided further support for Chapman's thesis: "it would appear that the emergence of corporate groups denotes a moderate to highly competitive environment for restricted essential or highly desired resources" (p.151).

A corollary of such a theory would be that unusual hunter-gatherer societies with a highly productive but very localized resource base might similarly evolve comparable social and ritual behaviour to that commonly found with fixed-plot agriculturalists (King 1978, Chapman 1981a). This point illustrates a general principle argued in the present paper, that the case being made for an evolutionary succession through various 'stages' in prehistoric European communities, rests upon what is believed to be the 'mode' of eco-social development for a particular era. It is suggested that the specific processes conditioning or favouring that mode may indeed operate in earlier and later eras, but irregularly in comparison to an alternative eco-social nexus which creates another 'mode'. In other words, a hunter-gatherer 'state', were one to be evidenced archaeologically, could be successfully accommodated within such an evolutionary theory, provided that it arose from a unique human ecology that had led to a 'mimicry' of the eco-social mode characteristic for highly complex agricultural systems.

Note 9
For the Lepenski Vir culture, cf. Srejović (1972), Boroneant (1970, 1973), J. Kozłowski (1973), Nemeskéri (1976) and Nandris (1977, 1978).

Note 10
This interpretation of developmental processes is the basis of the writer's analysis of European prehistory in this volume, although I am aware of its highly generalized nature that poses about as many questions as it seeks to resolve. An almost identical approach is adopted by Pat Phillips, as the following quotation reveals: "It seems likely that the larger populations of the Late Neolithic permitted more specialisation, that their density forced more complexity of social structure, and these complexities fuelled the demand for high-value goods to indicate their status. These goods might acquire value because of their rarity, or because of the length of time they took in manufacture" (1980, p.187).

Note 11
A number of 'core-land potential' studies exist for prehistoric Europe, such as the correlation obtained between tell-height and associated catchment potential in Bulgaria (Dennell and Webley 1975), between larger and more long-lived sites and exceptional arable productivity in the north western Balkans (Chapman 1981), and between the degree of settlement complexity and the fertility of associated 'Siedlungskammern' in Bronze Age Greece (Bintliff 1977a, vol. 2, appx. A). An obvious American parallel is the analysis of the ecology of the Moundville complex (Pebbles and Kus, 1977). Wider implications of the concept are discussed in Bintliff (1981).

Note 12
Characteristic FTN burials and those in the Early Aegean Neolithic are loosely dispersed within the settled area, lacking grave structures and with little or no gifts (Nandris 1970, Pavuk 1972, Comsa 1974a).

Note 13
At first sight, it is difficult to see why the LBK settlement pattern should be more conducive to land-population stress than that of the FTN, if we follow the Chapman thesis. But if we can generalize from detailed local studies of the probable land use for the two groups, it might be argued that in the FTN, exploitation was commonly carried out radially from a settlement located centrally to a large 'cell' of fertile land (Dennell and Webley 1975), whereas in the LBK, settlement was tied to a relatively narrow band of a particular quality of loess beside the smaller variety of regional stream systems (Kuper and Lüning 1975). It is conceivable that, although LBK communities are believed to have subsequently expanded into much more varied terrain, the seemingly 'confined economy' of the Early Neolithic may have created conditions of 'environmental circumscription' (Carneiro, 1970) favouring a new emphasis on the corporate group and the ancestral (burial) ties to particular strips of land (cf. for example, Bintliff, 1977a pt. 2, ch. 8; 1977b). LBK settlements throughout Europe concentrate on terrace land between the plateaux and river valley bottoms.

In contrast to traditional emphasis on the light, easily worked loess of this topography, J. Kruk (1980) and following him Sherratt (1981) and Howell (1982, 1983) believe that the agricultural economy was fundamentally one of fixed plot 'gardens' in the alluvial bottomlands themselves. A number of arguments make this reconstruction improbable. Firstly, there is growing evidence that the broad blanket of light alluvium over temperate European floodplains is proto-historic and historic in age, covering a far less hospitable mosaic of peat, sands and gravels. Secondly, an emphasis on root crops as opposed to the major cereals lacks any tangible support, and the well-evidenced significant cultivation of the tangible cereal crops such as wheat demand a well-drained environment above seasonal floods (as Howell (1983, p.134) concedes). A more feasible model would be to interpret the characteristic location of LBK sites as controlling freshwater supplies for men and herds, prime dry-farmed loess of the middle topography, excellent concentrated intensive grazing in the valley bottom lands and secondary extensive woodland grazing on the plateau above the site. Such a model fits very neatly for example to the pollen evidence from Villeneuve in the Aisne valley; the immediate alluvial environment below the site seems to be reflected in the dominance of pasture indicators, whilst cereal fields would have been higher upslope (Constantin et al. 1982). Howell's (1982, 1983) argument that valley-bottom cultivation in the French LBK was forced upon the local LBK settlers since the loesslands and rendzinas above this were 'unworkable' rests on an inappropriate transference of Kruk's model (based on the dry continental climate of Poland and its effect on interfluve soils) to the decidedly maritime climate of northern France. The recent analysis by Bakels (1978) of Dutch LBK human ecology also contradicts Kruk and places fields on the dry-farmed loess exposures well above the rivers.

Note 14
Childe considered the European Neolithic as characterized by relative 'self-sufficiency' and a lack of specialization, typical for a form of 'lower barbarism' as opposed to the 'higher barbarism' (nineteenth-century concepts) of the Bronze Age, when long distance dependence on mines and merchants enters the socio-economic system and transforms it. To some extent, Colin Renfrew's model for the development, or take-off, of the Aegean Bronze Age civilization (1972) envisages a major role for metal tools and prestige pieces that relied on inter-regional exchanges. Andrew Sherratt (1976) points out that although an inner core of communities could visit the source of good flint, obsidian or metal ore, most settlements on which such material occurs, (often in very considerable quantities and as a staple tool or common ornament), in prehistoric Europe during the Neolithic, Copper and Bronze Ages, must have relied on a regular and intricate network of raw material exchanges. Polish flint studies show that settlements closer to the mines contain finished tools and very plentiful debitage, whereas those further out in the distribution network have limited debitage to proportion of tools (Milisauskas 1978, p.150). Michelsberg Culture flint mines such as at Spiennes in Belgium show domestic debris betraying the activity of local, not distant communities, who are also demonstrated to be practising a balanced mixed farming/mining life in the region (Louwe Kooijmans 1976, pp.249-50). More recently (cf. this volume), Sherratt has suggested that control over such sources, in the case of copper, or the exchange routes radiating from them, might account for isolated nodes of 'prestige burials'. But to reverse his own earlier (1976) argument, one might reasonably expect a similar development from Early Neolithic times, given the great reliance of most communities investigated hitherto on exchanged items or materials. It is noteworthy that in Poland, where detailed study has been made of the widespread and vigorous mining and exchange of varieties of high quality flint (Tabaczynski 1972, Schild 1976) during the Neolithic, settlements believed to have been those especially concerned with the extraction process are still located on the nearest good agricultural land rather than at the mine site itself (as with the Michelsberg case, cited above). Sherratt has argued from ethnographic parallels that remote communities can share in the flow from such mining groups via participation in 'kula ring' networks cycling functional and symbolic or prestigious items, despite lacking an equivalent practical resource. Such exchange systems can operate successfully over large distances without the services of 'chiefs' and without giving rise to core-periphery dependency relations (1976). The mode of exchange would be a chain of short-step exchanges between adjacent communities, producing a distinct distance decay plot in quantity available from the source point, characterized as 'down-the-line' exchange (Renfrew 1975, 1977; for European Neolithic examples cf. Milisauskas 1978).

Note 15
Engels (1884) developed the Morgan matriarchy/patriarchy contrast and its evolutionary significance, and has been followed by a continuous succession of East European scholars to this day (Behrens, Häusler, Otto, Klejn). However, it is reassuring to find that some of their colleagues in the East can attack this totally spurious orthodoxy, particularly as regards the evidence of burials (Pavuk 1972), and the significance of 'fertility' figurines (Kaufmann 1976), as well as the general contradiction from modern ethnographic research (Pavuk 1972). It is of course a very different matter to consider whether Early Neolithic societies were matrilocal, patrilocal or bilocal. Although Western scholars have traditionally avoided confronting the Marxists on their own ground (though cf. Kurth and Röhrer-Ertl 1977), Piggott and Clark (1965) going no further than suggesting 'extended families' for the LBK social structure, pioneer attempts are being made, influenced by American research, to identify residential patterning and infer kinship rules (Van de Velde 1979, Sherratt this volume). But it must be borne in mind that the ethnographic record merely shows a **tendency** for matrilineal and matrilocal patterns to reflect the importance of female labour in the food quest. In the generally low role assigned to hunting and stock rearing in the

European Early Neolithic economy we must surely assume that male participation in the central task of hoe agriculture was at least equal to female.

Note 16
We now possess a growing number of thorough regional and micro-regional studies providing information on the density and locational preferences of LBK settlement. They all demonstrate the remarkable density of sites, generally within walking distance and inter-visible. But these close concentrations of settlement units cluster in discrete micro-regions defined by fairly clear soil, rainfall and humidity parameters (though including access to more varied micro-environments beyond the key arable land, for grazing and gathering activities). (Leciejewiczowa 1970, Sielmann 1971, 1972, 1976, Lies 1974, Mania and Preuss 1975, Kuper and Lüning 1975, Kooijmans 1976a, b, Pavuk 1976, Linke 1976, Kaufmann 1976, Van de Velde 1979, Kosse 1979, Kruk 1980, Howell 1983).

Note 17
In particular, a team of 12 men would be needed for setting the beams, although in general Startin (1978) considers a long house rather a daunting task for the single family who may have occupied it. The essential requirements of local population dynamics and gene pool health, however (Wobst 1974), would suggest that a number of contiguous hamlets would be tied by inter-marriage and social obligations, and it is possible that such loose communities were co-operating together on the small defensive enclosures that are now becoming a feature of the late phase of the LBK.

Note 18
The interpretation by the Aldenhoven team is presented as a working hypothesis, or model, for LBK settlement patterns, rather than a definitive statement from their study area (Kuper et al. 1974, Kuper and Lüning 1975, Lüning 1976a, Kuper et al. 1977). The larger settlements examined do indeed seem to contain pottery from all the main development phases of the Rhineland LBK, and this observation recurs at other larger sites elsewhere in the LBK distribution (Lies 1974, Kaufmann 1976, Leciejewiczowa 1970, Kruk 1980, Hamond 1981). In each phase, in the Aldenhoven area, a number of houses were in use in particular loci of each settlement, either to be replaced in the same loci or alternative loci in the next phase. Elsewhere the phasing of houseplans suggests rather a gradual drift of new houses from one zone of the site to another (Modderman 1971, Müller-Karpe 1968).

However, the pottery phases distinguished are on too long a timescale to mesh with the suspected lifespan of an LBK longhouse, 25-30 years. Presence of a group of people at site A, during a pottery style phase whose duration covers several house-lives, can neither prove nor disprove the opposing theories: of permanent residence at the site or cyclic occupation between site A and one or more near neighbours where pottery of the same phase is represented (cf. Czerniak and Piontek 1980). Further evidence from Poland does suggest that LBK settlers might operate long and short-term settlement systems (Bogucki 1979). Attempts by the Aldenhoven team to resolve this issue by computer seriation, wherein style evolution discontinuities might be revealed or disproved, yielded contradictory results. In fact the underlying theory of such an analysis is open to criticism as it makes the unwarranted assumption that each small district of the LBK should evolve its own smooth transformation series of styles, rather than being influenced at discontinuous points by the cultural diffusion of stylistic innovations from other LBK regions.

There is indeed some special pleading for low numbers of contemporary houses in the Aldenhoven settlements, probably to accommodate a necessary equation between the long life of regional LBK occupation (500 C14 years, more in calendar years), the short life of each LBK house, and the number of houses reconstructed for the area in total. The upper range of the estimates of contemporary houses, if generalized over the five settlements, might well create a credibility gap for the argument of absolute continuity in each site, as there do not seem to be enough house remains. It is indeed noteworthy that on other sites the average number of contemporary houses is generally larger than the low figure preferred for Aldenhoven, e.g. 5-15 at Elsloo (Modderman 1975), 7-8 at Olszanica (Milisauskas 1976) (cf. also Pavlu 1977). Furthermore it is noteworthy that at Langweiler 9 in the Merzbach valley, the phase of construction of the late LBK ringwork defence is contemporary to a final domestic use of the settlement site, despite abandonment of all house structures there; perhaps the suggestion of some kind of usage from another settlement site, that one might raise here, could also apply to earlier periods where such settlement shifts are obscured by later reoccupation and the coarse-meshed typology.

If this discussion leaves open the degree to which these closely-spaced sites represent genuine contemporaneous hamlets, suggesting that the Aldenhoven population range may be merely the upper limits of theoretical population, one is still in agreement that even if only half the known LBK sites per 'phase' **were** coexistent, the LBK population was still remarkably dense within its chosen environmental niche throughout Central and North Western Europe. Two obvious cautionary points naturally arise: firstly, whether such a concentration of people and exploitation in narrow strips of land was viable over millennia, given the problems of soil fertility maintenance in primitive agricultural conditions. Significantly, careful analysis of the macroflora from German and Dutch LBK sites suggests small cultivated fields associated with each site, surrounded by woods or hedges as 'infields' (Bakels 1979). Secondly, we must remind ourselves that the LBK deliberately selected the finest soils for hoe-agriculture, neglecting the sandier, clayier, more mountainous, drier or wetter landscapes that made up the greater part of the overall landsurface in continental Europe. Taken as a pioneer settlement of Central and North Western Europe as a whole, then, LBK densities are certainly low in comparison to later prehistoric periods, and as we shall see, it is unlikely that the LBK 'Least Effort' selectivity, though strikingly successful for 1000 years or so, could prevent a cumulative negative feedback on the soils thus exhaustively relied on. Indeed, if we accept the evidence for a significant movement of farmer-pioneers from the Near East into the Balkans, to act as a catalyst among local Mesolithic communities, we can hardly expect that the Near East had by the seventh millennium bc been filled 'to the brim' with expanding farming populations. Rather, we would likewise have to argue that early Neolithic settlement in the Near East was highly selective, and that the filling-up of the most desirable land led to continual expansion into new regions, leaving much of the landscape under-used or not used at all by Neolithic exploitation.

Note 19
Meyer-Christlein 1976, Lüning 1976a, Startin 1978, Van de Velde 1979.

Note 20
The role of these often exceptionally well-built, generally larger long houses is widely debated (Modderman 1970, 1975, Müller-Karpe 1968, Van de Velde 1979), but in the absence of preserved floor levels and their artifactual contents, their function is still obscure. It has been noted as significant that the walls are far stronger than ordinary domestic long houses. In borrowing the strengthening

technique applied to the proposed 'cattle stalls' sector of the long house some scholars have been led to the 'giant cattle shed' theory. However, the evidence for the customary domestic and storage subdivisions but on a much larger scale seems more appropriate for a privileged homestead, the residence perhaps of a district 'big man', chief or priest (Modderman 1975; cf. Milisauskas 1976). This function might not conflict with the view that the wall strengthening was intended to cope with communal gatherings.

Note 21
A recently published example from a site in the LBK long house tradition, though dating from the subsequent period, deploying the American 'household cluster' approach, is that of Bogucki (1981) for the Lengyel period Polish site of Brzesc Kujawski.

Note 22
Ihmig 1971, Tabaczynski 1972, Kooijmans 1976a, Kuper et al. 1977, Modderman 1976, Kaufmann 1977.

Note 23
See also note 13. Chapman (1981a) toys with the idea that known LBK cemeteries, which tend to be late LBK, reflect population rise and an intensification of land possessiveness paralleled by the LBK late fortifications. However, this hardly explains the numerous examples of formal cemeteries of early LBK date, and for the latter at least one might perhaps consider a localized 'environmental circumscription' model (cf. Note 13). In addition, the rise in gifts with the dead, in LBK compared to FTN burials, may also reflect a change towards more emphasis on social symbolism.

Note 24
About one quarter of the adult males at Nitra have no gifts, and around one third have the status hardstone celts (axes), usually with imported spondylus ornaments as well. This suggests a degree of 'ranking' within the class of adult males. Given the suggested life of the cemetery, 2-300 years, the estimated buried population might have been contributed by a community of three to five families (cf. Bintliff 1978). Per generation, therefore, we might be seeing a single 'big man' or lineage head for such a smallish group. If the clusters of graves represent separate phases (disregarding the debate about fixed base or cyclical agriculture in the area), they might represent the communal dead of one generation for such a social group (though with some age categories poorly represented and presumably buried elsewhere, such as very young infants).

It is curious that this possibility of ranking is absent in otherwise careful discussions of Neolithic social archaeology, such as that of Tabaczynski (1972). Moreover, when we consider occasional examples of supposed status accumulation in child or female burials e.g. at Rixheim (Gallay and Schweitzer 1971), it could be suggested that 'big man' ranking was creating 'reflected status' for close kin of the 'big man'. Pauli however, has warned us that sentimental factors commonly distort gift behaviour with infant burial.

Note 25
When typology alone and 'commonsense' inferences are employed to distinguish age and sex, as here, there is scope for re-interpretation, as the reviewers of Van de Velde's paper confirm (printed with his paper). His case that virtually all giftless graves are female is not borne out in other LBK cemeteries, nor his removal of a major contribution to the cemetery from children's burial. With 12 or so male 'big men' and a notable number claimed of 'reflected wealth' females, over four generations, we would have merely three individuals of top 'rank' in Modderman's community of 65-100 persons. But then, as

Modderman has earlier pointed out (1975), the burials with more than minimal or no gifts form a graduated scale to the 'richest', and the latter are never outstandingly prolific. In this context it is therefore helpful to introduce the Fried (1967) distinction between societies that are basically egalitarian, but contain a regular number of individuals with achieved status not normally formalized or inheritable (ranked), and, inegalitarian societies, in which ascribed status defines a distinct stratum of privileged kin (stratified).

Note 26
Early farming communities can be documented from the sixth millennium bc in Iberia, and during the succeeding 3000 years the archaeological record demonstrates a general trend to denser and more complex settlement, associated in many regions with megalithic tombs (symptoms of dense, well-organized societies tied to fertile land?). Increasingly in these communities the signs of status differentiation in terms of ranking become evident, until in several core regions by the first half of the third millennium bc we observe the crystallization out of a settlement hierarchy matched by notable burial stratification (Chapman 1977, 1981b, Gilman 1976, 1981, Arribas 1976, Savory 1968, Renfrew 1973a).

Note 27
Air photographs and surface survey reveal a density of Earlier Neolithic settlement in restricted lowland areas of southern Italy that is directly comparable to that of the LBK in Central Europe (Jarman and Webley 1975, Trump 1980, Tiné 1975, Delano-Smith 1979, Ammerman and Shaffer 1981). Although knowledge of domestic animals and plants was disseminated from the seventh millennium bc into the West Mediterranean coastlands, there is a hitherto unexplained period of very limited adoption of the full Neolithic economy - lasting up to 2000 years in some areas, before a striking take-off in settled village farming throughout the area during the fifth millennium bc (cf. note 2). Amongst the better explored regions where a dense network of hamlets and villages emerges at this time (such as south eastern Spain, southern Portugal, Provence), the expansion and contraction of the south Italian Earlier Neolithic deserves special attention. Around 1000 settlements are recorded from a limited part of the region, whilst recent survey in the Amendola area suggests a potential overall total four times that density (Whitehouse, 1981). On excavation they are generally found to be highly organized communities betraying significant community co-operation. At the giant village of Passo di Corvo, for example, it is estimated that the great ditch systems would have involved the removal of 100,000 cubic metres of rock with primitive tools, and, notably, nine tenths of the ditch systems served the village as a communal facility, only one tenth being associated with the individual 'farmsteads' (Tiné 1975). Whether these great ditches were truly defensive, or part of a water control system, they reveal the kind of social co-operation that is often linked to a chieftain society (Renfrew 1973a, b). Hitherto our knowledge of this culture is inadequate to verify a ranked or stratified base to these dense communities, with their co-operative and adaptive achievements in an exceedingly 'brittle' environment of rich, light soils but low and unpredictably fluctuating rainfall. But it is conceivable that the long survival of this tradition in these special environments witnessed enhanced social and craft differentiation. Recent analysis of village plans, primarily derived from air photographs, has isolated a number of unusually large household enclosures within these settlements which might represent the establishments of community leaders (B. Jones 1983).

However, as with the almost exactly contemporary expansion, long florescence and contraction of the temperate

European LBK of the fifth millennium bc, so the south Italian Earlier Neolithic appears to succumb to a widespread 'catastrophe' in which its core settled areas are almost entirely abandoned for a significant period of time, whilst their later re-occupation is at a far more confined and environmentally-sensitive level, at least until early historic times. Whitehouse has recently commented (1981, pp.163-164): "post-neolithic sites are extremely scarce ... The Tavoliere has a clear break in pattern in the later part of the Neolithic and was very sparsely occupied thereafter ... during the whole Bronze Age". The well-established climatic marginality of the region matched with such intensive exploitation under a primitive technology makes such a sequence or agricultural cycle a matter of no great surprise, and indeed recent research points to an agro-climatic crisis behind the radical settlement disjunction marking the collapse of the core areas (Winn and Shimbaku 1980).

Note 28

The data from all over continental Europe provide a very consistent picture of a dramatic process of adaptive change in Neolithic settlement patterns during the later Early Neolithic (second half of the fifth millennium bc) and by the beginning of the Middle Neolithic (by 4000 bc in both East and West, but with the West European MN soon running parallel to the Copper Age in the East through the mature and late fourth millennium bc). For the general population explosion off the loess and other early favoured soils into more varied soils, often poorer, or into moorland, waterlogged environments and onto uplands, cf. Tabaczynski (1972), Alexander (1978), Tringham (1978). A general tendency to broaden the economy with greater attention to hunting and gathering, or to locally native domesticates such as cattle and pig, is indicated by Milisauskas (1978).

For a more detailed presentation for Eastern Europe, in which it is suggested that population in early settled micro-environments expanded into new niches as listed above, cf. Lichardus (1974), Tringham (1980a,b,), Pavuk (1976), Sterud (1976), Sherratt (1976, 1982a, 1983) and J. Chapman (1981). An early development, or adoption, here, of the ox-drawn ard and dairy products may be highly relevant to the flourishing fourth-millennium societies of Eastern Europe (Ghetie and Mateesco 1977, Sherratt 1981, and especially J. Chapman 1981 pp.92, 115). In Central Europe, a number of detailed regional studies allow the changes to be analysed in detail. By late LBK times, a drop in site numbers seems to be matched by their retraction to a limited number of very fertile locations and the abandonment of large areas of formerly-settled loess. Arguably the remainder of the population is now to be found migrated into zones of the loess formerly not favoured due to their dry or waterlogged nature, or into new, non-loess locations (although local Mesolithic acculturation and integration with expanding Neolithic offshoots has to be a major additional element in the new, broader MN settlement picture) (cf. Leciejewiczowa 1970, Linke 1976, Kaufmann 1976, Sielmann 1976, Lies 1974, Mania and Preuss 1975, Kaufmann 1975, Kruk 1980). In Western Europe the same picture emerges of relocation within the loesslands into prime locations or poorer, hitherto unsettled loess zones, and of a particularly dramatic explosion of Neolithic settlement off the loess into more varied and generally more adaptively demanding terrain, involving more specialization in crops, animals, more hunting and gathering (cf. in general Sielmann 1971, Whittle 1977a). Most interest attaches to the tremendous expansion off the loess in France, Belgium and Holland, involving in the latter two countries virtual disappearance of settlement in the old LBK loesslands, and from which it is now possible to provide an appropriate demographic, ecological and cultural background to the almost contemporary Neolithic colonization of the British Isles (Bailloud 1974, Guilaine 1976, Kinnes 1982, Kooijmans 1976a, b, Van de Velde 1979, Moddermann 1976). The settlement of the Swiss lakesides and inter-lacustrine plains provides another case study of rapid adaptation to regional environments by incoming farmers of LBK tradition, merging with dense local Mesolithic communities to form a highly distinctive cultural and economic mosaic (Sauter 1976, Strahm 1977, Sakellaridis 1979). In the Rhineland, the detailed Aldenhoven Plateau Project reveals the familiar picture of contraction of settlement in the sectors of loess long occupied, coupled with relocations into less favourable loess and off the loess into lowland and upland habitats (Kuper and Lüning 1975). Environmental evidence suggests a progressive deterioration of the loess soils from the Neolithic clearance onwards, although the most violently erosive phase seems to be Iron Age and Roman era in date (Schalich 1973, 1977, Knörzer 1979). The decline of loessic soils in Eastern Europe is noticeable by the Bronze Age, often explicitly linked to human overuse (Kruk 1980, Kosse 1979). Resettlement of the European loess in later periods, despite its gradual decline, forms part of a pattern of intensification and contraction cycles for this rich but easily overworked soil, stretching up to the present day, with close parallels to the same cycles on the English chalklands. Easy to work, and very rich-yielding after a long fallow recovery, both environments can deteriorate rapidly from erosion and leaching, inadequate or lack of manuring or other fertilizers.

Finally, another great expansion zone for Neolithic settlement, once more with a clear LBK cultural inheritance but involving a considerable degree of integration with dense local Mesolithic peoples, occupies the great expanse of the North European Plain from north Germany across into Poland, then into the Ukraine, and further to the north the southern zone of Scandinavia amenable to the flourishing of the mixed farming economy. For the most part, the pioneer farming communities of the area belong to the TRB (Trichterbecherkultur = Funnel Beaker Culture), although other MN groups are represented (Piggott 1965, Tringham 1971, Lüning 1976b, Milisauskas 1978.) (But for an almost exclusive Mesolithic acculturation model for the TRB, cf. Kowalczyk 1970 and Madsen 1979).

Note 29

But see Newell (this volume) for a model of Mesolithic societies adopting the new lifestyle under no great stress and somewhat leisurely. Yet it is likely that in certain regions the integration of the two lifestyles, and arguably the two populations, occurred around the peak of the late Mesolithic florescence and at the crucial disjunction point (note 28) of Neolithic settlement and economy, e.g. in the Low Countries, the North European Plain and Scandinavia, perhaps also in Brittany and Portugal, and possibly in Eastern Europe if we can use the Lepenski Vir culture as a model (cf. Kooijmans 1976a, b, Gabriel 1976, Modderman 1976, Lüning 1976b, Schwabedissen 1979, Brinch Petersen 1973, Case 1976, Renfrew 1976, Chapman 1981a, Kinnes 1982, Nandris 1977 and 1978). And once such 'Mischkulturen' arise within the context of the expanding Neolithic lifestyle, evidence of late Mesolithic settlement and economy rapidly dwindles and dies.

An important discovery of recent years has been a new cultural group lying between and contemporary to the Linear Pottery settlement zones of the Lower Rhine and north eastern France - the Limbourg-Blicquy group (Moddermann 1982). Although the Dutch sites are in physical environments and with finds that might suggest acculturated Mesolithic groups, the Blicquy group is far closer to the LBK communities in house construction, site location and economy (Farrugia et al. 1982, Constantin et al. 1982). A hybrid population from both indigenous and

LBK sources may be the most appropriate explanation for the 'culture'.

Note 30
In south eastern Italy, as we have seen, cultural florescence and hints of organizational complexity are temporarily truncated by the fourth millennium bc, after the gradual evolution of a network of established village farming communities (which may commence by the sixth millennium bc) culminates in the flourishing of the ditched villages during the fifth millennium bc (supra). In Iberia, likewise, the progressive unfolding of more complex society can be traced as follows: we begin with a gradual sixth- and early fifth-millennium appearance (perhaps by diffusion amongst local Mesolithic populations), of pottery and domestic animals. This is followed by a key transformational phase from the fifth to early third millennium bc, which witnesses the appearance of mixed farming communities and then their expansion and socio-economic elaboration in terms of density, economic efficiency and the increasing effort devoted to mortuary structures (which with the evidence of symbolic, status artifacts may be suggested as indicative of increased communal organization and role differentiation). The culmination is the later fourth-millennium emergence of the prolific 'high culture' of the Iberian Copper Age, with its evidence for stratification of society and of a complex settlement hierarchy (Phillips 1975, Arribas 1976, Gilman 1976, Chapman 1975, Renfrew 1973a, Walker 1981). The expansion of farming settlement into the very arid southeasterly province of Almeria in Spain, the focal zone of the Spanish Copper Age high culture, appears to be relatively late. It may well reflect population pressure from adjacent regions of higher rainfall where dry farming was easier, and hence farming settlement earlier, whilst the peculiar potential of Almeria demanded a combination of farming the light, fertile hill soils (now highly eroded) and a process of adaptation to the more confined bands of valley-bottom land where unpredictable wet-season rainfall run-off offered unusual farming opportunities (cf. note 56, below; Bob Chapman, pers. comm.) The parallels to southern French colonization and putative socio-political elaboration seem noteworthy (cf. infra).

Note 31
Cf. Nandris (1977, 1978). For a similar picture of evolution towards a Copper Age climax in Eastern Europe, involving population rise, micro-environmental diversification, the elaboration of craftwork, the rise of a settlement hierarchy or of regularly spaced 'proto-urban' communities, and the hints of associated organizational hierarchies, cf. Tringham (1978, 1980 a, b,), Renfrew (1973a), Sherratt (1976), J. Chapman (1981), and further, below. The attraction of Nandris's presentation is enhanced by his recent (1976a, unpubl.) application of the ecological r- and K-strategy model (cf. Wilson, 1975). A pioneer colonizing species, entering a new habitat, may find exploitation space for its lifestyle without seeming limit, it therefore makes no major adaptation to its environment by behavioural shifts and goes through a rapid population boom (a generalizing r-strategy). But on approaching, eventually, finite limits to expansion within such a strategy, a behavioural shift may be enforced in which the species diversifies into a set of more specialized extractive activities that are finely attuned to the particular balance and variety of the regional micro-environments (K-strategy). The temporary or permanent resolution of population saturation under the r-strategy by specialization is however, commonly associated with a state of stress, territoriality and increased emphasis on behaviour to regulate group interactions. In the transference to the human situation, we would look for the observed gross changes in the economy, and greater emphasis on warfare and individual ranking (leadership roles). (For a parallel perspective on human social evolution in the Pacific Islands employing the r-and K-strategy model, cf. Kirch, 1980). Nandris himself underlines the cyclical nature of this bivariate mode of life by presenting the late Mesolithic Lepenski Vir culture of the Danube Gorges as a highly complex, K-strategy, climax to the mosaic of exploitative opportunities posed by the tiered micro-environments of the Gorges, the end-product of some four millennia of population growth and adaptation in the area (cf. also references in note 9). In contrast, the subsequent dominance of the Neolithic lifestyle in the north Balkans witnesses an initial r-strategy resting on the raising of the population ceiling via the enhanced productivity now possible, developing during later Neolithic and Copper Age times into a population-pressure induced K- strategy (cf. note 28).

J. Chapman (1981) stresses in addition the likelihood that an early use of the ard plough was a central factor in the takeoff of the East European Copper Age.

Note 32
The existence or otherwise of permanent ranking, or stratification, in fourth millennium Eastern Europe, is a controversial topic, even more hotly debated as a result of the discovery of the spectacular 'princely graves' within the Varna cemetery. Were we to ignore this site and the ambiguous 'treasures' and 'power symbols' found in very small quantities around the north Balkans in this period (cf. Renfrew 1973a), the combined settlement and cemetery evidence (which is fairly plentiful) presents a picture of large, well-organized communities but possessing little more than the traditional spectrum of statuses - child, male, female, adult male, 'big man' (Pavuk 1972, Comsa 1974 a, Sherratt 1976). In Colin Renfrew's intelligent probing of the data, we seem to sense that all the usual pre-requisites are there for chiefdoms, but the data obstinately refuse to indicate their unambiguous presence (cf. Evans 1978). With Varna they seem to be emerging with such spectacular style, and in such isolation, that most scholars are tempted towards special explanations that remove Varna from the normal processes of social change believed typical for the rest of the north Balkans, in particular by theories of 'special trading' or 'exchange' partnerships with communities in Turkey (Todorova 1978, 1980, Sherratt this volume). Alternative, and to this writer, more plausible interpretations are: a) we may soon recover a whole series of elite burial sites like Varna as archaeological research intensifies, allowing us to develop models of the rise of social strata that account for their appearance in terms of modifications in the internal social structure of the various regions of the north Balkans, especially as regards privileged access to surplus food, labour and raw materials within each region; b) social stratification or less formalized ranking is indeed far more prevalent than we have formerly accepted, but is generally symbolized in different and less obvious ways than by gold-covered burials (cf. Renfrew 1978). The latter abnormality might be seen as **one** means of emphasizing status individuals, practised by communities with special access to rare prestige materials. In other regions a different set of distinctions might be in operation. Take for example the Hamangia Culture cemeteries at Cernovoda, where in one burial zone some bodies had no gifts, others had a limited number; in another distinct burial zone, all bodies had gifts. Of these 600 or so formal burials, those with gifts showed little obvious internal ranking, although only a minority possessed the famous marble figurines. On the other hand, in yet a third subdivision of the burial territory, there is known to be a series of 'bone trenches' containing considerable numbers of human and animal bones, the former component probably numbering hundreds of individuals (Comsa 1974a) A potential is revealed for identifying a range of statuses that may well be at a more elaborate level than

the simple 'Early Neolithic spectrum' itemised earlier. John Chapman, in his study of the Vinca Culture of the north west Balkans (1981) points out that although few data are available for analysis from the cemeteries of this region, the Botos cemetery could be seen as evidencing a ranked society (pp.55, 58).

Note 33

If it is is widely suggested that temporary status had attached itself to 'big men' during the Earlier Neolithic (cf. above), it is often argued that during the Middle Neolithic, and certainly by the Late Neolithic/Copper Age of the later fourth and third millennia bc, genuine inherited rank had arrived amidst continental European Neolithic communities, i.e. a chiefdom society or the recognition by other kin groups of permanent privileges attached to a particular clan. Childe did not feel the need to subdivide Neolithic social evolution along these lines, for to him there had occurred no vital transformation in the mode of production, local agriculture and stone tools still prevailing in earlier as in later Neolithic times; instead it was the advent of the Bronze Age with the new conditions of community dependence on traders, craftsmen and chiefly retailers, that inaugurated the next major phase (cf. Sherratt 1976). A similar view of the quickening effect of the flow of metal and of the application of metal tools to everyday life, as well as its effect in stirring higher local surpluses to obtain such useful and prestigious material, can be found in Colin Renfrew's analysis of the development of the Aegean Early Bronze Age civilization (Renfrew 1972). But with the re-dating of the East European Copper Age (thanks largely to Renfrew's incisive arguments - cf. Renfrew 1969, 1973a) the possibility has opened up for a similar model to be applied to the rise of chieftains or chiefly clans in the context of the spread of copper working and copper exchange; on an east-west cline, this allows the metals' factor scope from the mid fourth millennium in the north Balkans, and the early then late third millennium bc as we move through Central into Western Europe. As we have seen (note 32), 'princely' burials at Varna and less obvious indications of salient ranking elsewhere unite Western scholars employing 'prestige-exchange' explanations for ranking (cf. Sherratt, this volume), with orthodox East European Marxist scholars. The latter invoke the customary model of the breakdown of matriarchal (hoe-agriculture) self-sufficient communities and the ascendance of patriarchal, trade-dependent communities via the rise of chiefly entrepreneurs who control the metal sources, the trade routes and the distribution of raw material and metal products (Todorova 1978). But with the widespread acceptance of the functional inadequacy of copper tools compared to traditional hardstone implements, and the ready comparison that may be made between the mining and distribution of copper and gold, and the remarkable flow of mined flint and hardstone during the earlier Neolithic (cf. Sherratt 1976, Renfrew 1978, and see below, note 53) it is difficult to sustain the transference of the Childe model back into the pre-Bronze Age era.

The alternative Marxist model of 'pastoral capitalism' is easier to reconcile with the undeniable economic transformation that characterizes Europe during the late fifth, and through the fourth millennium bc and beyond; the expansion of communities into landscapes where a far greater emphasis or even a dominance of the stock component may be both predicted and occasionally confirmed (cf. note 28). The new factor of mobile capital is, in this model, the reason for the Middle and Late Neolithic flourishing of fortified sites (to protect the valuable stock), the related elaboration during this era of stone 'battle axes' and the shift from female to male dominance in society (men as herders and protectors, of cattle) (cf. Tabaczynski 1972, and other authorities discussed by him such as Schlette, Neustupny). In actual fact, attachment

to dogma apart, there seems no logical reason why stock control should be divorced from land control, indeed privileged elites relying on such hoofed wealth would need preferential access to equivalent grazing land. There seems also no reason why landed wealth, in terms of cereals should not be equally important in such a postulated situation of scarcity of good land and pressure to carve out a viable set of new exploitation niches in varied and often difficult terrain for mixed farming. The inferred diffusion of ard-traction farming from a possible early centre of use in Copper Age Eastern Europe, into Central and Western Europe during the third millennium or local Late Neolithic (cf. J. Chapman 1981, Sherratt 1981), may be a vital element in increased productivity and related social elaboration.

In any case, it has to be admitted that our technical skills are as yet inadequate to detect clear proof of preferential access to stock or crops by those argued to be chiefs, or of a special clan, from their special treatment at death or other material culture indications.

The literature on 'chiefdoms' is very extensive, and it is too often assumed that such leaders can be squeezed into one overall model. Consider for example Renfrew's long checklist of 'things to look for when hunting chiefs in the archaeological record' (1973b). This is misleading to generalize from, because it reflects the rarer, very complex, chiefdoms in the anthropological literature and further is a portmanteau list culled from various chieftain societies and not necessarily valid for any one in particular. In fact, chiefs can be little more powerful than the Melanesian 'big man' and range from that end of the spectrum to the 'paramounts' with life and death powers over hundreds of thousands of people (Sahlins 1968). It is a vital weakness of European prehistory that outstandingly rich burials (the source of identification of 'chiefs' almost exclusively) are plausibly taken as being beyond the power of a 'big man', and lacking associated evidence for urban or palatial centres, or for bureaucracies, are seen equally reasonably as pre-state; then, however, they suffer the indignity of being alternately raised to the highest as sub-continental emperors or lowered to the depths as little more than petty, district chiefs (contrast e.g. Sherratt's placing of Bronze Age elites in the latter category, this volume, with the writer and Harding close behind him, and Maria Gimbutas's (1965) imaginative picture operating at the former scale of polity). Renfrew's correlation between central places and central people (1979b) is helpful, but only where the former exist, suggesting in themselves regional co-ordination. In later Neolithic Europe and through the Copper and Bronze Ages, elites detected are rarely provided with a clear settlement hierarchy, and this is indeed a reasonable reflection on the limitations to their sphere of operations and the complexity of such chiefdoms; such observations could open the way to an analytical spectrum in that plethora of chieftains bemoaned in this volume by Sherratt and Harding, parallel to the spectrum known from the ethnographic record. This also improves on Service's over-simplistic formulation that the 'chieftain stage' should include "centers which co-ordinate economic, social and religious activities" (1971, p.133).

Note 34

Renfrew 1973a, Tringham 1980a, b, Comsa 1974b, J. Chapman 1976. J. Chapman's important (1981) analysis of the Copper Age Vinca Culture of the north western Balkans identifies a three-tier settlement hierarchy with a small number of giant tells whose surface area and putative population rank more than favourably with small towns of the Aegean and Near Eastern Bronze Age (p.51). These key cultural foci developed in particularly advantageous agricultural situations and, he argues, played a central role for major regions of this extensive Vinca

Culture. Indications of a social elite are linked to a proliferation of exchange goods, prestige items and ceremonial behaviour centred on the larger communities (pp.133-37).

Note 35
As regional surveys of the individual cultural groupings demonstrate; cf., for example, the TRB culture covering much of Northern Europe (Davidsen 1978).

Note 36
In Western Europe, amidst many settlements lacking such a feature, one may mention the community of Aichbühl on Federsee (Tabaczynski 1972, p.42) with a central house. There are also, however, 'giant houses' of LBK derivation, which on analogy might represent local leaders - cf. for example the giant, 85m. long trapezoid at Bochum-Hiltrop (Müller-Karpe 1968, Fig. 234). In the east of Europe, the rise of Danubian 2 groups such as Tripolye has provided several good village plans, two of which have attracted much attention: Vladimirovka, and Kolomishchina. Here we find carefully planned house patterning, with concentric rings of structures around an open space and one or two isolated central houses. Not only have such central structures obtained the understandable label of 'chief's hut', but the additional planned layout has encouraged more detailed social speculation. For Kolomischina, for example, we can even be told that the two central houses are the chief's, then an inner ring of houses form his retinue's accommodation, finally the outer ring of houses represents the free peasantry (this despite the larger dimensions of the outer ring residences and the meagre scope of the inner ring structures for purposes other than a workshop or storage role!) (Tabaczynski 1972). Allowing for the purely hypothetical nature of any indentification of such settlement peculiarities as demonstrating an elite group or family, as opposed to other equally viable models (clubhouse, communal house etc), this state of uncertainty refers primarily to the independent use of settlement data to evince social stratification or ranking. If we accept the case suggested above for Early Neolithic ranking within the LBK tradition, and the continuity accepted between LBK burial and gift traditions and much of the Danubian 2 culture group that evolved from it, we may with more justification enlist the occasional support of settlement data to elaborate on a case for Danubian 2 ranking.

Note 37
In Eastern Europe the proliferation of defended sites, including definite village enclosures, is well-attested from the late fifth millennium to early fourth millennium bc/Danubian 2 phase and the Copper Age of the later fourth millennium, in such cultures as Boian, Cucuteni, Tripolye, Salcutsa, Gumelnitsa (cf. Comsa 1974b). It may be significant that they are particularly common in a mature phase of this eastern tradition, some time after the first burst of settlement expansion. In East-Central Europe, again in a mature phase of Danubian 2 (Lengyel Culture), throughout Czechoslovakia, the expansion and relocation of settlements, often onto poorer soils, leads to the erection of defended enclosures such as Hluboke Masuvky and Nitriansky Hradok. However, some of this series may have fulfilled a wider role: at Tesetice-Kyjovice for example, a large Lengyel site centres on a highpoint with a small but carefully constructed enclosure and evidence of cult activities. Here, in addition to the clearer cases of defended village sites in this region of Europe, we may be witnessing a further response to inter-community and community-environment stress, the elaboration of communal ritual behaviour. A late example in this tradition is the third-millennium 'woodhenge' at Quenstedt. (For Lengyel 'defenceworks' cf. Pavuk 1976, Podborsky 1976, Behrens 1981). A rather similar picture is emerging from Western Europe, with numerous

examples of enclosures on a scale compatible with defence, as well as a group of settlements with practical defences and claimed 'ritual enclosures', e.g. Köthing-eichendorf (cf. Lüning 1976b, Christlein and Schmotz 1977/8, Moddermann 1976a). In the Middle Neolithic populations of LBK derivation in northern France (Chassey-Pseudo Michelsberg), large ditched and defended sites are a characteristic feature of the later fourth and early third millennium bc, interpreted as the result of competition for favoured, long-occupied eco-niches (Howell 1983). In Northern Europe special attention is being given to recent evidence for defensive/ritual enclosures within the TRB Culture, especially in the light of the arguments from burial evidence (cf. below) for widespread ranking, often highly emphasized, perhaps reflecting genuine hereditary stratification. Although the examples cited tend to belong to the third millennium bc, or later phases of the TRB, (within the Late Neolithic or Copper Age properly speaking of north-west Europe), the earliest examples seem to belong to an important wider development within the mature TRB Culture (TRB C, the centuries following 3000 bc), being associated with the development of more complex burial structures of an arguably highly ranked or stratified society (megalithic dolmens). This tradition includes what appear to be genuine defended settlements, supposed ritual enclosures which are being compared to English causewayed camps and settlement-cum-cult centres: Wallendorf, Dölauer Heide, Salzmünde, Derenburg, Büdelsdorf, Sarup, Toftum (cf. Tabaczynski 1972, Lüning 1976b, Madsen 1978, 1979, Hingst 1971, Andersen 1975, Behrens 1975). Behrens suggests for some of these a possible territorial pattern at 10-20km. intervals, which may indicate a low-level set of political units comparable to those of the English chalk-land causewayed camps. In a recent detailed analysis of the Danish early third-millennium bc social and settlement landscape, Madsen (1982) documents a pattern of focal 'causewayed camps' surrounded by impressive mega-lithic tombs, both sets of monuments in his view reflecting elite organization (the tombs are complex and associated with elaborate ceremonial activity but were intended for only one or a very few persons): "the monumental tombs, especially with their outward display of pottery, ... served as symbolic expression of land rights ... the huge centres ... made up the frame for social interaction and rituals designed to regulate the patterns of access to resources and the inter-relationship of groups over a wider area" (p.222). Although it is clearly possible to consider ritual enclosures as a separate issue from purely defensive features around or beside villages (for communal refuge), the elaboration of supposed cult features both in terms of the living and of care for the dead, does appear to be inextricably linked into a nexus of change within European societies during the fourth millennium bc. With the radical shifts in settlement behaviour and economy, linked to greater pressure upon economic survival and adaptation, and hence, arguably upon the community's access to essential territory, the rapid spread of practical defence works requires no special pleading for explanation. More subtle must be our inferences regarding the evidence at this time for greater emphasis upon the symbolism or visible manifestation of ranking, and even more so for understanding the development of a much more elaborate ritual life. The role of leadership grew, and with it, that of ideological sanctions and community-enhancement behaviour of a formal kind - stressing group cohesion and reflecting a growing need for divine intercession in daily activities; these may rather speculatively be offered as elements in a preliminary model to relate these parallel developments in society.

Note 38
In Eastern Europe, the Danubian 2 tradition cultures from the late fifth millennium into the early fourth millennium bc witness the general adoption of formal cemeteries,

with the possible implication of more territorially-aware communities in the new conditions of enhanced need to corner a viable resource base (cf. above on both points, notes 8 and 28) (Pavuk 1972, Comsa 1974a). Both here and in the former LBK regions of Central and Western Europe, cemeteries offer strong parallels to LBK customs: thus we find gift richness concentrated with adult males at the expense of females and sub-adults in general. Likewise the contrast should not be overdrawn in supposed status intervals between these categories. Amongst the key items identified with status, stone axes continue but can be replaced by axes or axe-adzes in antler and, in the precocious Copper Age of Eastern Europe, which flourishes from the mid-fourth millennium bc parallel to the developed Neolithic elsewhere, copper axes and axe-adzes. Although it is customary to envisage age and sex as the major factors being underlined in variable gift quantity and quality, we may also, as with the LBK, point to the frequent evidence of ranking within the class of adult males, and furthermore to occasional child and female burials given unusual gift prominence (Pavuk 1972, Sherratt 1976, Kaufmann 1976). An interesting elaboration of the 'male status equipment' during the fourth millennium is the rise of perforated broad hardstone axes in Danubian 2 cultures. It has been suggested that a major role for these artifacts was as offensive weapons, and a developmental line drawn from this time through to the genuine 'battle-axes' that typify Late Neolithic Europe of the third millennium bc (Zapotocky 1966), although in origin they would seem to develop from the LBK woodworking axe and rare maceheads. Such a symbol as the 'armed man' has naturally attracted Marxist scholars seeking to pinpoint the crucial shift from matriarchal, hoe-farming centred communities to those of the patriarchal Gentile society dominated by male protectors of flocks and people (Tabaczynski 1972; Lüning 1976). It does seem far more plausible to emphasize the gradual shift from male status identification with the working celt to that of the warrior male, even more so in societies showing far greater attention to communal defenceworks on an increasingly time-consuming scale.

In an earlier discussion (notes 32-33) we have identified the possibility of ranking within a number of rather unusual East European cemeteries of the fourth millennium (Danubian 2/Copper Age), most particularly Varna, perhaps beyond the 'Early Neolithic spectrum' level of 'big man' into one of established chieftain families. Our data base, and the level of analysis hitherto practised on East European settlement and cemetery internal differentiation, prevent us from concluding whether a chieftain-like organizational level was a product of unusual local circumstances or widespread, as opposed to lower level ranking of the 'big man' variety. On the other hand, the nexus of societal elaborations of this 'high culture' (Renfrew) or 'climax economy' society (Nandris), involving very dense, well organized and planned communities with a flourishing craft specialization, intense regional exchange, a high level of symbolic activity (from the artwork and the Tordos script), have suggested to some all the hallmarks of a chieftain society **except** for the general absence of distinct high-status burials and prestigious monuments (Renfrew 1973a, 1978). Here the question is posed of a different set of activities and markers for a social elite from the case made for Western European Neolithic chiefdoms, although we may believe that both developments arose from a similar congruence of forces: from demography, economy and individual opportunism.

Note 39
Characteristic for the vast sphere of the TRB culture in Northern Europe, the context of the first general farming culture in the region, are simple earth graves or 'stone-packing' graves (shallow pits with bodies covered with piles of stones, sometimes amalgamated under later stone piles), and with few or no gifts. Both cemeteries and individual burials in these forms are known. This tradition accounts for the vast majority of TRB burials and in many areas no other burial type occurs (Tabaczynski 1972, Häusler 1975, Milisauskas 1978). In Denmark, however, from the first, (TRB A/B styles), there are known a small number of earthen barrows with wooden constructions within, and one to five bodies, reminiscent of English earthen long barrows (Liversage 1976, Madsen 1979, Chapman 1981a). By the early third millennium bc (TRB 'Megalithic' C style), there develop more elaborate tombs of megalithic and earth construction, dolmens, to which are to be added during the following centuries of the Nordic Middle Neolithic (actually the central third of the third millennium bc), grander megaliths of gallery and passage grave varieties. These elaborations remain however in the minority within each area of the TRB and are absent from large parts of the TRB distribution, although importantly there are plentiful examples of cemeteries with simple earth/stone packed graves amid one or more varieties of megalithic tomb (Hingst 1976). The number of bodies in megaliths is generally low, as with earthen/wood barrows, but the effort expended in the erection of these monuments and their greater degree of impressiveness has often led to interpretations stressing different tribes (Becker 1961), or different social classes (Häusler 1975). The sophisticated analysis of Danish burial customs of the TRB C era has provided satisfactory insights into the overall context of these mortuary practices (Randsborg 1975). An initial study of Neolithic population patterning over the landscape allowed Randsborg to correlate the distribution of earth graves and megaliths to both the overall density of inferred population and its degree of localized clustering. An important factor in comprehending the role of mortuary variability is the recognition that gift richness was rare and in any case found in both earth and megalith traditions, allowing two potential rank indicators, wealth and monumental prestige to be traced. Randsborg argues that where population was regionally dense, rich earth graves betrayed ranked individuals; where it was locally clustered, megaliths offered prestige for ranked persons and a visable communal focus. In conclusion, the society concerned had a characteristically small-scale but general level of ranking diffused through it.

In Sweden, four-fifths of the total passage graves are concentrated into a prosperous farming enclave of 500sq. km. Here the rich landscape seems to be divided into regular territories each focussing on a passage grave cemetery (Kaelas 1981).

Arguments for a higher level of ranking or 'chieftain statuses' have been advanced from the much more elaborate great tombs of selected areas of the TRB distribution, in TRB C and Middle Neolithic times. Most striking are the Polish 'Kujavian' graves, which are huge earth mounds with stone chambers that rarely contain more than one or two bodies, usually adult males, representing a massive communal effort and a permanent prestigious monument for those buried within. As in Randsborg's study, it is not gift richness but rather the monument itself that argues for high status (Tabaczynski 1972, Häusler 1975, Milisauskas 1978). On average in the Kujavian and Chelmno regions of Poland there is only one mound per community, and all things considered: "we may assume that only high-status persons were selected for interment in these mounds" (Milisauskas 1978, p.167). Similar unusually elaborate burial structures, chambered mounds of impressive proportions and human effort, are found in several other regions of the Central European TRB, e.g. tombs of the Baalberg and Salzmünde groups (Tabaczynski 1972).

Note 40

The initial identification of St. Michel and the similar site of Villeneuve as giant villages has had to be modified in the light of ongoing excavation of the endless alignments (at least 3-400) of rectangular and oval structures that fill their 20-30ha. expanses. Houses they generally do not seem to be, communal cooking and food preparation areas they may well be (amongst other roles). But in any case, they do represent large groups of people undertaking intensive domestic activity together at these locations (there are also major ditches, palisades, stock-enclosures, wells and grain-silos), associated at St. Michel with what might be seen as 'elite burials' (Phillips 1975, Clottes et al. 1979, Vaquer 1981).

The partial remains of two adults in a cobble-filled pit may not seem so obviously recognizable as evidence for social stratification or ranking, but the details and cultural context are convincing for this interpretation. The grave-pit at St. Michel was 80cms. deep and 7.4 by 4m. broad (C14 at 3490 bc). The bodies were probably exposed before a representative collection of bones was placed in a wooden structure beneath a great mass of cobbles. With the bodies was a large and varied collection of Chassey pottery. Pat Phillips, in a recent discussion of social developments in the French Middle Neolithic Chassey Culture (1982, p.61) comments: "Another aspect of differentiation is ranking. The most marked evidence for difference in treatment of individuals comes from burials ... The huge grave-pit at St. Michel-du-Touch represents an anomaly, but the relatively low numbers of burials that have been found throughout the Chasséen area suggest that probably only a few members of each group were buried in a structured grave, with grave goods; these burials may well reflect some degree of ranking in the local society". Phillips also argues that the remarkable size and density of the cobble structures at St. Michel and Villeneuve suggests communal social and ritual behaviour well beyond domestic activity and indicative of some kind of regional ceremonial focus role for these and other sites clustered relatively densely in the Toulouse region (op. cit. pp.17, 19). A contemporary population at the two major sites of several hundred is postulated (p.16).

Note 41

cf. above, note 14, contra Sherratt, this volume.

Note 42

The following calculations, though speculative, may indicate that a remarkable scale of flint axe production at source, including partial artifact preparation, and impressive distribution networks up to 1-200kms. long (accounting for a major part of local artifact needs), could have been in operation for long periods of time without anything more complicated than the workforces of several adjacent villages devoting half their labour to mining/preliminary working, connected to a chain of village-to-village, down-the-line exchanges. The calculations, or rather guesstimates (cf. Hopkins, 1978 for the heuristic value of such speculations), run as follows: a recently excavated Dutch flint mine at Rijckholt came into use in the fourth millennium bc, and for some 500 years out of about 5000 mineshafts may have produced some 150 million axe-roughouts (Bosch 1979). This would average at 300,000 axes a year. If we assume that the mining communities devoted half the year to their specialist activitiy, especially times free from concentrated agricultural work and the most severe weather, this would amount to around 2000 axes a day from the mine. Given this major restriction on a full commitment to providing their own sustenance, the workforce would require a major food input from axe-recipient communities surrounding them. Estimates of labour requirements and man-hours for the mining and preliminary axe-preparation are hard to come by, but Balcer claims that an experienced workman could produce a flint axe roughout from a nodule in no longer than ten minutes (Milisauskas 1978, p.147). In an eight-hour day, roughout preparation would therefore call for 40-plus workmen. If we allow for three times this effort to include men to mine and bring to the surface the flint nodules, we would be requiring 120 or so for the total workforce, or the mature male population of three or four medium to large villages. Axe demand is far more difficult to quantify, but we must surely cover ourselves by offering a range per family (i.e. per adult male in a group of four or five people) of 2 to 52 axes per year (a new one every six months **or** every week). Our yearly turnover of 300,000 axe roughouts in this range of demand would therefore satisfy between 30,000 and 750,000 people (or 6,000-150,000 adult males). One would suspect that two per year is far too low, one a week far too high, but we have now a reasonable range in the tens of thousands of adult males and perhaps the low hundreds of thousands of total population being serviced. A medium to large village would require on the same spectrum, per year, 70 to 1820 axes; somewhere in the middle of this range (1000 axes?) could probably be obtained in half a dozen village-to-village exchanges (each family obtaining five axes on each occasion for its own use, and a variable number to pass on) throughout the year. Such a vast human catchment fits the scale of distribution and the regular spread of down-the-line flint and hardstone exchange demonstrated for most regions of Europe (as calculations of the area enclosed within a 100-200kms. radius and its potential Neolithic population will reveal). And almost all of this vast, dispersed population supplied indirectly from the mine need not have had to concern itself with direct contact with or food support for the mining community, as the surplus required to supplement the miners' own diminished subsistence product could probably have been supplied by a small number of inner communities around the mining villages (Braudel informs us, for example, that the typical small medieval town could largely be fed locally by on average 10 rural villages' surplus; Braudel 1973, p.377). It is even possible that the above calculations underestimate the potential of such a small scale industry to service a vast region. Ethnographic data from New Guinea (Phillips, pers. comm.) suggest that stone axes may have a longer use than our maximum above of six months - up to several years in fact.

Note 43

The case is well-made in a number of recent publications by Whittle (1977a, 1978, 1980) and Bradley (1978a, b). In the early third millennium, now defined as the transition between an Earlier and Later British Neolithic in cultural terms, we can observe from environmental and settlement/burial evidence a very widespread decline in human activity in many regions of the British Isles. "Towards the middle of the third millennium BC a whole series of large agricultural clearances finally reverted to fallow ... and at about the same time the building of public monuments sharply declined. Communal burial sites became less impressive and causewayed enclosures were no longer built" (Bradley and Hodder 1979, p.96). In the remainder of the millennium two subsequent responses are observed to this arguable decline in settlement and economy. Firstly a renewed and prolonged phase of recovery and land intake (e.g. in Ulster, East Anglia and Cumbria) together with a first serious attack upon the mixed farming potential of upland areas such as Dartmoor, the Pennines, the North York Moors and parts of Cornwall, which will last into the Later Bronze Age (cf. below). Secondly, a response that seems to involve a reorganization of land use in old settled or exploited areas such as the southern chalklands, where grassland environments are now frequently encountered. The general interpretation offered is of ecological overkill by Early Neolithic populations, resulting in a widespread decline in soil productivity, followed by soil fertility recovery in some areas, a compensatory exploration of new and often rather marginal upland country, and a shift to more extensive grazing from mixed farming in the important chalkland environment of southern England -although Bradley has recently produced a controversial view that the chalk landscape was even in Early Neolithic times only a secondary resource area for farming exploitation (Barrett et al. 1981). Bradley (1978b) quotes with approval the earlier insight of Brothwell (1971,pp. 84-85): "when ... biosocial factors are taken into account our attempts to create a Neolithic population explosion are rather left in ruins. What is just as likely is that there were mini-cycles of population expansion and decrease with only a gradual trend to long-term increase". Bradley concludes (1978a, p.106): "It seems likely that Neolithic expansion had temporarily outstripped the capacity of the system to support it. Recovery when it did come was slow and rather distinctive". This suggestion of agrarian cycles in Britain is very much in harmony with the more widespread evidence for their operation in European prehistory already indicated in this chapter, and for which further possible examples will be offered below and in the writer's Iron Age chapter (this volume). Unexpected though it may be, the reality of the Neolithic population explosion is clearly evidenced from areas such as the outlying islands of Britain. Alisdair Whittle's conclusions from his research on the Neolithic settlement of the Shetlands "reinforce the impression of a period of rapid expansion and land-hunger before and around 3000 bc in the country as a whole" (Whittle 1980a p.47). John Howell has recently suggested that Brittany may form a close parallel to Whittle and Bradley's model for the British Neolithic (1983, pp.164-5). After a limited early farming occupation associated with the earliest megaliths, there is a remarkable expansion and florescence of human activity linked to the construction of the finest tombs in the Chassey or Middle Neolithic era. This process may have exceeded the productive capacity of the peninsula and there follows an apparent marked recession of human activity in the early third millennium bc, closely parallel to the British sequence, before a recovery later in the millennium which as in Britain may have a stronger pastoral component.

Note 44

"The initial step ... is to see in these monuments an expression of territorial behaviour in small-scale segmentary societies. The second step is to suggest that such forms of territorial behaviour may be particularly frequent in small-scale segmentary societies of this kind in circumstances of population stress. And finally it has been shown that there are grounds for thinking that such population stress was in fact experienced along the Atlantic/North Sea seaboard, but it was not felt among approximately contemporary communities in central or eastern Europe" (Renfrew 1976, p.200). Renfrew's initial evidence for the matching of megalith distributions to arable land followed an earlier study by Childe (cf. Renfrew 1973a, 1974). Recent regional analyses of megalith distributions show a strong link to the most favourable soil types in each area (cf. Cooney 1979; Holgate and Smith 1981, strangely ignorant of Grimes' pioneering contribution in the same area!).

Note 45

The relevance of the Mesolithic factor has grown in importance since Renfrew first raised it as the source of local stress, symbolized by 'group territory marker' megaliths. He was intrigued by the very simple funerary arrangements found with late Breton Mesolithic sites at Téviec and Hoëdic, since Brittany has from the beginning of its Neolithic era a series of impressive earthen and megalithic burial monuments. To this we may now add the argument that the importance of Mesolithic coastal activity in Brittany at this very time may well reflect food scarcity or 'climax' resource use (Bailey 1978, Chapman 1981a). Moreover, the earliest simple megalithic graves in Portugal may be contemporary to this early fourth-millennium bc Atlantic megalith rise (Whittle and Arnaud 1975), and here again we have a dense local late Mesolithic in the same general region with a developed coastal exploitation (cf. Chapman 1981a). (Bob Chapman, pers. comm., points out, however, that the early Portuguese megaliths are distinctly not in the same specific areas as the Mesolithic middens of the region). On the other hand, what happens to a community that splits from its parent village and settles in a new area with abundant land, when its parent village builds burial monuments and sends out surplus population because of local land shortage? Do the offspring foundations immediately drop the monument habit, or has it become a valuable cultural inheritance that serves to reinforce group cohesion in a foreign environment? Such questions are necessary if we turn to two recent studies of early burial monuments. Firstly, Ian Kinnes (1982) has excavated on the island of Guernsey a stone and earth burial mound dating from the Early Neolithic settlement on the Channel Islands, at Les Fouaillages. It overlies a Mesolithic domestic site, but the cultural material associated with the mound is derivative Linear Pottery, as typifies the spread of mixed farming across north and central France from the east at this time. Is this a Mesolithic 'pressurized group' rapidly adopting aspects of Neolithic culture from the mainland, or a re-use of the location by incoming Neolithic settlers? In any case, we have to ask ourselves if the monument could represent a degree of population stress because of dense Mesolithic/dense Mesolithic-plus-Neolithic settlement, or merely a cultural feature 'in the baggage' of westward spreading settlers of Linear Pottery origin, suitable to symbolize their cultural coherence as a community focus in this alien environment (and who are building megaliths now all over western and west-central France). Precisely the same set of issues arises with the recent dating of early Irish megaliths by a Swedish expedition (Daniel 1981) to around the beginning of the fourth millennium bc, contemporary with the first sporadic traces of the inception of farming in Ireland.

Note 46

Atkinson (1968) summarized the available data on the number, chronology and contents of earthen and megalithic long barrows in southern England. The average body count for earthen mounds was six, for megalithic long barrows, 15. On such a basis he calculated maximum population figures for southern England during the Neolithic of 70-140 people. This seemed at the time far less implausible than today with the subsequent great development of field studies and field survey in particular. It would now be impossible to conceive of such a low density, given the scale of Neolithic settlement and activity traces, even allowing for the recorded tombs being, say, a third or a quarter of the original number built. Also curious is the suggestion that half a dozen people could have constructed the earthen barrows, therefore they might represent a single family; one should rather envisage at least four or more families producing such an adult labour force. Furthermore, although Atkinson could reconcile himself both to the very low density estimates and the idea of a family-built and -used earthen barrow, he readily admitted that the labour involved in the stone-chambered long barrows was of a different order, and he suggested that this larger workforce was employed for the benefit of a minority of their number who were thus being honoured by interment within the monument. The higher body count in the megalithic mounds was largely a factor of their re-use over a longer interval by removal of blocking stones.

As the current estimates of Neolithic populations rose,

after this pioneer paper, it became increasingly obvious that despite Renfrew's adoption of the 'family tomb' model for long barrows, the interred population can only have been a small proportion of the total available for mortuary disposal. Curiously, Renfrew seemed to offer an alternative model that explicitly suggested a minority burial practice, when he raised his barrow-builders from the group size buried within, to a one in five ratio of workforce-buried group to total barrow 'owning' community (1973b). That such a minority should be seen as privileged was a logical step anticipated in Atkinson's discussion of the megalithic barrows, and by 1979 we find a general textbook confidently claiming: "Given, therefore, the possibility of a stratified society on the basis of the limited number of individuals buried beneath long barrows one might see in the Wessex region the grouping of long barrows into five major regional units as reflecting a social or tribal entity each controlled by a ruling aristocracy buried beneath the long barrows themselves" (Megaw and Simpson 1979, pp.95-6). What, then, of Renfrew's neat fit of c.20 long barrow construction groups to each causewayed camp manpower requirement? Firstly, the figure must now be seen as coincidental, as the regional totals are merely the accumulated contructions of a period of long barrow construction now estimated at 1000 C14 years (even longer in calendar years) i.e. 3400-2400 bc. Only at the end of this period can one reasonably claim that each region possessed c.20 'territorial markers'. Secondly, revised estimates of manpower requirements (Startin and Bradley 1981) suggest that long barrow manpower has been underestimated, with the larger examples requiring as many as 32-40 labourers, whereas causewayed camp and henge monument manpower may have been overestimated, requiring respectively 80 and 250-500. The physical anthropology of a few carefully studied tomb samples has provided several cases of skeletal peculiarities consistent with close kindred, e.g. Lanhill, West Kennet and others (Megaw and Simpson 1979), which should now be suggestive of an elite kin group in society.

However, an anomalous situation appears from the recent publication of Renfrew's researches in Orkney (Renfrew, C., 1979). Here the calculations derived from the excavation of the Quanterness chambered tomb are quite in line with the total dead of a small number of families, representing perhaps a living community of 20 people, or approximately the number originally argued by Renfrew (1973b) as required to build a typical mortuary barrow. Moreover, the pattern of chambered tombs on various islands of the Orkney group is dense enough to conform to small segmentary kin groups. Thus, in deliberate contrast to the 'elite' lobby, he reports of Quanterness: "the burials represent the mortality over many years of an entire human community, rather than of individuals selected instead for social reasons" (1979, p.162), and of the Orkney earlier Neolithic in general: "we shall be able to see the megalithic monuments not as a bizarre religious phenomenon, ... but as the exceptionally complete residue of a pattern of early territorial exploitation by small scale, autonomous societies which have their analogue in the early farming societies ... in many parts of the world" (1979, p.2).

One can raise a number of difficulties with the Orkney analysis to qualify the interpretation offered by Renfrew. Firstly, despite the continued use of the six manpower (note the important development from Atkinson's six workers equals a family, to six workers equals four or so families i.e. 20 people) as the yardstick for the theory of segmentary autonomy, it is now admitted, as Atkinson stated long before, that these large chambered tombs needed a greater labour force. Renfrew concedes that around ten men would be necessary (i.e. ten families or perhaps less if female labour were available = c. 40-50

people). Secondly, wherever in other Orkney megaliths we have body counts, they are far lower than Quanterness. This is especially important when we consider a third point, that the known tombs are very clustered in some districts of the islands, far more dispersed in others (the argument that destruction, burial, etc., has caused the disappearance of most megaliths and that very high densities prevailed generally, does not seem at all convincing to the present writer). Therefore we cannot use the small island of Rousay and its close packed tombs as a replicable module for the far more isolated Quanterness tomb. It might therefore by very significant that one of the Rousay cairns produced a mere 29 bodies compared to the minimum 157 claimed for the Quanterness cairn. Given the estimated period of use of the Rousay series of cairns, 400 years or more, the ideal four or so families believed associated with each tomb should have contributed four or five times the number recovered. This assumes of course that the tomb concerned was in continuous use throughout this period, indeed the idea of dense small kin groups is closely linked to a general contemporaneity of neighbouring tombs. If we were however to spread Rousay cairn building over the 400 plus years, we would either have to argue for a smaller population using the tombs for all their dead in sequence or alternation, or for a higher population in which only a minority received cairn interment. On the other hand, to be fair to Renfrew, the recent Quanterness bone analysis was carried out on different and more penetrating criteria than earlier studies utilized by Atkinson and by earlier workers on the Orkney material, and it has often been observed that recent bone counts produce higher minimum numbers than older reports. Yet we would have to argue generally for an error factor of four to five and often much more, to elevate the low counts normal for earthen and megalithic mounds in Britain to an acceptable total consistent with the total dead of four families over the use period of these monuments, and even then we would have to multiply the known tombs by a far greater factor than four to five to even approach the Neolithic population levels now being argued from the total archaeological and environmental data presently available. The mounting evidence for alternative and less prestigious modes of disposal makes such an exercise pointless in many regions, where de facto only a proportion of the population are now known to be interred in these monuments (cf. below). (Similar points are made, with further low counts for Rousay tombs, in a recent paper by Masters, 1981).

Quanterness poses therefore a problem case. In itself does its evidence support the Renfrew model? The body count might match the four-family unit for building a small earthen long barrow, but is far too small for the estimates of manpower required for its own more ambitious construction.

Significantly Stuart Piggott ranks Quanterness with Maes Howe as in the category of larger monuments when he comments: "the social system under which such monuments could be built must have involved some command of labour and technical skill concentrated in an individual - chieftain, priest or priest-chieftain - or in a ruling caste" (1982, p.41). And unless all the Orkney tombs are used continuously, we have to recognise in any case a large population not buried in the monuments. Moreover, in the context of the Orkneys as a whole and the British Neolithic evidence as a whole, the Quanterness model is inconsistent with the dominant evidence for burial differentiation. Two obvious alternative models present themselves as solutions: (a) we need not assume a 'monolithic' burial practice thoughout the British Isles; the densely packed tombs on some islands could indeed reflect small, autonomous kin groups burying all their dead, in contrast to the much more dispersed southern England long barrows which could represent a more highly differentiated society; (b) the large number of Quanterness dead may represent an elite drawn from a much wider area of Orkney · than the human/land catchment to be associated with the closely spaced Rousay cairns. Either model still allows us to follow the dominant present-day view that in the British Neolithic, from the first, burial monuments were normally reserved for a minority, arguably a privileged minority, of the total population. Significantly, the picture from early megaliths and earth mounds elsewhere around the 'Atlantic façade' of Europe, tends to confirm this view, and includes both older and recent bone counts. In the tumulus cemetery of Bougon, for example, in west-central France (Mohen 1977), Early Neolithic mounds comparable to contemporary examples in Brittany, and of very substantial proportions and work-investment, contain but a handful of bodies (C14 places the early tombs already in the first half of the fourth millennium bc - Giot 1981, p.88). Here also, in parallel to the Orkneys, we find a Late Neolithic giant megalithic tomb, with plentiful bodies, but considering the length of tomb use and the scale of the monument, probably representing a special prestigious monument for a few elite families within a wide district (cf. below, note 62).

This controversy has been taken a stage further in recent works by Darvill (1979) and Bradley (1982). Darvill suggests that Ireland conforms neatly to Renfrew's model of simple megalithic tombs (the court cairns) of the early Neolithic, being replaced by the complex passage-graves of the later Neolithic - suiting a shift from egalitarian communal burial to status monuments for an elite. However the territories he identifies for each court cairn, at 100-600sq. kms., are remarkably large for a few families. Moreover Bradley has pointed out that recent evidence could suggest that passage graves date back to the early Neolithic and in much of the settled area of Ireland may have been contemporary to neighbouring court cairns. One could suggest that we see here the elite and commoner monuments (to use Darvill's own hypothesis without the time difference). But since the court cairns could well represent burial foci for only a small part of the population we would have, alternatively, a three-tier hierarchy, with monuments for the upper two tiers: 'parish' monuments for the kin-heads or 'big men' of a village-sized area (court-cairns, average 4.5kms. apart), then 'district' monuments for regional chieftain families (passage-graves, cemeteries average 10.4kms. apart). Indeed, O'Kelly (1976) makes no major distinction between the elite role of smaller·and larger megaliths in Ireland, as well as providing important evidence concerning the court cairns: "When we look at ... megalithic tombs, the same points seem to emerge - a great effort was made to build a tomb to house only a few bodies ... the evidence suggests special people in all cases ... Fourknocks and the Mound of the Hostages have so far contained the largest numbers of people -Fourknocks 24 and the Mound of the Hostages many more. Apart from them, the number of persons are small in each case; and in several of the court cairns, only a single youth was found in the tomb" (p.129).

In the same fashion, Renfrew's Orkney sequence of simple to complex, which removes the most plausible elite monuments to the end of the Neolithic sequence, rests on insecure foundations. A revaluation of the chronology is forthcoming and: "There is a strong case that different stages of Renfrew's evolutionary scheme in fact occurred at the same time" (Bradley 1982, p.28).

Note 47
Briar Hill causewayed camp has a ditch silt date of 3490 bc (Bamford 1980).

Note 48
For Hambledon Hill see Mercer (1980, and subsequent Interim Reports, cyclostyled). The very important interpretation of the main causewayed camp as a locus for mass excarnation originates from two aspects of the fill of the camp ditches. Firstly, the 'ritual' deposition of parts of human bodies, especially skulls, supposedly selected from the camp interior mortuary area in connection with certain rites. Secondly, the unintentional washing in of body fragments into the silting ditches from the interior of the enclosure (perhaps also the dragging away by scavengers into the camp periphery, from bone wear indications). In all, this sample that found its way into the ditches, is estimated to amount to some 350 people, although it is suggested that the majority of bodies might have decomposed in the camp interior to leave no trace (medically quite feasible, and erosion has in any case removed the old landsurface). The high proportion of children in the ditch sample is consistent with a 'total population' exposure.

Note 49
For Hambledon Hill see above references; for Crickley Hill see Dixon and Borne (1977). Whittle has made the important point that the ditch sections of many of these causewayed sites, and adjacent linked camps, betray the former existence of a steep timber-strengthened rampart that is often known to have been surmounted by a substantial wooden superstructure (Whittle 1977b). A defensive function seems inescapable.

Note 50
Throughout Europe at this time, detailed regional studies demonstrate the further continuation of the process begun in Danubian 2 times, of settlement expansion into more varied and often more difficult and marginal soils, in which more extensive agriculture with longer fallow, high grazing emphasis, specialized crops, all may have played a significant role (cf. Machnik 1974, Lies 1974, Mania and Preuss 1975, Kruk 1980, Bradley 1978, Sherratt 1981, Starling 1983, and further regional studies cited below). For a clear broadening of the range of cultigens and wild resources from the Early to the Late Neolithic in Greece, cf. Renfrew, J. (1979) and Renfrew, C. (1972). The ard plough and dairy products now argued to be diffusing from a more limited Eastern European use in the preceding millennium, will have helped considerably in communities led or forced to adapt in this way (see below). In some regions, the Later Neolithic full use of the environment is linked to networks of megaliths, arguably emphasizing territorial claims where land has become precious e.g. the Magdeburg district of East Germany (Lies 1974). In northern France (Howell 1983), the third-millennium Late Neolithic SOM Culture marks a decisive break with preceding EN and MN traditions by expanding its sites over the entire landscape. A particularly broad range economy is evidenced, farming, herding, and hunting and gathering across a great variety of pedological and topographical contexts. Territorial marking of these newly established settlement niches is shown in the adoption or development in this phase of megalithic and rock-cut tombs.

Note 51
Not only could the ard plough break up the soil more efficiently, enabling tougher soils to be used and old fields to maintain tilth better, but combined with animal traction the area of land that a family could till would increase by about a factor of three. Of course there was now the problem of feeding traction animals; but the shift into poorer land would bring the new settlers into the proximity of extensive woodland fodder, and a larger acreage needed in poorer soil could both be covered by the plough in the time once taken by hoe for a smaller holding and at the same time offer a larger fallow zone supplying fodder. Furthermore, the development of dairy products would increase the benefit of greater stock investment. For a persuasive summary of the data

indicating these developments and their impact in third-millennium bc Europe, see Sherratt (1981). The dairy and traction-ard development may have been significant already in the fourth millennium in Eastern Europe, contributing to the Copper Age florescence (see note 28, above).

Note 52
A recent survey of settlement history in the Upper Rhine, Middle Rhine, Bavaria and Switzerland suggests that the prolonged Neolithic exploitation of the more obvious areas for mixed farming led to general overuse and a widespread pattern of Bronze Age relocation of settlement in far less promising zones of the landscape (Balkwill 1976). This carries to its most extreme the gradual tendency observed throughout the Neolithic in Europe towards such environments. Interestingly it is argued from these same regions, (and one can see parallels elsewhere, e.g. the English chalklands), that by the end of the Bronze Age the old core settled areas had recovered sufficiently, perhaps with the further advantage of better tools and crop practices, for a return to heavy settlement on the early farming landscape, a phenomenon that will last through the pre-Roman Iron Age.

Note 53
The gradual diffusion of copper artifacts and their local production or recycling, from a major inception in the north Balkans during the fourth millennium to general distribution throughout Europe by the end of the third millennium bc, is widely recognized as more indicative of the importance of status items in these societies than proof of an irreversible shift in the functional efficiency of workaday tools and weapons. Likewise (cf. above note 14) as our knowledge of flint and hardstone distribution networks grows the reliance of communities on distant sources and specialist miners for copper merges into equally extensive and older systems for stone. (For discussion of these points see Sherratt 1976, Pleslova-Stikova 1977, Renfrew 1978). Copper experimentation may have begun in the wider context of the flourishing 'climax economy' of Eastern Europe, in which the total resources of the landscape were being explored and tapped, copper first as a new kind of malleable stone of exotic and attractive ornamental potential. Its rise was initially primarily social, but as arsenic-rich ores were encountered, occasional bronzes were produced, leading to a precocious Early Bronze Age in the North Balkans and Greece by the third millennium bc, whereas the rest of temperate Europe only enters into an effective Bronze Age some centuries into the second millennium bc (with tin the key bronzeing agent) (Coles and Harding 1979).

Note 54
According to Bukowska-Gedigowa (1976), Milisauskas (1978) and Milisauskas and Kruk (1978) there are widespread indications from the later TRB culture in Poland and Czechoslovakia of regular settlement concentrations, which in detailed regional survey appear to be accompanied by two classes of smaller sites, suggesting a settlement hierarchy, and by inference, some kind of district chiefdom organization. At Bronocice, such a primitive 'central place' poses the question of the existence in parallel of 'central persons' (cf. Renfrew 1979b, p.114). Whereas in the northern lowland areas of Poland and adjacent regions of East Germany, prominent burials of Kujavian or similar style (cf. above, note 39) provide indications of high status individuals, the picture from the southern, upland areas of Poland where Bronocice and the detailed survey data are located is less clear. However, in later TRB times there does seem to be a local spectrum of burial practices which might suggest status, e.g. skull burial contrasted to single burial or multiple burial with a central adult male. We have already discussed the

growing evidence for putative ritual 'central places' from the end of the fourth millennium and continuing into this millennium, in TRB and contiguous central European cultures. A recently explored example is Quenstedt in East Germany, TRB culture and C14 dated to 2400 bc, suggested as a notable investment of communal effort (some 5000 trees were felled in its construction, for example) (Behrens 1981, and cf. note 37 above). At Makrotrasy, a TRB site in Bohemia, there are interesting claims for a major ritual site with signs of elaborate mathematical and astronomical activity, together with much imported material (Pleslova-Stikova 1977). When we know more about the function of the numerous impressive fortified hilltop enclosures of the West European Michelsberg 'culture' they may be recognized as a parallel territorial-ritual focus system (Boelicke 1976-77). Moddermann (1976) states that known Michelsberg defences are impressively functional, although he argues for non-defensive ritual enclosures elsewhere in third-millennium Western Europe comparable to contemporary henges in England e.g. Hienheim in Bavaria. A proto 'central place' role has been argued for third-millennium Baden sites in Moravia (Pavelcik 1973). John Nandris (pers. comm.) has kindly brought to my attention a most remarkable example of such large, highly planned communities -the recent excavation of the third-millennium, Copper Age, Tripolje Culture site at Majdanetskoe in the Ukraine, where some 1500 houses and perhaps 20,000 people were housed in a giant concentric layout reminiscent of other, smaller Tripolje sites (cf. note 36). Similar sites are known from air photography in the same region (preliminary report, Smaglij 1982). The agricultural basis of these 'towns' is clearly emphasized by the excavator and metal finds are insignificant.

Note 55
The 'defences' at Lébous and Boussargues are still somewhat questionable (P. Phillips pers. comm.). Lébous in particular has sometimes been regarded as a sheep enclosure. But there do seem to be other, more obviously defensive sites in Provence at this period.

With the Fontbouïsse Group of the third millennium bc there is a striking push of human settlement into the garrigue-covered limestone plateau of Languedoc. Adaptation to this specialized environment and its potential was probably aided by the contemporary spread of the ard plough into the area, but clearly the population was a dense one. The settlement pattern seems to have been based on largish village sites, dependent farms and temporary exploitation loci, and with one village for every 4sq. kms. (Gascó 1979). The spread of megalithic tombs and defended centres belongs to this widely evidenced advance of specialized adaptation into the more marginal limestone country of southern France (Arnal 1973, Chapman 1981a). According to Pat Phillips, commenting on this Late Neolithic/Copper Age expansion: "In Languedoc the increased population produced by the successful Chasséen subsistence economy split into large regional units, headed by highly-ranked kin groups or elites. The highly ranked kin groups adopted new ritual systems derived from neighbouring areas, involving communal burial with special grave-goods in stone built tombs or rock-cut chambers" (1982, p.65).

In the Balearic Islands of the West Mediterranean there is an exact parallel with the colonization of marginal land by the Pretalayotic Culture. It has recently been suggested that such extreme settlement decisions may even reflect directed colonization by a dominant elite rather than demographic overflow (Lewthwaite, in prep.) Also under investigation at present are a series of defended enclosures in west-central France of the Peu-Richard Culture, likewise of third-millennium bc date, associated perhaps with a specialized environment, a series of semi-waterlogged depressions (Scarre 1980).

Note 56

The case for an artificially-engineered, 'irrigation civilization' in south-east Spain appears little convincing to the
present writer, resting on the flimsiest and most ambiguous traces of one or two 'water-related' structures (cf.
also Walker 1981) and rather more hopeful inferences on
the fragility of the regional rainfall and the problem of
archaeological remains of water-demanding plants from
this environment (Chapman 1978). However, we are here
making an important distinction between the potential for
natural flood-farming and the physical creation of
channels and dams. As both Chapman and Gilman (1976)
have pointed out, many important Copper Age sites in
south eastern Spain lie adjacent to valley-bottom land
where seasonal rainfall flood run-off may have been
concentrated. The regular, **natural**, flooding and the high
watertable of this zone, could well have stimulated an
intensive cropping of such land, of great importance to
associated settlements. But as yet, evidence of water
control on any significant scale, as might be expected if
productivity was being notably affected by human interference, is lacking. It must further be pointed out that a
traditional emphasis made by these authors on valley land
that is often used today for irrigated, cash-crop agriculture in the Mediterranean, ignores the potential of the
light, lime-rich hill soils that are abundant in Iberia and
are elsewhere known to have been of central importance
to early farming in the Mediterranean (Bintliff 1977a). A
parallel being sought in the local rise of tree-cultivation
such as the olive, to that argued by Renfrew as critical to
the contemporary take-off of the Aegean Early Bronze
Age civilization (Renfrew 1972), awaits better samples of
Iberian Copper Age flora to be tested. At present it still
seems most likely that the flourishing settlement hierarchy and 'high culture', and the postulated complex social
hierarchy of Copper Age Spain and Portugal, arose from
increasing mastery of the dry-farmed and 'naturally-
irrigated' coastal and immediate hinterland landscapes of
these countries, encouraging denser and more organized
societies, emergent ranking and finally stratification.
Differential access to the most fruitful and reliable
farming resources might be a promising working hypothesis, or the indirect means of achieving the same end, a
developed patron-client system as has (incidentally?)
dominated Mediterranean rural societies through recorded
history (cf. Bintliff 1982).

Note 57

A congruence of leading theorists seems to have occurred
in considering the florescence and subsequent 'regressive'
transformation of the north Balkan Copper Age communities. During the fourth millennium bc, these societies,
variously categorized as Tiszapolgar-Bodrogkeresztur,
Vinca-Plocnik, Gumelnitsa-Salcutsa and more peripheral
groupings (Tringham 1971, Sherratt 1976, Renfrew 1969)
achieved a remarkable autonomous high culture, whose
basis has been argued to have been a maximizing, very wide-
ranging economy of high returns (Nandris 1976a). The
dense populations are reflected in large cemeteries and
clusters of straggling linear settlement loci (Sherratt
1982) or a regular network of large tell villages (Tringham
1980a, b, Renfrew 1973a).

By the third millennium bc, these societies, their characteristic settlement pattern and cultural complexity,
have been radically transformed and simplified, such that
the principal investigators deem this a cultural collapse.
For Renfrew (n.d.), the prolonged overuse of north Balkan
soils by dense and concentrated populations contained
within itself the seeds of destruction for any complex
socio-cultural edifice erected upon it, during an evolution
running from farming inception in the mid-sixth millennium bc for some two and a half thousand years. In the

south Balkans, or more precisely, in southern Greece, the
development of Mediterranean polyculture, or more real-
istically, of olive cultivation and the ard-plough combined, pushed the Aegean societies through this productivity
threshold into sustained take-off in the form of the Early
Bronze Age civilization. For Nandris (1976a, 1978), the
equally inevitable risk of the intense K-strategy economy
is one of the absence of a pressure valve or safety margin
in terms of alternative unexploited resources, hence the
Chalcolithic collapse. Ruth Tringham (1978) offers the
fullest discussion of the same general viewpoint. She
begins by reminding us that fourth-millennium bc Europe,
even in the advanced high culture of the north Balkans,
fell short of civilization, in terms of a truly elaborate
settlement hierarchy, specialized bureaucracy and large-
scale storage. Despite the viewpoint of more traditional
prehistorians that this lack of take-off is merely a progressive watering-down of Near Eastern civilization in
radiating circles, the more modern analysis of Renfrew
and of Tringham herself argues for internal causation. "If
one accepts this last viewpoint, then one may well ask:
what is it that prevented the Europeans, whose adoption
of agriculture and cultural development in many other
respects paralleled that of the Near East, from evolving
complex social systems and urban centres, characterizing
Childe's 'Urban Revolution'?" Pastoral steppe nomads
waiting in the wings to nip off emergent civilisation are
increasingly suspect, paving the way to a new explanation
stressing ecological limitations to state development.
One can see in south-east Europe "over-exploitation
during the fourth millennium bc, of both renewable and
non-renewable resources", including wood, and easily-
tilled land. "These long-term effects of short-term
benefits, combined with an increasing population, caused
a society, which, it has been suggested, was heading
during the fourth millennium bc for the 'Urban Revolution'
to undergo drastic socio-economic and technological
changes". Whereas other scholars such as Renfrew and
Sherratt have suggested that this collapse of the established Copper Age system was a catastrophe for civiliza-
tional growth, it may be quite wrong to see such societies
as 'unfulfilled', as it may reflect an essential adaptation
to local conditions. "The responses one sees more frequently in European prehistory include a preference for
more transitory settlement networks rather than vast
unwieldy urban centres, a preference for smaller scale
commodity exchange systems (although this does not
necessarily apply to communication networks) in contrast
to trade monopolies which could be managed only by a
bureaucracy, and finally a more moderate (although not
more conservative) aspiration level in terms of accumulation of wealth and political power". This pattern has
worldwide parallels as a specific response to the fundamental source of societal stress: population growth and
resource shortage (Tringham 1978, pp.59-60).

Excellent Hungarian Plain survey data have recently
allowed Andrew Sherratt (1982a, 1983) to examine the
background to the third-millennium settlement disjunction
in remarkable detail. After an Early Neolithic settlement
concentrating on limited preferred areas of the Plain
landscape, the Danubian 2, late fifth-fourth-millennium
settlement pattern is typified by a remarkable expansion
of settlement to the Plain edges and upland zones, mirroring a Europe-wide trend. Despite Sherratt's hypothesis of
archaeological population totals on the Plain itself staying
stable, 'imploding' into fewer, larger sites, this does not
seem justified by his published data which seem rather to
indicate a clear decline in population and areas farmed at
this time, in favour of population migration into more
varied land elsewhere. Subsequently in the early Copper
Age of the fourth millennium (Tiszapolgar era), a revival
of Plain settlement is attempted in areas formerly well-
settled during the Early Neolithic (possibly stimulated by
increased productivity available with ard-traction?). The

strategem seems to have been inadequate and the late Copper Age (Bodrog. era) sees resettlement on less attractive, higher zones of the Plain. The failure of this last adaptation (perhaps, it is suggested, due to soil decline), is marked by a total dislocation of settlement and the virtual abandonment of the Plain in favour of a concentration on the Plain edges and uplands with the succeeding Baden Culture of the third millennium. The new pattern will continue into the Bronze Age and is characterized by fortified tell sites. In conclusion: "the area rose to prominence and was then progressively reduced in importance" (1983, p.39).

We have quoted and summarized Tringham's analysis at length because of the close congruence with our own conclusions as regards the frequent cultural disjunctions in European prehistory, and we have already discussed several examples in the Neolithic of possible ecological/agrarian crises. In particular we might recall the case now made (cf. note 43) for cycles of agrarian decline in the Neolithic and later the Middle Bronze Age of large areas of Britain, about which, and with an eye to continental parallels (such as the LBK/Danubian 2 disjunction) Whittle has this to say: "Indeed it would be possible to view much of British prehistory in terms of the rise and fall of population and the efforts made to adapt to this" and "one important conclusion must be that it was extremely difficult for Neolithic communities to achieve a truly stable adjustment to their environment, a problem still with us today" (1978, p.40). The detailed problems of maintaining soil fertility without modern 'life-support systems' for plants are well discussed in the context of a similar model for prehistoric Sweden by Stig Welinder (1975). We shall have continual reason to refer to this overall Tringham model later in this chapter and in the writer's Iron Age chapter (this volume) for its explanatory value. For North American parallels to this ecological sequence cf. Braun and Plog (1982).

A different model, which could be an alternative explanation, or on the other hand could be used in combination with the 'agrarian crisis' model, would contrast regions with limited overall subsistence potential, with those much more fertile. Using Carneiro's concepts of environmental and social 'circumscription', we could posit initial farming populations in both kinds of landscape contemporaneously. As population rises, the less fertile landscape reaches crisis first; here population will be forced to decline and/or migrate to distant regions, unless it can adapt to stress by higher productivity or more efficient surplus storage and redistribution. In the more fertile region, eco-demographic stress may be reached in early settled areas due to the social pressure to maintain ancestral commitment to investment in the products of particular lands, but eventually the crisis may be removed by surplus population spilling out into adjacent land, which is more widely available in good quality than in our first, impoverished landscape.

If we were to consider some possible physical examples where these contrasted processes might have operated, the most obvious would be to contrast southern Greece with Italy during the prehistoric period. It is a commonplace and paradoxical observation that over the peninsula as a whole, Italian prehistory has very little indeed to offer in terms of population highs, monumental architecture, growth of regional centres, during the Bronze Age, compared to the Aegean high cultures and civilizations of the third to second millennia bc. Yet Italy is far more promising a country in terms of climate and soils for prehistoric farmers than is southern Greece. In the latter, perhaps, the stress of climate and limited soil resources would have been felt far earlier than in most regions of Italy (the extraordinarily arid Tavoliere being the Italian exception to prove the rule), and the potential

of olive cultivation and social elaboration as an ecological adaptation been exploited to the full. The apparent (?) lateness of significant olive cultivation in Italy and retarded population growth within most of its regions could be explained from the abundance of varied soils and a favourable climate, creating continual opportunities for further colonization and varied subsistence adaptations.

In Iberia, likewise, the apparent slowness of the evolution from early farming settlement to high culture may reflect the extensiveness of arable land and a milder climate than Greece. Significantly, the most important Spanish region for the rise of the third-millennium 'high culture' of fortified centres, is a part of Almeria that is exceptionally arid, and it is now being suggested (Bob Chapman, pers. comm.) that specific adaptations to local environmental stress are fundamentally tied to the rise of this Copper Age 'high culture'.

Note 58
Until quite recently, the wide distribution of material of these two complexes was readily viewed in terms of migrating nomads, warriors and/or metal prospectors (Sangmeister 1972, Fischer 1975). Less difficult to support today is the argument that these status kits, almost all found as burial assemblages, point to a general elite structure across Europe which is the direct ancestor of the chieftain and 'big man' societies typifying the Bronze Age (Fischer 1975). But the embarrassing problem of the relationship between these supposed migrating herders and the populous, preceding local Neolithic and Copper Age peoples was already exposed in a powerful critique by Neustupny (1969): here it became clear that whatever the Corded Ware-Battle Axe complex represented in ethnic terms, in economic terms the people involved continued with local practices, whether mixed farming, or alternative local subsistence specialization, just as earlier populations. However it is the special achievement of Stephen Shennan (1975, 1977, 1980, 1982) (in part pursuing unpublished ideas of the late David Clarke), to put forward the most recent view of Corded Ware and Bell Beaker 'cultures', and one which is gaining increasing acceptance amongst researchers in this period (Burgess and Shennan 1976, Whittle 1981), namely that these phenomena are of merely subcultural significance, representing a Europe-wide prestige kit used by a minority sector of every local community in special status contexts, especially burial. The communities concerned are the direct descendants of the earlier Neolithic/Copper Age inhabitants in each region (as is often shown by ancillary pottery and other items accompanying the prestige kit in both mortuary and other contexts).

In his most recent elaboration of this model, Shennan enlists the American concept of the 'cluster interaction sphere', as employed by Barbara Price in her analysis of prehistoric cultural systems (1977), and long influential from the eastern USA Hopewell Culture case study (Shennan 1975). Shennan summarizes the Price version of the model: "Starting from the observation that such major socio-economic developments as the appearance of agriculture and state formation" in the New World "occurred more or less contemporaneously over wide areas, she suggests that this is a significant regularity. Together individual regions form a cluster in which similar processes of cause and effect are operating to produce similar or convergent effects, enhanced by interaction between the cluster components. An important part of the cluster definition is that the members are comparable in size range, institutional structure, relative power and 'mode of production' " (Shennan, 1980; cf. now Shennan 1982).

The exact relationship between the wide spread of these putative prestige systems and ideological symbols across late third-millennium and early second-millennium bc

Europe, and the broad trends in land use and population discussed above, is likely to become a most fruitful area for future research. In Britain, the popularity of the Beaker sub-cultural assemblage has recently been seen in terms of elite identification with prestigious 'exotic' display of continental origin (Burgess and Shennan 1976). A native origin has been seen however for a contemporary widespread subcultural phenomenon found throughout the British Isles - Grooved Ware. Bradley (1982) has suggested that this distinctive pottery style represents an elite artifact type associated with ceremonial sites and ritual feasts, as well as status sectors of domestic sites.

Note 59

For further discussion cf. above (note 43) on the suggestion of cycles of Neolithic agriculture and population. An additional factor in the opening up of new zones of the landscape to mixed farming during the period around and after 2000 bc (the LaNEBA or Late Neolithic/Early Bronze Age transition) and on into the Later Bronze Age, may have been drier conditions in the new Subboreal era. There is substantial evidence for such an advantageous shift in the potential of low lying ground, and uplands with climatic limitations, in the evidence for drying out and extensive occupation in the fen country of eastern England (Pryor 1978, ch. 6; Manby 1980) and from the low-lying Somerset Levels of south-west England (Coles and Orme 1980), as well as from the palaeo-ecology and settlement expansion in the marginal uplands such as Dartmoor (Fleming 1978) and the North York Moors (Spratt and Simmons 1976, Spratt 1982). Equally important was a major broadening in the range of crops grown, allowing a wider spectrum of soil conditions to be utilized (Knörzer 1979). A model of ecological stress and close links between cycles of social elaboration and agrarian crises has been proposed for the British later Neolithic and Bronze Age by Bradley (cf. my Iron Age chapter, this volume, note 4). Growing evidence for formal field systems in Late Neolithic and perhaps even Early Neolithic Britain could reinforce the picture of land pressure (Whittle 1980a, p.49) and be seen to accompany and not just succeed the era of megalithic tomb makers.

A Copper Age/Bronze Age major expansion of settlement that can hardly be accounted for by increasing dryness of climate has been evidenced for Spain, where the arid interior Meseta lands are colonized at this time. A special interest in pastoralism and other adaptive changes may be responsible (Chapman 1981c).

For West European continental parallels to a major shift in zones of exploitation during the Bronze Age to counter the run-down of Neolithic landscapes, cf. Balkwill (1976).

Note 60

It seems unnecessary, therefore, to envisage Late Neolithic Britain as in an early stage of secular chiefly power; not only have we argued for widespread elites given special burial status from the Early Neolithic (see above), but the co-existence in many areas of Britain of major ceremonial monuments and a new, even more elaborate series of prestige tombs suggests a strengthening and perhaps widening of the secular power of certain chiefs. Hence Renfrew's (1974) contrast between 'group-orientated chiefdoms' of the Late Neolithic and 'individualizing chiefdoms' of the Early Bronze Age (based on the decline in ceremonial centre construction and the rise of rich barrow burials of a narrow elite, such as the Wessex 'culture') seems an unsupported distinction. It is sadly generally impossible to match the inferences drawn from British Neolithic tombs and other monuments with evidence from contemporary settlements, but recently Whittle (1980a, p.51) has suggested that a number of substantial domestic structures in the Shetlands might represent later Neolithic residences of high status families (e.g. the Stanydale 'temple').

Note 61

It is a regrettable tendency flourishing today, so to stress the regional perspective of monument-building that typological parallels are ignored and their relevance played down. It does not harm the hypothesis of 'local need' for monuments, to suggest that a suitable pattern or even ideology could be borrowed from elsewhere, and indeed it is too much of a coincidence that some 'psychic unity' process was able to produce sets of contemporaneous monuments of strikingly similar format in widely distant parts of Atlantic Europe. This unnecessary suggestion that each region evolved the same type of megalithic tomb detracts slightly from an otherwise excellent paper by Chapman (1981a) on megalithic burials. In another fine paper, by Waddell (1978), it is sad to find the sensible recognition that there were indeed flows of megalithic tomb and monument styles around Europe, matched with the unambitious conclusion: "whether or not the process of diffusion took the form of the spread of a concept or the spread of a cult ... is quite impossible to say" (p.124). Madsen has recently offered a solution similar to that proposed here by the writer, combining 'diffusionist' and 'autonomous' viewpoints along the lines of Clarke's concept of techno-complex, in other words for the diffusion of "structurally similar solutions to religious, ritual and sociopolitical problems" (Madsen 1979, p.319). Darvill's thorough analysis of the Cotswold-Severn chambered tombs brings out the obvious structural links between this region and Brittany and he states: "After such a long period of similarity in tomb type in Brittany it might be suggested that elaboration was a product of interaction" (1982, pp.18, 28). He concludes on a broader geographical canvas, that of Atlantic Europe (p.86): "While it is quite possible that the need for megalithic tombs developed independently in each of these areas ... it is difficult to substantiate the proposition that developments in northern Europe around the North Sea, English Channel and Irish Sea coastlines were totally autonomous ... If the question of origins is to be solved, then details of population dynamics and the transfer of information and goods between regions and between groups have to be considered".

One potential medium of communication across these waters could have been long-distance fishing. Although Grahame Clark is now generally cited for this suggestion as regards megaliths, may the present author be permitted (!) to draw attention to his (obviously) neglected prior discussion of 'megalithic transmerance' in his 1975 PhD thesis (published in modified form as 1977a, cf. pp.123-4)!

Note 62

A growing interest amongst prehistorians in continental Europe in the signs of socio-political diferentiation, especially stimulated by Renfrew's pioneer applications, is increasingly confirming the overall rise of elite complexity by the later Neolithic. Thus, for example, in the tumulus cemetery of Bougon, in west-central France, the Early Neolithic elite megaliths mentioned in an earlier context are replaced by the very large round mound A (a classic passage grave). This is in use for some 500 years and produced about 200 bodies, i.e. about a dozen per generation of continuous deposition in the monument. All ages and both sexes are well-represented and it is argued that the total dead of a number of elite families are involved: "on peut penser que les dix inhumés représentent une famille sans doute de haut rang. Cette supériorité de quelques-uns explique aussi une organisation sociale poussée, nécessaire à un travail collectif d'ampleur dont les tumulus sont les manifestations, aussi bien que les camps fortifiés de la même époque" (Mohen 1977, p.438). An indication of the work team required **at one time** for these monuments is provided by experiments conducted by Mohen to replicate the construction of the Bougon monuments (Giot 1981, p.91). A 32 ton concrete block comparable to the capstone of a local tomb was moved by about 200 people (170 pulling ropes and 30 moving wooden rollers).

Note 63

Overall, the indications for higher total population and a greater frequency of large nodal communities in the Bronze Age conforms to the model already suggested in this paper, of a series of flowing stages of greater overall population density linked to corresponding rises in the size of the elite sector and the complexity of human and settlement hierarchies. The reasons, however, for denser Bronze Age populations are not as simple as they might seem. Despite the general assumption that every peasant farmer could now wield the more efficient bronze tools, convincing proof of this situation is lacking and it may be that until the Late Bronze Age, (when most authorities recognize a remarkable circulation of bronze), this important material had a more restricted impact (cf. my Iron Age chapter, this volume, note 7). Perhaps the bronze equipment combined with the wider availability of ard ploughs and accumulated and improved crop expertise provided a crucial nexus allowing Bronze Age communities to expand into an even wider variety of environmental niches than the later Neolithic (cf. note 59 above).

Yet, once more reminding us of the technical and probably structural difficulties in maintaining regional high cultures, it is rare to be able to identify districts where 'central places' and very dense, long-lived communities occur in an unbroken sequence. Jockenhövel (1974) for example, in tracing some kind of continuity of central places in Europe from the third millennium bc in Eastern Europe down to the Western European Late Bronze Age, shows a phenomenon appearing then frequently disappearing, in any particular area, being especially patchy in Western Europe. The same picture emerges from the excellent synthesis of the European Bronze Age by Coles and Harding (1979). One example well-described is that of the Early Bronze Age communities in Moravia and Slovakia (Madarovce-Veterov and Otomani Cultures), where we have the suggestion of a network of small district centres, fortified settlements, associated with smaller and putative 'satellite' communities, and with each 'territory' encompassed by about a 10km. radius circle (Fig I) (cf. Milisauskas 1978, Fig. 8.9; Vladar 1974, Coles and Harding 1979). At the Spissky site, a strong case has been made for an elite dwelling area and a regional political and economic role. (Incidentally, the common appeal here and elsewhere in Europe north of the Alps, for a Mediterranean origin for these major settlements, does not stand up to chronological, typological or general theoretical analysis -cf. Coles and Harding 1979, Harding 1982, and comments on the Lausitz Culture in my Iron Age chapter, this volume). In Western Europe an interesting series of Late Bronze Age centres is often devoid of an appropriate local predecessor or successor, and probably reflects the generally ephemeral character of such regional co-ordination points and possibly the chiefdoms associated with them. Jockenhövel (1974) rightly points to their local origins and local functions, eschewing the traditional role of migrations, and in many cases discounting a limited, refuge enclosure (Fluchtburg) interpretation, preferring: "meine Ansicht, dass die befestigten Siedlungen als besonderer Niederlassungstyp vor allem mit dem allgemeinen Siedlungsablauf in entsprechendem Gebiet zu vergleichen und einzuordnen sind" and arguing "stellen die urnenfelderzeitlichen Befestigungen Süddeutschlands besonders geschützte 'Konzentrationsorte' (Coblenz) dar, in denen das politisch-soziale, wirtschaftliche und religiöse Leben der jeweils örtlichen Gemeinschaft bzw. des Siedlungsverbandes seinen gesich-

erten Mittelpunkt fand" (op. cit. pp.56, 59). The all-important attention to local origins will be taken up in the analysis of Hallstatt centres in my Iron Age chapter (this volume).

Note 64

Although a handful of cases can be itemized, where access to key ores could have given rise to local wealthy elites, e.g. with the ores and princely burials of Bronze Age Slovakia and the Ore Mountains region (Shennan 1980, 1982, Coles and Harding 1979), even here our poor knowledge of the agricultural correlates of such apparent high status is striking. The norm for Bronze Age status creation, at least as it is normally recognized from burial differentiation and prestige artifacts, far more rarely from elite residences, will almost certainly rest upon differential acces to agricultural surpluses, as may be inferred from the careful correlations between agricultural potential and wealthy burials in Bronze Age Denmark (Randsborg 1974a, b, c) and the evidence now coming in for the key role of that potential in settlement patterns and complexity elsewhere, e.g. southern England in the Later Bronze Age (Ellison 1981), northern England in the Neolithic and Bronze Age (Spratt 1982, pp.166, 183). For similar evidence in the Aegean Bronze Age see Bintliff (1977a, 1982).

Note 65

Summarizing their detailed analysis of the current data base, Coles and Harding report (1979, p.13): "Basically, the evidence of Bronze Age societies suggests a large number of small communities almost entirely self-sufficient and under little pressure. Within and between these societies there is a range of materials, mainly metal, which sometimes demonstrates long-distance distribution of raw material or finished products". And later (op. cit. p.60): "The Rhine valley and its neighbouring lands reflects the development of the earlier Bronze Age elsewhere in Central Europe, and as much as any area suggests small concentrations of population with relatively little desire, need or ability to participate in any wider issues of subsistence or tradition except that of increasing acquisition of copper ... and ... tin ... The quantities involved may not have been as great as we imagine; we might expect that re-use of metal reduced the necessity for constant major undertakings to acquire new material". Likewise Briard (1977, p.718) says of Bronze Age populations in Europe, the Aegean excepted: "restèrent encore des pasteurs et des paysans groupés en de modestes villages, au moins en Europe 'barbare' ". Milisauskas (1978, p.226) represents a growing viewpoint amongst younger prehistorians, when he describes the Bronze Age north of the Alps in terms of "hundreds of small independent sociopolitical units" through which goods moved, not via a merchant class, prospectors, or gypsies, but after Rowlands (1973), through 'interlocking regional exchange networks' with gift exchange and redistribution key, to a far lesser extent barter and trade.

For further examples of this picture on a regional basis, cf. Phillips (1980), Kristiansen (1980), Fleming (1978), Drewett (1979).

Note 66

The general picture of small-scale ranked and stratified societies, with 'big men' and village chiefs greatly outnumbering the discontinuous appearance of regional or 'paramount' chiefs, is brought out clearly in syntheses of the data base such as Coles and Harding (1979), and further illustrations are provided below (and see Harding and Sherratt, this volume). For a stimulating recent discussion of this general phenomenon see Gilman (1981), who correctly, in the writer's opinion (cf. notes 64, 65 above, and Bintliff 1981, 1982), argues for an agricultural power base as the dominant factor in status maintenance and creation.

112

For the Early Bronze Age, the over-emphasis on the limited occurrence of 'princely graves' amongst the large Central European Unetice Culture (not long ago elevated into 'imperial' status by Gimbutas (1965) in an approach now largely rejected by prehistorians), is criticized by Coles and Harding (1979, p.43) : "It seems necessary to see in these rich barrows the proof of social stratification, but it is notable that they are restricted to the latter part of the Early Bronze Age and are by no means typical of the whole". The implication is that only a limited part of the Unetice Culture was organized at such a higher social level, and this picture is indeed confirmed from consideration of the evidence from cemeteries and settlements in other areas of the Unetice and neighbouring cultural groups (cf. also Gallay 1972, Milisauskas 1978, pp.237-244; Phillips 1980, p.208). Rather neatly encapsulating this model, together with our stress on a more widespread pattern of district chiefdoms (linked to the now general occurrence of wealthy child and female burials), is the case study of the Magdeburg region by Lies (1974). As noted earlier, by the Late Neolithic there are definite traces of a simple settlement hierarchy and a network of 'territorial' megaliths, linked to a very wide use of the resources of the surrounding landscape. In the succeeding Early Bronze Age of Unetice culture tradition, it is suggested that the landscape is carved into three central villages or chiefdoms with associated satellite sites, dominating the best land but with good access to a variety of ecozones.

For the Early-Middle Bronze Age era, Bergmann (1967) has indicated a mosaic of regional cultures in north-west Germany, none very extensive, and each evidencing numbers of status individuals of small-scale chieftain kind. A similar picture emerges from several important studies in south Scandinavia (e.g. Randsborg 1974a, b, c, Strömberg 1974) where a mosaic of small independent communities associated with 'big men' and village chiefs is directly linked to agricultural wealth; rarely, and ephemerally, hints of regional 'paramounts' are observed.

In Central and Eastern Europe during the Middle and Late Bronze Age the general picture of small-scale district elites, and sporadic 'princely graves' of more regional importance, is clearly reflected in burials. Consider, for example, the well-studied situation in Czechoslovakia (Neustupny and Neustupny 1961, Bouzek et al. 1966, Paulik 1974, Milisauskas 1978, p.245), or the pattern in large cemeteries such as Cirna (Coles and Harding 1979, p.145). A similar model is emerging from recent work on the Scandinavian Late Bronze Age material (Levy 1978). Current research on the British 'Later Bronze Age' likewise points to a network of minor and major chiefs and an associated low-level settlement hierarchy (Ellison 1981, Barrett and Bradley 1980, Barrett et al. 1981). In the marginal landscape of the North York Moors, Spratt (1982) has identified a pattern of interlocking mixed farming 'estates', associated with territorial burial cairns of status individuals and major land boundaries.

Note 67
Without venturing far into the controversial topic of the origins and maintenance of Minoan and Mycenaean civilization in Greece, the writer would continue to affirm his conviction (cf. Bintliff 1977a) that this unique cultural florescence arose primarily from processes internal to the Balkans, many of which were persuasively isolated by Renfrew in his major synthesis (1972). Recently Harding (1982) has pointedly underlined the contrast between the small-scale chiefdom society suggested by pre-civilizational settlements and burials over much of southern Greece (so reminiscent of the norm for Bronze Age Europe north and west of the Aegean), with the dramatic changes in settlement form and hierarchy, and in burial content, that typify the mature Mycenaean civilization.

For some discussion of the reasons for this Aegean breakthrough in organizational complexity, see above (note 57).

Note 68
As argued earlier in this chapter, and cf. also Carneiro (1978) for a similar model.

ACKNOWLEDGEMENTS

The final version of this chapter has benefitted greatly from the detailed critical comments on an earlier draft kindly provided by Bob Chapman (Reading University), John Nandris (London University) and Pat Phillips (Sheffield University).

BIBLIOGRAPHY

ADAMS, R.E.W. 1978 - "Numerical Indices of Cultural Evolution: the Maya Case", pp.64-70 in D. Shimkin et al. (Eds.) Anthropology for the Future. University of Illinois, Dept. of Anthropology Res. Rep. 4.

ALEXANDER, J.A. 1978 - "Frontier studies and the earliest farmers in Europe", pp.13-29 in D. Green, C. Haselgrove, M. Spriggs, (Eds.) Social Organization and Settlement. British Archaeological Reports, Int. Ser. 47, Oxford.

AMMERMAN, A.J. and CAVALLI-SFORZA, L.L. 1973 -"A population model for the diffusion of early farming in Europe", pp.343-57 in C. Renfrew (Ed.) The Explanation of Culture Change. Duckworth, London.

AMMERMAN, A.J. and SHAFFER, G.D. 1981 - "Neolithic settlement patterns in Calabria", Current Anthropology vol. 22, pp.430-32.

ANDERSEN, N.H. 1975 - "Die neolithische Befestigungsanlage in Sarup auf Fünen (Dänemark)", Archäologisches Korrespondenzblatt, vol. 5, pp.11-14.

ARNAL, J. et. al. 1973 - "Le Lébous à Saint-Mathieu-de-Tréviers (Hérault)", Gallia Préhistoire, vol. 16, pp.131-200.

ARRIBAS, A. 1976 - "A new basis for the study of the Eneolithic and Bronze Age in south-east Spain", pp.154-162 in J.V. S. Megaw (Ed.) To Illustrate the Monuments. Thames and Hudson, London.

ATKINSON, R.J.C. 1968 - "Old Mortality: some aspects of burial and population in neolithic England", pp.83-94 in J.M. Coles and D.D.A. Simpson (Eds.) Studies in Ancient Europe. Leicester University Press.

AUSGRABUNGEN IN DEUTSCHLAND, TEIL I, 1975 - Röm.-Germ. Zentralmuseum, Mainz.

BACHOFEN, J.J. 1861 - Das Mutterrecht. Stuttgart.

BAILEY, G. 1978 - "Shell middens as indicators of postglacial economies: a territorial perspective", pp.37-63 in P. Mellars (Ed.) The Early Postglacial Settlement of Northern Europe: An Ecological Perspective. Duckworth, London.

BAILLOUD, G. 1974 - "The first agriculturalists: 4000-

1800 BC", pp.101-130 in S. Piggott, G. Daniel and C. McBurney (Eds.) France Before the Romans. Thames and Hudson, London.

BAKELS, C.C. 1978 - Four Linearbandkeramik Settlements and their Environment. Analecta Praehistorica Leidensia, 11 Leiden.

BAKELS, C.C. 1979 - "Linearbandkeramische Früchte und Samen aus den Niederlanden", pp.1-10 in Festschrift Maria Hopf, edited by U. Körber-Grohne. Rudolf Habelt Verlag, Bonn.

BALKWILL, C.J. 1976 - "The evidence of cemeteries for later prehistoric development in the Upper Rhine valley", Procs. of the Prehistoric Soc. vol. 42, pp.187-213.

BAMFORD, H. 1980 - "Briar Hill", Current Archaeology, vol. 6 no. 12, pp.358-63.

BARRETT, J. and BRADLEY, R. 1980 - (Eds.) The British Later Bronze Age. British Archaeological Reports, 83, Oxford.

BARRETT, J. et.al. 1981 - "The earlier prehistoric settlement of Cranborne Chase - the first results of current fieldwork", Antiquaries J., vol. 61, pp.203-25.

BECKER, C.J. 1961 - "Probleme der neolithischen Kulturen in Nordeuropa", pp.585-94 in J. Böhm and S. de Laet (Eds.) Europe à la Fin de l'Age de la Pierre. Czech Academy of Sciences, Prague.

BEHRENS, H. 1975 - "Wirtschaft und Gesellschaft im Neolithikum des Mittelelbe-Saale-Gebietes", Praehistorische Zeitschrift, vol. 50, pp.141-61.

BEHRENS, H. 1977 - "Matriarchat und Patriarchat in der Steinzeit?", Acta Praehistorica et Archaeologica vol. 7/8, 1976/7, pp.65-71.

BEHRENS, H. 1981 - "The first 'Woodhenge' in Middle Europe", Antiquity vol. 55, pp.172-78.

BERGMANN, J. 1967 - "Ethnosoziologische Untersuchungen an Grab- und Hortfundgruppen der älteren Bronzezeit in Nordwestdeutschland" Germania vol. 45, pp.224-40.

BINFORD, L.R. 1971 - "Mortuary practices: their study and potential", pp.6-29 in J. A. Brown (Ed.) Approaches to Social Dimensions of Mortuary Practices. Memoirs of the Society for American Archaeology, no. 25.

BINTLIFF, J.L. 1977a - Natural Environment and Human Settlement in Prehistoric Greece, British Archaeological Reports, Suppl. Series 28, 2 vols. , Oxford.

BINTLIFF, J.L. 1977b - "New approaches to human geography. Prehistoric Greece: a case-study", pp.59-114 in F.W. Carter (Ed.) An Historical Geography of the Balkans, Academic Press, London.

BINTLIFF, J.L. 1977c - "The Number of Burials in the Messara Tholoi", pp.83-84 in D.Blackman and K. Branigan, (Eds.) "An archaeological survey of the Ayiofarango valley". Annual of the British School at Athens, vol. 72, pp.1-84.

BINTLIFF, J.L. 1981 - "Theory and reality in Palaeoeconomy: some words of encouragement to the archaeologist", pp.35-50, in Economic Archaeology, edited by A. Sheridan and G. Bailey, British Archaeological Reports, Int. Series 96, Oxford.

BINTLIFF, J.L. 1982 - "Settlement patterns, land tenure and social structure: a diachronic model", pp.106-11 in Ranking, Resource and Exchange, edited by C.Renfrew and S. Shennan, Cambridge University Press.

BLANCE, B. 1961 - "Early Bronze Age colonists in Iberia", Antiquity vol. 35, pp.192-202.

BOELICKE, U. 1977 "Das neolithische Erdwerk Urmitz", Acta Praehistorica et archaeologica 7/8, 1976/7, pp.73-121.

BOGUCKI, P.I. 1979 - "Tactical and strategic settlements in the Early Neolithic of Lowland Poland", J. of Anthropological Research, vol. 35, pp.238-46.

BOGUCKI, P.I. 1981 - "The household cluster at Brzesc Kujawski 3: Small-site methodology in the Polish lowlands", World Archaeology vol. 13, pp.59-72.

BORONEANT, V. 1970 - "La période épipaléolithique sur la rive roumaine des Portes de Fer du Danube", Praehistorische Zeitschrift vol. 45, pp.1-25.

BORONEANT, V. 1973 - "Recherches archeologiques sur la culture Schela Cladovei de la zone des 'Portes de Fer'", Dacia N.S. vol. 17, pp.5-39.

BOSCH, P.W. 1979 - "A neolithic flint mine", Scientific American vol. 240, pp.98-194.

BOSERUP, E. 1965 - The Conditions for Agricultural Growth. Allen and Unwin, London.

BOUZEK, J., KOUTECKY, D. and NEUSTUPNY, E. 1966 - The Knoviz Settlement of North-West Bohemia. Fontes Archaeologici Pragenses vol. 10, Prague.

BRADLEY, R. 1978a - The Prehistoric Settlement of Britain. Routledge and Kegan Paul, London.

BRADLEY, R. 1978b - "Colonisation and land use in the Late Neolithic and Early Bronze Age", pp.95-103 in S.Limbrey and J.G. Evans (Eds.) The effect of man on the landscape: the Lowland Zone. CBA Research Report no. 21.

BRADLEY, R. 1982 - "Position and possession: assemblage variation in the British Neolithic", Oxford J. of Archaeology 1, pp.23-38.

BRADLEY, R. and HODDER, I. 1979 - "British Prehistory: an integrated view", Man vol. 14, pp.93-104.

BRANIGAN, K. 1975 - "The round graves of Levkas reconsidered", Annual of the British School at Athens vol. 70, pp.37-49.

BRAUDEL, F. 1973 - Capitalism and Material Life 1400-1800. Fontana, London.

BRAUN, D.P. and PLOG, S. 1982 - "Evolution of 'Tribal' social networks: theory and prehistoric North American evidence", American Antiquity vol. 47, pp.504-35.

BRIARD, J. 1977 - "Les premiers métallurgistes d'Europe", La Recherche, no. 81, Sept. 1977, pp.717-25.

BRINCH PETERSEN, E. 1973 - "A survey of the late Palaeolithic and the Mesolithic of Denmark", pp.77-127 in The Mesolithic in Europe, edited by S. Kozłowski, University Press, Warsaw.

BROTHWELL, D. 1971 - "Diet, economy and biosocial

114

change in late prehistoric Europe", pp.75-87 in D.D.A. Simpson (Ed.) Economy and Settlement in Neolithic and Early Bronze Age Britain and Europe. Leicester University Press, Leicester.

BRUMFIEL, E. 1976 - "Regional growth in the Eastern Valley of Mexico", pp.234-49 in K.V. Flannery (Ed.) The Early Mesoamerican Village. Academic Press, New York.

BUKOWSKA-GEDIGOWA, J. 1976 - "Die Trichterbecher-kultur im Flussgebiet der oberen Oder", Zeitschrift für Archäologie, vol. 10, pp.22-28.

BURGESS, C.B. and SHENNAN, S. 1976 - "The Beaker Phenomenon: some suggestions", pp.309-31 in C.B. Burgess and R. Miket (Eds.) Settlement and Economy in the Third and Second Millennia BC, Britain Archeological Reports 33, Oxford.

BURL, A. 1976 - The Stone Circles of the British Isles. Yale University Press.

CARNEIRO, R.L. 1970 - "A Theory of the Origins of the State", Nature, vol. 169, pp.733-38.

CARNEIRO, R.L. 1978 - "Political expansion as an expression of the principle of competitive exclusion", pp. 205-233 in R. Cohen and E.R. Service (Eds.) Origins of the State. Institute for the Study of Human Issues, Philadelphia.

CASE, H.J. 1976 - "Acculturation and the earlier Neolithic in Western Europe", pp.45-58 in S.J. De Laet (Ed.) Acculturation and Continuity in Atlantic Europe. Brugge, De Tempel.

CHAPMAN, J. 1976 - "Biosocial aspects of the Balkan Neolithic", Nice Congress of Pre and Proto-History, Abstract.

CHAPMAN, J. 1981 - The Vinca Culture of South-East Europe. Studies in Chronology, Economy and Society. British Arch. Reps. Int. Ser. 117, Oxford.

CHAPMAN, R.W. 1975 - Economy and Society within later prehistoric Iberia: a new framework. PhD thesis, Cambridge University.

CHAPMAN, R.W. 1977 - "Burial practices: an area of mutual interest", pp.19-33 in M. Spriggs (Ed.) Archaeology and Anthropology, British Archaeological Reports, Suppl. ser. 19, Oxford.

CHAPMAN, R.W. 1978 - "The evidence for prehistoric water control in south-east Spain", J. of Arid Environments, vol. 1. pp.261-74.

CHAPMAN, R.W. 1981 - "The megalithic tombs of Iberia", pp.93-106 in Antiquity and Man: Essays in Honour of Glyn Daniel, edited by J.D. Evans, B. Cunliffe and C. Renfrew, Thames and Hudson, London.

CHAPMAN, R.W. 1981a - "The emergence of formal disposal areas and the 'problem' of megalithic tombs in prehistoric Europe", pp.71-81, in Chapman, R. et al. (Eds.) The Archaeology of Death.

CHAPMAN, R.W. 1981b - "Archaeological theory and communal burial in prehistoric Europe", pp.387-411 in I. Hodder et. al. (Eds.) Pattern of the Past.

CHAPMAN, R., KINNES, I. and RANDSBORG, K. 1981 - (Eds.) The Archaeology of Death. Cambridge University Press, Cambridge.

CHILDE, V.G. 1950 (1969) - Prehistoric Migrations in Europe. Archaeological Publications, Oosterhout N.B. The Netherlands.

CHILDE, V.G. 1951 - Social Evolution. Watts and Co., London.

CHRISTLEIN, R. and SCHMOTZ, K. 1978 - "Zur Kenntnis des jungsteinzeitlichen Grabenwerks von Kothingeichendorf", Jahresbericht des historischen Vereins für Straubing und Umgebung, vol. 80, pp.43-56.

CLARK, G. and PIGGOTT, S. 1965 - Prehistoric Societies. Hutchinson, London.

CLARKE, D.L. 1968 - Analytical Archaeology. Methuen, London.

CLARKE, D.L. 1976 - "Mesolithic Europe: the economic basis", pp.449-81 in G. Sieveking et al. (Eds.) Problems in Economic and Social Archaeology.

CLOTTES, J. et. al. 1979 - "Le village néolithique de Villeneuve Tolosane", Archeologia (Paris) 130, pp.6-13.

COLES, J.M. and HARDING, A.F. 1979 - The Bronze Age in Europe. Methuen, London.

COLES, J.M. and ORME, B. 1980 - Prehistory of the Somerset Levels. Somerset Levels Project.

COMSA, E. 1974a - "Die Bestattungssitten im rumänischen Neolithikum", Jschr. mitteldt. Vorgesch. vol. 58, pp.113-56.

COMSA, E. 1974b - "Die Entwicklung, Periodisierung und relative Chronologie der jungsteinzeitlichen Kulturen Rumäniens", Zeitschrift für Archäologie, vol. 8, pp.1-44.

CONSTANTIN, C. et.al. 1982 - "Eléments non-Rubanées du Neolithique Ancien entre les vallees du Rhin inférieur et de la Seine: VI - Groupe de Villeneuve-St-Germain", Helinium vol. 22, pp.255-71.

COONEY, G. 1979 - "Some aspects of the siting of megalithic tombs in County Leitrim", J. of Roy. Soc. of Antiqus. of Ireland, vol. 109, pp.74-91.

CZERNIAK, L. and PIONTEK, J. 1980 - "The socio-economic system of European Neolithic populations", Current Anthropology vol. 21, pp.97-100.

DANIEL, G. 1981 - "Editorial", Antiquity vol. 55, July, pp.82-84.

DARVILL, T.C. 1979 - "Court cairns, passage graves and social change in Ireland", Man, vol. 14, pp.311-27.

DARVILL, T.C. 1982 - The Megalithic Chambered Tombs of the Cotswold-Severn Region. Vorda Publications, Highworth, Wilts.

DAVIDSEN, K. 1978 - The Final TRB Culture in Denmark. A Settlement Study. Akademisk Forlag, Denmark.

DELANO SMITH, C. 1979 - West Mediterranean Europe: a historical geography of Italy, Spain and Southern France since the Neolithic. Academic Press, London.

DENNELL, R.W. and WEBLEY, D. 1975 - "Prehistoric economy and land use in Southern Bulgaria", pp.97-109 in E.S. Higgs (Ed.) Palaeoeconomy. Cambridge University Press. Cambridge.

DIXON, P.W. and BORNE, P. 1977 - Crickley Hill and Gloucestershire Prehistory. Gloucs. County Council.

DRENNAN, R.D. 1976 - "Religion and social evolution in Formative Mesoamerica", pp.345-68 in K.V. Flannery (Ed.) The Early Mesoamerican Village. Academic Press, New York.

DREWETT, P. 1979 - "New evidence for the structure and function of Middle Bronze Age round houses in Sussex", Archaeol. J. vol. 136, pp.3-11.

ELLISON, A. 1981 - "Towards a socioeconomic model for the Middle Bronze Age in southern England", pp.413-38 in I. Hodder et al. (Eds.) Pattern of Past.

ENGELS, F. 1877/8 - Herrn Eugen Dührings Umwälzung der Wissenschaft (Anti-Dühring). Marx-Engels Werke 20. pp.5-303.

ENGELS, F. 1884 - Der Ursprung der Familie, des Privateigentums und des Staats. Zurich.

EVANS, J.D. 1971a - Prehistoric Antiquities of the Maltese Islands. Athlone Press, London.

EVANS, J.D. 1971b - "Neolithic Knossos - the growth of a settlement", Procs. of the Prehistoric Soc. vol. 37, pp.95-117.

EVANS, J.D. 1973 - "Priests and People - A note on evidence for social distinctions in Prehistoric Malta", pp.215-19 in Estudios Dedicados al Profesor Dr. Luis Pericot. Instituto de Arqueologia y Prehistoria, Universidad de Barcelona.

EVANS, R.K. 1978 - "Early craft specialization: an example from the Balkan Chalcolithic", pp.113-29 in C.L. Redman et.al. (Eds.) Social Archaeology: the Future of the Past. Academic Press, New York.

EVANS-PRITCHARD, E.E. 1940 - The Nuer. A description of the modes of livelihood and political institutions of a Nilotic people. Oxford University Press.

FARRUGIA, J.P. et al. 1982 - "Eléments non-Rubanées du Néolithique Ancien entre les vallées du Rhin inférieur et de la Seine: V - Excavations in the Blicquy Group", Helinium, vol.22, pp.105-34.

FISCHER, U. 1975 - "Zur Deutung der Glockenbecherkultur", Nassauische Annalen, vol. 86, pp.1-13.

FLEMING, A. 1978 - "The prehistoric landscape of Dartmoor. Part One. South Dartmoor", Procs. Prehistoric Soc. vol. 44, pp.97-124.

FOWLER, P.J. 1978 - "Lowland landscapes: culture, time, and Personality", pp.1-12 in S. Limbrey and J.G. Evans (Eds.) The effect of man on the landscape: the Lowland Zone. CBA Research Report no. 21.

FRANKENSTEIN, S. and ROWLANDS, M.J. 1978 - "The internal structure and regional context of early iron age society in south-western Germany", Bull. of the Institute of Archaeology, University of London, vol. 15, pp.73-112.

FRIED, M.H. 1967 - The Evolution of Political Society. Random House, New York.

GABRIEL, I. 1976 - "Die Limburger Gruppe", Offa vol. 33, pp.43-60.

GALLAY, G. 1972 - "Beigaben der Frühbronzezeit Süddeutschlands in ihrer Verteilung auf Männer- und Frauengräber", Homo vol. 23, pp.50-73.

GALLAY, G. and SCHWEITZER, R. 1971 - "Das Bandkeramische Gräberfeld von Rixheim (Dép. Haut-Rhin)", Archäologisches Korrespondenzblatt, vol. 1, pp.15-22.

GAMBLE, C. 1980 - "Information exchange in the Palaeolithic", Nature vol 283, pp.522-23.

GASCO, J. 1979 - "L'Organisation économique et spatiale d'une communaute paysanne préhistorique: le groupe de Fontbouisse en Bas-Languedoc, Etudes Rurales, vol. 75, pp.5-16.

GHETIE, B. and MATEESCO. C.N. 1977 - "L'Elevage et l'utilisation des bovins au Néolithique Moyen et Tardif du Bas-Danube et du Sud des Balkans", L'Anthropologie (Paris), vol. 81, pp.115-28.

GILMAN, A. 1976 - "Bronze Age dynamics in southeast Spain", Dialectical Anthropology vol. 1, pp.307-19.

GILMAN, A. 1981 - "The development of social stratification in Bronze Age Europe", Current Anthropology, vol. 22, no. 1, pp.1-23.

GIMBUTAS, M. 1965 - Bronze Age Cultures in Central and Eastern Europe. Mouton, The Hague.

GIOT, P.-H. 1981 - "The megaliths of France", pp.82-93 in Antiquity and Man: Essays in Honour of Glyn Daniel, edited by J.D. Evans, B. Cunliffe and C. Renfrew. Thames and Hudson, London.

GRAMSCH, B. 1973 - Das Mesolithikum im Flachland zwischen Elbe und Oder. Berlin.

GUILAINE, J. 1976 - La Préhistoire Française - t.2: Les Civilisations Néolithiques et Protohistoriques de la France. C.N.R.S. Paris.

GUILAINE, J. 1981 - "Les mégalithes de Malte", La Recherche vol. 12, pp.962-71.

HALSTEAD, P. 1977 - "Prehistoric Thessaly: the submergence of civilisation", pp.23-29 in J.L. Bintliff (Ed.) Mycenaean Geography. Cambridge University Library Press, British Association for Mycenaean Studies.

HAMOND, F. 1981 - "The colonisation of Europe: the analysis of settlement processes", pp.211-48 in I. Hodder et al. (Eds.) Pattern of the Past. Studies in honour of David Clarke. Cambridge University Press, Cambridge.

HARDING, A. 1982 - "Soziale Beziehungen und die Siedlungsform in der Europäischen Bronzezeit", pp.173-83 in Palast und Hütte. Beiträge zum Bauen und Wohnen im Altertum. Philipp von Zabern, Mainz.

HASELGROVE, C. 1982 - "Wealth, prestige and power: the dynamics of late iron age political centralisation in south-east England", pp.79-88 in C. Renfrew and S. Shennan (Eds.) Ranking, Resource and Exchange. Cambridge University Press, Cambridge.

HASSAN, F. 1978 - "Demographic Archaeology", pp.49-103 in M.B. Schiffer (Ed.) Advances in Archaeological Method and Theory, vol. 1. Academic Press, New York.

HAUSLER, A. 1975 - "Die Entstehung der Trichterbecherkultur nach Aussage ihrer Bestattungssitten", pp.91-122 in Symbolae Praehistoricae.

HAYDEN, B. and CANNON, A. 1982 - "The corporate group as an archaeological unit", J. of Anthrop. Arch-

116

aeology, vol. I, pp.132-58.

HINGST, H. 1971 - "Ein befestigtes Dorf aus der Jung-steinzeit in Büdelsdorf (Holstein)", Archäologisches Korrespondenzblatt, vol. I, pp.191-94.

HINGST, H. 1976 - "Neolithische Erdgräber auf der Tannenbergskoppel in Bordesholm, Kreis Rendsburg", Jschr. mitteldt. Vorgesch. vol 60, pp.189-96.

HODDER, I., ISAAC, G. and HAMMOND, N. 1981 - (Eds.) Pattern of the Past. Studies in honour of David Clarke. Cambridge University Press, Cambridge.

HOLGATE,R. and SMITH, P. 1981 - "Landscape studies in Prehistory: two examples from Western Britain", Bull. of Inst. of Archaeology, vol. 18, pp.171-89.

HOPKINS, K. 1978 - Conquerors and Slaves. Cambridge University Press, Cambridge.

HOWELL, J.M. 1982 - "Neolithic settlement and economy in Northern France", Oxf. J. of Archaeology, vol. I, pp.115-18.

HOWELL, J.M. 1983 - Settlement and Economy in Neo-lithic Northern France. British Arch. Reports, Int. Ser. 157, Oxford.

IHMIG, M. 1971 - "Ein Bandkeramischer Graben mit Einbau bei Langweiler, Kr. Jülich, und die zeitliche Stell-ung Bandkeramischer Gräben im westlichen Verbreitungs-gebiet", Archäologisches Korrespondenz-blatt, vol. I, pp.23-30.

JACOBI, R.M. 1978 - "Population and landscape in Meso-lithic lowland Britain", pp.75-85 in S. Limbrey and J.G. Evans (Eds.) The effect of man on the landscape: the Lowland Zone. CBA Research Reports no. 21.

JARMAN, H.N. and BAY-PETERSEN, J.L. 1977 -"Agri-culture in prehistoric Europe - the Lowlands", pp.275-86 in J. Hutchinson et al. (Eds.) The Early History of Agriculture. Oxford University Press, Oxford.

JARMAN, M.R. and WEBLEY, D. 1975 - "Settlement and Land Use in Capitanata, Italy", pp.177-221 in E. S. Higgs (Ed.) Palaeoeconomy. Cambridge University Press, Cam-bridge.

JOCKENHÖVEL, A. 1974 - "Zu befestigten Siedlungen der Urnenfelderzeit aus Süddeutschland", Fundberichte aus Hessen, vol. 14, pp.19-62.

JONES, B. 1983 - "Settlement analysis of the Tavoliere Neolithic villages", unpubl. lecture to the Northern Uni-versity Archaeologists' Seminar, Manchester June 1983.

KAELAS, L. 1981 - "Megaliths of the Funnel Beaker Culture in Germany and Scandinavia", pp.141-155 in Anti-quity and Man: Essays in Honour of Glyn Daniel, edited by J.D. Evans, B. Cunliffe and C. Renfrew. Thames and Hudson, London.

KAUFMANN, D. 1975 - "Waldverbreitung und frühneolith-ische Siedlungsräume im Saalegebiet", pp.69-83 in Sym-bolae Praehistoricae.

KAUFMANN, D. 1976 - Wirtschaft und Kultur der Stich-bandkeramiker im Saalegebiet. Veröff. des Landesmus. f. Vorgeschichte in Halle, Bd. 30, Berlin.

KAUFMANN, D. 1977 - "Entdeckung und Vermessung einer befestigten linienbandkeramischen Siedlung bei Eils-leben, Kr. Wanzleben", Zeitschrift für Archäologie, vol.

II, pp.93-100.

KING, T.F. 1978 - "Don't that beat the Band? Nonegal-itarian political organization in prehistoric Central Calif-ornia", pp.225-248 in C.L. Redman et al. (Eds.) Social Archaeology: the Future of the Past. Academic Press, New York.

KINNES, I. 1982 - "Les Fouaillages and megalithic origins", Antiquity vol. 56, pp.24-30.

KIRCH, P.V. 1980 - "Polynesian prehistory: cultural ad-aptation in island ecosystems", American Scientist vol. 68, pp.39-48.

KNÖRZER, K.-H. 1979 - "Über den Wandel der an-gebauten Körnerfruchte und ihrer Unkrautvegetation auf einer niederrheinischen Lössfläche seit dem Frühneolithi-kum", pp.147-163 in Festschrift Maria Hopf, edited by U. Körber-Grohne. Rudolf Habelt Verlag, Bonn.

KOOIJMANS see Louwe Kooijmans.

KOSSE, K. 1979 - Settlement Ecology of the Early and Middle Neolithic Körös and Linear Pottery Cultures in Hungary. British Archaeological Reports, Int. Ser. 64, Oxford.

KOWALCZYK, J. 1970 - "The Funnel Beaker Culture", pp.144-77 in T. Wislanski (Ed.) The Neolithic in Poland.

KOZŁOWSKI, J.K. 1973 - "The problem of the so-called Danubian Mesolithic", pp.315-28 in The Mesolithic in Europe, edited by S. Kozlowski, University Press, Warsaw.

KRISTIANSEN, K. 1980 - "Besiedlung, Wirtschaftsstrate-gie und Bodennutzung in der Bronzezeit Dänemarks", Praehistorische Zeits, vol. 55 (I), pp.1-37.

KRUK, J. 1980 - The Neolithic Settlement of Southern Poland. (Edited by J. M. Howell and N.J. Starling). British Archaeological Reports, Int. Ser. 93, Oxford.

KUPER, R. et al. 1974 - "Untersuchungen zur neolithi-schen Besiedlung der Aldenhovener Platte, IV", Bonner Jahrbücher vol. 174, pp.424-508.

KUPER, R. and LÜNING, J. 1975 - "Untersuchungen zur neolithischen Besiedlung der Aldenhovener Platte", pp.85-97 in Ausgrabungen in Deutschland.

KUPER, R. et al. 1975 - Bagger und Bandkeramiker. Köln.

KUPER, R. et al. 1977 - Der Bandkeramische Siedlungs-platz Langweiler 9. Rheinische Ausgrabungen 18.

KURTH, G. and ROHRER-ERTL, O. 1977 - "Bemerkungen zu: "Die Lokalgruppe-die sozialökonomische Grundeinheit in der Steinzeit" von Hermann Behrens", Archaeologia Austriaca vol. 61/62, pp.9-30.

LECIEJEWICZOWA, A.K. 1970 - "The Linear and Stroked Pottery Cultures", pp.14-75 in T. Wislanski (Ed.) The Neolithic in Poland.

LEVY, J. 1978 - "Evidence of social stratification in Bronze Age Denmark", J. of Field Archaeology, vol. 5, pp.49-56.

LEWIS, H.S. 1966 - "Origins of African Kingdoms", Cahiers d'Etudes Africaines vol. 23, pp.402-07.

LEWTHWAITE, J. 1981 - "Ambiguous first impressions: a survey of recent work on the Early Neolithic of the West Mediterranean", J. of Mediterranean Archaeology and

Anthropology vol. 1, pp.292-307.

LEWTHWAITE, J. (Unpubl.) - "Social factors and economic change in Balearic Prehistory, 3000-1000 bc".

LICHARDUS, J. 1974 - Studien zur Bükker Kultur. Saarbrücker Beiträge zur Altertumskunde Bd. 12. Rudolf Habelt Verlag, Bonn.

LIES, H. 1974 - "Zur neolithischen Siedlungsintensität im Magdeburger Raum", Jschr. mitteldt. Vorgesch. vol. 58, pp.57-111.

LINKE, W. 1976 - Frühestes Bauerntum und Geographische Umwelt. Ferdinand Schönigh, Paderborn.

LIVERSAGE, D. 1976 - "L'Origine de la sépulture en tertre en Europe septentrionale" Abstract, Résumés des communications, 9th Congress of the Pre- and Protohistoric Sciences Union, 13-18 Sept. 1976, Nice.

LOUWE KOOIJMANS, L.P. 1976a - "Local developments in a borderland", Oudheidkundige Medelingen Ait Het Rijksmuseum van Oudheden Te Leiden, 1976, pp.227-96.

LOUWE KOOIJMANS, L.P. 1976b - "The Neolithic at the Lower Rhine - Its structure in chronological and geographical respect", pp.150-73 in S.J. De Laet (Ed.) Acculturation and Continuity in Atlantic Europe. Brugge, De Tempel.

LÜNING, J. 1976a - "Ein neues Model zur Siedlungsweise der Bandkeramik", Abstracts pp.291-2, Résumés des communications, 9th Congress of the Pre- and Protohistoric Union, Nice, 13-18 Sept. 1976.

LÜNING, J. 1976b - "Zur Erforschung des Neolithikums (Alt-bis Jung-neolithikum) in der BRD seit dem Jahre 1960", Jschr. mitteldt. Vorgesch., vol. 60, pp.31-48.

MACHNIK, J. 1974 - "Die Siedlungsprobleme der Mierzanowice-Kultur in Kleinpolen", Zbornik Filozofickej Fakulty Univerzity Komenskeho, Musaica, 25 (14), pp.23-35.

MADSEN, T. 1978 - "Toftum -- Ein neues neolithisches Erdwerk bei Horsens, Ostjütland (Dänemark)", Archäologisches Korrespondenzblatt, vol. 8, pp.1-7.

MADSEN, T. 1979 - "Earthen Long Barrows and timber structures: aspects of the Early Neolithic mortuary practice in Denmark", Procs. of the Prehistoric Soc. vol. 45, pp.301-20.

MADSEN, T. 1982 - "Settlement systems of early agricultural societies in E. Jutland, Denmark: a regional study of change", J. of Anthrop. Archaeology, vol. 1. pp.197-236.

MANBY, T.G. 1980 - "Bronze Age settlement in Eastern Yorkshire", pp.307-70 in J. Barrett and R. Bradley (Eds.) The British Later Bronze Age. British Archaeological Reports, 83, Oxford.

MANIA, D. and PREUSS, J. 1975 - "Zur Methoden und Problemen ökologischer Untersuchungen in der Ur- und Frühgeschichte", pp.9-59 in Symbolae Praehistoricae.

MASTERS, L. 1981 - "Chambered tombs and non-megalithic barrows in Britain", pp.161-76 in Antiquity and Man: Essays in Honour of Glyn Daniel. Edited by J. D. Evans, B. Cunliffe and C. Renfrew. Thames and Hudson, London.

MEGAW, J.V.S. and SIMPSON, D.D.A. 1979 - (Eds.) Introduction to British Prehistory. Leicester University Press.

MEIKLEJOHN, C. 1978 - "Ecological aspects of population size and growth in late-glacial and early postglacial north-western Europe", pp.65-79 in P. Mellars (Ed.) The Early Postglacial Settlement of Northern Europe: An Ecological Perspective. Duckworth, London.

MEILLASSOUX, C. 1972 - "From reproduction to production", Economy and Society vol. 1, pp.93-105.

MERCER, R. 1980 - Hambledon Hill. A Neolithic landscape. Edinburgh University Press, Edinburgh.

MERCER, R. 1981 - The Stepleton Enclosure - 1981 Interim Report - Hambledon Hill Fieldwork and Excavation Project (cyclostyled).

MEYER-CHRISTLEIN, W. 1976 - "Die Y-Pfostenstellung in Häusern der Älteren Linearbandkeramik", Bonner Jahrbücher, vol. 176, pp.1-25.

MILISAUSKAS, S. 1976 - "Olszanica, an early farming village in Poland", Archaeology vol. 29, pp.30-41.

MILISAUKAS, S. 1978 - European Prehistory, Academic Press. New York.

MILISAUKAS, S. and KRUK, J. 1978 - "Bronocice - A Neolithic settlement in southeastern Poland", Archaeology vol. 31, pp.44-52.

MODDERMAN, P.J.R. 1970 - Linearbandkeramik aus Elsloo und Stein. Anal. Praeh. Leid. 3.

MODDERMAN, P.J.R. 1971 - "Bandkeramiker und Wanderbauerntum", Archäologisches Korrespondenzblatt vol. 1, pp.7-9.

MODDERMAN, P.J.R. 1972 -"The Aveburys and their continental counterparts", pp.99-106 in To Illustrate the Monuments, edited by J.V.S. Megaw. Thames and Hudson, London.

MODDERMAN, P.J.R. 1975 - "Elsloo, a Neolithic farming community in the Netherlands", pp.260-86 in R. Bruce-Mitford (Eds.) Recent Archaeological Excavations in Europe. Routledge and Kegan Paul, London.

MODDERMANN, P.J.R. 1976 - "Theorie und Praxis bei der Erforschung des Früh-neolithikums im Gebiet des Niederrheins und der Maas", Jschr. mitteldt. Vorgesch. vol. 60, pp.49-60.

MODDERMAN, P.J.R. 1982 - "Eléments non-Rubanées du Neolithique Ancien entre les vallées du Rhin inférieur et de la Seine: VII - Conclusion Générale", Helinium, vol. 22, pp.272-73.

MOHEN, J.P. 1977 - "Les tumulus de Bougon", Bull. Soc. Hist. et sc. des Deux-Sèvres, vol. 10, pp.397-440.

MORGAN. L.H. 1877 - Ancient Society. London.

MÜLLER-KARPE, H. 1968 - Handbuch der Vorgeschichte, Band 2, Jungsteinzeit. Beck Verlag, München.

NANDRIS, J. 1970 - "The development and relationships of the Earlier Greek Neolithic", Man vol. 5 (2), pp.192-213.

NANDRIS, J. 1976a "Changing premises of exploitation in r-and K- societies during the Early Neothermal Period in South-East Europe (c.10,000 - -3000bc)", Unpubl. lecture (cyclostyled) to the Brit. Assoc. for Advancement of Science at Lancaster, Sept. 1-8, 1976.

118

NANDRIS, J. 1976b - "Some factors in the Early Neo-thermal settlement of south-east Europe", pp.549-56 in G. Sieveking et al. (Eds.) Problems in Economic and Social Archaeology.

NANDRIS, J. 1977 - "The perspective of long-term change in South-East Europe", pp.25-57 in An Historical Geography of the Balkans, edited by F.W. Carter. Academic Press, London.

NANDRIS, J. 1978 - "Some features of Neolithic Climax Societies", Studia Praehistorica, Sofia, 1978, 1-2, pp.198-211.

NEMESKERI, J. 1976 - "La structure paléodémographique de la population Vlasac: Yougoslavie, (Epipaléolithique, Pre-Néolithique)", Abstract, p.262, Résumés des communications, 9th Congress of the Pre- and Proto-historic Union, Nice 13-18 Sept. 1976.

NEUSTUPNY, E. 1969 - "Economy of the Corded Ware cultures", Archaeologicke Rozhledy, vol. 21, pp.43-67.

NEUSTUPNY, E. and J. 1961 - Czechoslavakia Before the Slavs. Thames and Hudson, London.

NEWELL, R.A. 1973 - "The Postglacial adaptations of the indigenous population of the Northwest European Plain", pp.399-440 in S. Kozłowski (Ed.) The Mesolithic in Europe. University Press, Warsaw.

NORWEGIAN ARCHAEOLOGICAL REVIEW 1970 - vol. 3, pp. 4-34 "Analytical Archaeology", review papers.

O'KELLY, M.J. 1976 - "Some thoughts on the megalithic tombs of Ireland", pp.125-133 in To Illustrate the Monuments, edited by J.V.S. Megaw. Thames and Hudson, London.

OTTO, K.-H. 1960 - Deutschland in der Epoche der Urgesellschaft. Lehrbuch der dt. Gesch. Bd. I, Berlin.

PAULIK, J. 1974 - "Zur Bedeutung der jungbronzezeitlichen Hügelgräber in der urzeitlichen Entwicklung der Slowakei", Slovenska Archeologia, vol. 22, pp.73-81.

PAVELCIK, J. 1973 - "Befestigte Industriezentern der Träger Badener Kultur und ihr Platz in der gesellschaftlich-ökonomischen Entwicklung des östlichen Teiles Mitteleuropas". Zbornik Filozofickej Univerzity Komenskeho, Musaica, vol. 24(13), pp.41-49.

PAVLU, I. 1977 - "To the methods of Linear Pottery Settlement Analysis", Pamatky Archeologicke vol. 68, pp.5-55.

PAVUK, J. 1972 - "Neolithisches Gräberfeld in Nitra", Slovenska Archeologia vol. 22, pp.5-105.

PAVUK, J. 1976 - "Zur einigen Fragen der Entwicklung der neolithischen Besiedlung in der Westslowakei", Jschr. mitteldt. Vorgesch. vol. 60, pp.331-42.

PEACOCK, D.P.S. 1969 - "Neolithic pottery production in Cornwall", Antiquity vol. 43, pp.145-49.

PEEBLES, C.S. and KUS, S.M. 1977 - "Some archaeological correlates of ranked societies", American Antiquity vol. 42, pp.421-448.

PEQUART, M. et al. 1937 - Téviec, station-nécropole mésolithique du Morbihan. Archives de l'Institut de paleontologie humaine, 18. Masson, Paris.

PEQUART, M. and S.-J. 1954 - Hoëdic, deuxième station-nécropole du Mésolithique cotiér armoricain. De Sikkel, Antwerp.

PHILLIPS, P. 1975 - Early Farmers of West Mediterranean Europe. Hutchinson University Library, London.

PHILLIPS, P. 1980 - The Prehistory of Europe. Allen Lane, London.

PHILLIPS, P. 1982 - The Middle Neolithic in Southern France - Chasséen Farming and Culture Process. British Arch. Reports, Int. Ser. 142, Oxford.

PHILLIPS, A.P. and MOORE, A.M.T. 1981 - "The origins of farming in the Mediterranean", paper delivered at the 10th Congress of the Union of Pre- and Protohistoric Sciences, Oct. 19-24, 1981, Mexico.

PIGGOTT, S. 1965 - Ancient Europe. Edinburgh University Press.

PIGGOTT, S. 1982 - Scotland Before the Scots. Edinburgh University Press.

PLESLOVA-STIKOVA, E. 1977 - "Die Entstehung der Metallurgie auf dem Balkan, im Karpatenbecken und in Mitteleuropa, unter besonderer Berücksichtigung der Kupferproduktion im Ostalpenländischen Zentrum (Kultur-Ökonomische Interpretation)", Pamatky Archeologicke, vol. 68, pp.56-73.

PODBORSKY, V. 1976 - "Erkenntnisse auf Grund der bisherigen Ausgrabungen in der Siedlung mit mährischer bemalter Keramik bei Tesetice-Kyjovice", Jsch. mitteldt. Vorgesch. vol. 60. pp.129-48.

POLGAR, S. 1975 - "Population, evolution, and theoretical paradigms", pp.1-25 in S. Polgar (Ed.) Population, Ecology and Social Evolution. Mouton, the Hague.

PRICE, B.J. 1977 - "Shifts in production and organisation: a Cluster-Interaction model", Current Anthropology, vol. 18, pp.209-33.

PRYOR, F. 1978 - Excavation at Fengate, Peterborough, England: The Second Report. Archaeology Monograph 5, Royal Ontario Museum.

RANDSBORG, K. 1974a - "Social stratification in Early Bronze Age Denmark: a study in the regulation of cultural systems", Praehistorische Zeitschrift. vol. 49, pp.38-61.

RANDSBORG, K. 1974b - "Population and social variation in Early Bronze Age Denmark", Kuml 1973/4, pp.197-208.

RANDSBORG, K. 1974c - "Prehistoric populations and social regulation: the case of Early Bronze Age Denmark", Homo vol. 25, pp.59-67.

RANDSBORG, K. 1975 - "Social Dimensions of Early Neolithic Denmark", Procs. of the Prehistoric Soc. vol. 41, pp.105-18.

RANDSBORG, K. 1982 - "Rank, rights and resources - an archaeological perspective from Denmark", pp.132-139 in Renfrew and Shennan (Eds.) Ranking, Resource and Exchange.

RENFREW, C. n.d. - "Settlement organisation and resource exploitation in South-East Europe and the Aegean, 6000 to 1000 BC" unpubl. paper delivered to the Anglo-Russion Colloquium, Cambridge.

RENFREW, C. 1967 - "Colonialism and megalithismus", Antiquity vol. 41, pp.276-88.

RENFREW, C. 1969 - "The autonomy of the South-East European Copper Age", Procs. of the Prehistoric Soc. vol. 35, pp.12-47.

RENFREW, C. 1972 - The Emergence of Civilisation: the Cyclades and the Aegean in the Third Millennium BC. Methuen, London.

RENFREW, C. 1973a - Before Civilisation. Jonathan Cape, London.

RENFREW, C. 1973b - "Monuments, mobilization and social organization in neolithic Wessex", pp.539-58 in C. Renfrew (Ed.) The Explanation of Culture Change. Duckworth, London.

RENFREW, C. 1974 - "Beyond a subsistence economy: the evolution of social organisation in prehistoric Europe", pp. 69-95 in C.B. Moore (Ed.) Reconstructing Complex Societies. Bulletin of the American Schools of Oriental Research 20, Suppl.

RENFREW, C. 1975 - "Trade as action at a distance: questions of integration and communication", pp.3-59 in Ancient Civilisation and Trade edited by J.A. Sabloff and C.C. Lamberg-Karlovsky. University of New Mexico Press, Albuquerque.

RENFREW, C. 1976 - "Megaliths, territories and populations", pp.198-220 in S.J. de Laet (Eds.) Acculturation and Continuity in Atlantic Europe. Brugge, De Tempel.

RENFREW, C. 1977 - "Alternative models for exchange and spatial distribution", pp.71-90 in Exchange Systems in Prehistory, edited by T.K. Earle and J.E. Ericson. Academic Press, New York.

RENFREW, C. 1978 - "Varna and the social context of early metallurgy", Antiquity vol. 52, pp.199-202.

RENFREW, C. 1979a - Investigations in Orkney. Thames and Hudson, London.

RENFREW. C. 1979b - "Transformations", pp.3-44 in C. Renfrew and K.L. Cooke (Eds.) Transformations: Mathematical Approaches to Culture Change. Academic Press, New York.

RENFREW, C. and SHENNAN, S. 1982 - (Eds.) Ranking, Resource and Exchange. Cambridge University Press, Cambridge.

RENFREW, J.M. 1979 - "The first farmers in South East Europe", pp.243-65 in Festschrift Maria Hopf, edited by U. Körber-Grohne. Rudolf Habelt Verlag, Bonn.

ROWLANDS, M.J. 1973 - "Modes of exchange and the incentives for trade, with reference to later European prehistory", pp.589-600 in The Explanation of Culture Change, edited by C.Renfrew, Duckworth, London.

RUGGLES, C.N.L. and WHITTLE, A.W.R. 1981 - (Eds.) Astronomy and Society in Britain during the period 400 - 1500 BC. British Archaeological Reports 88, Oxford.

SAHLINS, M.D. 1963 - "Poor man, rich man, big man, chief: political types in Melanesia and Polynesia", Comp. Studies in Society and History, vol. 5, pp.285-303.

SAHLINS, M.D. 1968 - Tribesmen. Prentice-Hall, Englewood Cliffs.

SAHLINS, M.D. 1974 - Stone Age Economics. Tavistock Publications, London.

SAKELLARIDIS, M. 1979 - The Mesolithic and Neolithic of the Swiss Area. British Archaeological Reports, Int. Ser. 67, Oxford.

SANGMEISTER, E. 1972 - "Sozial-ökonomische Aspekte der Glockenbecherkultur", Homo, vol .23, pp. 188-203.

SAUTER, M.-R. 1976 - Switzerland. Thames and Hudson, London.

SAVORY, H.N. 1968 - Spain and Portugal. Thames and Hudson, London.

SAXE, A.A. 1970 - Social Dimensions of Mortuary Practices. Ph.D. Dissertation, University of Michigan (unpubl.)

SCARRE, C. 1980 - "Neolithic camps around the Marais Poitevin", Current Archaeology, no. 72, pp.23-5.

SCHACHERMEYR, F. 1976 - Die Agäische Frühzeit. Band I: Die Vormykenischen Perioden. Verlag der Osterreichishen Akademie der Wissenschaften, Wien.

SCHALICH, J. 1973 - "Geologische und bodenkundliche Befunde", pp.292-296 in W. Göbel et al. Naturwissenschaftliche Untersuchungen an einer späthallstattzeitlichen Fundstelle bei Langweiler, Kr. Düren, Bonner Jahrbücher vol. 173, pp.289-315.

SCHILD, R. 1976 - "Flint mining and trade in Polish prehistory as seen from the perspective of the chocolate flint of Central Poland. A second approach" Acta Archaeologica Carpathica vol. 16, pp.147-77.

SCHRÖTER., P. 1975 - "Zur Besiedlung des Goldbergs in Nordlinger Ries" pp.147-77 in Ausgrabungen in Deutschland

SCHWABEDISSEN, H. 1979 - "Die 'Rosenhof-Gruppe', Ein Neuer Fundkomplex des Frühneolithikums in Schleswig-Holstein", Archäologisches Korrespondenzblatt, vol. 9 pp.167-72.

SERVICE, E.R. 1962 - Primitive Social Organization. Random House, New York.

SERVICE, E.R. 1971 - Primitive Social Organisation. 2nd Edition, Random house, New York.

SHENNAN, S.J. 1975 - "Die soziale Bedeutung der Glockenbecker in Mitteleuropa". Acta Archaeologica Carpathica vol. 15, pp.173-80.

SHENNAN, S.J. 1977 - "The appearance of the Bell Beaker assemblage in central Europe", pp.51-70 in R. Mercer (Ed.) Beakers in Britain and Europe. British Archaeological Reports, Int. Ser. 26, Oxford.

SHENNAN, S.J. 1980 - "Cluster Interaction and the European Early Bronze Age", paper delivered at the Conference on Relations between the Near East, the Mediterranean World and Europe, 3rd-1st mill. BC, Aarhus 17-22 August 1980 (Unpubl.).

SHENNAN, S.J. 1982 - "Ideology, change and the European Early Bronze Age", pp.155-161 in I. Hodder (Ed.) Symbolic and Structural Archaeology. Cambridge University Press.

SHERRATT, A.G. 1976 - "Resources, technology and trade", pp.557-81 in Sieveking, G. et al. (Eds.) Problems in Economic and Social Archaeology.

SHERRATT, A.G. 1981 - "Plough and pastoralism: aspects of the secondary products revolution", pp.261-305 in I.

120

Hodder et al. (Eds.) Pattern of the Past.

SHERRATT, A.G. 1982 - "Mobile resources: settlement and exchange in early agricultural Europe", pp.13-26 in C. Renfrew and S. Shennan (Eds.) Ranking, Resource and Exchange. Cambridge University Press, Cambridge.

SHERRATT, A.G. 1982a - "The development of Neolithic and Copper Age settlement in the Great Hungarian Plain. Part I: the regional setting", Oxf. J. of Archaeology, vol 1, pp.287-316.

SHERRATT, A.G. 1983 - "The development of Neolithic and Copper Age settlement in the Great Hungarian Plain. Part II: site survey and settlement dynamics", Oxf. J. of Archaeology, vol. 2, pp.13-41.

SIELMANN, B. 1971 - "Zum Verhältnis von Ackerbau und Viehzucht im Neolithikum Südwestdeutschlands", Archäologisches Korrespondenzblatt, vol. 1, pp.65-8.

SIELMANN, B. 1972 - "Die frühneolithische Besiedlung Mitteleuropas", pp.1-65 in J. Lüning (Ed.) Die Anfänge des Neolithikums vom Orient bis Nordeuropa: Westliches Mitteleuropa. Fundamenta Va. Bühlau Verlag, Koln.

SIELMANN, B. 1976 - "Der Einfluss der geographischen Umwelt auf die linien-und stichbandkeramische Besiedlung des Mittelelbe-Saale-Gebietes", Jschr. Mitteldt. Vorgesch . vol. 60, pp.305-29.

SIEVEKING, G. de G., LONGWORTH, I.H. and WILSON, K.E. 1976 - (Eds.) Problems in Economic and Social Archaeology. Duckworth, London.

SMAGLIJ, N.M. 1982 - "Grosse Tripolje-Siedlungen zwischen Dnepr und Südlichem Bug", Das Altertum, vol. 28, pp.118-25.

SOUDSKY, B. 1962 - "The Neolithic site of Bylany", Antiquity vol. 36, pp.190-200.

SOUDSKY, B. and PAVLU, I. 1971 - "The Linear Pottery Culture, settlement patterns of Central Europe", pp.317-328 in Man, Settlement and Urbanism, edited by P. Ucko et al., Duckworth, London.

SPRATT, D.A. and SIMMONS, I.G. 1976 - "Prehistoric activity and environment on the North York Moors", J. of Arch. Science vol. 3, pp.193-210.

SREJOVIC, D. 1972 - Lepenski Vir. Thames and Hudson, London.

STARLING, N.J. 1983 - "Neolithic settlement patterns of Germany", Oxf. J. of Archaeology, vol. 2, pp.1-7.

STARTIN, W. 1978 - "Linear Pottery Culture houses: reconstruction and manpower", Proceedings of the Prehistoric Soc., vol. 44, pp.143-159.

STARTIN, W. and BRADLEY, R. 1981 - "Some notes on work organization and society in prehistoric Wessex", pp.289-96 in C.L.N. Ruggles and A.W.R. Whittle (Eds.) Astronomy and Society.

STERUD, E.L. 1976 - "Obre and the question of Butmir origins: a quantitative evaluation", Abstracts p.354, Résumés des communications, 9th Congress of the Pre-and Protohistoric Union, Nice, 13-18 Sept. 1976.

STEWARD, J.H. 1969 - "Postscript to bands: on taxonomy, processes and causes", pp.228-95 in D. Damas (Ed.) Contributions to anthropology: Band societies. National Museums of Canada, Bull. no. 228.

STRAHM, C. 1977 - "Kontinuität und Kulturwandel im Neolithikum der Westschweiz", Fundberichte aus Baden-Württemberg vol. 3, pp.115-43.

STRÖMBERG, M. 1974 - "Soziale Schichtungen in der älteren Bronzezeit Südschwedens", Die Kunde, vol. 25 (N.F.), pp.89-101.

SYMBOLAE PRAEHISTORICAE 1975 - Festschrift Schlette. Wiss. Beitr. Martin-Luther Univ., Halle.

TABACZYNSKI, S. 1972 - "Gesellschaftsordnung und Güteraustausch im Neolithikum Mitteleuropas", Neolithische Studien I, pp.31-96.

TAINTER, J.A. 1978 - "Mortuary practices and the study of prehistoric social systems", pp. 106-143 in M.B. Schiffer (Ed.) Advances in Archaeological Method and Theory, I. Academic Press, New York.

THEOCHARIS, D.R. 1973 - "The Neolithic Civilisation. A brief survey", pp.17-110 in D.R. Theocharis (Ed.) Neolithic Greece, National Bank of Greece, Athens.

TINE, S. 1975 - "Passo di Corvo - Ausgrabungen in einem neolithischem Dorf auf dem Tavoliere della Puglia", Antike Welt vol. 3, pp.27-32.

TODOROVA, H. 1978 - "Die Nekropole bei Varna und die sozialökonomischen Probleme am Ende des Aneolithikums Bulgariens", Zeitschrift fur Archäologie, vol. 12, pp.87-97.

TODOROVA, H. 1980 - Review of I.S. Ivanov 'Die Schätze der Warnaer chalkolithischen Nekropole', Germania, vol. 58, pp.169-174.

TRINGHAM, R. 1971 - Hunters, Fishers and Farmers of Eastern Europe, 6000-3000 BC, Hutchinson University Library, London.

TRINGHAM, R. 1978 - "A re-appraisal of Gordon Childe's concepts of the Agricultural and the Urban Revolution: recent research in Europe and the European USSR", pp.57-70 in D. Shimkin et al. (Eds.) Anthropology for the Future. University of Illinois, Dept. of Anthropology Res. Rep. 4.

TRINGHAM, R. et al. 1980a - "The early agricultural site of Selevac, Yugoslavia", Archaeology, 1980, March-April, pp.24-32.

TRINGHAM, R. 1980b - "Research design and planning behavioural analysis", paper given at the 45th Annual Meeting of the Society for American Archaeology, Philadelphia, April-May, 1980.

TRUMP. D. 1976 - "The collapse of the Maltese temples", pp.605-609 in Sieveking, G. et al. (Eds.) Problems in Economic and Social Archaeology.

TRUMP, D. 1980 - The Prehistory of the Mediterranean. Allen Lane, London.

TRUMP, D. 1981 - "Megalithic architecture in Malta", pp.128-140 in Antiquity and Man: Essays in Honour of Glyn Daniel, edited by J.D. Evans, B. Cunliffe and C. Renfrew. Thames and Hudson, London.

UCKO, P.J. 1969 - "Ethnography and archaeological interpretation of funerary remains", World Archaeology, vol. 1, pp.262-277.

VAN DE VELDE, P. 1979 - "The Social Anthropology of a Neolithic cemetery in the Netherlands", Current Anthropology, vol. 20, pp.37-58.

VAQUER, J. 1981 - "D'étranges fosses néolithiques", La Recherche, vol. 12, no. 124, pp.882-3.

VITA-FINZI, C. and HIGGS, E.S. 1970 - "Prehistoric economy in the Mt. Carmel area of Palestine: site catchment analysis", Procs. Prehistoric Soc. vol. 36, pp.1-37.

VLADAR, J. 1974 - "Mediterrane Einflüsse auf die Kulturentwicklung des nördlichen Karpatenbeckens in der älteren Bronzezeit", Preist. Alp., vol. 10, pp.219-36.

WADDELL, J. 1978 - "The invasion hypothesis in Irish prehistory", Antiquity vol. 52, pp.121-28.

WALKER, M.J. 1981 - "Climate, economy and cultural change: the S.E. Spanish Copper Age", pp.171-97 in Miscelanea -Abstracts, 10th Congress of the Pre- and Protohistoric Union. Mexico, 19-24 Oct. 1981.

WARREN, P. 1975 - The Aegean Civilisations. Elsevier-Phaidon, London.

WELINDER, S. 1975 - Prehistoric Agriculture in Eastern Middle Sweden. Acta Archaeologica Lundensia series in 8 Minore No. 4, Lund.

WHITEHOUSE, R. 1981 - "Prehistoric setlement patterns in Southeast Italy", pp.157-65 in Archaeology and Italian Society, Ed. G. Barker and R. Hodges. British Arch. Reports, Int. Ser. 102.

WHITTLE, A.W.R. 1977a - The Earlier Neolithic of Southern England and its Continental Background. British Archaeological Reports, Suppl. Ser. 35. Oxford.

WHITTLE, A.W.R. 1977b - "Earlier neolithic enclosures in north-west Europe", Procs. of the Prehistoric Soc. vol. 43, pp.329-48.

WHITTLE, A.W.R. 1978 - "Resources and population in the British Neolithic", Antiquity vol. 52, pp.34-42.

WHITTLE, A.W.R. 1980 - "Two Neolithics?", Current Archaeology Nos. 70-1, pp.329-34 and 371-73.

WHITTLE, A.W.R. 1980a - "Scord of Brouster and early settlement in Shetland", Arch. Atlantica vol. 3, pp.35-55.

WHITTLE, A.W.R. 1981 - "Later Neolithic society in Britain: a realignment", pp.297-342 in C.L.N. Ruggles and A.W.R. Whittle (Eds.) Astronomy and Society.

WHITTLE, E.H. and ARNAUD, J.M. 1975 - "TL dating of Neolithic and Chalcolithic pottery from sites in Central Portugal", Archaeometry vol. 17, pp.5-24.

WILSON, E.O. 1975 - Sociobiology: the new synthesis. Harvard University Press.

WINN, S.M. and SHIMABUKU, D. 1980 - "Responses to deteriorating agricultural conditions at Grotta Scaloria, Southeastern Italy, during the Neolithic", Unpubl. paper delivered at the 45th Annual Meeting of the Society for Anerican Archaeology, Philadelphia, May 1-3, 1980.

WISLANSKI, T. 1970 - (Ed.) The Neolithic in Poland. Wrocław.

WOBST, H.M. 1974 - "Boundary conditions for Palaeolithic social systems: a simulation approach", American Antiquity vol. 39, pp.147-78.

ZAPOTOCKY, M. 1966 - "Streitäxte und Streitaxtkulturen", Pamatky Archeologicke vol. 57, pp. 172-209.

4

SOCIAL EVOLUTION:
EUROPE IN THE
LATER NEOLITHIC AND COPPER AGES

Andrew Sherratt

Introduction: reconstructing prehistoric societies

Although archaeological information about the later Neolithic and Copper Ages[1] has increased enormously since the later part of the last century, its interpretation in social terms has remained at a relatively primitive level. While the need to deal with underlying social processes has been increasingly stressed in recent years, many of the concepts employed have been no more than revivals of nineteenth-century schemes. Technological change and the unilinear development of increasingly hierarchical forms of society still lie at the base of many current interpretations.

One symptom of this is the frequent appearance of the term 'chiefdom', covering a wide range of social forms from the groups encountered by the Romans in the later Iron Age to the Copper Age inhabitants of Bulgaria or the megalith-building Neolithic farmers of western Europe. Looking for 'the indian behind the artifact' (in Robert Braidwood's phrase) has become increasingly difficult when there is nothing to be seen but chiefs.

This uncertainty as to when social stratification actually arose is symptomatic of the problems of describing European prehistory by comparison, say, with that of the Near East. While we have a fairly refined vocabulary for dealing with the various stages in the emergence of complex urban societies, Europe's stubborn failure to organize itself until just before the arrival of the Romans leaves us with some 6,000 years of social development for which a simple division into 'tribal' or 'chiefly' seems hopelessly inadequate. It is especially primitive by comparison with the sophistication of our typological and chronological analyses, which allow us to divide this same period into nearly 20 major cultural divisions, many themselves subdivided into three or four phases.

The temptation in interpreting the archaeological record of the later Neolithic and Copper Ages is thus to see some sort of cumulative growth of social complexity, with evidence such as monument-building or minority burial reflecting emerging hierarchies. Terms such as 'chiefdom' have become stretched to include earlier and earlier examples of prehistoric societies. The account presented here takes a different point of view: it tries to explore the variety in early agricultural societies in terms of non-hierarchical forms of social organization. Although social change did not benefit all sections of the population equally, it is misleading to see prehistory simply in terms of the increasing domination of an elite. We need to look more closely at the problems faced by communities in different circumstances and the sorts of power relations that emerged in each case. While such societies may demonstrate a considerable degree of cultural complexity, this does not necessarily take the form of centralization, ranking and stratification.

Recent debates on social evolution

A problem common to many discussions of 'social evolution' is the use of categories derived from contemporary ethnography and their application to long-term archaeological sequences. From Lewis Henry Morgan (1877) onwards evolutionary writers have put forward schemes defining successive 'stages of culture': savagery-barbarism-civilization (Clark 1946) ; band-tribe-chiefdom-state (Service 1962); egalitarian-ranked-state (Fried 1967); and so forth. While differing in detail, they share the same logic: they attempt to convert static snapshots into a dynamic sequence. Such schemes are now increasingly under attack. The band to state sequence - that most used by archaeologists - has now been trenchantly criticized by its own author (Service 1968, p.169). Recent bands, he noted, were often the smashed remnants of more complex systems dislocated by western colonial impact. Tribes, in the sense of discrete political units, were often created by interaction with more organized units (Fried 1978); chiefdoms and simple states frequently arose in reaction to slave-raiding and the trading opportunities offered by contact with the west (Stevenson 1968). Even if we do not treat the whole band-tribe-chiefdom-state continuum simply as a reflection of the differential impact of colonial contact, these arguments at least point to differing degrees of social complexity in the ethnographic record as being largely related to positions within the 'macro von Thünen rings' of a recent world system - a geographical zonation as a result of historical interaction around a few major centres.

The difficulty of interpreting archaeological sequences in social terms is thus that of mapping an observed spatial variability onto an inferred chronological sequence of social forms reconstructed from artifactual remains. Not only do the two bodies of evidence -ethnographic and archaeological observations - differ in their raw material, but they also reflect different parts of the process of global development. Many of the 'chiefdoms' of the ethnographic record reflect secondary consequences of the existence of states that cannot be projected back into periods before the emergence of the state. The time has now come to re-assert the independent validity of archaeological data, which offer too multivariate a pattern to be constrained within arbitrary partitions of a homogenized universal succession. For this reason the following discussion takes a more inductive view of the archaeological evidence, in searching for internal contrasts before seeking external comparisons in world ethnography.

This point of view coincides with that of a number of recent commentators (e.g. Yoffee 1979) who have criticized the association of 'social evolution' with unilinear schemes and the failure to deal with individual examples of social change. The current search for 'ideological' contrasts between prehistoric European societies (Shennan 1982, Hodder 1982b) represents an attempt to define the particular properties of social groups that otherwise escape gross characterization as 'stages of development'. However, an immediate appeal to the intangible bypasses precisely those areas of social analysis which recent fieldwork has done most to illuminate: the interaction between communities and their landscape through time. While an awareness of the symbolic organization through which social contrasts are expressed is an improvement on a simplified social ecology, it is in itself insufficient as an explanation of the course of change.[2]

Another recent set of approaches which by stressing the dynamics of inter-group competition may be said to have a primary concern with social change, have their inspiration in recent Marxist thought (Friedman and Rowlands 1977; cf. Godelier 1977). Even these, however, have been most successful in defining the processes which precede and accompany the onset of urbanization, and set up the structures of interaction and dependence around the core areas of established states (Friedman and Rowlands 1977, Nash 1978, Rowlands et al. in press). While these help to make sense both of classic areas of ethnographic work (e.g. in Africa) and many aspects of later Bronze and Iron Age Europe, they lose much of their force when projected backwards to earlier periods of European prehistory, when these kinds of interaction did not take place, at least outside the Mediterranean.

Central to Service's (1962) definition of the 'chiefdom' was the idea of redistribution. Within the general wave of Marxist reaction to 'stages of culture' models and the 'modernization theory' which they imply (e.g. Renfrew 1972) has been an attack on the idea of redistribution as the function of emerging elites. By incorporating Polanyi's typology of exchange (reciprocity, redistribution, markets) into his sequence of tribes, chiefdoms and states, Service tied the neo-evolutionary view to a specific interpretation of economic anthropology. Much of Polanyi's work has now been discredited, both within those parts of the ancient world which were its inspiration (Adams 1974; Yoffee 1982), and also in its application to ethnographic examples of chiefdoms such as Polynesia, where control of critical resources is now seen as the basis of elite power rather than a benevolent concern with the re-distribution of scattered commodities (Earle 1977). This interpretation has been applied to European prehistory by Antonio Gilman (1981), who has characterized the increasing evidence for social stratification in later European prehistory as a consequence of the advantages which accrued to powerful groups able to seize control of capital investment in fixed facilities - olive groves, fishing grounds and ploughs. The application of this principle, however, is not simple - as will be seen below - for technological innovations such as the scratch-plough often served to release constraints rather than rigidify them, and scarcity of basic resources was a cyclical rather than a unilinear phenomenon. Moreover this process was relative to the opportunities of particular landscapes, whose individual properties emerged at different times in the filling-up of the continent (Sherratt 1972). Nevertheless Gilman's suggestion is timely, in

emphasizing the motivation of specific groups as the source of change, rather than the well-being of society as a whole. While these recent contributions to the debate on 'social evolution' have widened the range of factors to be considered, they have not yet been applied to the full range of the archaeological record, and in particular have still to make use of the great regional variety which is a striking feature of later Neolithic and Copper Age societies in Europe. A full understanding of these phenomena can only come from the conjunction of general principles with the opportunities of specific landscapes and the patterns of interaction which can be traced between them. The present contribution thus seeks to define the nature of some of the observed variability on a continental scale, and so to sketch how the interpretation of local sequences may be articulated in a wider context.

Some principles of interpretation

A characteristic feature of the agrarian societies under discussion is their propensity for continuing change, at a faster rate than contemporary non-agrarian societies in southern Africa or North America, for instance, though slower than that of farming groups in many parts of the Near East. While we need not resort to single-factor explanations such as that of 'population pressure' (Spooner 1972) or 'social competition' (Bender 1978), this constant alteration is a necessary assumption for the present level of discussion. It relates to the introduction of agricultural resources into a temperate woodland zone, and in a wider context is characteristic of the Holocene as a whole, irrespective of the particular resources concerned, as a function of the long-term building-up of population densities through the late Quaternary (Cohen 1977). The relative slowness of change in Europe relates both to the high friction of distance in a forested landscape, and the relative homogeneity of the temperate European environment. In both these respects Europe contrasts with the Near East, with its easier contacts across steppe landscapes and the marked local ecological diversity resulting from exotic water sources within a semi-arid zone. These factors lead to a faster rate of development in the Near East, where urban societies were already emerging at the time under discussion. Yet the different ecological conditions of temperate Europe resisted the reproduction of such advanced social structures for another two millennia, and European societies were able to absorb selected elements of higher technology without themselves being incorporated into the chain of secondary states reaching back to Egypt and Mesopotamia. The relative isolation of Europe from the increasingly interlinked societies of the Near East is illustrated for instance by the individual and generally primitive nature of early copperworking traditions, by comparison with the alloy-based complex moulding techniques which had already appeared over a wide area from Anatolia to southern Iran. European societies were not linked to this wider network until the third millennium BC, when the opening up of northern Europe, the linkage of Mediterranean coastal networks, and the expansion of steppe populations created a chain of emerging elites along which innovations could travel. Even so it was only in the Aegean during the second millennium BC that direct influences from the commercial core areas of the Near East had a significant effect on the course of social development (Sherratt and Sherratt in press). Variability within the continent of Europe during the Neolithic and Copper Age does not have the simple character of core and periphery which can be detected in the later Bronze Age around the expanding commercial networks of the Mediterranean.

Other reasons must thus be sought for contrasts within European societies in the later Neolithic and Copper Ages, and a number of factors may be suggested.

1   Regional adaptation   Perhaps the most obvious factor is the diversity of environmental zones which make up the continent of Europe. Early agricultural settlers selected only a fraction of the available landscapes and created a series of more or less uniform regions which contrast one with another. Thus south east Europe formed an entity which contrasts both with the Mediterranean and with the loess-covered plains of central Europe. Further expansion added the areas of sandy outwash sheets and morainic lakes in the North European Plain, and the scarplands and coastal areas of Western Europe. Settlement of these areas brought an additional element of diversity through the continuing existence there of substantial native (Mesolithic) populations.

This diversity increased again as internal colonization took place and the full range of landscapes was encountered in each region. Environmental changes consequent upon agricultural land-use also further enhanced regional contrasts, through processes such as podsolization and bog-formation which occurred more rapidly in the areas of higher rainfall in the west. In addition, economic differentiation occurred as particular forms of land-use emerged in response to local conditions; in the Mediterranean the use of tree-crops, extensive sheep-rearing and fishing added new areas of limestone uplands, islands and coasts, giving this region an increasingly distinctive character. The addition of new zones of settlement reduced the importance of some previously nodal areas, like Thessaly in the south or some of the loess areas next to the North European Plain, creating a new topology of inter-regional links.

2   Succession   Related to the existence of a range of environmental opportunities is the idea of a succession of types of social organization as a consequence of the gradual filling up of the landscape. Each area thus has its local trajectory, with specific problems at each stage of expansion and particular forms of territorial demarcation in relation to critical areas of land under a given system of land-use. This principle also applies to the manipulation of non-subsistence commodities in response to shifting patterns of demand. The opportunities for exchange depend on the structural position of a given area in relation to the resources and requirements of its neighbours. Supplies of domestic animals, hard rocks or metal ores may at different times have given a trading advantage to particular areas within a wider network, so that even within a zone of uniform settlement type the differential flows of material created contrasts in wealth. A shifting pattern of local florescences, related to changing patterns of demand for particular commodities may thus be expected and helps to explain why certain areas appear to occupy nodal positions at certain times and not at others (Sherratt 1982).

The pattern of growth predicted from this principle consists not only in successive stages of exploitation of particular landscape zones, but also of characteristic cycles of colonization and territorial demarcation within them, in which certain types of site (e.g. settlement or burial mound) may have a temporary role in particular phases of expansion. Social organization in specific areas may similarly become temporarily more complex and then devolve, as the context changes, as well as manifesting a sequence of regional stages.

Although this principle is primarily chronological, it may be manifested in spatial terms if there is a time-lag in its operation from one area to another. This is, indeed, the case in Europe, where agricultural settlement spread basically from east to west and the local successions were initiated at times which differed by up to three millennia.

3   Interaction   The sequences discussed above did not take place in isolation, even if initially the patterns of interaction were mainly local in scale. While 'intercontinental' relationships between European and Near Eastern societies did not occur in a continuous way until the Bronze Age, there was nevertheless an increasing scale of interaction among the component regions of later Neolithic and Copper Age Europe. The wider structures which defined the role of particular areas thus became successively larger in size. The earlier Neolithic exchange systems, as defined by distribution areas for items like Breton dolerite, Sardinian obsidian, or Krzemionki banded flint in the early fourth millennium were characteristically limited in scale with a radius of 200kms; by the later Neolithic and Copper Age such commodities as jadeite, copper, Grand Pressigny flint or Krzemionki flint in the later fourth millennium had a radius of up to 800kms. (Sherratt 1976, Lech and Leligdowicz 1980). The contrast is well exemplified in the Carpathian Basin, where Neolithic flint supplies were predominantly from within the Basin, while in the Copper Age there were considerable imports from Little Poland and Wolhynia (Kaczanowska 1980).

Moreover the character of traded goods shows an increasing use of items whose principal interest was their exotic character, rather than their use value - for instance copper ornaments, hammer-headed pins, or carved bone plaques. This increasing exploration of the cultures of adjacent regions coincided with a significant transfer of features which formerly had a role only in local systems: horses, woolly sheep, alloy metallurgy, single graves, which were capable of transforming existing systems by the injections of new elements. This process produced 'corridors' within the wider inter-regional structure - the North European Plain, the Mediterranan, the Atlantic facade - and new nodal areas within this larger network. Yet there is no inevitably unilinear element even in the expanding range of exchange linkages. The Beaker network represents a peak of inter-regional interaction which was a temporary episode within a specific structural context - the culmination of a cycle rather than a stage within a cumulative process of growth.

These three principles may be used to order and perhaps partly explain some of the features of the archaeological record of this time. Even in combination, however, they are insufficient to explain the observed pattern of later Neolithic and Copper Age variability. Their uniformitarian and deterministic character fails to deal with contrasts such as that between the British Isles and adjacent areas of the continent, or the individual character of the Maltese islands within the Mediterranean. To approach this problem, a fourth principle is required.

4   Trajectory maintenance and discontinuity   Many apparently stadial phenomena result from the rapid imposition of systems developed in nuclear areas on less fast-moving peripheries. For instance the contrast between 'Mesolithic' and 'Neolithic' ways of life is in fact as much geographical as chronological, as economies based on cereals increasingly intruded into neighbouring areas whose subsistence was based on the increasingly intensive cropping of local resources. In other parts of the world, this process was less abrupt and indigenous sequences were able to develop further before being radically restructured by outside contact. Temperate North America offers a relevant example, where the florescence of monument-building and trading in exotica that characterizes phenomena such as Hopewell, for instance, preceded rather than resulted from the spread of cereal cultivation from further south. Indeed it is now suggested that the apparent 'cultural decline' of the later Woodland period in fact represents a period of increased stability and security in food supplies, with cereal cultivation requiring a less complex and certainly less spectacular socio-cultural system.

There are two points to note here. One is the way in which a 'Mesolithic' system, if preserved from outside interference, may manifest far more complex properties than would be inferred from the truncated sequence of early postglacial Europe. The other is the way in which new subsistence elements that may actually raise popula-tion levels and energy flows can at the same time cause a simplification or decentralization of social structures.

While this has a direct bearing on specific features of the European sequence, such as the contribution of Mesolithic communities to the megalithic phenomenon, or the likely effect of the introduction of the plough on the social systems of temperate horticulturalists, it also raises a more general issue. In interpreting the appear-ance of phenomena such as monument-building horizons and local 'florescences', it is the specific local situation and its structural problems that are relevant, not some hypothetical average sequence of stages of complexity. We should expect rather than be surprised by divergences from the general pattern - especially where relative isolation allows a greater degree of trajectory mainten-ance and even the emergence of new properties with an established framework. Conversely, in areas which are axially placed in relation to corridors of contact, dis-continuities in cultural development should be evident which cannot be explained purely by their position in local successions.

It is this kind of variability which characterizes semi-isolated regions such as the woodlands of Europe and North America. Structural principles which were rapidly superseded in nuclear areas may have continued to be important in the more drawn-out sequences of social change where urbanization was a relatively late feature. Rather than trying to see in the European prehistoric sequence an increasingly ranked series of societies in which successively more powerful chiefdoms succeeded one another at each opportunity, it may be more profit-able to explore alternative descriptions of social organ-ization.

One of the striking features of the west European archaeological record is the abundant evidence of ritual monuments which are not accompanied by elaborate individual burials or residences. Instead of always looking for hierarchization, it may become appropriate in such contexts to look for a different principle, that of ritual formalization as the basis of social order. To equate certain artifacts - monumental tombs, rare or craft-made items (Renfrew 1973) in the later Neolithic of western Europe - with 'chieftainship' may be to miss the essential character of such societies, and to obscure both their essential similarity to earlier Neolithic societies and their contrast with contemporary groups further east.

It is clear that this approach requires European prehistory to be treated as a whole, and that it is necessary to go beyond the artifactual manifestations to postulate underlying similarities in social organization which may cross-cut conventional divisions. Such social forms may have no direct correspondence to that of any particular group within the ethnographic record; but while this makes the task of such reconstruction more difficult, it also makes the attempt more worthwhile as a contribu-tion to the general study of pre-literate societies.

Evolutionary pathways

The basic regional structure of Neolithic and Copper Age societies was established by the arrival of agricultural groups and their interaction with native communities.[3] Along the main axis of agricultural spread, in the Balkans and the central European loesslands, the dominant process was one of colonization. By 5000 BC the unity of 'Danubian' cultures across the loess, from western Hungary in the south to the Low Countries and the western Ukraine in the north, was already established. Cultures of the Balkan group with a core area of tell settlements in Bulgaria and southern Jugoslavia extended northwards into Romania and eastern Hungary. In the central and west Mediterranean (Lewthwaite 1982), the successive adoption of sheep and pottery by native littoral groups was increasingly supplemented by cultivation as the complex expanded from its coastal base. The main surviving zone of hunting and collecting groups lay in a broad arc from the British Isles, across Scandinavia and the north European Plain, to the marshes of eastern Europe which drain into the Black Sea. As the Atlantic forests thickened and the climax trees of the mixed oak forest shaded out pioneer species such as hazel, the nuts and game resources of forest areas declined in product-ivity and concentrated the attention of native groups on coasts, lakes and rivers where fish and molluscs provided a substantial part of the diet.

Two processes, therefore, dominated the develop-ment of European societies in the period following this initial establishment of agriculture: one was the differ-entiation and linkage of the increasingly copper-using groups of south-east and south-central Europe; the other was the expansion of agricultural groups and their inter-action with native populations in the outer arc. As a result of these processes, the relative regional homo-geneity of the first agricultural communities gave way to a diversity both within and between regions, that reached its climax during the fourth millennium BC before giving way to a degree of uniformity within the new corridors of contact which were opened up - the Mediterranean, the North European Plain, the Steppes and the Atlantic Sea-board.

The first question, therefore, is the nature of the changes that were taking place in south east Europe during the fifth millennium BC. This period encompasses the climax of the pattern established in the Balkans during the seventh and sixth millennium, and illustrates a relatively pure 'successional' change in that these societ-ies then underwent an important transformation without interference from adjacent zones.

The climax of the tell cultures is represented by a variety of groups whose ceramic distinctiveness is a hallmark of the period. There is a profusion of substantial settlement sites, rich in the imported materials of everyday life: obsidian, greenstone axes, shell beads. Female figurines, often in elaborate settings of painted clay altars and shrines, are a characteristic feature; though burials (often still in household clusters within settlements rather than in formal cemeteries) are not marked by large accumula-tions of grave goods. I have tried elsewhere (Sherratt 1982) to sketch how these systems may have operated. There is no reason to suppose that these groups were composed of anything other than autonomous communities and lineages. What is evident is an elaboration of material culture, particularly the decorative elements, at the same time as an increase in **regional** trade: an intensive production of locally specific pottery types, the production of local specialities like salt and perhaps linen textiles, and a massive transfer of materials like obsidian and flint between adjacent highland and lowland zones. There is also a special emphasis on ritual elements - figurines and house decoration, in south east Europe, and also some of the first ritual monuments like Kyjovice Tesetice (Moravia), Schalkenburg (central Germany) or Kothingeichendorf (Bavaria) in the related area of the central European loess belt (Höckmann 1972).

These two elements, regional trade and ritual, give a clue to the social mechanisms that organized and linked such communities. The wealth of everyday objects, manufactured to high standards of craftsmanship, represent more than satisfaction of material needs. The flow of such items was clearly vital to social reproduction as much as material survival. This would explain the large quantities of items at the top end of the range of utilitarian goods - well-finished axes, fine pottery, good flint or obsidian tools - that occur in such profusion. Such quantities of valuables were generated by social rather than economic needs (cf. Douglas and Isherwood 1978). Anyone who has a small child is familiar with this principle: every visitor or relative sends another toy digger, fire engine or teddy bear on social occasions, quite beyond the propensity of the child to consume such wealth (he has boxes full upstairs). Similarly with these Neolithic settlements: every site is a bonanza to the archaeologist, who finds great quantities of museum-worthy objects (stored in boxes downstairs) that originally circulated to cement alliances, to purchase wives, or to compensate for offences.

If relations between communities rested on alliances and the flow of material valuables, the proliferation of items with ritual associations suggests that this was important in regulating social life within the community. The common forms of figurines suggests that these ritual codes were widely shared between groups. Indeed the contrasts between archaeological cultures in this context (e.g. Vinca and Tisza, to take two classic Childean examples), which are evident in their figurine designs and decorative styles but not in their more mundane objects, are likely to reflect not breaks in social interaction (Hodder 1982a) but the limits of particular, consciously held, ideological systems. The general form of these ideologies was probably very similar in the different areas in which they were expressed, since the typical female figurines are all variations on a theme. The basic features of this cult may even be reproduced in very different cultural contexts, though similar social circumstances, in other parts of Europe for which the shadowy presence of a mother goddess has been inferred. We shall return later to the megalithic temples of Malta, but it is perhaps worth noting the association of such Neolithic societies with the worship of female deities or earth spirits. It is this kind of association that lies behind older views - going back to Lewis Henry Morgan and surviving in the canon of Marxist orthodoxy - which describe Neolithic society as 'matriarchal' (e.g. Neustupny and Neustupny 1961).

In settlement terms, this phase was characterized by big sites - large communities of several lineage groups with their own burial areas - aggregating for co-operation and defence. In such acephalous groups, intensification of warfare is the other side of the coin from the intensification of trading and ritual activity, and competition between communities for the acquisition of material goods involved both alliance and hostility (Sherratt 1982).

This, then, is what I mean by ritual formalization in an east European context. The actual social structures that underlay these archaeological manifestations remain to be defined, but we may bear in mind the elaboration of cross-cutting ties - clans and sub-clans, moieties and ceremonial associations - that ethnography suggests may

be relevant, and that do not involve hierarchy. Their material evidence, in the form of ceremonial houses, dancing grounds, symbolic oppositions or totemic signs, should not be beyond the perception of archaeology.

The hallmark of this type of system - which archaeologically we may term the 'mature' Neolithic, to respect its time-transgressive character and avoid regional terminologies - is the presence of an abundance of material items, mostly of an unspectacular kind, that are imported but not rare, moved by active regional trading networks and circulating as small valuables. Allied to this is the pervasive ritual and symbolic character of material culture in general, which nevertheless lacks the marks of individual rank and achievement.

Some time around the middle of the fifth millennium BC this system was radically changed, marking the beginning of what is locally termed the 'Copper Age' (Sherratt 1982). The tight regional groupings disappeared; settlements dispersed or became less continuously occupied; burials received greater emphasis (often being easier to find than the settlement); the bulk of regionally traded products was replaced by smaller quantities of exotic items (notably copper and gold); objects symbolizing individual status appeared (shafthole axes); the figurines became more schematic and less overtly female; and there are greater contrasts in these new forms of wealth both within regions and in individual cemeteries. The use of ritual within established and long-lived communities was thus replaced by an apparently more fluid system in which more explicit statements about rank were necessary, and a wider range of competition was possible. Even so there is little indication of hierarchy: the rich burials are the end of a continuum, and occur within the same cemeteries as the others - there was no mobilization of labour for a Fürstengrab like Helmsdorf or Łeki Małe. Nor are there hoards in the same way as in the Bronze Age.

This pattern continued into the fourth millennium when agricultural settlement was expanding onto the Steppes and the North European Plain. These movements of expansion on the periphery did not take place in isolation: for the increasing scale of inter-regional trade from the Carpathian Basin and the Balkans reached even the outer margins, in Denmark and the Ukraine. These long-distance links were associated with shifts in the centres of prosperity within south east Europe. Instead of the central agricultural areas, in Thrace or the Körös depression for instance, the areas which rose to prominence were on the edges, at nodal positions between regional systems: in east Slovakia, at Tibava by the critical passes through to the Ukraine (modern frontier crossing-point at Uzgorod); on the Black Sea coast at Varna, with its spectacular, gold-filled graves perhaps indicating access to the Anatolian gold; in Kujavia (Brzesc Kujavski) on the interface with the North European Plain. Access to metal sources and control of the trade routes was the key to economic and social success, as the rich graves in these areas testify, and the products which crossed regional boundaries included Wolhynian flint in eastern Hungary (Kaczanowska 1980) - especially the long flint dagger blades - and also the first hoards (Bökönyi 1978), in return for the Balkan/Carpathian copper objects which appeared at this time as far afield as Ukraine and in Early Neolithic contexts in Denmark.

Although this theme is clearly relevant to the developing picture in northern Europe, we will follow through the sequence in south east Europe down to the end of the fourth millennium BC; for there follows a classic example of a discontinuity caused by the incorporation of new features from a neighbouring region. That region was the Steppes, where major developments were now occurring. The expansion of population into the dry interfluves altered the economic role of this region in a fundamental way. It now came to act as a bridge between the peripheral Near Eastern cultures of the Caucasus and those of south east Europe: and many of the features involved in adaptation to the steppe landscape were also relevant to the increasingly open parts of temperate Europe. The early transfer of horses has already been mentioned, though these early specimens -doubtless objects of wonder and curiosity - did not survive as a local breeding stock. Equally important (though contacts with Anatolia may have been equally relevant here) were new breeds of sheep that are evident from the increased size of European stocks at this time (Bökönyi 1974). I personally believe, though cannot prove, that the plough was also introduced through these new contacts (Sherratt 1981).

In any case, a radical change in the settlement structure of south east Europe took place at this time, which accelerated the divergence of truly Mediterranean areas (where tree crops now became important) from inland areas. In the Carpathian Basin, the change is manifested in a major shift of population to previously marginal areas both on the edges of the Basin and the surrounding valleys penetrating into the uplands, and on the sandy interfluves within it like the area between the Danube and Tisza (Sherratt 1982). Within the interstices created by this shift, some actual penetration of Steppe tribes seems to have occurred (Ecsedy 1979), for example on the Tisza and lower Danube. As with the Late Woodland phenomenon mentioned above, the effect of a more secure subsistence base was to render some of the spectacular efforts of the previous period largely unnecessary: there is no later-fourth-millennium equivalent to the Varna cemetery, and indeed a relative recession in the copper industry. Social differences were now perhaps evident in more basic ways - between village headmen buried with their draught oxen and their local followers in the Alsonemedi cemetery for instance - than between generally wealthy communities in nodal regions and poorer populations in the hinterlands. Such a foundation had the potential for a taller edifice of social structure, in which hierarchical divisions could cut deeper than ever before - the beginning of the Bronze Age pattern - though it was another millennium before these divisions were to become evident in the rich, fortified centres of Early Bronze Age Hungary, Romania and Slovakia.

And so back to central and northern Europe. While the south east had a protracted early agrarian sequence unaffected by neighbouring developments, north west Europe was from the beginning in contact with a wider network. It was also an area of greater diversity, from the relatively dense coastal native populations to the pioneer farmers of the loess bridgehead. Inevitably, therefore, it did not simply replicate the stages defined for Balkan and Carpathian Europe; though at a deeper level there are some significant resemblances.

The sequence on the loess corridor of central Europe has something of a transitional character: it reflected some of the developments of the south east, but its limited area rather reduced its importance in the fourth and third millennia when the surrounding regions were opened up. This change in role makes it difficult to treat as an independent entity and it will therefore be considered in conjunction with its northern and western hinterlands. The increasing aggregation of settlement that was characteristic of the early fifth millennium in the Carpathian Basin (Sherratt 1982) was repeated during the later fifth and early fourth millennia in the central European zone. The clusters of hamlets that were characteristic of the pioneer phase, for example in the Rhineland, were replaced by nucleated, enclosed villages of

long-houses. Already, however, small groups were penetrating northwards into the interstices of established Mesolithic groups around the lakes of the North European Plain, and a complex pattern of interaction was beginning.

The origins of the northern Neolithic cultures (TRB) have conventionally been sought either in continuity from local Mesolithic groups or in some fresh wave of agricultural population from further south (e.g. Troels Smith 1952; Becker 1954). The present picture suggests that the new pattern of farming cultures that united both the North European Plain and the northern loesslands, actually originated from interaction on the interface between the two. In some areas, such as Scandinavia, the expansion of farming seems to have followed a relative collapse of local resources (Rowley-Conwy in press); in others, such as Brittany, some kind of fusion seems to have occurred; in the British Isles, colonization into empty niches seems more likely. Despite these diverse origins, a strongly convergent pattern came about, in which scattered hamlets were focussed on small burial-monuments and enclosures that provided continuing points of integration between a diversity of exploited zones. Already, however, there were significant regional exchange systems, which at certain points articulated with long distance chains reaching back to central and south east Europe; though these imported objects did not serve to mark an elite in the same way as in Hungary or Bulgaria (Randsborg 1979).

These relatively small-scale systems, limited in territorial extent, were greatly enlarged at the same time as the radical shift which transformed Balkan and Carpathian Copper Age groups. The appearance of plough-marks in northern Europe suggests that these phenomena had a common cause, and that in both areas the use of plough cultivation greatly enlarged the area which could be exploited for agriculture. The effect of this technological innovation, on two contrasting socio-economic systems, was very different: rather than changing the direction of development, as in the south east, this more extensive form of agriculture actually intensified propensities already present in north western Europe.

One effect was greatly to extend the area under cultivation, absorbing in the process many of the remnant communities of hunters and fishers. This was accomplished, however, within the existing framework: the megalithic tombs became larger and more elaborate, taking the form of passage-graves rather than simple burial-chambers; the enclosures which seem to represent a level of local integration above that of the monumental tombs reached a peak and then declined; and existing methods of exploiting raw materials either for tools (e.g. flint) or ornaments (e.g. amber) were greatly enlarged. In the loess area this progress was manifested in a shift from the riverine strip to the edge of the inter-fluvial zone (Kruk 1973, 1980); though since this area lacked the local diversity of the north western landscape the foci of this process were nucleated (and now often defended) villages (Bronocice, Dölauer Heide) rather than burial monuments. The common basis of all these societies, however, was an attachment to place and the rituals which were performed there, rather than to individuals of a particular rank.

How were these societies integrated, and in particular how do they compare in this respect with the various stages defined for south east Europe? My impression is that despite their contemporaneity with the Copper Age and Early Bronze Age groups of that area, they were fundamentally more similar to those of the late Neolithic tell climax, in which ritual (manifested both in the monuments and the artifacts), rather than rank, was the organizing principle. As with these earlier 'mature' Neolithic communities, the artifactual repertoire does not distinguish symbols of individual rank, but rather offers a broad range of often finely-made domestic items - such as decorated pottery, stone axes and amber beads - which did not themselves act as sumptuary markers of a particular rank, but served to structure social relations through their use as valuables. Burials were not accompanied by impressive quantities of wealth objects associated with particular individuals, although burial itself was a focus of ritual which involved both monumental construction and the disposal of wealth. The tombs are usually communal, and convey meaning by the arrangement of the bones, rather than by varying quantities of personal grave-goods, which often take the form of offerings at the monument as a whole. Emphasis was on the community rather than the individual, and effort was expended not to commemorate powerful leaders but to enhance corporate prestige and territorial integrity.

Moreover burials in monumental tombs probably represent only a part of the total population; though this in itself does not imply a system of social stratification. The tombs should not be considered as a means of disposing of the dead, but rather of giving significance to selected people whose death was of importance to the groups involved. There was often a considerable interval between death (and exposure of the corpse, which was perhaps the usual means of disposal) and interment in a tomb. The remains selected for such treatment were probably not those of people who occupied a particular rank in their own lifetime, but venerated ancestors who stood in critical genealogical positions in relation to group fissioning.

The main contrast between 'mature Neolithic' groups in south east and north west Europe, then, is the elaboration of mortuary ritual which characterizes the latter. It can be argued that this is more an expression of local ecology than of fundamental differences in social organization. Funerary monuments are typical of areas of early agricultural settlement beyond the loess, and are associated with the particular conditions of the North European Plain and the Atlantic coastlands - unlike the defended centres, which also occur on the loess. Monumental tombs are characteristic of areas where settlement was still constrained - note their occurrence in clusters and linear arrangements in relation to river-valleys - but where large aggregated communities were not possible. They represent foci and territorial markers for an expanded (though not dispersed) pattern of settlement, particularly in core areas like the Danish islands where settlement was relatively dense. Other types of non-monumental 'earth-graves' occur in less densely settled zones like western Jutland (Randsborg 1975), where a seasonally mobile way of life may have persisted, that was perhaps also characteristic of the earliest phase of settlement in the core area. The monuments thus mark a phase of saturation and the crystallization of defined territorial units.

Such monumental tombs served not only to legitimate rights to particular territories, but were also agents of social control within the groups. One striking feature, both of long barrows and 'causewayed' enclosures, is the composite nature of their construction - reflected in discontinuous quarry ditches as well as constructional compartments[4] that seem to relate to corporate work-groups involved in their construction. Rather than simply representing the tombs of different lineages, therefore, the tombs may be the products of cross-cutting local associations which provided a focus of political allegiance. This would be particularly important if surviving Mesolithic groups retained a corporate existence within the agrarian territorial structure, and such monuments would thus be particularly developed in areas where native populations were integrated into Neolithic societies at a local level.

This interpretation of the social basis of the megalith-building groups of north west Europe does not imply that such groups were essentially egalitarian - in the sense that there was no conflict of interests between different status- and kinship-groups - for it is basic to the idea of such ritual-centred organizations that competition took place between (probably exogamous) local units, and that certain sections of the population (notably senior men) exercise dominance within them. But authority was localized, and there was no hierarchy in the sense of successive tiers of authority: rather, dominant groups promoted a common ideology which supported their own interests within the unit, and left them free to engage in competition for prestige between units. This probably took the form of competitive feasting - 'fighting with wealth' - involving both consumption of subsistence goods and the ritual destruction of material items, e.g. pot-smashing. Differences in wealth between units (whether communities or lineages) are therefore to be expected and are indeed manifested in the different quantities of offerings associated with communal tombs, just as there are notably 'wealthy' settlements among the Neolithic villages of south east Europe. Such differences in wealth, however, do not add up to a conical pattern of ranking between communities and these must still be considered as largely autonomous.

This parallelism with the 'mature Neolithic' phase of the south eastern sequence is even more striking in its transition to a pattern which reversed many of these elements - the disappearance of large, central sites and the dispersal of population; the decline in ritual elements and the appearance of status-symbolic artifacts; the development of long-distance trade (especially in metal) rather than in common regional items. These new features characterize the Corded Ware cultures that succeeded the variety of megalith-building groups throughout the North European Plain and initiated the pattern than was to characterize the second millennium BC; and in this sense, it may still be useful to describe the Corded Ware and Beaker periods as 'Copper Age'.

One evident feature of this period was a major phase of internal colonization penetrating more deeply into the inter-fluvial areas of the loess and cover sands, and extending agrarian occupation to the outwash sands of the North European Plain. Settlement had a greater fluidity, with less substantial and long-lived sites, and a shorter-term investment in burial monuments: single graves under round barrows[5] rather than long megalithic or earth-built structures. Material culture had a more segmentary character; a consistently replicated series of status-kits comprising a personal drinking vessel and weapon (battle axe) which accompanied a large number of males to the grave. These symbols became internationalized to a much larger extent, even integrating neighbouring hunting and fishing groups within a single framework of status codes, as in central Scandinavia and the Baltic regions.

This pattern did not emerge in a uniform way over the whole of the North European Plain. It seems to have crystallized earlier in the east, perhaps in central Germany and eastern Poland, and to have spread like a domino effect westwards into the megalithic heartlands, as far as the North Sea. This complex seems to have penetrated within and around the established TRB communities of the Low Countries and Scandinavia, before absorbing them into the new pattern. It opened up a new east-west corridor that articulated at its eastern end with the expanding Steppe groups, transmitting horses and woolly sheep (as well as artifacts such as hammer-headed bone pins) directly across the open landscape of northern Europe, and restructuring the communities of the adjacent loess belt. It did not, however, penetrate westwards as far as the British Isles or large parts of northern France (Seine-Oise-Marne culture), where the earlier pattern of territorially focussed communities persisted (Howell 1982).

This linkage, from the forest Steppe to the Atlantic sea-board, was a manifestation of the speed of forest clearance on the lighter soils of the North European Plain. The increased size of cultivated area allowed a greater development of the pastoral sector of a mixed farming economy based on light plough agriculture, with an emphasis on the male role in warfare and protection of an acquired territory. It produced a similar, segmentary social structure over a large interconnected area, with the ability to penetrate and corrode the more static structures of surrounding groups. In the following centuries, this pattern was to spread, and be further enriched, by contact along the Atlantic coast, the Rhone, and across the western Alps: the Bell Beaker network.

It is now time to consider the third major geographical division, the central and western Mediterranean. During the earlier fourth millennium there was no major opening up of new areas for settlement as in northern Europe, and a relatively stable pattern of large villages with stone or rock-cut tombs occupied the more fertile zones within it, at a relatively low overall density. Exchange networks carrying material such as obsidian linked islands such as Sardinia with the adjacent mainland, but these had a limited, regional scope. Some signs of the elaboration of territorial foci were in evidence, in the beginning of megalithic construction in Iberia and in the prototypes of the trefoil-shaped temples in Malta.

As in north west Europe, the mid-fourth millennium saw an increase in the scale of these activities, without a discontinuity of developmental trajectory. Tomb and temple construction became more elaborate, with a concomitant appearance of small cult objects such as female figurines. Craft production developed, with copper axes supplementing stone ones and pottery bearing a profusion of ornamental and symbolic signs including the 'oculus' motif.

These features bear a general resemblance to those of the megalithic cultures of north west Europe and they probably shared a similar form of social organization. Increasingly, however, a further process of spatial expansion and inter-regional linkage introduced new elements, both from northern Europe and from the east Mediterranean. This expansion can plausibly be attributed to the use of the light plough, which assisted in the opening up of the interfluves in the same way as in other areas of Europe at this time, and to specific features of the drier Mediterranean environment: the cultivation of tree crops along with an expansion of sheep rearing, and also fishing. An important outcome was the colonization of new areas, particularly high-lands like the limestone plateaux of Languedoc and islands like Lipari, which acted as nodal points in inter-regional contacts. Fortification was a notable feature of Mediterranean settlement patterns, both at large villages such as Los Millares (Almeria)[6] and smaller fortified enclosures like Zambujal (Portugal) and Lébous (southern France). The new external links promoted the rapid spread of particular features such as bastion fortification which can be traced throughout the length of the Mediterranean. These contacts can also be seen in portable artifacts, like the distribution of Castelluccio bone plaques.

This growing network of regional links within the Mediterranean began to be articulated with the long distance routes reaching down from northern Europe. The characteristic combination of drinking vessel (sometimes a beaker but often a local form of handled cup) and

personal weapons (now a dagger and arrows rather than a battleaxe) began to appear in male graves, though normally these were rock cut tombs more appropriate to a Mediterranean environment than the earthen barrows of the north. This emphasis on the male warrior began to replace that on the female figure in representations, stelae and rock engraving.[7] The transition was most rapid in Italy and southern France, with their more direct northward connections, but also penetrated to the islands (e.g. Corsica). In Iberia the change was less clear-cut, and was only fully complete in the second millennium with the appearance of the Argaric culture with its male warrior burials. The pattern of settlement in the Mediterranean, however, continued to be based on defended centres now often positioned on spectacular heights.

As with the British Isles in relation to the North European Plain, there were spatial limits to this penetration, and in peripheral areas an older stratum survived and continued to develop along its own lines. In Malta the temples serving a female divinity reached a peak of elaboration in the earlier third millennium, culminating in the massive structures of Tarxien and the nearby Hypogeum. The stability of these temple-centres, of which over a dozen are known, is indicated by their cumulative re-building and extension, and this territorial stability must be related to the finite size and relative isolation of the island; these laboratory conditions allowed the undisturbed growth of perhaps the most complex of these ritual-centred organizations.

Britain itself must also be considered as part of the archaic fringe to which continental innovations were introduced at a relatively late stage, and which continued to develop along its existing trajectory to take an older pattern to new heights of elaboration. While large enclosures and other monuments to territorial stability largely disappeared in adjacent areas of the continent during the third millennium BC, many parts of the British Isles saw a renewed phase of monumental construction, either of large passage graves like Maes Howe or Newgrange in northern and western Britain in the later fourth millennium, or of henges like Avebury or Durrington Walls - the latter being significantly close to earlier territorial foci - in the south in the third millennium BC. The scale of such construction, however, was entirely new; and the ritual landscapes of the British chalklands - for instance the triangle of Avebury and its avenues, the 'Sanctuary' and Silbury Hill - represent a concentration of effort unparalleled before. In this case, the relative isolation from the Corded Ware 'domino effect' was reinforced by the local setting of continued territorial expansion, which was internally focussed within the chalk-lands and adjacent gravel terraces, rather than externally directed to the large areas of outwash sands as it was in the North European Plain. This elaboration of ritual and territorial foci seems to have been an alternative to the segmentary organization reflected in Beaker 'status-kits', which began to be represented in parts of Britain, outside the main henge areas. This 'Beaker' pattern led to the formation of rich individual burials in Wessex itself shortly before 2000 BC, associated with the erection of stone settings in the earlier earth and timber henges, e.g. at Avebury and Stonehenge. The 'Beaker' pottery lost its role as a status item and merged with the rest of the domestic pottery assemblage to form the basis of the Bronze Age wares of the second millennium. These were associated with a major spatial expansion into more marginal areas outside the earlier chalkland foci, in the manner of Corded Ware and Early Bronze Age expansion on the Continent.

This third-millennium phase of ritual monuments represented by henges, like the Maltese temples discussed above, clearly went beyond the simple, relatively autonomous character of earlier ritual-centred forms of social organization. They may well have been associated with a specialized ritual caste with access to esoteric (e.g. astronomical) knowledge, rather than simply being run by lineage heads or village elders in the way that may be imagined for earlier Neolithic ritual monuments. But although they were able to mobilize impressive quantities of labour, this apparently did not extend to the accumulation of surplus produce or the extensive patronage of manufacturing operations based upon it. These properties and the 'conical' patterns of ranking that underlay them, only emerged from the more explicitly individualizing warrior-centred form of organization associated with Corded Ware and Beakers.

Conclusion: space, time and social structure

This brief review of the contrasts between successive and contemporary groups in different parts of Europe demonstrates the difficulty of applying any simple scheme of social evolution to this phase of maximum diversification. Nevertheless, some common elements have been identified, as well as trends which were to result in a much greater degree of convergence during the Bronze Age.

A basic theme of discussion has been the contrast between east and west. Many of the most conspicuous artifacts of this phase - the megalithic and earthen monuments of western Europe - have no direct parallels in the east. Yet the types of society which they represent may, at a deeper level, have a fundamental resemblance to already superseded stages of social development in those parts of Europe which had been settled by agricultural communities at an earlier date. The evident contrasts stem from the historical and environmental setting of their respective developments, and the relative isolation of the western periphery which allowed a further elaboration of social forms which in other areas had been rapidly extinguished.

These contrasting trajectories determined the different reactions of the various areas to the major technological and economic innovations of the period, the secondary products complex (Sherratt 1981). The rapid spread of features like the plough and woolly sheep crosscut local successions of social development, and they were integrated into local systems in different ways. In the east, they caused something of a recession in the production of spectacular elite items such as the goldwork of Varna; in the west they accelerated and increased the scale of monument construction and territorial demarcation, giving a further twist to the elaboration of ritual integration. In this way the effect of these innovations was to increase regional contrasts, even though in the longer term it was to provide a more uniform basis for convergent development.

Although elites of different kinds were produced by the various processes which have been defined, with a measure of ranking both within and between communities, there are no signs of substantial contrasts between different levels of society that would deserve the term 'stratification'; nor of the cumulative addition of levels of executive authority that could be described as a hierarchy. The basic building block of Neolithic and Copper Age societies was the community or lineage, and the bonds between them were the fragile ones of exogamy and alliance.

Within this framework, however, there was a variety of ways in which social relation might be organized. An important variable was the layout of settlement on the ground. Although Europe went through a protracted process of 'filling up', this did not produce a simple linear increase in population pressure and stress on land: instead, we can observe small cycles of infilling within particular

zones, followed by the unlocking of further zones either within or beyond the region. The plough in particular opened up extensive areas for cultivation (incidentally increasing the pastoral component of agricultural economies) which allowed a more rapid process of spatial expansion than was characteristic of the often river-based patterns of initial land-taking. Paradoxically, therefore, analogies with slash-and-burn farmers in the tropics may be more relevant to the later Neolithic than the early Neolithic, whose constrained commitment to zones of primary productivity is perhaps more analogous to that of the lowland rice farmers.

The implication of these patterns of expansion can be taken further. In an illuminating article on stateless societies in West Africa, Horton (1976) has discussed the circumstances under which lineages and corporations based on principles other than descent, become important media of social organization. He contrasts the conditions of unconstrained expansion, in which dispersed settlement is the norm and spatial and genealogical distance maintain an approximate equivalence, with constrained expansion where 'leapfrogging' and disjunctive migration become necessary. In the former case, segmentary lineages can occur in which a single genealogical scheme can embrace many thousands of people; in the latter, aggregates composed of several lineages are formed, which must be integrated by cross-cutting ties and a genealogical definition of landholding rights is replaced by a territorial one. Co-residence, rather than common descent, becomes the focus of political allegiance.

Such territorally-based societies may be of two kinds: those where the political community coincides with a large, nucleated village, and those where its members are scattered in a number of smaller settlements. In the former case, the role of lineages is subordinated to crosscutting institutions based on age grades, secret societies, and especially ritual groupings -"a cluster of adaptations to the problem posed by the presence in the community of strong and rivalrous lineages" (ibid, p.96). In the latter, the lineages maintain their importance as social groupings within the territorial unit, whose role in this potentially fissiparous situation is stressed by the cult of an earth spirit that unites the constituent descent groups. In this case, the head of the leading lineage usually acts as cult priest and presides over internal affairs.

Now these distinctions correspond in a rough way to some of the contrasts which have emerged in discussing the societies of later Neolithic and Copper Age Europe. While there are no equivalents here to the pioneer societies of the earlier Neolithic, there are striking resemblances between the institutions that have been inferred for the large Neolithic villages of south east Europe and the loess area, for instance, and those of stateless groups in West Africa such as the Kalabari. The problems of scattered, but territorially defined, groups like the Lodagaa are paralleled by the megalith-building communities of north west Europe, and were apparently solved in a similar way, through a focus in territorial ritual.

Can the properties inferred for 'Copper Age' societies (both the fourth-millennium examples from south east Europe and third-millennium examples from the North European Plain) be related to a pattern of segmentary lineages (Kristiansen 1982)? Settlement was both dispersed and expanding in space, producing the (temporary) conditions under which genealogical reckoning was an effective way of maintaining an expanding series of relationships, and reducing the emphasis on territorial definition. In such a system there is no permanent political community, but rather adventitious combinations for particular threats, drawing on as large a kinship range as necessary. This equivalence of segments and relativity of political grouping -overlapping ego-centred units - leads to a predominance of leadership over authority: political position is a matter of external negotiation rather than internal control. In such circumstances, the role of individual lineage heads becomes crucial, both as a widespread status position (marked by an appropriate set of sumptuary artifacts?) and as a potential focus for wider allegiances in a shifting configuration of political structures (with the possibility of achieving individual prominence in the process). In this context, we can understand the emergence both of inter-regional symbols of rank, such as stone or copper battle axes or decorated drinking vessels. The deposition of these items in graves (as Shennan, 1982, remarks) was important in the process of defining succession to these ranks and their acquired prestige. Moreover this type of organization has the property of being able to spread at the expense of surrounding groups - Marshall Sahlins (1961) has called it an "organisation of predatory expansion". This seems a particularly appropriate description of the spread of Corded Ware and its impact on the ritually focussed megalith-builders.

The main contrast in the European succession is thus between two sorts of societies. The first was characterized by stable flows of regionally-acquired goods, and was organized on an established territorial basis, with public rituals and symbolic analogies based on female images. The societies which superseded them were characterized by a greater emphasis on exotic goods and longer distance trading contacts often of a less stable and more adventitious kind, in which information-carrying items took precedence over more basic commodities. Their territorial basis was less stable, their ethos was a competitive and self-aggrandizing one, with sumptuary codes of artifact use and symbolic analogies based on the image of the warrior male. More generally, we can perhaps discern in these European sequences an underlying shift from societies organized primarily on the basis of **community** (whether a single settlement of several sites with a common focus) to an increased emphasis on the potential of **kinship** for forming wider networks of alliance than had hitherto been realized.[8] This is perhaps the clue to the new properties which emerged in Copper Age systems in temperate Europe.

This latter type of social structure provided the basis for Bronze Age development, in which the scale of inter-regional exchange was expanded from a primary concern with symbolic items to include a greater volume of 'consumer durables' like textiles and bronze tools. This involved a greater organization of local production for inter-regional exchange, with regional specialization in commodities and manufactured products which were more widely available but still supplied through an elite. With the gradual filling-up of the continent during the second millennium, differential access to productive land became more significant and provided preconditions for the emergence of true stratification. At the same time the expansion of urban trading networks from the east Mediterranean started a process of interaction with indigenous European communities, to produce the core-periphery pattern of the first-millennium Iron Age (Frankenstein and Rowlands 1978).

The societies of later prehistoric Europe thus provide an extended series of examples of the processes operating in the early stages of social differentiation. Such societies are arguably poorly represented both in the ethnographic record, and in the archaeological evidence from nuclear regions where these types of society were rapidly superseded. European Neolithic and Bronze Age archaeology thus represents a prime source for the study of such phenomena. It may be complemented by the study of other areas - for instance Polynesia - whose relative remoteness from expanding core areas of states and empires allowed indigenous sequences to achieve a measure of social complexity. An understanding of social change requires a continuing dialogue between the evidence of ethnography and archaeology. By a better definition of their own material, archaeologists will be in a better position to understand the relevance of other branches of anthropology to it.

ACKNOWLEDGEMENTS

The picture presented here is a personal one, but reflects ideas which have been put forward by Richard Bradley, Ian Hodder, Kristian Kristiansen, Jim Lewthwaite, Klavs Randsborg, Mike Rowlands and Steve Shennan, and incorporates suggestions by John Bintliff.

NOTES

Note 1
The terminology of period divisions in European prehistory has been elaborated over more than a century and is still inconsistent. 'Neolithic' was first defined as the later part of the Stone Age in opposition to 'Palaeolithic'; the idea of a 'Copper Age' before the beginning of the Bronze Age grew up as a local concept both in Ireland and Hungary in the 1870s. National terminologies have incorporated this usage (often in the form 'Chalcolithic' or 'Eneolithic'), but these usages are often mutually inconsistent and in any case do not precisely conform to the beginning of copper use in any particular area. This article uses calibrated radiocarbon dates (following Clark, Antiquity 1975, vol. 49, pp.252-75) to give absolute ages. The terms 'mature Neolithic' and 'Copper Age' are used in a descriptive sense to denote particular types of social systems that are defined in the text. 'Copper Age' thus denotes a system in which copper objects are used in a particular way, rather than a period defined by the first use of metal.

Note 2
Recent social theories (Giddens, A. 1979, Central Problems in Social Theory, London, Macmillan; Harré, R. 1979, Social Being, Oxford, Blackwell) have attempted to overcome the essentially static nature of conceptions of social structure based on fixed roles and functions, determined by efficient adaptation to external (usually economic) circumstances. Instead they have proposed a more dynamic view in which individuals and groups manipulate their shifting advantages in a continuous process of negotiation (called 'structuration' by Giddens) which itself creates and defines the patterns of social life. While this overcomes some of the problems associated with the endless search for a 'prime mover' of social change, it has yet to be formulated in a way which is relevant to changes on an archaeological ('evolutionary') timescale.

Note 3
For a systematic general account of European prehistory and that of adjacent areas (with references), see Sherratt, A.G. (Ed.) Cambridge Encyclopaedia of Archaeology, Cambridge University Press 1980.

Note 4
Such compartments are seen both in earthen long barrows, where they are defined by hurdling, and cairns like the Severn-Cotswold barrows where the mound was construct-

ed of dry-stone cells filled with material from the quarry-ditches, themselves dug in a series of intersecting pits. This suggests an organization of several co-operating groups, perhaps on the scale postulated by W. Startin (PPS 1978, vol. 44, pp.143-59), for construction of a Band-keramik longhouse. Such a co-operating unit, itself segmentary in character, would represent a political community but not necessarily a co-resident group. This may be the logic behind the settlement clusters definable in Neolithic settlement patterns in several areas.

Note 5
Such tombs still had a 'monumental' aspect in that they were covered with earth mounds, which might form small cemeteries through the accumulation of satellite and secondary burials. A role as territorial markers is evident from their occurrence on interfluves and on sight-lines, but not all such burials were marked by mounds. In some areas where spatial expansion was not occurring, flat graves are found - sometimes in large cemeteries -e.g. Vikletice, Bohemia.

Note 6
The Almerian collective burials in tholoi (nearly 90 at Los Millares) differ from other European megalithic tombs in their direct associations with a large adjacent settlement: in this case the tombs may directly reflect lineages within the community. These appear to be ranked in wealth and this pattern is probably associated with the continuing importance of limited areas of wet bottomlands in this arid environment.

Note 7
This occurs on menhirs in the West Mediterranean, and also on Cycladic figurines.

Note 8
This is not to deny the existence of extensive kinship networks in earlier times, especially among Upper Palaeolithic hunters in open environments; but it suggests that an initial effect of the introduction of agriculture (or other forms of existence involving large, sedentary communities) was to place the emphasis of social organization foremost on community. This would be the case both in the large settlements of the Neolithic of central and south east Europe, and in the Neolithic of western Europe where 'big monuments' replaced 'big sites'. The formation of more extensive kinship networks would then represent a shift to forms of social organisation that were less tied to patterns of residence and the existence of large, stable settlements.

This kind of change is well exemplified in eastern Europe in the later fifth millennium BC (Sherratt 1982) with the declining importance of settlements and the rising prominence of cemeteries, which mapped social relations symbolically (in the rows of graves, varying positions and quantities of grave goods) since these were no longer evident from residence patterns. The simultaneous effects of wider kinship links on exchange networks is dramatically demonstrated in the coalescence of regional systems ('network linkage' - Sherratt 1972, p.529) that culminated in the cultural chaining linking Bulgaria and the North European Plain in Late Gumelnitsa/Bodrog-keresztur/Lengyel. This kind of shift was apparently repeated in western Europe with the rise of Corded Ware.

BIBLIOGRAPHY

ADAMS, R.M. 1974 - "Anthropological perspectives on ancient trade", Current Anthropology, (vol. 15, pp.239-58).

BECKER, C.J. 1954 - "Stenalderbebyggelsen ved Store Valby i Vestsjaelland: Probleme omkring Tragbaeger-kulturens aeldste og yngste Fase", Aarboger fra Nordisk Oldkyndighed og Historie 1954, pp.127-97.

BENDER, B. 1978 - "Gatherer-hunter to farmer", World Archaeology, vol. 10, pp.204-22.

BOKONYI, S. 1974 - History of Domestic Mammals in central and eastern Europe, Budapest, Akademiai Kiado.

BOKONYI, S. 1978 - "The earliest waves of domestic horses in East Europe", Journal of Indo-European Studies vol. 6, pp.17-76.

CLARK, J.G.D. 1946 - From Savagery to Civilisation, London, Cobbett Press.

COHEN, M.N. 1977 - The Food Crisis in Prehistory, Yale Univ. Press.

DOUGLAS, M. & ISHERWOOD, B. 1979 - The World of Goods, Penguin, Harmondsworth.

EARLE, T.K. 1977 - "A reappraisal of redistribution: complex Hawaian chiefdoms", pp.213-29 in Earle, T.K. and Ericson, J. (Eds.) Exchange Systems in Prehistory, Academic Press, N.Y.

ECSEDY, I. 1979 - The People of the Pit-Grave Kurgans in Eastern Hungary, Budapest, Akademiai Kiado.

FRANKENSTEIN, S. and ROWLANDS, M.J. 1978 - "The internal structure and regional context of early Iron Age society in south-western Germany". Bulletin of the Institute of Archaeology, (London) vol. 15, pp.73-112.

FRIED, M. 1967 - The Evolution of Political Society, Random House, N.Y.

FRIED, M. 1978 - The Concept of Tribe, Cummings Publishing Co. Menlo Park California.

FRIEDMAN, J. and ROWLANDS, M.J. 1977 - "Notes towards an epigenetic model of the evolution of 'civilisation' ", in Friedman, J. and Rowlands, M.J. (Eds.), The Evolution of Social Systems London, Duckworth, pp.201-76.

GILMAN, A. 1981 - "The development of social stratification in Bronze Age Europe", Current Anthropology, vol. 22, pp.1-24.

GODELIER, M. 1977 - Perspectives in Marxist Anthropology, C.U.P.

HODDER, I.A. 1982a - Symbols in Action, C.U.P.

HODDER, I.A. 1982b - "Sequences of structural change in the Dutch Neolithic", pp.162-77 in Hodder, I.A. (Ed.) Symbolic and structural Archaeology, C.U.P.

HOCKMANN, O. 1972 - "Andeutungen zu Religion und Kultus in der Bandkeramischen Kultur", Alba Regia vol. 12, pp.187-209.

HORTON, R. 1976 - "Stateless societies in the history of

134

West Africa" in J.F.A. Ajayi and M. Crowder, History of West Africa, I, pp.72-113.

HOWELL, J.M. 1982 - "Neolithic Settlement and Economy in Northern France", Oxford Journal of Archaeology, vol. 1, pp.115-18.

KACZANOWSKA, M. 1980 - "Uwagi o surowcach, technice i typologii przemysłu krzemiennego kultury Bodrogkerszturskieji i grupy Laznany", Acta Archaeologia Carpathica, vol. 20, pp.19-56.

KRISTIANSEN, K. 1982 - "The formation of tribal systems in later European prehistory: Northern Europe 4000 - 500 BC", pp.241-80 in C. Renfrew, M.J. Rowlands and B.A. Seagrave (Eds.) Theory and Explanation in Archaeology, Academic Press. New York.

KRUK, J. 1973 - Studia Oszadnicze nad Neolitem Wyzyn Lessowych, Ossolineum, Warsaw.

KRUK, J. 1980 - Gospodarka w Polsce Południowowschodniej w V-III Tysiacleciu PNE, Ossolineum, Warsaw.

LECH, J. and LELIGDOWICZ, A. 1980 - "Die Methoden der Versorgung mit Feuerstein und die lokalen Beziehungen zwischen den Siedlungen und Bergwerken im Weichselgebiet während des 5. bis 2. Jt. v.u.Z.", pp.151-84 in Schlette, F. (Ed.) Urgeschichtliche Besiedlung in ihrer Beziehung zur natürlichen Umwelt, (Wissenschaftliche Beiträge der Martin-Luther Universität) Halle/Saale.

LEWTHWAITE, J. 1981 - "Ambiguous first impressions: a survey of recent work on the early Neolithic of the west Mediterranean", Journal of Mediterranean Archaeology, vol. 1, pp.292-307.

MORGAN, L.H. 1977 - Ancient Society. New York.

NASH, D.M. 1978 - "Territory and state formation in central Gaul", pp.455-76 in D. Green, C. Haselgrove and M. Spriggs, Social Organisation & Settlement, Oxford BAR Int. Ser. 47.

NEUSTUPNY, E. and NEUSTUPNY, J. 1961 -Czechoslovakia before the Slavs, London, Thames and Hudson.

POLANYI, K., ARENSBERG, K. and PEARSON, H. 1957 - Trade and Market in the Early Empires, New York, The Free Press.

RANDSBORG, K. 1975 - "Social dimensions in Neolithic Denmark", Proceedings of the Prehistoric Society, vol. 41, pp.105-18.

RANDSBORG, K. 1979 - "Resource distribution and the function of copper in Early Neolithic Denmark", pp.303-18 in Ryan, M. (Ed.) Proceedings of the fifth Atlantic Colloquium, Dublin.

RENFREW,A.C. 1972 - The Emergence of Civilisation, London, Methuen.

RENFREW, A.C. 1973 - "Monuments, mobilisation and social organisation in Neolithic Wessex", pp.539-58 in Renfrew, A.C. (Ed.) The Explanation of Culture Change,

London, Duckworth.

ROWLANDS, M.J., KRISTIANSEN, K. and LARSEN, M.T. (in press) Core and Periphery in the Ancient World, C.U.P.

ROWLEY-CONWY, P. (in press) - "The laziness of the short-distance hunter: final hunters and first farmers in Denmark", New Directions in Scandinavian Archaeology, 3.

SAHLINS, M. 1961 - "The segmentary lineage: an organisation of predatory expansion", American Anthropologist, vol. 63, pp.322-45.

SERVICE, E.R. 1962 - Primitive Social Organisation: an Evolutionary Perspective, Random House, NY.

SERVICE, E.R. 1968 - "War and our contemporary ancestors", pp.160-7 in M. Fried, M. Harris and R. Murphy (Eds.) War: the Anthropology of Armed Conflict and Aggression, Doubleday, NY.

SHENNAN, S.J. 1982 - "Ideology, change and the European Early Bronze Age", pp.155-61 in Hodder, I.A., Symbolic and Structural Archaeology, C.U.P.

SHERRATT, A.G. 1972 - "Socioeconomic and demographic models for the Neolithic and Bronze Ages of Europe", pp.477-542 in Clarke, D.L. Models in Archaeology, London, Methuen.

SHERRATT,A.G. 1976 - "Resources, technology & trade: an essay in early European Metallurgy". pp.557-81, in G. Sieveking, I. Longworth, K. Wilson (Eds.) Problems in Economic & Social Archaeology, London, Duckworth.

SHERRATT, A.G. 1981 - "Plough and pastoralism: aspects of the Secondary Products Revolution" pp.261-305 in I. Hodder, G. Isaac, N. Hammond Pattern of the Past, C.U.P.

SHERRATT, A.G. 1982 - "Mobile resources: settlement and exchange in early agricultural Europe", pp.13-26 in A.C. Renfrew and S.J. Shennan, Ranking Resources and Exchange. C.U.P.

SHERRATT, E.S. and SHERRATT, A.G. (in press) - "The Aegean Bronze Age and the east Mediterranean: political structures and external trade" in Rowlands et al. in press.

SPOONER, B. (Ed.) 1972 - Population Growth : Anthropological Implications, M.I.T. Press.

STEVENSON, R.F. 1968 - Population & Political Systems in Tropical Africa. Columbia U.P.

TROELS-SMITH, J. 1952 - "Ertebøllekulture-Bondekultur: Resultater af de sidste 10 Aars Untersogelse i Aamosen, Vestsjaelland", Aarboger fra Nordisk Oldkyndighed og Historie, 1952, pp.5-62.

YOFFEE, N. 1979 - "The Decline and rise of Mesopotamian civilisation; an ethnoarchaeological perspective on the evolution of social complexity", American Antiquity, vol. 44, pp.5-35.

YOFFEE, N. 1982 - "Explaining trade in western Asia". Monographs on the Ancient Near East, 2.

5

ASPECTS OF SOCIAL EVOLUTION
IN THE BRONZE AGE

Anthony Harding

In the early development of social distinction in pre-history, it is clear that certain periods and areas played key roles. The European Bronze Age was one of these. During its course, archaeological evidence for wealth differentials, in the form of grave goods, production of luxury items, and the scale and range of both domestic and funerary sites, appears to increase. There is direct evidence of long-distance, highly specific trade to and from known source and reception areas, particularly in materials like gold and amber which are related to wealth display and accumulation. There is abundant evidence for intensifying industrial production, a fact which would be hard to attribute simply to personal initiative. There is also evidence for warfare on an increasing scale: not just weapons for skirmishing between groups of archers but heavy duty weapons for regularized battle procedures from fortified centres. All these things attest increasing hierarchization during the course of the period, and it is therefore clear that these years were especially forma-tive ones. The quantity of material and range of sites from the Bronze Age is greater than in the Neolithic and Copper Age and enables a rather more elaborate formula-tion of models to account for this development.

For present purposes the term 'Bronze Age' is taken in its traditional sense, namely the period following the Copper Age (i.e. after Beakers, Corded Ware and their analogues) and preceding the Iron Age (defined as the first regular local production of iron). The period is thus roughly that from 2000 to 700 BC in Europe, or 3000 to 1000 BC in Greece (calendar years).

If one examines the evidence for social division at either end of the Bronze Age, one can see the nature of the problem with which we are dealing. Broadly speaking, the cemeteries of continental Europe around 2000 BC consist of flat inhumations, or in some areas inurned cremations, not notable for the wealth of their grave goods. By the Urnfield period the sporadic occurrence of extremely rich graves, interspersed with thousands of mediocre ones, is attested. In between, there are various areas and periods where noticeable wealth relative to other graves occurs, especially where barrow graves were popular. It is hardly surprising that most authorities have viewed the period as one in which social divisions, or at any rate the outward expression of such divisions, increas-ed markedly, going from a situation where some people may have held favoured positions but not markedly so, to one where a few individuals, by amassing material posses-sions, achieved pre-eminent status. The most favoured terminology to describe the nature of Bronze Age societ-ies has been that of chiefdoms, and the explanatory

mechanisms invoked are, as we shall shortly see, many and varied. Before we pass on to consider some of these factors, we should first pause to take note of the main approaches to Bronze Age social evolution manifested in the past.

Main approaches to the study of Bronze Age social evolution

Until recently, views on the nature of Bronze Age society were implied rather than expressed: little or no discussion took place and the preoccupations of most scholars were with description and ordering of material culture rather than with its social significance. All the main authorities have characterized the Bronze Age as a period in which chieftains can for the first time be clearly recognized, and left it at that. A few speculated on the possible economic background to such social differentiation, but there has never been an extended or wide-ranging review of the subject. Most scholars have been content to receive and transmit again the standard model - which is not to say it is inapplicable, merely that other models can also be devised.

Inevitably when dealing with synthesizing views of European prehistory, one returns to Gordon Childe, who combined a deep knowledge of the material with a close interest in the social status of prehistoric stages. This is something that cannot be said for scholars preceding him, like Montelius. Perhaps not surprisingly, in view of his political and philosophical leanings, he followed Marx and Engels in maintaining the terminology proposed by Tylor and Morgan, that is, three successive stages labelled 'savagery,' barbarism' and 'civilization'. Childe proposed food-production and writing as the distinguishing features of respectively the latter two stages. On this basis the European Bronze Age falls in the second stage, with the Near Eastern cultures (and to a small extent the Aegean area) coming into the third. Childe also viewed the Bronze Age as a major economic as well as a technolo-gical stage, as shown by incipient specialization of labour, by the organization of trade and by particular inventions and discoveries which greatly increased man's control over nature. He did not talk of chiefdoms as such but frequently of chiefs, whom he saw as apparent already in the Neolithic (1963, p.59ff.). "In general", he remarked, "the most that an archaeologist can mean by 'chiefs' is persons who monopolise an appreciable fraction at least of the social surplus. But even if these were chiefs exercising political functions, they were not necessarily specialists living entirely on the reward of leadership" (1963 p.62). Recognizing an aristocracy is said to be still harder than recognizing chiefs, though ethnographic cases show plenty of examples of pastoral-based aristocracies ruling agricultural subjects. The Wessex culture Childe called an "aristocracy of petty chieftains" (1963 p.102); at other times he referred to "ruling classes, extracting from a vanquished peasantry a surplus". In this connection it is important that Childe was adamant that Bronze Age smiths were full-time specialists: this notion he derived ultimately from Marx and Engels as part of the package involving craft specialization. Childe also took into account, though does not seem to have subscribed to, the pre-War Soviet division of history into pre-clan, clan and class society: the Bronze Age falls in the clan stage, when matrilineal was gradually replaced by patrilineal organization (1963, p.37).

Some modern assessments of the position with European social evolution of the Bronze Age are not dissimilar. Milisauskas (1978), for example, combines knowledge of the central European material with an approach founded in American-style anthropology. He speaks of the "flowering of complex chiefdoms, some of which, such as Mycenae in the Aegean region, may have attained the status of state societies" (1978, p.208). He distinguishes between "high-status individuals" and the "ordinary members of a society" or "lower-status members" of the chiefdom. He also refers, in talking of the Urnfield period, to "spectacular burial mounds ... which reflect increasing social differences among the members of Bronze Age chiefdoms". This is admittedly in a general book, but it is apparent that the conceptual framework is essentially similar to that of Gordon Childe - and the same could be said of many other works, including the general review by Coles and Harding (1979).

The dogmas of Marxism-Leninism concerning the materialist view of history have naturally also played a role in these matters, though it is doubtful if the practical effects of this have been very great. The concern of Marxists with the forces of production and the relations of production have led to a preoccupation by Marxist archaeologists with artifacts of all sorts and specifically tools. "Instruments of labour not only supply a standard of the degree of development to which human labour has attained, but they are also indicators of the social conditions under which that labour is carried on" (Marx 1954, pp.175-6). This is one reason why typological studies have loomed so large in central and eastern Europe: material culture is considered more objective and truthful than spiritual. The other dominating conceptual force in Marxist archaeology is the Morgan sequence already alluded to. Engels followed Morgan almost precisely in The Origin of the Family, Private Property and the State, published in 1884, and this work is the one most commonly quoted with approval by socialist archaeologists today. Paulik, for instance, (1974, p.76) favours the Engels-Morgan idea of a military democracy to explain the rich Late Bronze Age barrows of Slovakia; Dusek (1973) discusses the matter generally. In this model, power is concentrated in the hands of a warrior elite for whom warfare is a means of accumulating prestige, material wealth and slaves and through which come privileges that distinguish the elite from other members of the family or clan. Furmanek (1977 p.332) debates whether the Engels division of types of labour can be applied to the Piliny culture (Middle Bronze Age), and stresses the importance of the economic basis in the Marxist materialist conception of history. Another aspect is the 'philosophical-historical category' of early societies: in this case the view that the Bronze Age was 'patriarchal' (cf. Neustupny 1967), as shown above all by the developing ability of individuals to concentrate wealth in their hands, presumably by means of social manipulation of increased economic capacity.

A major influence on the development of thought concerning the social status of prehistoric organization has been the American anthropological school, as typified for example by Service (1962, 1975). Initially a tripartite division into band, tribe and state was proposed. Among those who have applied the idea to European prehistory has been Renfrew (e.g. 1972 pp.363-4; 1973), who found that the Aegean Bronze Age did not fit neatly into either 'tribe' or 'state', though many of Service's criteria for 'chiefdom' were applicable, such as the existence of the office of chief (visible in dress, conduct, activities etc.), significant degrees of personal ranking, increase in population density, increase in craft specialization, development of religion, execution of public works and the rise of warfare. Later (1974) Renfrew tried to tie down the concept of chiefdom more firmly by distinguishing between 'group-oriented' ("societies where personal wealth in terms of valuable possessions is not impressively documented, but where the solidarity of the social unit was expressed most effectively in communal or group activities", examples: Neolithic Wessex or prehistoric Malta) and 'individualizing' ("societies where a marked disparity in personal possessions and in other material indications of prestige appears to document a salient personal ranking, yet often without evidence of large communal meetings or activities", examples: the Celtic Iron Age or Mycenaean Greece). This model has been criticized as being over-typological and based on categories (i.e. Service's) that may in any case be inappropriate.

Much attention has also been paid to the question of the origin of the state, and the criteria of 'statedom'. This problem, which other contributors to this volume consider in detail, impinges only marginally on us here, since it is only in the eastern Mediterranean that social entities dignifiable by the term 'state' (or 'proto-state') can be claimed in the Bronze Age. This fact serves to underline the great disparity between 'barbarian' Europe, where evidence for the existence of larger political units, of administrative activity, and of communal works other than for religious purposes is almost totally lacking in the Bronze Age; and the polities of the Aegean and Near East where social, economic and political activity is historically documented, and decision-making and public works can thus be seen to have been initiated by specific individuals for the furtherance of aims within specific political units. The scale of possible political, or at any rate economic, units in the barbarian world is touched on below; here we may note for the Aegean Late Bronze Age the existence of regional centres, even possibly supra-regional centres, administered by professionals, controlled by aristocrats and serviced by craftsmen, labourers and slaves, with defined geographical limits, and procedures for setting in motion works of communal concern (e.g. defence). The question of statedom will not be further considered in this paper, but these remarks may serve to demonstrate that it is no insignificant question in the context of the Aegean and East Mediterranean Bronze Age.

Description and explanation of Bronze Age social evolution

It is possible to distinguish various phases in the development of models to describe and explain the process of social evolution in the Bronze Age. By far the longest-lived and most prevalent is the notion that social evolution follows a progressive course much like physical evolution and that the natural course of events was for increasing social complexity and developing stratification. I have alluded already to the 'stages' of social evolution so beloved of nineteenth-century anthropologists and adopted, with modifications, by Engels and others. Less formalized notions can be found in many introductory works at the present day. Basically, we are conditioned to expect a higher degree of stratification at the end of the Bronze Age than at its beginning. This is, of course, only an assumption and stating it has no explanatory or predictive force - beyond the observed fact that many societies do move through various stages of social complexity from simpler to more developed. To what extent any other societies in world history are genuine analogues to the European Bronze Age is a matter for speculation.

A second type of explanation which has become increasingly prevalent is to take an observed shift in social complexity (as it might be the rise of Mycenaean civilization) and seek accompanying changes in some other part of the system than that showing the principal change. Environmental change, economic shifts, or technological developments have been most popular as causal (or at any rate contributory) factors, in such major shifts. Environmental explanations have involved climatic change, deforestation, soil impoverishment, resource depletion, famine, disease and other factors. Economic shifts have been concerned with new configurations in trade orientation, cropping practice and the like. Technological developments include such obvious factors as the origin and spread of metallurgy but also more subtle ones like the use of irrigation to "increase and stabilise agricultural yields" (Gilman 1976, p.316). Gilman's recent (1981) attempt to turn the process of reasoning on its head by asking not what functions elites serve, but how they maintain their hold on society in spite of being a factor at variance with the common good, must also be considered under this heading. For in spite of his assertions to the contrary, Gilman is concerned with external factors leading to internal shifts, with activities leading to "capital-intensification of subsistence": plough agriculture, Mediterranean polyculture, irrigation and off-shore fishing, each of which he sees as capable of transforming the subsistence base of the economy, and, therefore, of society.

The third main type of explanation may be termed organic or internal and grew up essentially as a reaction to particular kinds of functionalist explanation - particularly to the model which suggested that external trade or migration was responsible for changes in societies. This type of explanation relies instead on the internal dynamics of human groups to achieve social change, bringing about rather than brought about by technological and economic change, and related only coincidentally to other stimuli, like those of the natural environment. Lastly, analogue explanations seek answers to problems through the study of analogical situations. Obvious candidates for study are socially or technologically comparable groups in different areas or periods, preferably historically documented. In the case of the Bronze Age, these might stem from the contemporaneous Near East or Egypt, from early Celtic society, from the early Greek world, or from various historical or ethnographical groups. The latter two explanatory models have not been systematically employed in Bronze Age studies. The preoccupations of the rest of this paper may serve to demonstrate my own view that certain fields of research can be more profitably employed in the study of social evolution than others.

GENERAL SURVEY

The transformations in material culture that occurred between the Copper Age and the Iron Age must to some degree reflect transformations in society and economy. The archaeologist naturally finds it easier to document the material culture, and though it is fashionable to belittle this approach it remains the basis by means of which statements about society and economy can be made. In the present case two major transformations have to be accounted for: the rise of clearly marked social division, which occurs early in the second millennium bc, and the great increase in population, with attendant easier access to material goods, which marks the second half of the Bronze Age, from about 1100 BC onwards.

Rise of social division

One might expect that the progression from Copper to Bronze Ages would be understood most clearly in those areas of Europe where the most remarkable monuments of each period are visible, for instance in Britain or Brittany. Stonehenge, for example, can be seen as exemplifying the transition from a relatively undifferentiated ritual monument, in a cleared but as yet sparsely built-up landscape, to an elaborate complex at the centre of a huge spread of monuments, mainly but by no means exclusively funerary. In fact, the most impressive sites are in some ways also the hardest to understand, because the scale of monument-building was not backed up by equivalent wealth of material culture or by monumentality in other activities. In funerary terms, individual burials start with the Copper Age and continue through into the Bronze Age without a significant break. It is rather the nature of the grave-goods which separate the two periods, with the first major signs of differentiation only appearing in the Early Bronze Age.

There are various possible approaches to this problem. The evidence could be a reflection of various archaeological situations. It may genuinely mean that social division did now start to exist. It may mean, on the other hand, that such divisions only started to be marked at this time, although they had existed long before. It may, again, reflect purely fortuitous effects which have little to do with social stratification. This last view can and has been argued for various areas and periods but is essentially an abrogation of responsibility; it seems helpful to assume that grave-goods do reflect status in life in some manner.

Other transformations also occurred at approximately the same time, but it is important to avoid assuming that they are necessarily connected with the rise of social division. Among them we may list:

1   Probably from an early stage of the Bronze Age, interest in dividing up blocks of agricultural land. The evidence for this is restricted to the extreme west of Europe.

2   'Re-emergence' of established settlement forms: settlements of post-built houses on areas settled densely in the Neolithic but only sparsely in the Copper Age.

3   A gradual cessation of interest in megalithic monuments, with increasing use of barrow burial.

4   Regular and widespread use of metals, with deep mining, the use of more complex moulds, leading to more elaborate metal types, and the start of single-type hoards (hoards consisting predominantly of one type).

From the start of the second millennium bc, it is possible to envisage an increasing intensification of land and resource usage. The evidence from pollen diagrams suggests regular clearance of woodland on a medium scale, with subsequent recolonization by pioneer species. Numerous Bronze Age monuments are situated on soils that are today impoverished or poor and may have been tending in that direction already. Bradley (1978) has suggested that the first land division took place in areas where soil impoverishment had led to pressure on land.

Since the main preoccupation of most people in the Bronze Age continued, we may assume, to be subsistence agriculture, such factors would be powerful agents for change. Whether they do in fact relate to known aspects of social change remains to be seen.

The re-establishment of 'visible' settlement may be related to these factors, but probably only rather vaguely. For a spell during the Copper Age we temporarily lose sight of the regular and dense settlement patterns and types known from the Neolithic. In well-documented areas the number of recovered settlement sites falls to a very low figure (e.g. north-west Bohemia, Bouzek, 1982) during the Copper Age, though the population is unlikely to have fallen, to judge from the size of cemeteries. One possible reason for this change may have been a shift away from the most archaeologically 'visible' situations, e.g. loess river terraces, to those where recovery is bound to be more haphazard, e.g. clays and marls.

It is hard to date the earliest evidence for land division. The well-known old land surface under the South Street long barrow preserves a line of stake-holes tentatively interpreted as a fence; this evidence is much earlier than the bulk of that known from upland Britain, but Caulfield's findings (1978) at Belderg Beg, Co. Mayo, may lend support to the idea. The Bronze Age, however, seems to have seen a great increase in the scale and scope of land division, many of the present-day moorland areas of the country being treated in this way as well as such other areas as are capable of providing evidence (e.g. Wessex downlands). We will return to the significance of these matters below.

In the Early Bronze Age, on the other hand, many areas recover their settlements which typically (in central Europe) lie again on the loess terraces. If the cause of their earlier desertion was agricultural, we should bear in mind that Middle Bronze Age settlements are again poorly known, i.e. the same process might have occurred again. Only with the Late Bronze Age does large-scale settlement over a wider area re-appear and, apparently, stay for a longer period: certainly reflecting a larger population but possibly also more stable management of the land.

A factor of considerable interest in western Europe is the loss of appeal of megalithic monuments to Early Bronze Age communities ('breakdown of ritual formalisation'). Whereas Beaker pottery occurs quite commonly in megalithic complexes (both tombs and ceremonial sites) very few sites apart from British stone circles (and not a lot of those) have Bronze Age find associations. Discussion of these sites is inevitably bound up with one's view of their significance to the people who erected them, a controversy already alluded to by Bintliff. While it is possible that a functionalist explanation of the type favoured by Chapman (1977) is relevant, the symbolic attributes of megaliths seem to me far more persuasive as raisons d'être for the monuments. What is important, therefore, is that the symbolic view of the population changed, and did so just at the time we are here concerned with, the start of the Bronze Age. This mental shift is presumably to be seen in conjunction with other shifts that we are considering.

Metal extraction and technology also demand consideration: the problems may be put as questions. (1) Was metal widely available in the Early Bronze Age (as compared with the Chalcolithic)? (2) Was the technology really abstruse and restricted to a few people only? (3) Who were the main customers for smithing products? (4) What was the status and life-syle of the smith? (5) What was the status and life-style of those who acquired

prestige objects, notably gold and elaborate copper ornaments?

Metals were doubtless never so plentiful that they became devalued. At the same time they were not rare, so that most areas of Europe stood a reasonable chance of getting hold of them. There are obvious exceptions to this: the metal-less areas of northern Europe, for example, and the many parts of the continent far removed from gold sources. We cannot here discuss these matters, but it is clear that the range of tools available, and not just ornaments and weapons, strongly suggests a relative abundance of the material in at least some areas and phases. On the other hand Kristiansen has demonstrated (1977) in a sophisticated manner that, in the Nordic area at least, supplies were erratic or demand variable, because of the different lengths of time over which objects circulated. The same might also be deduced from the imitation of southern forms, or actual exports from southeastern central Europe, that are found in the Early Bronze Age of the north (Hachmann 1957).

Secure information is lacking on smiths and smithing. We may assume that detailed knowledge of the intricate processes of smelting and casting was restricted to very few people, but at the same time the smith would have need of a number of helpers to carry on his work. Only long experience would give a person adequate knowledge of the processes involved for successful casting to be carried out. The technology was thus theoretically available to all but in fact can hardly have been used by more than a small number of people. Of the status of the smith, and of his customers, nothing is known for the 'barbarian' world. An Egyptian text denigrating the trade is often quoted, but since its context is that of praise for the art of the scribe it may not be typical (Forbes 1964, p.85). Ethnographic examples can be quoted of cases where the smith possessed considerable status. It is evident that the great bulk of objects produced was of everyday items, though tours de force could also be executed for the satisfaction of particular patrons. We shall return to these problems later.

The economy of the Bronze Age was 'pre-industrial', but enough evidence for industrial activity survives for us to be sure that it played an important overall role. The evidence for mass-production of metal objects on an increasing scale through the period, and equally the clear signs of strain on the metal supply (alloying with lead, inadequate rations of bronze to smiths at Pylos) suggest that industrial production had a marked impact on the economic system as a whole. It would be naive to seek too close a correlation between these facts and observed social shifts without much more detailed information, but the building up of the economic picture must be a prerequisite for understanding the social picture.

Burial data

In contradistinction to some other periods, a very large proportion of the available data for the Bronze Age stems from burials. It is estimated, for example, that Denmark alone (area 43,000sq. kms.) once contained between 25,000 and 50,000 barrow mounds, most of them of Bronze Age date. A study of Late Bronze Age Lausitz culture cemeteries (Malinowski 1961) was concerned with 2832 published cemeteries in the modern territory of Poland (more have turned up since). These cemeteries are rarely known in toto since they are usually discovered by accident: that at Przeczyce contained 874 burials, by no means an exceptional figure. The buried population of Bronze Age Poland alone could easily be 3 million or more. By contrast, knowledge of other types of site, notably settlements, remains extremely scanty.

A straight correlation between wealth in death and wealth in life has long been popular. Helmsdorf and Leubingen barrows, for instance, have always been regarded as chieftains' graves; the great mound of Haga outside Uppsala, excavated in 1902-3, has long been known as Kung Björns Hög and on excavation produced rich grave-goods which reinforce this name; the great mound at Seddin in Brandenburg is known as the Königsgrab because of its rich finds on its discovery in 1899; rich Wessex culture graves have been described as intrusive warrior-aristocrats from Brittany (Piggott, 1938 p.94): indeed, Stukeley's judgement (1740, p.43) has remained current: "They are assuredly the single sepulchres of kings and great personages, buried during a considerable space of time, and that in peace". Similarly Otto in 1955 distinguished various categories of burial in the central European Bronze Age: chieftains' graves, outstandingly rich, isolated (Helmsdorf, Leubingen); very rich male graves within a cemetery, including gold (Łeki Małe 1); rich graves with metal but no gold or display items; poor graves, with the odd pot or nothing at all. Gimbutas (1965, p.267) takes this further: the "chieftains" are assumed to have been patriarchal tribal heads with the ability to marshall the labour resources of society. The very rich graves would, on her analysis, be "members of the nobility, the most powerful and influential next to the king", who could have formed a council, the Indo-European tauta. Other similar interpretations have already been mentioned.

The best-known case-study in detailed cemetery analysis in the Bronze Age is that of Susan Shennan on the Early Bronze Age inhumation cemetery at Branc, to provide an objective assessment of the excavator's assumption about social ordering in the period. These were expressed as follows: "The concentration of more poorly and richly furnished graves reflects here the relations of a developed patriarchal social organisation with demonstrable social ranking. This is attested too by the structure of the find complexes from single graves and their comparison with the quality of the grave-goods in the framework of their grave-group" (Vladar, 1973, pp.132-218). In this cemetery the actual rite - single inhumation in a pit, with different orientation of males and females - was relatively undifferentiated, and in only a few cases did grave form itself stand out, as for instance with grave 31 with its wooden chamber, or grave 62 with its encircling ditch. Number 31 was reasonably well provided with grave-goods, but 62 was robbed. (In fact over 10% of the graves had been robbed, which is itself a worrying fact if one assumes that rich graves might, like no. 62, have been marked on the surface). Vladar here boldly describes these two graves as "Chieftains' graves" (1973 p.217), and points out that rich graves surround them, in some cases having the typical "Warrior assemblage" (daggers etc).

Shennan, by proceeding from the obvious fact that grave-goods were provided differentially at Branc, and on the basis of good anthropological observation of age and sex, was able to suggest interesting possibilities concerning the distribution of wealth through society, in particular as certain children and infants - notably girls - were unusually well provided for. The interest of these results transcends the difficulties experienced by Shennan in overcoming the fact that some graves had been robbed. The assignation of values to given grave-goods must always contain a subjective element and the provision of grave-goods to children is an imponderable which may not be governed by the usual rules because of sentimental factors. Yet the large number of adult females with 'rich' grave-goods clearly reflects wealth plausibly to be connected with marriage. Comparable data, with the potential for comparable results, have been given for south Germany and Austria by Rückdeschel (1968) and Gallay (1972).

Shennan has since observed (1982) that the situation in Early Bronze Age Slovakia reflects a progression from "minimal to moderate ranking", a limited degree of ranking in the earlier part of the period giving way to much more marked distinctions in the middle part. Developments at the end of the period are still more dramatic: the rise of fortified sites and suggestions of pressure on metal resources (grave-robbing, deposition of metal hoards in fortified sites), but not, however, much evidence for increased cemetery differentiation. This interplay between differentiation within communities and within regions in the Early Bronze Age is clearly a matter that needs critical attention.

The analysis of Early Bronze Age burials in Denmark by Randsborg (1974) also showed clearly the variability in grave-good provision (but also the different ways of exhibiting high status at different periods), and demonstrated a good correlation between population density (i.e. number of graves) and degree of social stratification (number of graves over a certain level of wealth divided by number of graves below it), the idea being that a denser population would need greater social complexity to articulate it. Also of significance is the evidence for the increasing status of women with increasing population density, which may relate to their changing role in the economy as new areas were brought into intensive exploitation and, perhaps, new cropping and other practices were introduced.

It is assumed for the Bronze Age that social hierarchies, although without doubt present in the Early Bronze Age, were of a relatively undeveloped or crude form, and conversely that in the Late Bronze Age such divisions were much more evolved, even conspicuously visible. In view of the fact that by Hallstatt D spectacularly rich graves occur, our image is really of incipient 'paramounts' in the Frankenstein and Rowlands sense (1978). Until analysis of later Bronze Age material is carried out, however, such a hypothesis cannot be tested.

It is therefore worth looking at least at one large Late Bronze Age cemetery for comparative purposes. To make it worthwhile carrying out such an investigation, such a cemetery should contain aged and sexed individuals, complete excavation recovery and a negligible archaeological loss rate. It should also come from an area well-known in other respects (e.g. hoard deposition, settlement types etc.)

Such a cemetery is Przeczyce, district Zawiercie, in Little Poland (Szydłowska 1968-1972). Rescue excavations here in 1961-2 revealed no less than 874 graves of the Lausitz culture, including 727 inhumations and 132 cremations. In 650 cases the sex and age were determinable. One hundred and four had no grave-goods at all. By far the commonest class of object put in graves was pottery, usually low cups or jugs. The commonest practice was to put one pot in the grave (155 occurrences), but no pots, 2 or 3 were almost as common; in fact 82.69% of all undisturbed graves had from 0 -4 pots and a mere 4.57% had six or more pots. However, if one hoped that these might be the 'rich' burials one would be disappointed: they often contain nothing else but the pots or else a single finger-ring, button or rattle. Even grave 262, containing no less than 15 pots, only had a bronze button with its male inhumation. If pottery is inherently unlikely to be a sign of marked wealth, it may of course indicate the number of people owing kinship or status obligations to the deceased; it may simply indicate large families. Few other objects occur in more than a very few graves. The commonest object apart from pottery is the small bronze button (321 pieces), appearing in large numbers in some graves (e.g. 49 in grave 598), but only in 25 or so graves in total. But these trivial ornaments seem far too small and insignificant to have carried much prestige with them when one knows that fine weapons and ornaments were being produced and were deposited in certain graves of the period. Other items which might indicate higher status in their owners occur at Przeczyce very infrequently; there is no gold at all. The single knife (grave 481, adult male) was found with a fish-hook, one of the two razors on the site, one button, three finger-rings and five pots. The other razor (grave 113, adult male) was with a spindle-shaped ornament, three buttons and six pots. The single sickle (grave 624, adult male) was with a fish-hook and seven pots. The only object for which this cemetery is famous, the set of pan-pipes (grave 89, adult male), accompanied a pin, a pendant, a bracelet, a leg-ring, four pots and animal bones. A handful of other graves might also be considered 'abnormally rich', but really one's overriding impression is of a uniform mediocrity of grave-good provision. The variations described indicate, as did those at Branc, considerable variability in the provision of grave-goods, but the recipients were not 'rich' viewed on a global scale. Given the fact that luxury goods were available in the period, we can deduce little more than that family or group size were variable. A Late Bronze Age cemetery like Przeczyce is thus unlikely to make a suitable subject for Shennan-type analysis, though a recent study has attempted to demonstrate that the Przeczyce society was patriarchal, with patrilineal succession and patrilocal residences: this on the basis mainly of the superior position of men according to their grave-goods (Rysiewska 1980). My reservations about this conclusion will be apparent from the foregoing.

Where, then, do such cemeteries fit in our picture of Bronze Age social evolution? What was the nature of social organization at Przeczyce? We could explain the data we have been examining in several different ways. First, we could say that the distribution of wealth in graves was an accurate reflection of that in the living population. (This population is reconstructed as having consisted of 100 people over 250 years (Period V and the beginning of Period VI), made up of around 20 families, and containing 60 adolescents and adults and 40 children under 14.) This would effectively mean that there was very little, if any, differentiation present in society, with such few 'rich' graves as there were being restricted to adult males. It need hardly be pointed out that such an idea ill accords with what we know of the eighth and seventh centuries BC from other regions, e.g. Austria, southern Germany or Bohemia.

Second, it could be that however society was organized, in death all were treated alike and everyone ended up with rather little in the way of grave-goods. Here it is worth remarking that there appears to be no significant correlation between types of grave-goods and types of burial, both inhumations and cremations sharing in all forms of grave-goods. There is thus no correlation between wealth (as expressed in grave-goods) and treatment of the body after death, and this latter is presumably to be seen as being related to mental states and attitudes that are not deducible from archaeological material alone. This lends support to the hypothesis that society was ranked but that the ranking was not discernible after death.

A third possibility might be that other things (e.g. archaeological recovery) being equal, the whole Bronze Age population is not present. Those members of society who were not marked out by special wealth are represented, but the rich are not. If they did indeed exist, they should on this view be somewhere else; so that the matter

cannot be decided by reference to this one cemetery alone.

Now certain burials or groups of burials **can** be seen as clear evidence of ranking in the Late Bronze Age, and specifically in Period V. Individual instances of rich graves are in any case known from various areas and periods of the Late Bronze Age. Graves such as Ockov, Velatice, Caka, or Hart-an-der-Alz are commonly quoted and certainly contain grave-goods of well above average quality and quantity, including specifically weapons, body armour, and fine bronze drinking services. All these examples occurred in barrows, though they were not usually inhumations. It is thus possible that barrow burial itself at this late stage of the Bronze Age - as often in the Early Iron Age - was indicative of special treatment of special individuals, and various authors have pointed out the similarity of some of these processes to what Homer tells us of the funeral and burial of Patroclus.

An area containing a variety of graves of period V that has been studied for its differential richness (Wüstemann, 1974) is the Prignitz, that is a small part in the west of the former province of Brandenburg just north of the Elbe at Wittenberge (today in Bezirk Schwerin). The region has its normal quota of Urnfield cemeteries, but also an unusual number of barrow graves of Periods IV to VI (320 burials in c.240 barrows, and around 1,000 urn-graves). The Urnfields are typically rather poor in bronzes: only 170, that is 17%, contain metal grave-goods, and the average Urnfield cemetery in the area is seen as representing a "socially undifferentiated layer of the population" (Wüstemann, 1974 p.71). By contrast the barrow graves, themselves of several constructional types, are richer in metal: 150 of the 320 graves (47%) contain metal, though even here some graves have no grave-goods at all: some of these are urn-graves. The graves containing metal can themselves be divided into groups according to what exactly they contained. A mere ten can be assigned to the highest wealth level, as defined by the presence of a sword and usually other rich goods as well. Chief among these rich graves was the 'King's Grave' at Seddin itself, with metal vessels, knife, socketed axes, razor, tweezers, neck-ring, arm-ring, finger-ring, spiral beads, comb, bracelet and other ornaments. The barrow itself is unusually elaborate: over 80m. in diameter and 11m. high, it contains a central stone cairn with polygonal slab-lined chamber 2m. across and 1.60m. high, with painted plaster on the walls. This and some of the other barrows stand apart from the remaining graves. The second group of graves is characterized by the presence of a knife and sometimes two or three other ornaments or toilet articles, but never in great quantities. Thirdly, there are graves with only one of a number of possible artifact types present: socketed axe, spearhead, bridle gear or sheet bronze vessel. In order to make full use of these facts, one must also know the chronological and geographical parameters within which they operated. The Urnfield cemeteries span the three Periods IV, V and VI, but by far the majority, including most of the richest graves, fall in V, and many cemeteries stop in V. Certainly very few continue through and beyond Period VI. As far as distribution is concerned, the rich graves of this area cluster in four main zones, which could well be taken as having a territorial significance. The variability of grave-good provision in Nordic Late Bronze Age graves has also been the subject of study by Thrane (1981).

Another detailed analysis of a north European Late Bronze Age cemetery is that by Bergmann (1982) on the cemetery of Vollmarshausen (Kassel). Here attention focussed not only on differential grave-good provision but also on the existence of clusters or 'zones' of graves, in simultaneous use and interpreted as family burial-places: specific depositional practices varied from zone to zone (for instance the provision of a covering slab over the urn). A basis of family-sized kinship units, as alleged for Vollmarshausen, is also seen by Ellison (1980) and by Petersen (1981) in the urn cemeteries of southern England, where burial clusters are to be seen, though not significant correlations between age/sex and grave-goods or form.

We may perhaps reasonably conclude from this discussion that the similarity of grave-goods in Urnfield cemeteries in northern Europe reflects an 'equality' that is more apparent than real. At certain periods and in certain areas clear signs of wealth differentials are present, though the individuals thus marked must be contrasted with the situation in the Early Bronze Age, and were relatively few in number. These general conclusions agree broadly with those of Levy in her sane and thorough study of Bronze Age Denmark, where among other things she distinguished the highest number of levels of rank differentiation in Period V, an 'elite' being most visible in Periods IV-V (1977, 1979, 1982).

Both these studies and Levy's more recent work (1983) have also emphasized the role of religion as a means of maintaining ranked societies or chiefdoms, for instance through "the elite's ability to control the items needed for offerings in fertility ritual".

Settlements

The study of Bronze Age settlement data has been much hampered by the lack of material in those areas - the majority - where stone was not used for house construction. Nonetheless, improved recognition and recovery techniques have resulted in the accumulation of quite a large body of evidence. The treatment accorded it has, in social terms, been rather haphazard. Consider for instance, the case of the Late Bronze Age settlement at Dampierre-sur-le-Doubs in the French Jura: houses of different sizes and shapes were found (visible as postholes cut in the subsoil) and the excavators concluded, after a brief mention of one or two other sites: "There exists then a certain social hierarchy among the people practising cremation in 'Urnfields'" (Pétrequin et al. 1969, p.32). True enough, but what? Various authors have attempted to interpret settlement plans in social terms, and in our period the most notorious case is that of the Wasserburg near Bad Buchau on the Federseemoor, where a stockade contained 38 houses in the first phase, nine in the second; in both phases one of the houses had an extra piece added on to it - a porch or ante-room - which has led to its being dubbed a "chieftain's house" (Reinerth 1928).

House size and village layout seem very poor guides to social organization, however. Levi-Strauss, indeed, showed many years ago how dangerous such interpretations can be without an understanding of the mental states that created such layouts (1956/1977). Add to this the further difficulty that so few settlement plans recovered archaeologically in temperate Europe are anywhere near complete, and the whole flimsy edifice erected by excavators over the years collapses. On the other hand, Drewett's (1980) analysis of the settlement at Black Patch, Sussex, does clearly hold out possibilities for the future, possibilities already exploited by Ellison (1981). Her discussion of Middle Bronze Age settlements makes a convincing case for modular units in the settlements of southern England, consisting of a major residential structure, an ancillary structure, and capacity for storage, shelter and open-air activities. Such modular units are taken to suggest standard social units of 10-20 individuals, linked in extended family units and having patrilineal and patrilocal kinship organization.

In fact it is only in the Mediterranean area that the expected signs of increasing organization are clearly visible, with the culmination in palaces, complete with their administrative systems and social hierarchies. With the aid of the Linear B tablets we can point to Messenia as one example of a known case of the development of settlement form concomitant with the development of social organization. Another area of increasing settlement regularity and complexity is Sicily, where complete village plans with undifferentiated round or oval houses of the Early and Middle Bronze Ages give way to a regular rectilinear type of site (Thapsos) in the Late Bronze Age.

In contrast to the situation with settlement layout, settlement patterning is often highly suggestive, notably in the case of hill-forts. Fortified sites on hill-tops in both Early and Late Bronze Age in central Europe and elsewhere show a distinctly 'territorial' distribution which must be related to group organization and therefore indirectly to social division. Indeed, the very existence of such sites would indicate social conditions, including the prevalence of antagonistic territorial groupings, that would readily allow exploitation by elites.

BRONZE AGE ECONOMICS IN RELATION TO SOCIAL ORGANIZATION

Since elites have to rely on production to achieve, or at any rate manifest, their dominant status, consideration of the economic base and organization is clearly of importance. There are two contrasting aspects of this Bronze Age production: industry (principally metal production) and subsistence (mainly food production). Ignore for present purposes labour directed to non-productive ends, e.g. the erection of religious monuments (though a site like Stonehenge shows that this aspect of labour expenditure must have played a considerable part in the whole).

Let us first consider the question of metal production, the principal industrial component of the Bronze Age. There are various possible approaches to this matter. We can remark first of all that generally through the Bronze Age the range of objects produced increased very markedly. Early Bronze Age hoards and other finds in central Europe, for instance, contain some 18 to 20 different types of object (e.g. Tihelka 1965, von Brunn 1959). An analysis of the bronze industry of the middle Danubian Tumulus culture (Furmanek 1973) distinguishes 25 main categories of material, with no less than 65 main types being represented. A typical catalogue of Late Bronze Age material, like that of Vinski-Gasparini (1973) for Croatia, lists over 40 main categories of material, and around 226 different types - some admittedly restricted to particular parts of the Urnfield period. The general picture is therefore clear: during the course of the Bronze Age the bronze-smith indulged in increasing experimentation with his materials. Metal, being capable of being both plastic and solid, naturally gave the smith almost unlimited scope, which he apparently used to the full.

Next we can consider the composition of hoards at various periods. Of the various types of hoard, scrap hoards are least informative for present purposes and will not be considered further. Some hoards contained mainly or entirely a single class of object, while others contained several or many classes of object in equal or unequal proportions. Each relates to technological factors, to specialization, to local depositional circumstances and to socio-economic context. Mould technology, for instance, would affect hoard type if the same mould was capable of being used again and again to produce identical objects, whereas clay moulds that might be broken up after a single casting might tend to produce less uniformity. Specialization might tend to have the effect of smiths concentrating on particular types at the expense of others. Depositional circumstances clearly played a part in influencing hoard composition, but it is hard to say what unless we know the precise position of the hoard in the customer/supplier network.

As examples of the two hoard types we may take the well-known hoards 2 and 3 from Dieskau (Saalkreis), as shown in Table 1. It is clear that the two hoards emanate from the same smithing background, yet are qualitatively and quantitatively different. One can find comparable concentration on various classes of object, and not just tools either: ornament hoards (rings and bracelets) are one well-known category of the Late Bronze Age. Two quite different types of demand - and therefore supply - are present. One is of a general nature: a smith equips himself with a broad range of objects to dispose of, perhaps not expecting a heavy run on any one type. The other is specialized: either through commissioning, or by the chance that he happens to have run a casting of a particular type not long previously, or - conceivably -because there is a specialized demand for a particular product in a particular area. With tools this would presumably reflect the ability to procure metal among artisan classes - itself a fact of some importance. With weapons (rather unusual in hoards) and ornaments, it is possible to envisage a demand that was distinctly 'up-market' from the artisan classes. (This argument cannot be taken too far, however, as both Leubingen and Helmsdorf contained axes.) Regardless of the precise interpretation one chooses to put on single-type hoards, it is clear that the massive production of single types reflects a demand for both utilitarian and display items on a large scale.

Table 1

Contents of hoards 2 and 3 from Dieskau, Saalkreis

Hoard 2	Hoard 3
10 ring ingots	3 heavy oval open rings
4 heavy oval open rings	1 heavy oval closed ring
4 heavy oval closed rings	6 arm-spirals and one
2 leech-shaped rings	fragment
7 open arm-rings	2 double-axes
2 arm-spirals	1 large halberd blade
1 flanged axe	with rivets
2 double-axes	293 flanged axes
2 hafted "Saxon" halberds	
1 other halberd with rivets	
11 halberd blades	
23 spiral tube beads	
106 amber beads	
Total: 175 objects (69 bronze)	Total: 307 objects (all bronze)

The two aspects of hoard composition taken together indicate that the productive capacity of Bronze Age smiths increased enormously over the period. Both the skills of the artisan and the tastes of his customer diversified, and the range of people able to acquire metal objects must - in spite of fluctuation - have gained. It is also increasingly possible to spot the production of one-off, custom-built objects. Commissions were thus possible; society contained groups of at least a few people able to command the necessary resources.

But how exactly could these resources have been acquired? At this point we may turn to subsistence activities. Work on the land must have been the main preoccupation of most people in the Bronze Age world outside the few palatial centres that we know of. Few areas of Europe have produced no traces of Bronze Age activity at all, and even if we do not wish to imagine the whole of Europe under plough or pasture at any one time, we can legitimately envisage a landscape essentially devoted to arable and pastoral activities. Of crucial importance is the question of land division and control. Agricultural technology, important though it is, does not - in my view - show marked differences in the Bronze Age from the Neolithic, so that the general range of implements available, and therefore presumably the methods employed, were the same in both periods. What changes is the relationship of labourer and land. Here the great bulk of our evidence comes from the British Isles, in the form of Bronze Age land divisions. It does now seem that such division of the land was indeed under way in Ireland in the Neolithic (Caulfield 1978), but it is in the Bronze Age that the majority of our evidence falls. In the case of Dartmoor, such dating evidence as there is suggests that the stone walls or reaves date to a period well into the Bronze Age, perhaps fourteenth to thirteenth centuries bc (Fleming 1978, pp.110-11; Wainwright and Smith 1980, pp.117-18). The first such land divisions were not built of stone; excavation has revealed traces of fences underlying later stone walls, and puzzling gaps in the walls may be explained by imagining fences or hedgerows at these spots. The stone land-divisions represent, in fact, the fossilized final product of the division process, presumably after a considerable period of organic growth that had gone on since at least the start of the Bronze Age. Land divisions in Wessex probably date to much the same period. The combined evidence suggests strongly that during the second millennium bc the agricultural landscape was divided up on a large scale. This situation is especially interesting in the light of fieldwork on Hawaii which has suggested that major land units, in the form of long strips from the coast into the inland forests, are associated with community social groups, and indeed with specific local residence groups situated on the coast (Cordy and Kaschko 1980). Several possible development patterns are suggested, based on either the infilling of a dispersed system, or the subdivision of communal land. Fluctuations in settlement patterns have been explored by many authors, of whom Bintliff (1982) may be specifically cited. In this model, "cyclical alternation of population ... must reflect **intensification** and **deintensification** of land use ... a cyclical shift from ... small infield round the low population centres, surrounded by extensive outfield, to ... a vigorous pushing back of outfield to minimal proportions and a massive intake into extensive cultivation of the outer lands. With clear evidence that much of moorland Britain was taken into cultivation in the Bronze Age, but abandoned thereafter, a cyclical pattern certainly seems indicated".

The resulting fields tend to be of different sizes and shapes (even allowing for geographical variability), while long linear divisions, often several kilometres long, play an important role. Neither of these two facts would indicate a landscape controlled simply by those who worked on the land. Yet such settlements as accompany these land divisions do not contain obvious signs of ranking in terms of housing (but cf. the work of Drewett, above): that is left to the grave finds. Graves like Bush Barrow drive home the idea that work on the land was not a universal chore. That point accepted, one has opened the way to admitting the existence of a peasant class, perhaps toiling on land formally annexed by someone else in return for a share in the produce. If land division was as widespread as it appears to be, and took place particularly on those areas that were already under pressure (Bradley 1978), a mechanism can be seen by which land labourers could acquire an inferior position -and, therefore, by which 'others' could acquire a superior one. This mechanism could, other things (like environmental conditions) being equal, reinforce itself with time, the familiar syndrome of serfdom being near at hand in any land-based labour-dependent hierarchy. It is interesting to note in this connection the class system known from the Linear B archives at Pylos, though it is striking in that context that farmers are dependent on, but not subservient to, the palace administration.

It need not have been restricted to land-based hierarchies, either. Apart from in corpore examples of boats (mostly canoes or other short-haul craft) we have countless depictions of boats in the rock art of Scandinavia. Many of these, being miles inland, have been connected with ritual activities, but this is hardly the point: what we need to know is, whose boats were these? Not, one imagines, the community's, but the possession of individuals or families. A boat clearly represents a considerable amount of labour input and is thus inherently valuable in itself: how universally available were they? On some of these depictions, moreover, there appears a row of vertical or oblique strokes above the gunwales which are plausibly taken to be oarsmen; these can number up to 40 or more (are they shown on one side only, or in false perspective?). Other depictions, perhaps more 'realistic', show only six strokes, sometimes in paired groups. If these are privately owned vessels containing substantial numbers of oarsmen, hierarchization had already proceeded to a considerable length. The purposes of the ships should also be considered: possibilities include fishing, transport and warfare. Either the first (favoured by Gilman) or the last would imply the existence of organization processes designed to maximize the degree of convenience for a small elite body.

It is instructive to compare this situation with that known from Iron Age Greece, a suggestion for which I thank Dr. J. Bintliff. Snodgrass (1980 pp.137-8) has recently sketched the development of ship-building in Greece, from the first oared longships in use down to the later sixth century BC, to the large sail-driven merchantmen seen thereafter. In the early period he supposes that the ships were sailed by "other kinds of men than professional merchants", a situation that gave way to the rise of "independent ship-masters" and the evidence of "agents and dependents of the ship-owners and exporters, rather than being self-employed merchants". The existence of such a class is clearly to be related to the land and labour relations which Snodgrass and others discuss.

SUMMARY: THE REGIONAL ECONOMY

The several lines of approach followed here provide abundant evidence that elites existed in the Bronze Age. It remains to ask how they achieved that elite status. I have already hinted at what I believe to be the crucial importance of economic factors in this development, but one cannot ignore the role of political factors. That is to say, economic production may enable status differentiation to take place; it may not necessarily cause it. There does not seem to be any easy way open at present to distinguish political power from other types of ostentation known archaeologically; yet early records and archives demonstrate the existence of such political power. Material wealth, furthermore, can be 'achieved' or 'ascribed', and both - but particularly achieved wealth -can come about in a variety of ways. The means by which elites achieve their dominance, whether by physical prowess, by leadership, by intelligence or by some other means are essentially unknowable to the prehistorian, though it has been suggested, for example, that the unusually robust male skeletons in the Shaft Graves betoken special physical eminence in life. What one can speculate on is the nature of the economy operating in the Bronze Age and

the size of the socio-political units which the elites controlled or acted on.

Here a crucial role is played by the nature of the Bronze Age economy. There were of course, in the Bronze Age as now, several different components of economic activity and production, which we may conveniently divide into primary (food procurement, shelter etc.) and secondary (industrial and manufacturing production - most notably metal extraction and working). There is evidence for the extensive nature of the distribution of secondary products in the form of large-scale dispersal of both metal types and finished objects. Workshop areas can be suggested, as can regions to which such distribution was primarily directed. On the other hand, there is little or no evidence for entrepôts through which such trade passed, suggesting that it was carried out on a rather casual basis perhaps by independent individuals or groups. But while secondary production shows abundant signs of movement, primary production (for which little information is available), although it can by its very nature tell us little of such matters, can be assumed to have been a much more localized affair. When one considers the nature of Bronze Age settlement sites, and the evidence in favourable areas for territoriality, there can be no presumption of the creation of agricultural surpluses. The very concept of the agricultural surplus is, moreover, an unlikely one in prehistoric Europe. Bronze Age settlements, apart from their capacity to produce grain, had very limited ability to store it: the only attested type was the pit cut in the ground, unreliable for storage over more than one winter. The 'Genesis strategy' was here impossible: grain yields and population size and health must have borne a relationship to one another, even if not a direct Malthusian one (it is hardly surprising that Shennan found far less rich female infants than demographically expected if differential access to food, shelter and clothing was involved). The area from which grain was gathered can thus be assumed to be very limited, plausibly the 5km. radius used by the Higgs school for site catchment analysis of agricultural sites. If this is the case, agricultural settlements in Bronze Age Europe (and outside Greece these preponderate) can be demonstrated to be concerned not with large-scale or long-distance movement of foodstuffs but with production for feeding local mouths or at the most for exchange on a district level for other comparable commodities. This picture is in fact confirmed by cemetery analysis, where the great majority of the dead throughout the Bronze Age are not conspicuously provided for.

Where, then, do the few who **were** so provided for fit in? In the absence of substantial settlement structures the sway these people held must have been visible only in material possessions and clothing; it could therefore relate principally to success at acquisition. Such success is, however, most likely to be derived from political sources, as already described. What it is unlikely to have been based on, in the light of the foregoing, is agricultural surpluses, at any rate in those areas of Europe where settlement networks were well developed. But this immediately raises the question of the 'ranches' known from various parts of the British Isles. I have indicated already that both in this case and in that of the Scandinavian boat-owners control of people - people who depended on the fruits of their own labours for their continued existence, but who nevertheless were not at liberty to dispose of those fruits - may have been the determining factor.

This does not solve the problem of the missing link, namely how control of people was initially achieved, but it does suggest how elite status continued to be maintained. Why certain elites should have chosen to manifest their status in special ways at death may have to be answered as much in terms of secondary production

144

(particular favourable combinations of raw material distribution, trade routes in finished products, movements of smiths etc.) as in terms of people owing allegiance and therefore marking the death by acts signifying corporate involvement. Production of 'invisibles' like salt and textiles may have contributed -the former almost certainly in the East Alpine Early Iron Age, to take the best-known example.

Bronze Age territories, then, show little sign of having transcended the district level, outside the Mycenaean world. Even at the end of the Bronze Age, with the rise of hill-forts, the size of the putative territories does not rise above regional level and the number of those involved in conspicuous grave deposition never becomes large.

These considerations naturally have an impact on our appreciation of long-distance exchange, especially exchange in exotic objects or substances, where this can be demonstrated. The prevalent notion of benighted barbarians gratefully receiving the next batch of faience beads or Aegean-imitating spirally-decorated pots is quite unrealistic. In economic terms exchange of exotica over long distances - whether direct or via a 'prestige chain' - was essentially irrelevant. Only those whose privileged position enabled the acquisition of exotic goods by means of gift exchange or the like were involved, and what (if anything) they provided in return may equally have had little to do with the economic system. The fact that such goods were traded over long distances thus says nothing about the economy, but potentially a great deal about society.

CONCLUSION

That social divisions were marked in the Bronze Age is clear from several lines of approach. That the nature of the divisions differed at different stages is suggested by the circumstantial evidence available in the later Bronze Age for population increase, greater production of metalwork, physical partitioning of land, and differential access to exotic trade-goods. Various ways of modelling these social and economic changes are possible. The Bronze Age thus saw the development of two contrasting but related trends: on the one hand, village or even proto-urban life in which a sizeable population lived side by side, unmarked (at least in death) by a notably disparate outward display of wealth; on the other, the role of the individual which achieved new proportions, marking what we may call, to adapt a connotation coined by Professor Sahlins, the era of the 'big man'.

BIBLIOGRAPHY

BERGMANN, J. 1982 - Ein Gräberfeld der jüngeren Bronze-und älteren Eisenzeit bei Vollmarshausen, Kr. Kassel. Marburg (Kasseler Beitrage zur Vor- und Fruhgeschichte, Band 5).

BINTLIFF, J. L. 1982 - "Settlement patterns, land tenure and social structure: a diachronic model", in C. Renfrew and S. Shennan (eds.) Ranking, Resource and Exchange. Aspects of the Archaeology of Early European Society, pp.106-111

BOUZEK, J. 1982 - "Climate changes and central European prehistory", in A.F. Harding (Ed.) Climate Change in Later Prehistory, pp.178-91.

BRADLEY, R. 1978 - "Prehistoric field systems in Britain and north-west Europe - a review of some recent work",

World Archaeology vol. 9 (3), pp.265-80.

BRUNN, A.W. von 1959 - Bronzezeitliche Hortfunde. Teil I: Die Hortfunde der frühen Bronzezeit aus Sachsen-Anhalt, Sachsen, Thüringen. Berlin: Akademie-Verlag.

CAULFIELD, S. 1978 - "Neolithic fields: the Irish evidence", in H.C. Bowen & P.J. Fowler (Eds.) Early Land Allotment, BAR 48, pp.137-43.

CHAPMAN, R.W. 1977 - "Burial practices: an area of mutual interest", in M. Spriggs (Ed) Archaeology and Anthropology: Areas of Mutual Interest, BAR S19, pp.19-33.

CHILDE, V.G. 1963 - Social Evolution. London: Fontana Library.

COLES, J.M. & A.F. HARDING 1979 - The Bronze Age in Europe, An Introduction to the Prehistory of Europe, ca. 2000 B.C. to ca. 700 B.C. London: Methuen.

CORDY, R. & M.W. KASCHKO, 1980 - "Prehistoric archaeology in the Hawaiian Islands: land units associated with social groups". Journal of Field Archaeology vol. 7, pp.403-16.

DREWETT, P. 1979 - "New evidence for the structure and function of Middle Bronze Age round houses in Sussex", Archaeol. J. vol. 136, pp.3-11.

DUSEK, S. 1973 - "Kotazke vojenskej demokracie v pravekom vyvoji Slovenska," Slovenska archeologia vol. 21, pp.409-42.

ELLISON, A. 1980 - "Deverel-Rimbury urn cemeteries: the evidence for social organisation" in J. Barrett & R. Bradley (eds.) Settlement and Society in the British Later Bronze Age, BAR 83, pp.115-26.

ELLISON, A. 1981 - "Towards a socioeconomic model for the Middle Bronze Age in southern England", in I. Hodder, G. Isaac, N. Hammond (Eds.) Pattern of the Past. Studies in Honour of David Clarke, pp.413-38.

FLEMING, A. 1978 - "The prehistoric landscape of Dartmoor. Part I: South Dartmoor", Proc. Prehist. Soc. vol. 44, pp.97-123.

FORBES, R.J. 1964 - Studies in Ancient Technology, vol VIII. Leiden: Brill.

FRANKENSTEIN, S. and ROWLANDS, M.J. 1978 - "The internal structure and regional context of early Iron Age society in south-west Germany", Bull. Inst. Archaeol. London vol. 15, pp.73-112.

FURMANEK, V. 1973 - "Bronzova industrie stredodunajske mohylove kultury na Morave", Slovenska Archeologia vol. 20, pp.25-145.

FURMANEK, V. 1977 - "Pilinyer Kultur", Slovenska Archaeologia vol. 25, pp.251-370.

GALLAY, G. 1972 - "Beigaben der Frühbronzezeit Süddeutschlands in ihrer Verteilung auf Männer- und Frauengräber", Homo vol. 20, pp.50-73.

GILMAN, A. 1976 - "Bronze Age dynamics in south-east Spain", Dialectical Anthropology vol. 1, pp.307-19.

GILMAN, A. 1981 - "The development of social stratification in Bronze Age Europe", Current Anthropology vol. 22, 1, pp.1-23.

GIMBUTAS, M. 1965 - Bronze Age Cultures in Central and Eastern Europe. The Hague: Mouton.

HACHMANN, R. 1957 - Die frühe Bronzezeit im westlichen Ostseegebiet und ihre mittel- und südosteuropäischen Beziehungen. Atlas der Urgeschichte. Hamburg: Kartographisches Institut.

KRISTIANSEN, K. 1977 - "The circulation of ornaments and weapons in Bronze Age Denmark", Archaeol. Baltica vol. 2, pp.77-91.

KRISTIANSEN, K. 1980 - "Besiedlung, Wirtschaftsstrategie und Bodennutzung in der Bronzezeit Dänemarks", Praehist. Z. vol. 55, pp.1-37.

LEVI-STRAUSS, C. 1977 - "Do dual organisations exist?" in Structural Anthropology, London: Peregrine Books (article first published 1956).

LEVY, J.E. 1977 - Social and Religious Change in Bronze Age Denmark, Ann Arbor: University Microfilms.

LEVY, J.E. 1979 - "Evidence of social stratification in Bronze Age Denmark", Journal of Field Archaeology vol. 6, pp.49-56.

LEVY, J.E. 1982 - Social and Religious Organisation in Bronze Age Denmark. An Analysis of Ritual Hoard Finds. BAR S 124.

LEVY, J.E. 1983 Rank and religion in prehistoric chiefdoms. Lecture given to the Society for American Archaeology, Pittsburgh, April 1983.

MALINOWSKI, T.1961 - "Obrzadek pogrzebowy kultury łuzyckiej w Polsce", Przeg. Archeologiczny vol. 14, pp.5-135.

MARX, K. 1954 - Capital Moscow: Progress Publishers.

MILISAUSKAS, S. 1978 - European Prehistory. London/New York: Academic Press.

NEUSTUPNY, E. 1967 - "K pocatkum patriarchatu ve stredni Evrope", Rozpravy ceskoslovenske akademie ved vol. 77, p.2.

PAULIK, J. 1974 - "K vyznamu mohyl z mladsej doby bronzovej v pravekom vyvoji Slovenska", Slovenska archeologia vol. 22, pp.73-81.

PETERSEN, F.F. 1981 - The Excavation of a Bronze Age Cemetery on Knighton Heath, Dorset. BAR 98.

PETREQUIN, P., J.-P. URLACHER, and D. VUAILLAT 1969 -"Habitat et sepultures de l'âge du bronze final à Dampierre-sur-le-Doubs (Doubs)", Gallia Préhistoire vol. 12, pp.1-35.

PIGGOTT, S. 1938 - "The early Bronze Age in Wessex", Proc. Prehist. Soc. vol. 4, pp.52-106.

RANDSBORG, K. 1974 - "Social stratification in Early Bronze Age Denmark: a study in the regulation of cultural systems", Praehistorische Zeitschrift vol. 49, pp.38-61.

REINERTH, H. 1928 - Die Wasserburg Buchau. Führer zur Urgeschichte 6.

RENFREW, A.C. 1972 - The Emergence of Civilisation: the Cyclades and the Aegean in the Third Millennium B.C. London: Methuen.

RENFREW, A.C. 1973 - "Monuments, mobilisation and social organisation in Neolithic Wessex", in A.C. Renfrew (ed.) The Explanation of Culture Change, pp. 539-58. London: Duckworth.

RENFREW, A.C. 1974 - "Beyond a subsistence economy: the evolution of social organisation in prehistoric Europe", in C.B. Moore (ed.) Reconstructing Complex Societies, pp. 69-95. Cambridge (Mass): American Schools of Oriental Research.

RUCKDESCHEL, W. 1968 - "Geschlechtsdifferenzierte Bestattungssitten in frühbronzezeitlichen Gräbern Südbayerns", Bayerische Vorgeschichtsblätter vol. 33, pp. 18-44.

RYSIEWSKA, T. 1980 - "La structure patriarchale des clans comme type hypothétique de la structure sociale des groups humains dans la culture lusacienne. Essai de vérification de l'hypothèse d'après la necropole de Przeczyce", Archaeologia Polona vol 19, pp.7-48.

SERVICE, E.R. 1962 - Primitive Social Organisation. New York: Random House.

SERVICE, E.R. 1975 - The Origins of the State and Civilisation. The Process of Cultural Evolution. New York: W.W. Norton.

SHENNAN, S. 1975 - "The social organisation at Branc", Antiquity vol. 49, pp.279-88.

SHENNAN, S. 1982 - "From minimal to moderate ranking", In C. Renfrew and S. Shennan (Eds.) Ranking, Resource and Exchange. Aspects of the Archaeology of Early European Society, pp.27-32.

SNODGRASS, A.M. 1980 - Archaic Greece: the Age of Experiment. London: Dent.

STUKELEY, W. 1740 - Stonehenge: a Temple restor'd to the British Druids.

SZYDŁOWSKA, E. 1968 - Cmentarzysko kultury łuzyckiej w Przeczycach, pow. Zawiercie (Rocznik Muzeum Gornoslaskiego w Bytomiu 5,8,9).

THRANE, H. 1981 - "Late Bronze Age graves in Denmark seen as expressions of social ranking - an initial report", in H. Lorenz (ed) Studien zur Bronzezeit. Festschrift für W.A. von Brunn, pp.475-88.

TIHELKA, K. 1965 - Hort- und Einzelfunde der Uneticer Kultur und des Veterover Typus in Mähren. Fontes Archaeologicae Moravicae 4, Brno.

VINSKI-GASPARINI, Z. 1973 - Kultura polja sa zarama u sjevernoj Hrvatskoj. Zadar: Filozofski fakultet.

VLADAR, J. 1973 - "Osteuropäische und Mediterrane Einflüsse im Gebiet der Slowakei während der Bronzezeit", Slovenska Archeologia vol. 21, pp.253-357.

WAINWRIGHT, G.J. and K. SMITH 1980 - "The Shaugh Moor project: second report - the enclosure", Proc. Prehist. Soc. vol. 46, pp.65-122.

WUSTEMANN, H. 1974 - "Zur Sozialstruktur in Seddiner Kulturgebiet", Z. für Archäologie, vol. 8, pp.67-107.

6

CONCEPTUALIZING THE EUROPEAN BRONZE AND EARLY IRON AGES

Mike Rowlands

"It seems to me axiomatic that where neighbouring communities have demonstrable economic, political and military relations with each other then the field of any useful sociological analysis must override cultural boundaries" from E.R. Leach 1954 Political Systems of Highland Burma p.292. London, Bell.

A 'Western' sense of history has been defined as a mode of consciousness that assumes social change to be inevitable, continuous and linear (Levi Strauss 1966). The idea that societies 'evolve' is therefore deeply rooted in European thought as a rationalization of a period of recent social change which perhaps inevitably, has been considered the most disruptive in world history. Whilst European philosophy may therefore be accused of exaggerating its own sense of loss, it is a unique feature of Western intellectual life that it has come to terms with its own experience by conducting one of the longest and most detailed historical investigations into its own genesis ever attempted. In order to avoid endless historical regression and to put some kind of order into what could be seen as an endless series of disasters, Western historians have chosen to select three major periods of social change for special attention: the beginning of classical antiquity, the fall of the western Roman Empire and the transition from feudalism to capitalism. All three 'events' are unified at a higher level since they all claim to answer a single question: what was so distinctive about Europe that encouraged the development of modern capitalism there and nowhere else and what were the origins of this distinctive developmental sequence?

A concern with understanding the uniqueness of the European experience has been the leitmotif of social and philosophical thought since the eighteenth century. The search for 'the other' as alien comparison motivated an earlier anthropology to see the world in simple binary terms of the primitive/civilized variety. Perhaps more than the social sciences, history and prehistory have been concerned with studying uniqueness, rather than the comparison of cultural difference, as their particular contribution to constructing a European identity. The historical method differs quite fundamentally from the anthropological in this respect. Comparison to elucidate difference is replaced by the construction of a particular developmental sequence in order to detect those points in time when certain events had the unintended consequence of diverting the European sequence of social change from the rest of world history. Hence, the anthropological mode of treating ethnographies as cases for elucidating some general principle is inverted in the case of history where general concepts are useful only to the extent they

facilitate our reconstruction of a particular past. History as the conscious search for cultural identity is therefore humanity whilst anthropology as the interpreter of cultural difference becomes social science. Some practitioners in both disciplines have disagreed vehemently with such a characterization of their respective disciplines and give the uncomfortable impression of trains passing each other in a rather dark tunnel, (contrast Evans Pritchard 1961 and Binford 1962). But otherwise few in European archaeology have inquired into the reasons why their work is so deeply enmeshed in the complexities of reconstructing a particular cultural sequence. According to Whallon they should be off subsuming their particular case as illustrative of some more general comparative principle (Whallon 1982). This paper is an essay in why this has not been the case and yet why the results of such work are still of general significance.

Over the last century the answer to when did a distinctively European form of society diverge from the rest of the world, has been moved further back in time. To avoid endless historical regression and recognizing the probable arbitrariness of the decision anyway, Marx and Weber favoured the Medieval notion that a benchmark could be set at the decay of later antiquity and the emergence of Europe as a moral and cultural synthesis of Romano-Germanic elements, ethnically unified in its opposition to Byzantine and Arab imperial aspirations, (Anderson P. 1974). The classical tradition, consistent with a wider view of what constituted western civilization, emphasized the appearance of the Greek city state system as the 'event' which initiated the divergence of the West from that of the ancient Near East. Recent debates betray a related assumption that the character of modern Europe can be projected back into classical antiquity and its origins established as a kind of negative mirror reflection of the present e.g. the Polanyi characterization of market and non-market economies in ancient Athens (Polanyi 1977), the role of commerce and the use of class versus status group to define stratification in the ancient world (Finley 1975). Finally, European prehistory provided an alternative rationalization that required regression into a more remote past, stressing the autonomous development of Europe from a much earlier period than hitherto conceived. The Bronze Age became prehistory's answer to the question when and how a distinctive European society emerged in world history.

Defining the European Bronze Age

By exposing our motivations for studying the past, we lay bare the guiding principles that lead us to assume certain

148

periods in prehistory to be of greater interest than others. As is well known, the Bronze Age was defined in the nineteenth century as part of a general scheme that combined a glorification of technological progress with millennial expectations of the kinds of human freedom this would produce in the future. The Bronze Age was therefore a period of 'primitive science', the achievements of which would be measured unproblematically with those of the modern age. Like many other historical schemes which segment time into blocks that are opposed to each other by qualitative differences in the characteristics common to them all (in the case of the Three Age system these were qualitative differences in the forces of production characteristic of each of these periods), emphasis is placed on the transitions between the segments rather than the segments themselves. Gordon Childe, for instance, was able to sustain the Three Age system for a while by proposing certain socio-economic correlates to the technological criteria that defined the segments (Childe 1957). But as a more rigorous sociological approach has begun to show that change at the economic, political and ideological levels are not 'all of apiece' we have come to realize that time may be segmented in as many ways as convenient to the researcher concerned.

Gordon Childe retained the traditional Three Age system primarily because his arguments for the relationship between the political, the ideological and the economic were of a highly determinist nature. As is well known his case invoked the utilitarian thesis that bronze metallurgy introduced a more efficient technology. This required an international trade for the acquisition of copper and tin and the complex nature of metalworking skills fostered the creation of a stratum of full time metalworkers, existing on the boundaries of tribal societies as itinerant craftsmen (Childe 1957, 1958). Now if Childe was simply arguing for the primacy of technology thesis and drew the wrong social 'facts', then his model for the Bronze Age has probably been rightly dismissed as a set of conjectures refuted by subsequent 'facts'. But it seems to me that Childe was attempting to say something else which, even if the precise arguments about bronze metallurgy don't apply, still lurks in the background as a set of unrefuted prepositions.

For instance, Childe was as equally concerned with the development of copper and bronze metallurgy in the Near East and Egypt (Childe 1944). Moreover, he was fully aware that metallurgy did not serve the same purpose in all three areas nor did similar technologies necessarily result in the same social facts. In the ancient Near East, metalworkers like other craftsmen were tied to palace and temple; in Europe they had a semi-autonomous political and economic status. In Mesopotamia, craftsmen produced under duress for the luxury and warlike needs of aristocracies. In Europe, they produced on demand and were 'free' of political constraint. Hence, in the Near East, metallurgy was harnessed to non-utilitarian needs and in Europe to the utilitarian. In the Near East, metals had to be acquired by tribute and administered trade, in Europe they were acquired through commerce.

In other words we have two sociological models lurking in the background here which tend to characterize Europe and the Near East as polar opposites of each other. One of these conceptualizes ancient Near Eastern societies as totalitarian and despotic, lacking in personal liberty and leading to endless cycles of empire formation and stagnation; and the other defines Europe as ranked but never stratified, (i.e. empires have never developed indigenously in Europe), with greater personal freedom and a more dynamic tendency for economic growth and development.

But what were the origins of these two social models that Childe used to contextualize the different functions of bronze metallurgy in Europe and the Near East? The characterization of the Near East as a despotic society under the control of temple and palace, derives its inspiration from Hegel's description of Oriental Society and Marx's conceptualization of the Asiatic mode of production ('AMP' cf. Anderson 1974, Appendix B). Influences upon both of these thinkers can be traced back to the philosophical debates concerning the nature of social inequality in the French and Scottish schools of Enlightenment. In De l'esprit des lois (1748), Montesquieu made despotic society one of his three basic types of government, the others being monarchic and republican. He maintained that Asia, for most of its history, had been characterized by the rule of despots, by slavery and by the state control of land and other natural resources. Europe by contrast was characterized by the rule of law, and a spirit of liberty and the relative dominance of society over the state. As an explanation for this contrast, Montesquieu stressed geographical differences between the two areas and initiated the hydraulic irrigation debate by arguing that despotic government was most suited to societies in large, hot, desert areas where the maintenance of order was difficult and the state had to undertake special managerial tasks. Adam Smith took the next step by contrasting Europe and Asia as two different kinds of political economy. In Asia, agrarian production dominated over manufacture, the countryside inhibited the growth of a manufacturing urban base, and tribute and tax prevented the growth of free trade. Hence, Europe and Asia were conceptualized as mirror images of each other. To these, Marx added his concept of the AMP, including for Asia the absence of private ownership of land, the self sufficiency of village communities in combining agriculture with craft production so that there was no need to participate in external exchange, and the dominating role of the state over society. But in answer to a question from Engels, Marx emphasized that it was the absence of private property in land and the predominance of the 'self sustaining village community' that was the key to understanding oriental society - "The absence of private property in land ... is the real keystone of the Oriental vault" (Marx-Engels Selected Correspondence p.82).

As for the reasons for this contrast between a stagnant East and a dynamic West, Hegel, Marx and Weber went little further than agreeing with Montesquieu's original emphasis on environmental and geographical circumstances and, in particular, the importance of irrigation (Weber 1976, pp.37-8). Hence it is of no surprise that as far as the Near East was concerned, Childe adopted the AMP model with little modification, although in later years the discoveries at Jericho and elsewhere led him to begin to modify the irrigation hypothesis.

But in the case of Europe, Childe consistently believed archaeology would provide the answer to why European society diverged from that of the Near East and the origins of the social conditions that encouraged the development of those virtues of individualism, entrepreneurial skill and inventiveness which he believed were the progressive features of modern European society. These virtues he believed to be not of recent origin. Instead they could be traced back into prehistory and in particular to the inception of the Bronze Age with the first appearance of free craftsmen who could develop their skills and accumulate wealth untrammelled by religion or by servitude to a despotic ruling class. In the preface to The Dawn of European Civilization, Childe summed up the major theme of the book as the "foundation of European civilization as a peculiar and individual manifestation of the human spirit" (1947 p.XIII). Elsewhere he maintained "Among the Early Bronze Age peoples of the Aegean, the Danube Valley, Scandinavia and Britain, we can recognize already these very qualities of energy, independence and inventiveness which distinguish the western world from Egypt, India and China" (Childe 1925, pp.XIII, XIV). In other words Europe had been capitalist since the Middle Bronze Age and the growth of the economic and moral forces unleashed at this early time were finally, in his own day, about to transform the face of the earth. A Braudellian 'longue durée' of quite gigantic proportions, which incidentally allowed him to embed the past in the present and intellectually justify the existence of archaeology as an academic discipline to his own satisfaction.

To substantiate this interpretation of the European Bronze Age, as a form of primitive capitalism, Childe concentrated his work on the Neolithic and Early-Middle Bronze Age since he believed this to be the major period of transition which established the unique course of later European prehistory and history to have been perpetuated from then on. For him, the Neolithic in Europe was simply an extension of Near Eastern Orientalism. He described 'Megalithic builders' absorbed in the cult of the dead, with superstitious observances paralysing all their activities. In later works, the emphasis is placed on the self-sustaining nature of the Neolithic community, the insignificance of trade and the absence of technological development (which in Childe's eyes was the equivalent of science) (1958, pp.75-7). This stagnant variant of Asiatic society was changed irreversibly by the introduction of bronze metallurgy from outside which served to burst open the self-sufficiency of the European Neolithic community. More than this it was the external derivation of bronze metallurgy that determined the peripheral manner of its incorporation. "European metalworkers were free. They were not tied to any one patron or even to a single tribal society. They were producing for an inter-tribal if not an international market" (Childe, 1958, p.169). And it was this freedom which encouraged the development of 'native genius' and the growth of scientific knowledge that classical, medieval and modern European societies were to capitalize upon and extend. Technology had served the needs of production and exchange rather than status requirements at least since the Bronze Age and in this respect the Industrial Revolution was only different in degree from previous stages of European technological achievement.

The fact that Childe subsequently came to be characterized as the diffusionist who could not detect any originality in European development is ironic considering the philosophical origins which determined his empirical interests. One can only describe Childe's view of the relation of Europe to the Near East as a form of Hegelian dialectic (Childe 1957, p.15). Apparent dependency of Europe on Near Eastern innovation is negated by the mode in which the latter was incorporated, which in turn led to irreversible changes and differences in the conditions of existence of Europe from those of the Ancient Near East. At this point Childe again uses bronze metallurgy as an indicator of how unconstrained relations of production led to a dramatic growth of technology in Europe in contrast to stagnant forms of bronze technology and functional -variation in the Near East (Childe 1942). By stressing the role of innovation, Childe provided an alternative explanation of the divergence of Europe and the Near East from the ecological determinism of Montesquieu which had been accepted by all subsequent writers up to and including, in his own day, Julian Steward, (Steward 1955). By denying the significance of geographical conditions, Childe inadvertently shifted from an ecological determinist position as far as the Near East was concerned to an economic determinist view of European prehistory.

Redefining the Neolithic/Bronze Age transition

We have seen that in his characterization of the European Bronze Age, Childe relied on a number of commonly accepted eighteenth- and nineteenth-century generalizations about the difference between Oriental and Western society. He projected this contrast back into European prehistory. The European Neolithic was a variant of a more generalized form of Oriental society that elsewhere evolved into the more highly bureaucratized forms of empires which Europeans were to encounter in modern times (India, Persia, China etc.). Childe was one of those of Enlightenment sympathies whose macro-view of world history was firmly rooted in the primacy of the West and in understanding the origin of those dynamic forces that were, in his own time, transforming the world around him.

We are left with several legacies due to the manner in which the contrast between the Neolithic and the Bronze Age had to be conceptualized in order to fit this wider world view; many of which we still operate with although we may no longer understand their genesis. The image of a Neolithic economically self-sustaining community immured from trade and stagnating under the dead hand of religion, probably has undergone most change (Sherratt 1976). The role of bronze metallurgy and its mode of incorporation into European society, has retained its significance, although the prestige functions of the earliest metalwork would now be stressed rather than Childe's utilitarian model. Childe's portrayal of the emergence of wealth based aristocracies from the dissolution of Neolithic quasi-theocratic communities has not been radically altered although conceptualized in more sophisticated forms (e.g. Renfrew 1973, p.242; Shennan 1982).

The root of the problem lies, of course, in the extent to which the periodization of European prehistory rests on such received wisdom and thus obscures contradictory patterns emerging from more concrete empirical analyses. For instance, discussing the Late Neolithic/Early Bronze Age transition in western Europe, Renfrew has distinguished a pattern of group oriented chiefdoms from a succeeding pattern of individualizing chiefdoms (Renfrew 1973, 1974). Gilman proposed a similar dichotomy for the Late Copper Age/Early Bronze Age of south east Iberia and more recently attributed this to contemporary processes of agricultural intensification (Gilman 1976, 1981). Shennan has generalized the distinction to central and western Europe, allowing for a time lag between the two, in which 'Neolithic' hoe cultivators, egalitarian in social relations and ritually defined in communal relations and ideology move into contrast with more hierarchical, prestige good oriented systems in the late Neolithic and Early Bronze Age (Shennan 1982a, b). Although conceptually far more sophisticated and precise, this would in broad terms fit the general picture described by Childe and retains an implicit faith in the significance of bronze metallurgy as a disruptive innovation.

However, both Shennan and Sherratt (this volume) have recently elaborated a more gradual and regionally diverse description which permits the transformation of a description that was in danger of drifting into epochal stages, to a millennial-long process of subcontinental proportions. In the case of western Europe, only in southern Britain and particularly Wessex have more fine grained analyses begun to show a more complex pattern than the simple replacement of one social form by another. Barrett and Bradley, for instance, have described the change from mid third- to mid second-millennium BC in Wessex as the slow separation of ritual and secular power in which both structures coexist as part of a single dual system in the Late Neolithic. New forms of wealth accumulation provided by the latter structure are embedded in and serve to elaborate existing ceremonial practices into hyper-ritualized forms which continue well into the Early Bronze Age (Barrett and Bradley 1980, chs. 3 and 4). No such long term elaboration and gradual decomposition of traditional principles seems to have occurred in northern and central Europe. In the former area, the sudden flourish in megalithic tomb building in the EN/MN transition decomposes rapidly into the Funnel Beaker/Battle Axe series of the MN/LN with an emphasis on local regional styles in material culture and exchange networks (Randsborg 1975, Kristiansen 1982). The decline of earlier ritualized forms of social integration is therefore extremely rapid. New forms of status principles become established based on direct control of local resources which are developed further by the late Early Bronze Age in a phase of increasing trade with Central Europe.

Sherratt (this volume) has summarized his own interpretation of the contrast between central and eastern Europe, emphasizing that similarities between the sequences tend to be obscured by the obvious chronological disparity. Two points need to be emphasized. Firstly, as Sherratt argues, no necessary dependence upon the introduction of bronze metallurgy is implied. On the contrary, it is the east-west clinal process covering more than a millennium that is the determinant of the relative value attached over time to metalwork and other categories of valuables in circulation. Secondly, apart from the western peripheral areas, where as Sherratt emphasizes, traditional ritualization could be maintained and elaborated rather than being disrupted by expanding exchange networks, the maintenance of monopoly control over circulation appears to have been extremely difficult. This would presumably explain the relative absence of status differentiation prior to the end of the Early Bronze Age, when bronze production and circulation attained sufficient velocity to achieve some degree of dominance over other spheres of production and exchange. Even in these cases, we should remember that areas where this may have occurred (signified by the presence of 'rich' burials) were marginal (e.g. on the northern periphery of the Unetice area) and its duration short lived.

By adopting a macro-spatial and temporal approach to Europe from the late fourth to early second millennium, a pattern has been detected which could never have been built up through the painstaking comparison of local sequences (where essentially complexity is being reduced by emphasizing time scale within the confines of an arbitrarily defined territorial unit). The fact is that starting in south east Europe in the later fourth millennium and extending to the most western fringes by the mid second millennium, a series of profound and structurally similar changes occurred in subsistence, settlement, burial rite and attribution of personal status, technology and craft production, (Shennan, S.J. 1982a, p.10). The simplest explanation would be to view them as the consequence of a long cycle of expansion in exchange networks and trade density that began in south east Europe and followed a north west direction, weakening and dissipating in intensity along its westernmost extension. All of this suggests that a long term tendency existed for an increase in the density of exchange and alliance networks in eastern Europe, which had expanded into parts of central and western Europe by the end of the third millennium. Elsewhere, Rathje has suggested that there is a more general tendency for large scale exchange systems to establish themselves initially over extensive areas, (applying Sahlin's reciprocal exchange principle, 1972, pp.294-312), and then subsequently to decompose into more economically specialized and regionally differentiated networks (Rathje 1978). Friedman has applied a similar principle to Oceania and would associate the first

mode of exchange with a political principle of limiting access to strategic items and the second with situations where competition for status depends on the circulation of such items and hence serves to intensify their production and exchange. In the case of Oceania, the first mode would correspond generally with societies of broadly Polynesian type and the second with those of Melanesian type, with the latter as essentially decomposed or elaborated versions of the former (Friedman 1981, 1982). Gledhill has described a similar pattern of expanding and contracting exchange networks centered on the Meso-american heartland, and has related these to events in the American south west and mid-west, (Gledhill 1978).

In the European context, the additional factor of intensification in subsistence economy requires a special mention. Gilman, Shennan and Sherratt have laid great emphasis on changes in subsistence economy and settlement associated with what Sherratt has termed the secondary products revolution (Sherratt 1981). In all the comparative cases cited, intensification of the subsistence economy is involved because foodstuffs enter directly into circulation (cf. Friedman's discussion of western Polynesia, 1982). This is particularly so in more marginal areas where access to strategic items may be limited and political competition may itself involve the accumulation and circulation of foodstuffs. It would be most unfortunate if we continued to assume that there is something called a subsistence sector, (i.e. food/agriculture) and something else called production for exchange (i.e. craft production). Such differentiation is most uncharacteristic of such social situations and ignores completely the often high symbolic value that is attached to the consumption of particular kinds of foodstuffs in these ceremonial exchange systems. Sherratt makes much the same point in emphasizing that the technical and expressive role of livestock cannot be separated in European prehistoric contexts (Sherratt 1982). This is even more so, when large scale regional networks decompose into more intense and specialized systems since circulation takes on a more 'economic' character and all surpluses will be undifferentiated in exchange rather than being differentiated through withdrawal from circulation for ceremonial purposes. Moreover, the logic of the argument presented here would argue against the separation of technical items like ploughs and animal traction or consumption items like wool and milk from the more general system of circulation simply because they have 'subsistence connotations'. In fact it seems most unlikely that they could have 'diffused' as a separate technological category but are intimately connected with the whole gamut of change that characterizes the later fourth to late third millennium in Europe.

In what way does this new synthesis, recently provided for us, alter our conception of the beginning of the 'Bronze Age'? In the first instance, it serves to emphasize once again that the role of bronze metallurgy has been seriously overestimated and that bronze production as a separate sphere in the political economy scarcely needs to be isolated until the later phases of the Early Bronze Age at least in each particular area. It suggests instead that a different periodization is needed in which roughly an Early/Middle Neolithic may be contrasted to a Late Neolithic/Early Bronze Age and the latter in turn contrasted with a Later Bronze Age/ Early Iron Age unity, in central and western Europe. By reorganizing our time segments in this way, we also have to keep the process at work firmly in mind rather than the discontinuities it generated in different regional sequences at different time periods. Figure 1 thus attempts to diagram the changing sequences of political and economic forms in different sectors of central and western Europe. Finally, there is no reason to assume this intensification process operates within a 'closed system'. Without requiring any model of imperialism or direct economic intervention, the dates of these major changes in the European sub-continent correspond too closely with the major period of urban origins and commercialization of the Near Eastern regional system of the later fourth and particularly third millennium BC, for this correspondence between the two areas to be coincidental. Comparative cases of sudden inter-regional bursts of economic activity usually associated with breakdowns in distant pre-existing core systems of political control and stratification are too well known to require much elaboration here (cf Rathje 1975 on Classic/Post Classic Maya; or Allen 1977 on the Lapita horizon in Melanesia; or Gledhill and Larsen 1982 on the Old Babylonian period in Assyria). That the consequences of such bursts of activity may spread far outside the original cognized domain of the actors involved, illustrates once again how archaeology can record the unintended consequences of essentially blind historical processes.

Conceptualizing the Later Bronze Age and Early Iron Age

The first half of the first millennium BC was once described by Jaspers, correctly, as an axial age. By this he meant the emergence of major religious and intellectual 'breakthroughs' within the orbit of the major civilizations. The rise of classical Judaism, Zoroastrianism in Persia, Confucianism in China, the transition from the Vedas to Buddhism, Jainism and other sects in India, accompanied the change from pre-Homeric mythical thought to philosophy in classical Greece. The beginning of classical antiquity has thus been a focus for research for over a hundred years precisely because it was viewed as the period in which a distinctively 'European' form of society diverged from that of the Ancient Near East. What constitutes the distinctive features of this uniqueness depends on one's conceptual orientation but at least, in the hands of Marx, Weber and Polanyi, there was a consistent emphasis on the freeing of economic forces from political constraint. Polanyi's purpose in studying the genesis of archaic Greece was to contrast the age of Homer to the age of Hesiod as the consequence of a period of major political and economic disruption, (Polanyi 1977, p.147). The freeing of economic forces for the pursuit of gain was contingent therefore on the destruction of the Late Bronze Age palace systems and their regulation of administered trade. In the case of northern Syria, Liverani has explained the collapse of the Late Bronze Age palace systems as the result of internal processes of social and economic differentiation of palace personnel and the increasing ability of such segments, (merchants/landowning aristocracy), to disengage from the palace and continue their activities in a different framework, (Liverani 1978 and forthcoming). The restructuring of the regional economy after the 'collapse' required technical innovations in transport (both land transport, pack animals and larger ships) to facilitate more directional long distance trade; a change in settlement to smaller and more diffuse urban centres requiring technical innovations such as water storage, and terracing, irrigation, new fallowing techniques and use of iron ploughs, to facilitate intensification of agricultural productivity in a more limited territory. A similar pattern of urban growth, short distance migration, technical innovation to sustain settled population in more limited territories and the expansion of nomadic populations in interstitial zones has been described for the Palestine coast in the eleventh and tenth centuries by Frankenstein (1977). It may seem rather arbitrary to limit the period of crisis to the traditional twelfth-century date and the restructuring of the regional economy to the eleventh and tenth centuries and certainly in some areas, e.g. north Syria, central and south Anatolia, palace centres continued alongside these urban developments (more properly commercial city states). Moreover to limit the crisis to the twelfth century would ignore what was probably a

longer process of gradual destabilization of the palace economies during the thirteenth century which culminated in the decentralization of the palace systems and a break-up of pre-existing monopolies in production and inter-palatial control of material flows via gift exchange and royal agreements. This, of course, requires further investigation as a particular case exemplifying a more general principle concerning the relationship between status hierarchies and their ability to maintain monopoly control over the circulation of goods and services (Douglas 1967, Rowlands 1982 p.168). Whilst analogous cases may be cited from the Old Assyrian period in the Near East (Gledhill and Larsen 1982) or post classic Maya in Mesoamerica (Rathje 1975), the distinctive feature of our particular case lies in the inability of Near Eastern empires to extend political control over these developments in the outer periphery of their sphere of influence. The long term result is thus the birth of the 'Mediterranean world' as a semi-autonomous political and economic system which diverges in basic structure from the Near East of the first millennium B.C.

The situation on mainland Greece is obscure, in large part due to the fact that the ancient prejudice against speaking of banausic matters has led to a superficial view that stratification could be based on either landed or commercial wealth. Although the debate on the scale of commerce and manufacturing in the eighth century threatens to continue (Snodgrass 1980), even moderate expansion in a wealth accumulating secondary sector is likely to have increased rather than undermined opportunities for investment of wealth, from whatever source, in status building activities such as land investment, temple building and religious festivals. The fact that this may have led to the semi-commercialization of land holding and the reification of land from a kinship right into a status principle, makes it even less easy to claim a separation between landed and commercial wealth. A wider regional perspective, allows the speculation that the growth of commercial city states on the Syro-Palestine coast and possibly Ionia in the tenth to ninth century generated in turn a secondary and subordinated commercial sector of the agrarian dominated territorial states of the Greek mainland by the eighth century. The resulting ideological (but not real) cleavage between landed and commercial wealth could thus be manipulated as a stratification principle in order to control the disruptive influence of free flows of wealth.

The response to the restructuring of the regional economy appears to have taken a different course in north Syria and Palestine. There is a shift from conventional gift exchange to transactions of a more formally commercial pattern. In the cases of Phoenicia and north Syria, the merchant is removed from indigenous status hierarchies and plays a more interstitial role in which the supply of raw materials is pursued for its own sake and profits accrued are not cycled back into local status competition. The description of the Phoenicians by Homer as pirate-sailors who were not averse to kidnapping strangers to sell as slaves and the similar opprobium attributed to the Phocaeans is an apt representation of the activities of these mercantile groups. Liverani has described how the entire terminology of trade in Syro-Palestine underwent semantic change in the first millennium to a more overtly commercial usage and how the ideological representation of profit came to be highly prized in contrast to Late Bronze Age ideals of generosity and disinterest (Liverani, forthcoming). The situation in Greece was almost certainly more variable than in north Syria or Phoenicia and a contrast between the Ionian Greeks and the Greek mainland should be borne firmly in mind, particularly as the relatively exceptional case of Athens, where a land based aristocracy retained control, is our primary source.

152

But it is the extent of new contacts and the stimulus to trading that are most important. The Phoenicians, for example, were clearly as much concerned with encouraging the production of manufactured items for sale as in the carrying of raw materials. Their activities were typically mercantile in the sense of buying cheap and selling dear and avoiding the cost of production themselves. Moreover, they were no longer limited to the regions they could contact, by the necessity for formal political relations due to the control of local rulers over their activities. They could operate in a more far-flung and extensive manner, establish contacts to their own advantage and where necessary operate from autonomous trading stations. The collapse of Egyptian control over the Red Sea, Mycenaean control of the Aegean and further west and the freeing of overland routes to Assyria and Babylonia also expanded enormously the opportunities for profitable long distance trading. We can also assume that these opportunities were taken up relatively soon after the collapse of the Late Bronze Age regional system. Even in the case of Phoenician involvement in the Western Mediterranean, whilst the traditional date for Cadiz (Gades) to the eleventh century is too early, there is no reason why the initial exploration of trading opportunities should not have occurred by then. Moreover there is every reason to suppose that initial Greek colonization of the Black Sea coast and the west had been preceded for some time by renewed trading activities of both Greeks and Phoenicians in former Mycenaean areas of influence.

For some reason these destabilizing tendencies on the western Asiatic periphery were a considerable threat to the stability of the Assyrian/Babylonian core areas. We witness a brief attempt by Tiglathpilesar I at the end of the twelfth century to restore control over the north Syrian area and then a gap of two centuries before the more successful campaigns of Assur-nasir-pal II and Shalmanesar III who successfully imposed control over the trading cities of the Levantine coast. The effects of Assyrian expansion are threefold. Firstly, it resulted in the destruction of the Aramaean states in north Syria as a conscious and directed piece of Assyrian policy and excluded the Greeks from the entrepôts that they had established there. Secondly, the Ionian Greeks were excluded from the Anatolian overland trade, particularly after the destruction of the Urartrian-North Syrian axis by Assyria in the late eighth century. Thirdly, the incorporation of the Phoenician states by Assyria resulted in their being allowed to maintain a commercial role under favourable treaty terms and at the same time be relieved of competition from north Syrians and Greek access to the overland trade to Mesopotamia. On the other hand, it implied that they would be locked into a particular clientship cum commercial role within a larger regional empire with consequent effects upon their political evolution. It is insufficient at this point to simply emphasize the effects of Assyrian military pressure and tributary demands on Phoenicia since an extensive commercial base to the neo-Assyrian empire can scarcely be in doubt (Winter 1973). The exact nature of the role of the Levantine city states after the eighth century is, therefore, unclear but the largely mercantile role they played in the central and western Mediterranean in the following 200 years without evidence for territorial annexation or the extension of tribute relations at the expense of trading monopolies, implies the continuation and expansion of a specialized commercial role.

The same can scarcely be said for Greek colonization in the west. The fact that it was the Thessalian-Euboean-Cycladic network which previously dominated the Near Eastern trade that was also precocious in the trade with the west, implies a rapid redeployment of trading activity as a consequence of their exclusion from

the Syro-Palestine coast, at the latest by the first half of the eighth century. In certain specific instances, it could be argued that the motivation was clearly the replacement of raw materials now denied to them from the Near East, (e.g. iron from Elba and central Italy or Sardinian copper). It is sufficient for our purposes here, however, to point out the significant effect that non-incorporation into the regional empires of the first millennium had for the development of the Greek city states in contrast to those of north Syria and Phoenicia. The elaboration of a commercial sector that was a characteristic feature of much of the eastern Mediterranean at the start of the first millennium BC could only develop on the Greek mainland within an evolving agrarian based city state structure. And here, in a different relation to land holding defined oligarchic elites to that characteristic in Ionia and the Syro-Palestine coast. This should be sufficient to remind us that the evolution of the classical Greek city state is not to be understood simply by the presence or absence of commercial relations with the Near East.

What bearing do these 'events' in western Asia and the eastern Mediterranean have on our characterization of the Later Bronze Age and Early Iron Age of temperate Europe? An initial premise would be that the unity of Reinecke's Hallstatt chronology is a more certain guide to our understanding of this period than the traditional Bronze/Iron Age dichotomy. A second would be to agree conveniently with the emerging orthodoxy that large parts of Europe underwent fundamental change towards the end of the second millennium BC (Renfrew and Shennan 1982, p.57). At least one view of what this significant change constituted emphasizes decomposition of established status hierarchies and the perdurance of more unstable principles of status acquisition and maintenance, (Rowlands 1980, Bradley 1982). The most striking indicator of such a state of affairs is the extension of the Urnfield cremation rite from a centre on the Middle Danube to most areas of central and western Europe by the ninth century. Obviously no universal meaning can be attached to cremation as such (there is no reason to assume it even evoked its earlier Bronze Age meaning in the first millennium) but the fact that in the few instances where stable hierarchies were able to emerge for a time, there was a constant struggle to return to a traditional form of legitimation based ideally on inhumation, tumulus burial, personal weaponry and access to prestige items, suggests that these represent two principles of status ordering (fluid and competitive ranking versus fixed hereditary succession to status) that were in constant tension during the Later Bronze Age. Significantly this apparent dissolution of stable mechanisms of status acquisition and succession, appears to correspond broadly with increasing competition for control over land, agricultural intensification and a more rigorous definition of land holding (e.g. Bradley 1978 and 1981). In contrast to what might be predicted by some this unstable state of affairs was apparently a major stimulus to deep mining of copper, metalwork production, salt extraction and the production and supply of other raw materials. Bronze becomes more widely available, particularly in parts of eastern and central Europe where basic agricultural implements are consistently made of bronze (see Harding, this volume, for summary). In other words, apparent devolution towards more competitive and antagonistic political relations (which incidentally does not imply lack of complexity but quite the reverse) implies reorganization and intensification of production in all sectors as well as a massive increase in the velocity of circulation.

Even in Urnfield contexts there is some evidence that under certain conditions more stable, ordered hierarchies could develop, for example in the early and late phases of the Urnfield sequence. The reappearance of rich burials, usually in marginal areas with either cremation or inhumation practice and categories of high status grave goods suggests that more coherent and extensive hierarchies could develop under special conditions in the Later Bronze Age. It is, however, the late Hallstatt C-D period in central Europe which provides us with the clearest indicator of the conditions for the emergence of this kind of stable ranking structure. It might well be significant that dominant Hallstatt B centres in south west Germany or east France were located in areas where occupation from Hallstatt B-early Hallstatt C is less apparent. In the eastern Alpine region, on the other hand Hallstatt B occupation was radically altered due to the development of trade with the south. But other areas, that were strong Urnfield centres in Hallstatt B, for example south Bavaria, were peripheralized in the ensuing Hallstatt C-D periods. In other words, the strong regional shifts detected in political dominance which characterize Hallstatt C-D development may not only be to do with reorientation to the Mediterranean world but also to do with resistance or avoidance of these new contacts either by late Urnfield strongholds or by Mediterranean trading partners wishing to avoid relatively well-organized polities and wanting instead to stimulate or transform weaker local societies to serve their needs (cf. Harke 1979 on Hallstatt C-D settlement relocation).

The arguments concerning the internal structuring of the Hallstatt D chiefdoms have already been rehearsed elsewhere (Frankenstein and Rowlands 1978). Control of monopoly advantage in external sources of wealth inputs into the local systems were crucial for understanding the set of conditions which permitted, for a brief period, a phase of stabilized ranking in certain areas of central-western Europe. This requires that such external conditions have to be related to existing internal circumstances; the different responses of the eastern versus the western Hallstatt regions is a case in point. In the latter case, these internal circumstances appear to be a pre-existing but weakly developed alliance and exchange network. This was of a highly fragmented and competitive nature that, under an external stimulus, could be cohered by certain powerful households into a more stable ranking structure. The archaeological evidence of centralized craft manufacture in a range of status items (necessary to define access to rank position) and prestige objects (needed at all social levels for transactions such as payment of bridewealth) is indicative of the form of control exercised, i.e. over gift giving, marriage alliance and 'tributary relations'. I would also argue that this 'superstructure' of a status hierarchy emerges out of and leaves relatively intact an extended household domestic economy although conditions would exist for an intensification of agricultural production for exchange.

Moreover, we emphasized the relative instability and fragility of these kinds of structure. When the monopoly is broken, the political arena quickly fragments and returns to previously existing competitive cycles of status rivalry, competition and display. Hence, the emphasis on warfare, raiding for plunder, the emergence of warrior age grades or retinues under some kind of chiefly or aristocratic patronage in Early/Middle La Tène, with warfare directed toward the acquisition of cattle, gold ornaments, weapons and probably slaves (i.e. locally socially constituted wealth items) may differ only in degree rather than kind from a more long term and still prevailing Later Bronze Age pattern.

The relative stability of the Hallstatt D phase may also, to a certain extent, be illusory, since raiding/trading are really two strategies for acquiring the same thing - wealth to use for internal circulation and exchange in competitive status rivalry (Nash pers.comm.). If certain areas were, for a short period, able to gain access to sources of wealth of a consistent and enduring character,

then quite exceptional conditions for the maintenance of stable hierarchies may be expected to develop. As Daphne Nash has explained, one of the really significant differences between Late Hallstatt and La Tène is the manner in which wealth could be acquired from the Mediterranean world. In the earlier period by regular trade and in the later period as a return on demand for Celtic warriors as mercenaries (Nash, pers. comm.).

The question is can we relate any of these developments in the Later Bronze Age/Early Iron Age north of the Alps to contemporary change in the Mediterranean, or are we only to consider such situations when evidence of direct contact can be established? It must of course be stated quite firmly that here we are only concerned with the conditions controlling the reproduction of these 'societies' and not the particular local forms adopted. The cultural idioms manipulated in status competition and the actors' representation of their own particular political arena do not concern us here. In fact it is quite likely there would be a number of different local systems in operation that could not be viewed as transforms of each other and would have their own distinctive properties and evolutionary potential. Our point instead is to stress that their capacity to function in a locally appropriate manner depends on conditions that are not included within these local ethnically defined circumstances. It has been argued that we have evidence of relatively stable status hierarchies in the European Early and Middle Bronze Age contemporaneous with palace regulated economies and elaborate title systems in the western Asiatic (including the Aegean) Later Bronze Age. There is also evidence for the growth of unstable competitive status systems in the European Later Bronze Age occurring in the same period as the semi-commercialization of the eastern Mediterranean in the early first millennium. The principle that underlines both situations is the presence or absence of the conditions for maintaining monopoly advantage over internal distribution and external exchange. Here we could follow both Friedman's arguments about relative trade density or scarcity, which really involves velocity of circulation and Douglas's more general principle of differentiation of hierarchies and the difficulties these conditions create for established status holders to maintain control over material flows (Friedman 1981, Douglas 1967, Rowlands 1982). Hence we need not be limited to the presence of prospectors, traders or other such human agencies to be the conscious instigators of these conditions. Such correlations indicate only that we are dealing with open regional systems. In other words that Europe was always part of a larger whole. The conditions necessary for direct intervention and even control of parts of temperate Europe in the later first millennium can only be properly conceptionalized as due to the presence of longer term processes which apparent discontinuity would encourage us to deny.

CONCLUSION

Over the last hundred years, the 'prehistory of Europe' has been conceptualized in terms of two sets of opposed principles: discontinuity/continuity; dependency/autonomy. The first of these principles stems from a nineteenth-century positivistic faith that methodological rigour would reveal the objective truth of historical development. In this paradigm, the key to understanding the origins of modern Europe lay in tracing the genesis of its contemporary character to a period of short term disruption and discontinuity, the unintended consequences of which were only to be revealed in a longer term process of continuous change. The second is derived from the role historical consciousness has played in European nationalism. Each European nation state has made claim to a unique history and has sought evidence in the past for its cultural autonomy and continuity. A sense of past is thus used to promote social closure whilst dependency and change are de-emphasized and externalized as factors existing outside of a social system defined in basically ethnic terms.

Discontinuity, change, innovation and dependency as outside thus become opposed to continuity, tradition, autonomy and inside as the often implicit organizing principles of much narrative prehistory. Up until the Second World War, the former principle was emphasized in British archaeology, probably as a reaction to the obvious dominance of the latter in central European work. Shorn of its particular nationalistic overtones, the continuity/autonomy principle has been revived in recent years utilizing arbitrarily defined spatial units in place of the culture area concept. An implicit sense of European pan-nationalism seems to lie behind this revival. An autonomous 'prehistory of Europe' emerges as a cultural vision which acts as a motivating force to achieve a degree of political and economic unity in Europe in the face of competing claims to domination by outside forces (an interesting modern parallel to the conditions in the eighth century AD which first promoted the use of the term 'Europe' to describe the emergence of a sense of ethnic consciousness in the face of external aggression, Hay 1968).

All of this teaches us that such principles are not abstract theoretical devices for constructing objective historical 'truths' but relate to contemporary interest. A paper which appears to stress a 'dependency view' is scarcely likely to be well received in the current ethos. Moreover, it is quite unsatisfactory since it remains locked within a distinctively eurocentric view of the nature of social change, the validity of which the author has been at some pains to question. Whilst the solution may not be entirely satisfactory, it may still retain some merit if one is clear as to what one is trying to avoid. This is quite simply to deny that one has any a priori knowledge of the unit whose 'history' is to be constructed or within which change is said to occur. If one accepts that social bounded-ness is a relative and shifting concept of emic proportions, then the conditions promoting such closure cannot be viewed a priori. Put simply, a prehistory of Europe cannot be assumed (except ideologically) and it is the conclusion of this paper that it does not exist except as the presentist projection into prehistory of current interests in establishing a unified sense of a 'European' past.

No doubt this will be viewed as an unsatisfactory answer to the 'uniqueness of Europe' question. But if one does not start with the assumption that one is dealing with the prehistory of some ethnically bounded unit, then the processes one describes cannot be expressed in terms of the autonomy/dependency opposition. (A linguistic packing model may be more appropriate). Europe as an ethnically defined unit did not exist prior to the eighth century AD when chroniclers first used the term to refer to the Romano-Germanic populations (Hay 1968, p.25). Understanding how this state of affairs emerged is scarcely helped by projecting it or its sub-units back into prehistory as a unifying frame of reference. In this manner we learn once again that understanding our own particular historical development - as a necessary component of creating a sense of identity - is founded on a more open-minded attitude to comparison. In this regard the societies that have occupied the European landmass have played a structurally similar role in world history as other 'blocked areas' such as sub-Saharan Africa and Oceania. The situation changed in Europe in the sixteenth century AD when the wealth crises experienced by European feudal aristocracies encouraged them to gain access to independent sources of revenue from the New World and the Far East. By thus breaking their dependence on

long distance trade with the Mediterranean and the Near East, the societies of the European sub-continent unwittingly achieved an autonomy of action, the results of which are only too visible at the present day. Since a few hundred years out of several millennia is like a drop in the ocean, we may be unwise in assuming this recent shift to autonomous 'core status' to be a permanent state of affairs.

ACKNOWLEDGEMENT

I am most grateful to Andrew Sherratt for his comments and advice on this paper.

BIBLIOGRAPHY

ALLEN, J. 1977 - "Sea traffic, trade and expanding horizons," in Allen J, Golson J. & Jones, R. (Eds.) Sunda and Sahul, pp.387-418. Academic Press, London.

ANDERSON, P. 1974 - From Antiquity to Feudalism. NLB, London.

BARRETT, J. AND BRADLEY, R. (Eds.) 1980 - The British Later Bronze Age. BAR 83, Oxford.

BINFORD, L. 1962 - "Archaeology as anthropology" American Antiquity vol. 28 (2) pp.217-25.

BRADLEY, R. 1978 - The Prehistoric Settlement of Britain. RKP.

BRADLEY, R. 1981 - "Economic growth and social change: two examples from prehistoric Europe", in Sheridan A. & Bailey G. (Eds.) Economic Archaeology, BAR, Oxford, pp.231-37.

BRADLEY, R. 1982 - "The destruction of wealth in later European prehistory", Man (NS) vol. 17, pp.108-22.

CHILDE, V.G. 1925 - The Dawn of European Civilisation. 1st edition. RKP.

CHILDE, V.G. 1942 - What Happened in History. Harmondsworth.

CHILDE, V.G. 1944 - "Archaeological ages as technological stages", J.R.A.I. vol. VXXIV, pp.7-24.

CHILDE, V.G. 1947 - The Dawn of European Civilisation. 6th edition. RKP.

CHILDE, V.G. 1957 - "The Bronze Age ", Past and Present vol. 12, pp.2-15.

CHILDE, V.G. 1958 - The Prehistory of European Society. Harmondsworth.

DOUGLAS, M. 1967 - "Primitive rationing : A study in controlled exchange", in Firth, R. (ed.) Themes in Economic Anthropology. Tavistock, London, pp,129-47.

EVANS-PRITCHARD, E. 1961 - Anthropology and History Manchester University Press.

FINLEY, M.I. 1975 - The Ancient Economy, Chatto and Windus.

FRANKENSTEIN, S. 1977 - "The Impact of Phoenicians and

Greek Expansion in the Early Iron Age of Southern Iberia and South Western Germany' - Unpublished Ph.D Thesis, London University.

FRANKENSTEIN, S. AND ROWLANDS, M.J. 1978 - "The internal structure and regional context of Early Iron Age society in South West Germany", Bull. Institute of Archaeology, London 15, pp.73-112.

FRIEDMAN, J. 1981 - "Notes on structure and history in Oceania", FOLK vol. 23, pp.278-95.

FRIEDMAN, J. 1982 - "Catastrophe and continuity in social evolution", in Renfrew et al. Theory and explanation in Archaeology. Academic Press, New York, pp.175-96.

GILMAN, A. 1976 - "Bronze Age Dynamics in Southeast Spain", Dialectical Anthropology, vol. 1, pp.307-19.

GILMAN, A. 1981 - "The development of social stratification in Bronze Age Europe", Current Anthropology, vol. 22, pp.1-23.

GLEDHILL, J. 1978 - "Formative development in the North American South-west", in Green, D. Haselgrove, C. & Spriggs, M. (Eds.). Social Organisation and Settlement BAR, Oxford, pp.241-90

GLEDHILL, J. AND LARSEN, M. 1982 - "The Polanyi paradigm and a dynamic analysis of Archaic states", in Renfrew, et al. Theory and Explanation in Archaeology Academic Press, New York, pp.197-229.

HARKE, M.G.H. 1979 - Settlement types and settlement patterns in the West Hallstatt province. BAR, Oxford.

HAY, D. 1968 - Europe: the emergence of an idea. Edinburgh University Press.

KRISTIANSEN, K. 1982 - "The formation of tribal systems in later European prehistory: Northern Europe 4000-500" in Theory and explanation in archaeology Eds. Renfrew, C. et al. Academic Press, New York, pp.241-80.

LEVI-STRAUSS, C. 1966 - The Savage Mind. Weidenfeld and Nicholson.

LIVERANI, M. 1978 - "Non slave labour in Syria (Bronze Age)", in Proc. 7th Int. Economic History Congress, Edinburgh.

LIVERANI, M. (forthcoming) "The collapse of the Bronze Age regional system at the end of the 2nd millennium, BC," in Rowlands, Larsen & Kristiansen Centre/periphery relations in the Ancient World. CUP

MARX, K. AND ENGELS, F. 1965 - Selected Correspondence. London & Moscow, Progress Publishers.

MCNAIRN, B. 1980 - The Method and Theory of V. Gordon Childe. Edinburgh.

NASH, D. 1978 - "Territory and state formation in Central Gaul", in Green, Haselgrove and Spriggs (Eds.) Social Organisation and Settlement. BAR, pp.455-75.

POLANYI, K. 1977 - The Livelihood of Man Academic Press, New York.

RANDSBORG, K. 1975 - "Social dimensions of early Neolithic Denmark", Proc. Prehist. Soc. vol. 41, pp.105-18.

RATHJE, W. 1975 - "Last tango in Mayapan", in Sabloff, J. and Lamberg-Karlovsky, C. (Eds.) Ancient Civilisation and Trade Albuquerque University of New Mexico Press, pp.409-48.

RATHJE, W. 1978 - "Melanesian and Australian exchange systems: a view from Mesoamerica", in Specht, J. and White, P. Trade and exchange in Oceania. Mankind 21, p.3.

RENFREW, C. 1973 - Before Civilisation. Cape, London.

RENFREW, C. 1974 - "Beyond a subsistence economy, the evolution of social organisation in Europe", in Reconstruction Complex Societies. (Ed.) Moore, C.B. MIT, Cambridge, pp.69-85.

RENFREW, C. AND SHENNAN, S.J. (Eds.) 1982 -Ranking, Resources and Exchange. CUP

ROWLANDS, M. 1980 - "Kinship, alliance and exchange in the European Bronze Age", pp.15-55 in J. Barrett and R. Bradley (Eds.) The British Later Bronze Age, BAR 83, Oxford.

ROWLANDS, M. 1982 - "Processual archaeology as historical social science", in Renfrew et al. Theory and explanation in archaeology. Academic Press, New York, pp.155-74.

SAHLINS, M. 1972 - Stone Age Economics. Tavistock, London.

SHENNAN, S.J. 1982 a - "The development of salient ranking", in Renfrew and Shennan (Eds.) Ranking, resources and exchange. CUP, pp.57-60.

SHENNAN, S.J. 1982b - "Ideology, change and the European Bronze Age", in Hodder I (ed) Symbolic and Structural Archaeology. CUP, pp.155-161.

SHERRATT, A. 1976 - "Resources, technology and trade", in G. Sieveking, I.H. Longworth and K.E. Wilson (Eds). Problems in Economic and Social Archaeology London, Duckworth, pp.557-81.

SHERRATT, A. 1981 - "Plough and pastoralism: aspects of the secondary products revolution" in Hodder I., Isaac, G. and Hammond, N. Patterns of the Past: studies in honour of David Clarke. CUP, pp.261-305.

SHERRATT, A. 1982 - "Mobile resources : settlement and exchange in early agricultural Europe", in Ranking, resources and exchange, Eds. Renfrew A.C. and Shennan S. CUP. Cambridge, pp.13-26.

SNODGRASS, A. 1980 - Archaic Greece. Dent, London.

STEWARD, J. 1955 - "Cultural causality and law: a trial formulation of the development of early civilisations" in Theory of Culture Change. Illinois, U.P., pp.178-209.

WEBER, M. 1976 - The Agrarian Sociology of Ancient Civilisations. NLB, London.

WHALLON, R. 1982 - "Comments on explanation", in Renfrew and Shennan (Eds.) Ranking, resources and exchange, CUP, pp.155-58.

WINTER, I. 1973 - North Syria in the early 1st millennium BC, with special reference to ivory carving. PHD. Columbia Univ.

156

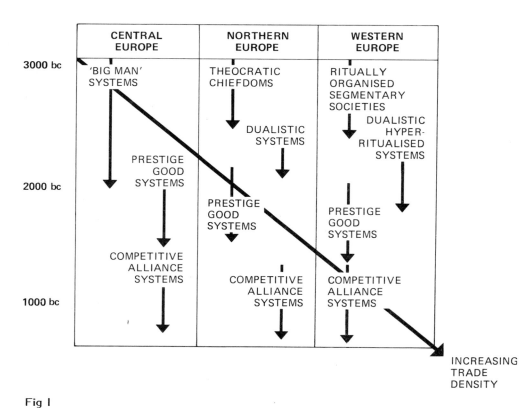

Fig I

Succession of social types (generalized).

7

IRON AGE EUROPE, IN THE CONTEXT OF SOCIAL EVOLUTION FROM THE BRONZE AGE THROUGH TO HISTORIC TIMES

John Bintliff

In my Neolithic contribution (this volume) I have characterized Bronze Age Europe as a landscape dominated by villages and hamlets. Occasionally, and never lastingly, (Crete and perhaps Iberia excepted), a favourable balance of dense population and ecological opportunity sponsors proto-urban nucleations, which may develop rudimentary regional functions in servicing surrounding populations. Even here, however, there is little evidence for local chiefs developing palatial residences and none for a burgeoning group of administrators, in comparison to the more natural concentration of regional craftwork and industry that is a function of scale economy (cf. Harding, this volume). In fact it is frequently difficult to identify leadership at all in these larger than average settlements. For the most part, therefore, we seem to be witnessing a sub-continent fragmented into innumerable, arguably autonomous units, each consisting of one or several communities recognizing a common leader (perhaps now hereditary ?) whose presence is inferred primarily on burial differentiation and, to a far lesser extent, structural differences within settlements.[1]   The continual pressure on the land, and the larger population units arising from more efficient artifacts and intensive mixed farming,[2] seem reflected in communal erection of land divisions and impressive hillfort refuges. The greater concentration, now possible, of subsistence and craft surpluses, is clearly reflected in the considerable flow of imports into these societies, especially metal, whilst the privileged position of the elite seems evident from the inclusion of luxury dining equipment and 'show' armour and weaponry. That a similar diversion of resources is occurring on the **intra**-regional scale may be inferred from the nature of local craftwork (with a strong elite-centred sector) and the special human effort and gift wastage associated with status burials. Nonetheless, it is not clear whether these correlates denote ascribed privilege draining from the communal surplus, or the expenditure of the personal household economy of the elite, who have either used their position to differentiate their productivity from the rest of the community or arose from such initial economic priority. The rarity of proto-urban communities and of regional elite structures, may to a considerable extent be due to the inability of these early farming communities to maintain the arable soils and the woodland/open pasture grazing land in good health, i.e. to create a stable long-term foundation upon which could arise the reliable surpluses required for a permanent superstructure of professional craftsmen, priests, administrators and perhaps warriors who were only part-time farmers. One can demonstrate this failure countless times in the environmental and archaeological record from all over Europe,[3] and it must be significant

that the largest and most complex communities are generally to be found in Eastern-Central Europe, where the mixed farming economy first appeared after Greece, and where a typical tell site exhibits centuries and sometimes millennia of stable and successful adaptation supporting unusually large densities of population; in the rest of Europe such settlement continuity is remarkably rare. But even here in the East, the archaeological record shows clear traces of cultural and demographic collapse over wide regions, for example, the later Copper Age or Middle Bronze Age,[4] that truncates high points of proto-urbanism when one might be tempted to envisage an imminent takeoff into small states or centralized tribes. It is also surely no surprise to find that Europe's first civilization, the Minoan, found its most impressive manifestation in the giant palace at Knossos, a site that had been occupied continuously by a large community for 4000 years before the first palace was constructed. It is undeniable that the early and persistent presence of states in Egypt and Mesopotamia was intimately associated with the natural renewal of fertility in the core agricultural areas during the annual floods.

All these considerations are of prime importance for our understanding of social evolution in the Iron Age. Firstly, and most importantly, we find once more the phenomenon observed with previous eras: the **general** presence of a socio-economic level of complexity previously a **rare and localized** feature. Here we are dealing with the emergence in areas of dense population of centres servicing a region of villages and hamlets, farmsteads, and in various ways, often and increasingly in combination: security, with the far wider spread and on a larger scale of defended refuges; craft production and distribution of imported material; administrative functions and arguably regional judicial and cult roles.

There has been throughout Europe a quite substantial rise in population density, and primarily arising from a major shift in local agricultural productivity. The population rise will continue up into and beyond the extension of Roman power across much of Europe, and those most qualified to pronounce on the data consider late Iron Age southern Britain, for example, to be at the level of the early Medieval Domesday population (i.e. one to two million). Similar levels over large parts of Europe seem plausible.[5] Bulk foodstuff imports from beyond Europe are hardly responsible, and we cannot discuss the phenomenon merely in terms of an elite stimulus to grow more for exchange with exotic tableware to decorate their feasting tables. One has to account for the general creation of demographic conditions over much of the subcontinent where previously only limited favoured regions had achieved as much. There are changes argued in crops, in their range and adaptability, that may have contributed; climatic improvements are relevant, at least in some areas;[6] but far more significant must be deemed the widespread adoption of iron technology. The diffusion of the traction-drawn ard plough and farm waggon from the later Neolithic period, the increasingly wider availability of bronze tools throughout the mature and late Bronze Age, can be seen to alter the parameters of regional population densities and of individual productivity. Yet bronze, for all but a few, was arguably a rare commodity, carefully recycled; nor could it tip the ard plough and improve on its performance over stone and wood shares.[7] Iron on the other hand was available in virtually every region of Europe, and could provide an efficient plough-share to tackle a much wider range of heavier soils and improve the aeration and moisture retention of the lighter soils already in use.[8]

These and other factors can be seen as operative over most of Europe. In some regions, over-expansion in the later Bronze Age had brought previous populations to very low densities (parts of the Nordic sphere, perhaps Greece - cf. Renfrew 1979, Bintliff 1982), whilst in other areas there is a continuity from dense later Bronze Age communities into even denser early Iron Age settlement patterns. It must be stressed that the numerous fertile regions of Europe, with or without iron, may be expected to undergo cyclical growth and decline of population, from inadequate population control and the inherent potential of the land, and the subsequent (rarely avoided) ecological mismanagement and density dependent destructive warfare that ensues. In many of these regions, proto-urban centres and other marks of regional centralization are apparent in Bronze Age and even sometimes Neolithic contexts.[9] The recurrence of such developments may thus be predicted for some regions as a function of their natural resources. But the far wider spread of the proto-urban phenomenon must indeed reflect a general raising of productivity in the Iron Age concomitant on agricultural and technological advances. If we step aside from the traditional contrast between the Mediterranean 'civilized' world and 'Barbarian' Europe north of the Alps, we see in fact the same development at this time in both spheres, whether in late Geometric Attica (Snodgrass 1980) or Villanovan central Italy (Potter 1979), or Central Europe.[10]

The marks of the new adaptation are visible in the thousands of hillforts that spring up over early Iron Age Europe, the efforts of co-ordinated supra-community labour. Inside many of them, it seems, an important part of the agricultural surplus was stored; but increasingly, we find evidence for craft specialization and (at times) the domestic residences of a sector of the regional population who may be hypothesized to include communal functionaries. A similar and better documented rise of nucleated regional centres with central cult, craft and elite quarters (and ultimately circuit walls) has been argued for contemporary Archaic Greece and central Italy (Potter, Snodgrass, op. cit.). Initially, in almost all areas, the scale of the hillfort territories is small, perhaps the achievement of less than half a dozen hamlet/villages or equivalent dispersed population (Fig. 1). Often these develop into territories several times as large, as one centre grows and its neighbours drop out of use; at the same time the surviving centre seems to grow concomitantly in its range of functions.[11] One can fruitfully observe the same process in Greece and Italy during the rise of the larger Archaic states.[12]

Just as we have seen in earlier eras, it need not be assumed that considerable regional density of population and the emergence of regional centres were entirely dependent upon a strongly emphasized social hierarchy. Economic conditions were clearly widespread for the maintained growth of a superstructure for each region, and for provisioning communal activity on the construction and repair of regional refuges. The alternative to an elite 'forcing' role on the economy is to envisage pre-existing ranked structures 'riding the wave' of population and surplus growth.[13] Leadership and organization there must have been, and the production and exchange of costly showpieces for the chieftain's table and military parade is a sustained flow. Less widespread are accentuated differences in the treatment of the dead, the elite being considered identifiable throughout a wide swathe of West-Central Europe during the early Iron Age (Hallstatt era) from their well provided waggon and tumulus burials (Piggott 1965). Very much rarer are any structures resembling a mansion or palace. It is possible therefore that the scale of the contemporary regional centres, and their complexity of function, was still generally low enough not to require a bureaucracy. This low level of centres reinforces the 'riding the wave' model, i.e. widespread and parallel local stimuli to growth.

THE HALLSTATT CULTURE: BACKGROUND

It is a curious fact, that one frequently encounters analyses of striking cultural phenomena that seek to interpret such development with little or no reference to a longer time perspective, emphasizing not surprisingly from such an intentionally confined approach, the need for dramatic 'deus ex machina' factors to account for these notable occurrences at a particular point. The European Iron Age has been particularly prone to such abuses, especially since the existence of historic records from contemporary Mediterranean and Near Eastern civilizations - contrasted to the mute and generally scrappy archaeological data from 'barbarian' Europe - has made the option of explaining developments amongst the barbarians as the effect of direct or indirect interference from the 'civilized world' an especially inviting (if not least effort) one. All the signs are that this return to the kind of approach notorious from the diffusionists and hyper-diffusionists of the first few decades of this century, is a fast-growing trend (though dressed in new clothes of 'prestige goods economy' and 'world systems' - cf. Frankenstein and Rowlands 1978, Frankenstein 1979, Rowlands 1980 and this volume, Wells 1980a, Haselgrove 1982, and for an earlier era, Sherratt this volume). In this chapter we shall attempt to indicate the serious failings of this movement, particularly as regards the origins and development of the Western Hallstatt Culture and the climax 'oppidum' era of the subsequent La Tène Culture.

The initial point to stress, in studying the development of the Iron Age Hallstatt Culture (Hallstatt C-D), is that the florescence of Western Europe in Hallstatt D (Ha D) has to be understood, not just in terms of contemporary sixth-century BC developments in the Mediterranean world, but as a clear outgrowth from very similar and often identical phenomena in Hallstatt C times in Central Europe. Further, this Hallstatt C (Ha C) florescence, and less striking activity at this time in Western Europe, must be understood as developing quite naturally out of characteristic phenomena of the preceding Late Bronze Age or Urnfield period (Bronze Age D, Hallstatt A-B) in continental Europe. Let us begin by underlining some of the more important aspects of Late Bronze Age background to the Hallstatt Culture.

Chieftain statuses: As we have briefly discussed above, (and cf. Harding, this volume), the totality of archaeological data for the European Bronze Age points to the dominance of small scale chiefdom organization throughout Europe. Occasionally, especially rich burials may indicate a regional 'paramount' chief, but it seems plausible to argue for instability in such wider power bases. The evidence for status at this level is argued to be least ambiguous in the context of burial distinctions, but increasingly it is being shown that a more widely applicable approach is the analysis of status kits within the bronze industry (for Britain e.g. we may note the excellent work of Burgess, Rowlands and Ehrenberg). It does seem more than likely that the symbolic expression of rank is more generally and continuously to be found in metal equipment than in differentiation in burial rites (a fact proven beyond doubt by the total dichotomy in much of Europe between historic sources and burial data for the late Iron Age, cf. below). Even less valuable is the evidence from settlement archaeology for the Bronze Age. Clearly our sample of well-excavated sites is very poor, and the sophistication of analysis open to criticism (cf. Harding this volume) and only in a small number of cases is it possible to **suggest** that the residence of an elite family (as is inferred from contemporary burial and status-kit studies) is identifiable amongst less impressive dwellings.

Despite these drawbacks, a number of more positive points may be made. Firstly, there are still plenty of rich or even 'princely' burials from most areas of Europe in all phases of the Bronze Age, providing a clear basis for the manifestations of elites during the succeeding Hallstatt Culture. Often the more striking graves are to be found during the Late Bronze Age within areas prominent in wealthy burials during succeeding Hallstatt C and/or D. Even where such status burials are less common or even lacking, modern study of the plentiful and diverse finds of the bronze industry indicates for all areas of Europe the existence of a distinct stratum of status individuals. Levy (1978) and others have pointed out that the widespread shift in large regions of Europe during the later Bronze Age towards urn cremation burial, often without a prominent covering mound, from the tumulus plus inhumation chamber of earlier centuries, regularly coincides with a marked decline in offerings to the dead, and an apparent 'levelling' of burial distinctions (districts with continuing wealthy graves or tumuli excepted). Nonetheless, the products of the bronze industry make clear that the same kind of elite-centred societies continued to exist across Europe throughout this period.[14] We seem to be dealing with a major change in ritual practice, perhaps part of a very widespread religious transformation (Alexander 1979), as was to occur again during the Iron Age, where in final pre-Roman centuries status indications are largely absent from burials despite clear indications of highly stratified societies. It has been argued cogently that the great proliferation of bronze hoards during this Urnfield era offered an alternative mode of elite prestige to replace that formerly played by burial ritual. In Hallstatt Iron Age times distinctive burials for the elite return progressively across Europe, and hoard deposition declines dramatically. Indeed in some areas e.g. south Germany (which will be especially notable for elite burials from Hallstatt C to early La Tène times), the evidence for distinctive rites for the elite already begins in late Urnfield times (i.e. Hallstatt B) (Jockenhövel 1974).[15]

It is therefore little disputed that during the Late Bronze Age much of continental Europe was characterized by localized smallscale chiefdom societies, whose elite may be picked out readily from prestige bronze kits of weapons, fine tableware, dress ornament, and rarely armour, deposited largely in hoards, less commonly in distinctive elite burials. In many cases the older tradition of tumulus chamber with wealthy burials survives through the urn cremation era, to be revived for the normal elite rite in the Hallstatt Culture;[16] but more often status is obscured in the giant cremation cemeteries of large parts of Europe (although sometimes the general, unpretentious

rite **is** accompanied by high status offerings, which may be burnt as well).

But where do the elite reside? Is there any Late Bronze Age background to the fortified princely seats (Fürstensitze) of the Hallstatt Culture? It is generally acknowledged that the fortified hilltop site typical of the early centuries of the Iron Age has its origins in similar sites found throughout Europe during Urnfield times.[17] Often the Iron Age site has Bronze Age occupation and defences, and even if not, the typical defences of the Iron Age hillfort are the box rampart and derivative types of its Urnfield ancestor. However, if we can point to an indisputable continuity in the erection and use of fortified hill sites from Late Bronze Age into Hallstatt times, it is rare that direct occupational continuity can be shown for any one particular site.[18] It is inferred from this that local power was unstable, and that individual elite families were unable to establish lasting authority over rival chieftains. The seat of local power hence moved from phase to phase. We do come up against the usual lack of information about possible rival centres in terms of type of occupation and chronological span, but the kind of regional study offered by Haerke (1979) for parts of the Western Hallstatt sphere (where some of these shifts of power base are suggested) offers the potential in future for analysing political fragmentation of this type. Haerke also offers us an even more intriguing pathway for investigation. It now seems likely that some of the elite burials (Fürstengräber) of the Hallstatt Culture in the west of Europe, though adjacent to typical settlements of 'princely seat' type, in fact antedate those settlements. In the absence of direct local continuity between other obvious major settlements in the region, Haerke suggests that there may be phases where status individuals lived in discrete 'estate-like' rural homesteads amid a landscape of dispersed farms of varying rank. There is indeed some fragmentary evidence he adduces in support, apart from the obvious negative argument of the gap in use of major nucleated sites, and a similar pattern is becoming increasingly likely for much if not all of the La Tène period in Europe. These individual rural 'villa' type sites would of course be even less researched than the poorly understood hillforts of the Iron Age whose presence is so much easier to document. Once again, therefore, whilst Bronze Age chieftains are often to be related to major earthwork sites, they may as often, or more frequently, have resided in a settlement type least recorded by fieldwork up to the present. Yet it is generally admitted that in all areas where prominent elites are displayed during Hallstatt times, they were already present in muted or obscured form in the same areas during the preceding Urnfield era.

Notwithstanding these contextual and local difficulties of interpretation of the archaeological record, it is rather striking that commentators have long agreed that the most vigorous and wealthy zone of Europe north of the Alps during the Late Bronze Age, the Middle Danube/eastern Alp/west Carpathian region, is precisely that within which by a combination of demonstrable local continuity and internal transformation, arose the first flowering of the Hallstatt Culture, that of the Eastern Hallstatt sphere (E Ha) of Hallstatt C period date (c. 750-600 BC) (Filip 1977, Gabrovec 1974, 1980). In this great region comprising much of Austria, Czechoslovakia, and north and western parts of Yugoslavia and Hungary, we find the most flourishing expression during Late Bronze Age times of chiefly elites, whether in bronze status kits, burial differentiation or defended district foci.[19] In other regions the picture is of the incomplete jigsaw variety discussed earlier. For large areas of West Germany for example, where major princely seats and graves will arise during Hallstatt D and Early La Tène times, distinctively elite burials and hillfort centres appear discontinuously in time and space across the landscape and the many subphases of the Urnfield era. Yet Jockenhövel (1974) is surely correct in seeing, for example, the rich burials such as the Steinkistengräber, and the Hallstatt B2-3 series of complex defended sites of south Germany as belonging to 'ancestral lords' (Ahnherren) of the later Hallstatt 'princes' of the area.[20] That the hilltop site of the Heuneburg is arguably an important local community with impressive defences during late Middle Bronze Age and early Urnfield times, then is abandoned for many centuries, until Hallstatt D1 in fact, when a key princely seat is founded upon it (Kimmig 1975), need not deceive us into thinking that local society sank into a classless peasant democracy of family farms in the intervening period.[21] It is postulated here that local chiefdoms continued throughout this period, at rival seats (as Haerke has indicated) and from 'estate' centres dispersed across the landscape. In late Hallstatt times, elite settlements return to the nucleated community form, at the same time as fashion and/or ritual shifts revive the custom of lavish status-indicating burial. However, amongst the numerous local chieftains of this later era, some are plausibly of paramount status over their neighbours, supporting the idea of a network of large territorial cells over the Western Hallstatt sphere (Haerke 1979, Frankenstein and Rowlands 1978). There is, to match our case for local elite continuity, an obvious requirement that we should account for the **elaboration** of chiefdoms at this time, a point that will be dealt with below.[22]

A final aspect of Late Bronze Age society that offers a firm and generally ignored basis for subsequent Hallstatt developments, is that of long distance exchange. A central part of the new 'Mediterranean interference' model for the rise of the Hallstatt chieftain society is played by imports of luxury goods into elite circles of barbarian Europe. This exchange system is closely linked to the expanding commerce of the Etruscan cities of northern Italy and other communities of the north-east of Italy, and even more so to the early Greek colonies of the West Mediterranean such as Massilia. All this, though firmly rooted in the historic record of these Mediterranean peoples, takes absolutely no account of exchange systems and cultural interactions between the Mediterranean and the Urnfield regions during the Late Bronze Age. In that preceding era, study of bronze styles, status kits, actual imports and exports, and in some areas, identity of burial custom, all indicate a very active exchange system and flow of cultural ideas between those regions around the west, north and east of the Alps which are to be central to the florescence of the Hallstatt Culture, and north and central Italy (Proto-Villanovan and Villanovan traditions) (Müller-Karpe 1959, Hencken 1968, Gabrovec 1974, Pauli 1980b). Indeed, if the apparent physical obstacles to such a semi-koine give pause for thought, we may consider the future potential of studies such as that of Pauli (1980a) on the Golasecca Culture of the north-west Italian Alps, suggesting a Celtic population here as early as the Late Bronze Age, forming one element in what may have been a whole series of trans-Alpine bridges through which the strong interactions (between elites in particular) took place. In Urnfield times, it is generally considered that the dominant current of influence was from north to south, a situation reversed in Iron Age times with the more rapid development of complex societies south of the Alps. But arguably the nature and importance of this great zone of interaction was already formed in Late Bronze Age times. (A parallel worth adducing is that of the 'Cluster Interaction Sphere' of Shennan and Price, developed in the context of the earlier Corded Ware and Bell Beaker international elite-orientated phenomena - cf. my Neolithic Chapter, this volume). Likewise, in contrast to the undue significance given to Black Sea steppe influences and even 'migrations' upon the development of the Hallstatt Culture, it has to

be stressed that there existed a long preceding tradition of mutual influences between Eastern Europe and that region, with ideas, forms, and objects widely exchanged. Yet the exotica coming into Europe remained foreign within the continuity of local Bronze Age traditions (Angeli 1980), a situation arguably repeated in the context of the Hallstatt Culture (see below).

THE HALLSTATT C ERA

The Hallstatt Culture of the Early Iron Age is primarily distinguished by the first general usage of iron artifacts over much of Europe north of the Alps, but also by characteristic and widespread burial traditions (especially for the elite of society) and shared artistic styles. Iron tools were indeed known well back into the later Bronze Age of Central Europe, but only now became a major force for change in the efficiency of agricultural and craft tools, and weaponry. This transformation in technology was hastened, if not created, by strong contacts between Central Europe and other 'barbarian' peoples around the Black Sea, and between Italy and the expanding Greek colonies and Greek Mainland. This advantageous diffusion of practice during the eighth century BC and onwards, altered what had been primarily hitherto in barbarian Europe a technique for decorating aristocratic prestige pieces, into a powerful force for change in economy and social organization (cf. earlier discussion). The elaboration of the network of Bronze Age chieftains into a mosaic including major areas of more complex paramount or 'princely' territorial blocs (Fig. 4), alongside a continuation of simpler political units of the older model (cf. for example Haerke 1979), surely reflects the great rise in local populations, in the potential of the local resource base, and new opportunities for inter-community friction and peaceable interactions. Such conditions - which we have earlier suggested had been created more sporadically during the Bronze Age, with its lesser economic potential - now became general in Europe, and a growing sophistication in settlement and political systems seems to be indicated from different areas widely scattered over Europe north and south of the Alps.

The region that appears to be most especially flourishing and complex in Hallstatt times (750-500/400 BC), as we have seen, added the vital force of everyday iron technology to its existing pre-eminence in development from the Bronze Age, the Middle Danube/eastern and south-eastern Alps region (Czechoslovakia, Austria, part of Hungary and north-west Yugoslavia) - known as the Eastern Hallstatt sphere. In this broad region, the invigorated elite stratum, its status enhanced as it rode on the crest of the economic boom, adopted some striking prestige behaviour via easterly contacts to express its new power and influence, though merging it with older, Urnfield prestige customs (Angeli 1980). The custom of tumulus burial, still surviving in many places of Urnfield Europe, often for elite burials, but a commonplace striking memorial amongst the peoples around the Black Sea ('Thraco-Kimmerians'), is revived as a characteristic aristocratic burial form for the Hallstatt Culture. The association of the elite with warfare from horseback (contrasted to plebeian footsoldiers) is closely linked to the great tradition of mounted warfare on and beside the Black Sea steppes.[23] Likewise a key aspect of life around the Black Sea since the third millennium bc had been transport in four-wheeled waggons, but at this time the prestigious custom of burial of the noble dead on such a vehicle, as a hearse, is also prevalent in this area adjacent to Eastern Europe. Both customs make their mark on the Hallstatt Culture as means adopted by the elites of the Eastern Hallstatt sphere to enhance the visible status symbolism in Hallstatt C times (c. 750-600 BC), i.e. the appearance in their burials of showy equipment for horse-riding (clearly in Thraco-Kimmerian styles), and in many areas of hearses of four-wheeled waggon type. The new longsword of Hallstatt C type, however, is an iron version of the Urnfield swords, and prestige armour is very much a series of elaborations on local Bronze Age forms.

It is now widely accepted that the 'Steppe factor' is merely another episode in a very long development of mutual influence between the indigenous cultures of Central and Eastern Europe, and peoples inhabiting the lands bordering the Black Sea. Little support is now given to theories of waves of horse-riding nomads from the true Steppes flowing through Europe and establishing local Hallstatt dynasties.[24]

These crucial transformations of Urnfield, or Bronze Age, into Hallstatt (or later, La Tène) Iron Age societies appear to be time-transgressive. In Hallstatt C, already complex societies of the Eastern Hallstatt sphere evidence settlement relocations, a new spawning of district foci (defended hillfort communities primarily), and the new status symbolism in aristocratic equipment and burial rites (elite tumulus burial with cavalry and/or waggon equipment). Areas thus affected reach as far west as Bohemia and parts of West Germany (Bavaria) (cf. Filip 1977, Pauli 1980b). But in general, Germany, Switzerland and eastern France, while providing evidence for a local continuity of chieftain societies and minor foci during this time, are moving forwards from a much less developed Bronze Age tradition during this first stage of the Early Iron Age, although individual high-status burials comparable to those typical for the East do already appear in exceptional areas (Hodson and Rowlett 1974, Filip 1977, Haerke 1979). This Western Hallstatt sphere will peak later, in Hallstatt D times (sixth century BC and later). In the Nordic sphere, where the progress of the Bronze Age was associated with severe ecological problems (see below, this chapter), and full iron-using is a feature only from a period contemporary to the La Tène age further south, not surprisingly no major socio-political developments stand out for the time of the Hallstatt culture. But significantly, in regions of Europe that can only with difficulty be linked into the tight nexus of a Hallstatt 'Culture', such as Britain and Poland, the contemporary take-off of full iron-using is associated with a major florescence in the construction of district foci and new raised population densities. Here, also, the later Bronze Age is now considered in both areas to be a time of heightened organization of communities and land use, preparing without discontinuity for greater elaboration during the subsequent Iron Age.

In the core region of the Hallstatt C culture, with sporadic outliers amongst the less developed areas further west, Urnfield period chiefly and rarer paramount graves are transformed into the more numerous 'princely graves' (Fürstengräber) and chieftains' graves, typified by the expanding Thraco-Kimmerian status kit and the revival of inhumation tumulus burials for the local elites cf. Koutecky 1968, Filip 1977). District hillforts are often relocated or founded from less notable preceding elite foci, the most striking referred to as 'princely residences' (Fürstensitze). This heightened development of the settlement hierarchy and its associated socio-political hierarchy will spread throughout the Western Hallstatt sphere in Hallstatt D, then into a wider region of France and Germany in Early La Tène times (cf. Filip 1978). Increasingly, as the movement shifts westward from its original Middle Danube core, and over time, as the power and influence of the Archaic Mediterranean city-states increases, the 'interaction sphere' from the Black Sea is joined by the diffusion of status items from the south, from the Greek colonies of the West Mediterranean and the indigenous north and central Italian states and confederacies. By Hallstatt D and La Tène A, this alternative

source of prestige material is more important in the Western Hallstatt region, and in the south-eastern Alps, likewise with easy access to the Mediterranean world via the Adriatic.[25] But in the central, linking region of Czechoslovakia, Mediterranean prestige material and interaction is understandably rare, though both this and the rest of the Eastern Hallstatt sphere is strongly affected by a renewed popularity for Black Sea warrior prestige equipment diffused from the new Scythian presence (there by late Hallstatt times). Indeed, Scythian cultural and status symbol influences, including weaponry, are a notable component in the nascent La Tène culture of West-Central Europe, alongside native Hallstatt and Mediterranean Classical styles, symbols and equipment.

The indigenous basis for the Hallstatt Culture is not only clear from the locally orientated artifactual record accompanying the international prestige items, but also from regional variation in the elite burial forms.[26]

Perhaps the most spectacular regional development in Hallstatt C times is that of the Yugoslav province of Slovenia, where the Early Iron Age transformation is marked by settlement changes and the elaboration of a whole series of fortified 'central-places' around which are found vast numbers of tumuli including very impressive 'princely mounds' (such as Sticna, Brezje, Magdalenska Gora, Vace and Novo Mesto; Filip 1977). A particular variety of high-status burial within this region is the 'Sippenhügel' or 'clan-mound', where the rank of the central burial in a particularly impressive tumulus is clearly exhibited from the secondary burial of up to several hundred 'dependents' in satellite graves encircling the central grave, all within a great covering mound which may have a striking stone perimeter.[27] The origin of this flourishing society lies indisputably within the local highly-developed culture of the Late Bronze Age, and the geographical position of the region between Mediterranean and continental worlds, and between East and West, allows it to borrow and adapt to its own uses a wide range of diverse cultural influences. The Thraco-Kimmerian prestige kit is rapidly and widely adopted, but the long-nourished exchange of ideas and actual objects of warfare and ornament between the east and south-east Alps and northern Italy is never broken (Gabrovec 1980). Indeed as Hallstatt C progressess into D, the common culture of communities around the head of the Adriatic, at least as far as elite styles, develops into a regular koine, reaching notable artistic heights in the fine metal-ware of the Situla Style (Gabrovec 1980). More perhaps here than anywhere else, the traditional scholarly dichotomy or 'fault-line' between the 'Mediterranean Classical Culture' and that of the continental 'barbarians' seems to be a product less of the evidence than of the diverse educational backgrounds of prehistorians and Classical archaeologists. On both sides of the Alps, and in the fringe-hinge world of Slovenia, chieftain societies of Urnfield tradition origin receive a vital impetus from the new potential of iron technology. Their interactions intensify, their socio-political structures grow increasingly more elaborate, denser populations crystallize around more numerous and generally more complex central foci. This process occurs at different rates in different regions of Europe, and this push towards proto- and full urbanism, and political units of larger territorial scale and tauter central authority (princedoms, archaic states) is most lasting and successful south of the Alps, in Italy and Greece (Archaic city-states and expansive colonies).

A major part of neighbouring Austria has a closely comparable regional culture to Slovenia (cf. the cemeteries of Frög, Klein Klein and fortified sites (Ringwälle) - Gabrovec 1980), but in the westerly Salzburg region we move into a more central Hallstatt sphere that forms a cultural bridge to Czechoslovakia and the Western Hallstatt variants. Naturally great attention continues to be paid to the two cemetery sites here of Hallstatt and Hallein, whilst analysis of the burial data has frequently been carried out for reconstructions of contemporary social systems at this stage of the Iron Age. Both cemeteries are very large, that of Hallein being much less investigated than Hallstatt (where a recent study was able to analyse 734 graves of an estimated total of over 2000; Hodson 1977). Between them, their period of use helpfully runs right through traditional Hallstatt C and D, but then continues into a final Hallstatt D3 and Early La Tène as in West-Central Europe (fifth century BC to mid fourth) (Maier 1974, Pauli 1978, Barth 1980). The theories and interpretations offered since the last century concerning the society represented by these burials are varied and often strikingly contradictory, but it does seem possible to indicate a modern tendency in interpretation that is highly important to our general understanding of Hallstatt and indeed all pre-Roman Iron Age society and economy in 'barbarian Europe'. Firstly, there is little doubt that the communities burying at these locations were rather unusual in being highly active in the mining, processing and exchange of key salt deposits of the Salzburg region. The local wealth of copper ores must also have been significant, most obviously in terms of privileged easy access to the main ingredient of bronze (still used in the Iron Age for most prestige table and dress equipment and display armour, for technical reasons), but perhaps also these communities had some role to play in the metals trade. This special geographical factor has reasonably been seen as accounting for the much higher level of wealth items (e.g. bronze vessels developed from Urnfield types) in the average grave, compared to Hallstatt era cemeteries elsewhere (both elaborate prestige items typical for production from this region, and imports from outside) (Barth 1980). Allowing for a general raising in status indicators, it is still rather striking that the burials tend to fall into clusters of graves each comprising a spectrum of rich, moderately wealthy and poor assemblages, and a mixture of men, women and children. Although in the past it has been argued that the Hallstatt cemetery represents a clear 'class society' with poorer miners' graves and warrior protector graves, more recent research suggests convincingly that these two cemeteries probably represent status distinctions within small local communities, all of whose members were actively involved in the salt industry. None of the burials, till Final Hallstatt times, seem to stand out as 'Princely', and a view that sees the overall numbers of bodies and their relative proportions by wealth as indicating little more than village communities with internal distinctions along extended family or clan lines, is supported by the evidence at present available. The minority wealthier graves would therefore point to 'big men' or clan-heads within one or two villages (or a series of local hamlets) in themselves wealthier than the norm for this time and region. The small scale nature of these status distinctions and overall organization suggested can be seen from the recognition at Hallein of eight or nine discrete main burial zones matched to a possible male miner workforce of a mere 50 at any one time.[28]

The implications of this new interpretation cannot be overemphasized. Firstly, it suggests that even one of the arguably most important industrial and trade centres of Europe, the rich salt mines of the Salzburg region, by this late stage in prehistoric development was nonetheless still organized on a staggeringly small scale, by a small number of villages (or hamlet groups) under the direction of leading families or perhaps just extended-family heads. These 'elite' individuals, although from burial statistics they must have been active in the industry (if not necessarily swinging heavy tools themselves), are indicated by characteristic Hallstatt status gear, i.e. as

'warriors', just as in Archaic Greek society the wealthier members of the population were defined as the 'armoured ones' (hoplites) or 'cavalrymen' (hippeis). A well-known parallel from La Tène times is the doctor's burial with warrior-status equipment (Piggott 1965, Fig. 129). The palaeodemographic analysis by Schwidetzky (in Pauli 1978, cf. also Pauli's discussion p.505 ff.), for the Hallein community, suggests very strongly a life common to all ranks: hard work, unhealthy working and living conditions, and an unusually short lifespan. All this to achieve display wealth which the community could not convert to any more practical use in contemporary socio-economic conditions.

Secondly, we must note that this major 'industrial centre' of the Salzburg area, did not apparently lead (until perhaps in a final phase, see below), to the creation of a powerful princedom based on industry and commerce with the rest of the Hallstatt world or with the related north and central Italian sphere, despite demonstrably strong cultural and material exchange between Hallstatt and Hallein society and this wider world. This must give serious pause for thought, for those who ignore the arguments of the Polanyi-Finley school of ancient economic history in favour of a later prehistoric Europe where major settlements and 'princedoms' rise and fall due to the dictates of a market economy or specific long-distance arrangements for the supply of raw materials or finished products (cf. above). Thirdly, the conclusions regarding the size of the salt-mining community are highly pertinent to the importance of industry and trade relative to other occupations and means of achieving wealth and status. If a major salt industry exists with a mere handful of core villages employed in mining and preparation and presumably initial despatch along the exchange network, then the remarkably dense populations presently being posited for Iron Age Europe on the basis of field archaeology and ancient sources, cannot in any way be assigned in any significant proportion to an 'industrial' or 'commercial' profession for regional and inter-regional 'markets'. However high we place the number of alternative salt mines, copper mines, iron workings and other raw material sources, their workforce and active distributors cannot conceivably make even a noticeable bite into the kind of population density over the land that gives Britain some 1-2 million Iron Age inhabitants. These vast populations, and the great development of wealth categories and leadership hierarchies that we find within them during the course of the Iron Age, grew from that far more universal economic base of land, agricultural produce, and small scale craftwork for local consumption, operating as forcing agents within each separate region of Europe. Such a conclusion should come as no surprise to anyone familiar with the supposedly far more complex and diverse economy of the Classical world. [29]

Czechoslovakia, like areas to the south-east, has a flourishing high culture from the Bronze Age through the Hallstatt Culture and into Early La Tène. Local settlement relocations and discontinuous use of obvious hill-centres cannot disguise the continuity of dense population, rural crafts and elite-centred fine arts, and a chieftain/paramount chieftain political organization, in this country rich in farming, quality grazing and metal sources.[30]

During the first phase of the Hallstatt Culture, C, as we have seen, the Western sphere is only gradually adopting the new modes of elite prestige burial and display from the East, and the region is far less developed in terms of settlement hierarchy and apparent population density during the preceding Late Bronze Age. A degree of settlement and territorial elaboration comparable to the situation in East and Central Europe will only be achieved after a longer maturation period, during Hallstatt D. Nonetheless, there are examples where the elites already appear in 'steppe trappings', and it has been clear for some time that the gradual movement is a direct importation from the Eastern Hallstatt world (cf. Gabrovec 1980b, Pauli 1980, Freidin 1983, Stead 1979). There are also occasional finds of luxury imports from the East, or the Mediterranean world, which anticipate the following era when more powerful and internationally-orientated chieftain/princes in the West will symbolize their aloofness from the rest of their society by the display in the ceremonies of life and death of such exotica (Frey 1980a).[31] Our appalling ignorance of the development of the overall settlement pattern during this period has naturally reinforced the impression of a dramatic rise, almost from nothing, of the network of Hallstatt D regional foci. However, the inadequacies of 'revolutionary stimulus' theories, which purport to create complex institutions such as proto-states or urbanism in a generation, as a result of trade links between lowly barbarians and Mediterranean city-state societies, have recently prompted a recognition of, and research into, the necessary local antecedent growth of complex political and settlement structure (cf. particularly the excellent work of Haerke discussed above, and Wamser 1975). One can now begin to see a possible preparatory stage in the West, spanning both Urnfield and Hallstatt C periods (see earlier), which will develop onto a higher plane of sophistication by D. The retarded effects of the socio-economic forcing factor of iron technology in the West, compared to the East, require careful investigation which has yet to be begun in the field, yet it must be significant that a similar dichotomy prevails during the Bronze and Copper Ages for these regions. But it is sufficient to say that this preparatory stage reflects the general continental picture for the Bronze Age, of characteristic small scale chiefdom societies and episodic occurrences of 'paramounts' and 'central-places'. Despite this, the new factor of possible 'estate centres' in periods without regular nucleated foci makes it necessary to consider the possibility of gradual political elaboration during Hallstatt C in the West, which only secondarily results in an obvious revival of central places and regional 'princely burials'. As we shall see, there is good reason to support such a scenario.[32]

THE EASTERN HALLSTATT SPHERE IN HALLSTATT D AND EARLY LA TENE TIMES

Whilst in the Western sphere we find the spectacular establishment of a network of regional foci and 'paramount' princely burials closely modelled along long established East Hallstatt lines, the East sees at this time both strong elements of continuity and important transformations in the symbolic repertoire, together with changes in settlement and burial form and location that vary by region and in their timing. Not surprisingly, the new focus of high culture in the West has tended to overshadow the East, particularly when the latter is in many respects less innovative and less directly linked to the Greek colonies and rising power of the Etruscans (i.e. less amenable to historical treatment). Moreover, there are further changes in burial behaviour which once more tend to obscure relationships of status and ethnic continuity. It must therefore be stressed again that specialists refer to the Hallstatt D (1-2) century (c. 6-500 BC) and the succeeding Hallstatt D3 to Early La Tène (LT A) era, (c. 500-c. 350 BC) as the final flourishing of the East Hallstatt sphere, before the spread of the true 'Celtic' culture of La Tène B (=1b-c) to supplant it throughout East and Central Europe. This means that over much of the area, major foci and elite burials continue through this period, though in many ways distinctive from the parallel institutions in the West.

During Hallstatt D1-2 there is little change over most of the East Hallstatt sphere, apart from new contacts in its western zone with the rising Etruscan exchange pattern, a faint echo of the stronger links of the true West Hallstatt sphere. In the crucial fifth century BC, the last half-century of florescence for both East and traditional West Hallstatt cultures, followed by the first half-century of the new cultural florescence of the La Tène culture (originating in the region north of West Hallstatt), princely burials and centres continue in the East (Bretz-Mahler 1971). Generally they continue with the dichotomy between elite tumulus burials (often inhumation) and the rest of the community (flat graves and usually cremations), and as in the West, the four-wheeled waggon is being replaced by the two-wheeled chariot. The luxury goods of the Hallstatt art style are still confined to the elite contexts; in several areas of East Hallstatt, however, elite and specialist craft circles are receptive to the new elite style of the La Tène 'Early Style' emanating from the core region of Marne-Middle Rhine (Schwappach 1973, Lessing and Kruta 1979). At the same time, in Hallstatt D 1-2 and the D3/Early La Tène fifth century, an invigorated Black Sea cultural sphere (that of the indigenous Thraco-Kimmerian culture transformed by the arrival of Central Asian Scythian populations) provides an attractive new package of elite display and art style elements that spreads rapidly to enliven the symbolic repertoire of the East Hallstatt circle of nobles and their attendant craftsmen (Neustupny and Neustupny 1961). This same 'Scythian' package is indeed an important element in the creation of the new Western La Tène style, along with the more accessible Classical Mediterranean artistic borrowings. But already during the fifth century the pattern of burial behaviour is changing throughout Europe. The Hallstatt tumulus rite is giving way to what had hitherto been the 'plebeian' rite, flat burial, at first generally in the traditional cremation form, but increasingly the elite inhumation rite appears in the new dominance of flat grave cemeteries (Saldova 1971, Filip 1977). In some areas indeed, inhumation had been common for all ranks throughout Hallstatt, but the general shift seems to have had some wider significance at this time that we cannot as yet interpret. The changeover is clear in several areas of both the former West Hallstatt sphere and core La Tène region during the fifth century, and in some areas of the East now (e.g. Slovakia). But generally, it is with the fourth century and La Tène B (1b/c) and C (2) times that we find the new rite of flat inhumation cemeteries, including all ranks, sweeping through the whole of West, Central and East-Central Europe (Filip 1977). To some scholars, the displacement, progressively, in both east and west, of the traditional elite burial distributions, reflects socio-political upheaval and the rise of the yeoman 'middle class' to power in society (represented by the characteristic significant proportion of warrior burials in these new cemeteries) - a military democracy (cf Collis 1973a, Filip 1977). A related argument sees the disappearance of the West Hallstatt centres and princely tombs of this time, and serious decline over much of the Eastern sphere in such phenomena, as indicating political collapse, due respectively to internal warfare/trade dislocation with the Mediterranean (for the West), and the attacks of nomadic Scythians (for the east). However, the return of inhumation graves is likely to indicate a revival of the earlier Bronze age attitude towards greater burial display (Neustupny and Neustupny 1961, Saldova 1971), in which both the corpse and its body ornaments and accompanying gifts are interred, giving what may be a quite illusory appearance of a levelling out of wealth in favour of a **new** middle class (as contrasted to the old 'rich' plus gifts versus 'poor' with few or none). In general therefore, graves now become more stocked with artifacts with the new rite, enabling us to see what must previously have been the case in Hallstatt and Urnfield times, that the chiefs and princes rested upon wealthier and poorer farming strata rather than an undifferentiated class of humble peasants.

On the other hand the class of 'princes' is perhaps on the decline during the fifth century, in favour of rich but less distinctive 'chieftain burials' now generally found amidst the flat graves and primarily distinguished from less important personages by gifts rather than tomb form and burial rite (Neustupny and Neustupny 1961). Whilst the last century of West Hallstatt region princely burials (Hallstatt D3 to La Tène A, formally) runs parallel to the penultimate phase of such in the East (where it is often the fourth century where they and their foci cease), in the new core La Tène zone there is both a final survival of princely pomp in the Middle Rhine and already the dominance of chiefs and yeomen (alongside occasional 'princely graves') in the other, Marne region in flat cemeteries (Filip 1977). It seems, therefore, reasonable to agree with previous opinions on this point and suggest that apart from long-lasting traditional areas such as the South-East Hallstatt, the top level of power and centralization may have collapsed between 450-400 BC, at the same time as (doubtless a closely linked phenomenon) lower level district leaders and clan heads/big men express their greater political and social importance through the revived 'inhumation with gifts' rite (cf. Lessing and Kruta 1979, 50 ff.)[33]

Imp.
If in
the
earlier
period
the
princely
graves
are
collects
or law
not
been
found,
Then there
was no
collapse
of
centralization
but
simply
a
broadening
of power
even
further.

That the West Hallstatt world underwent some crippling crisis is a topic we shall investigate shortly, but it seems little likely that the gradual transformation of the East (earliest in Czechoslovakia, later in Austria and later still in Slovenia) reflects Scythian onslaughts. Internal breakdown of the Hallstatt princedoms in the former area (see below) and the same factor and/or the spread of 'princeless' Celtic groups from the West (Neustupny and Neustupny 1961, Lessing and Kruta 1979) for the latter, seem at present the more likely explanatory factors. There is additional support from the very fragmentary contemporary and later, 'archive based', records of the literate Mediterranean, for a general transformation of Celtic society from one based on centralized kingship to one based on a broader chieftain-plus-wealthy yeoman power structure (see later). In the process, the works and style of the finer craftsmen, hitherto usually confined to the princely elite class with Hallstatt and Early La Tène art, become far wider diffused amongst the broader ranks of the new leadership strata, in the 'democratization' of La Tène or Celtic art by Middle La Tène times (La Tène B/C, or later fourth century onwards) (Lessing and Kruta, 1979, p.53).

If we turn to some detailed comments on the situation in the various regions of the East Hallstatt sphere, Bohemia is especially notable for its 'hinge' role between East and West. Indeed, because it reflects the general shift in Hallstatt D towards West Mediterranean prestige imports more than other areas of East Hallstatt it is rather misleadingly often assigned to Western Hallstatt from this phase (Saldova 1974). In actuality a more significant fact is thus obscured, namely that we have strong continuity here of the elite superstructure from Hallstatt C (and well back into the Bronze Age) into Early La Tène, but fluctuations in the relative importance of exotic influences adopted by the elites in their display.[34] The custom of impressive tumulus burial fades by the end of the fifth century, and during the fourth the more communal flat inhumation graves begin to dominate, with their clear ranks from chiefly family to commoner (Saldova 1971). Whether this change marks a further stage in the adoption by indigenous communities of wider trends or reflects a dominant new population group, (Celtic warriors arriving from the West)is a matter still

under debate; possibly both factors are at work. But before the transformation of burial and, arguably, society, the final phase of Bohemian Hallstatt and the initial phase of Early La Tène society demonstrate a development more than equal to the overemphasized Hallstatt D central places of Western Hallstatt. Our information is all but confined to one well-explored site, the giant hillfort of Zavist near Prague, but the implications for the sophistication and centralization of late Hallstatt/Early La Tène society in Bohemia are unambiguous. We have earlier noted the importance of the site in the Urnfield period as a putative regional focus; this becomes even clearer in the time range of the fifth to fourth centuries BC. On the acropolis of this gigantic defended site there is erected a massive stone platform with additional stone foundation features. Subsequently an even larger platform is constructed on a truly remarkable scale, composed of stone and earth. Around this special area a rock-hewn perimeter comparable to later Celtic ritual enclosures or Viereckschanzen is dug.

It is perhaps not surprising, if disappointing, that the explanation of these major indigenous monumental activities should confine itself to bizarre theories involving 'barbarian' attempts to build a Classical Greek altar, and later a foundation platform for a pseudo-Greek temple (Motykova 1978).[35]

Far more important, therefore, is this evidence that in the heart of Europe, within the undisputed context of well-established elite communities, one or several powerful figures brought together on a major regional centre a great force of labourers and erected a hitherto unparalleled monument, doubtless both to symbolize elite status and power but also as a central focus for local communities to identify with.

In Moravia the transformation towards new social expression and related settlement changes is gradual but early in commencement. During Hallstatt D2, latter sixth century, the custom of princely burials declines, leaving the indigenous cremation cemeteries, whilst the settlement pattern is increasingly modified. These changes provide a natural transition for participation in the more general shift towards flat inhumation 'warrior cemeteries' that will dominate Central Europe by Middle La Tène times (Podborsky 1974). The development in Slovakia is particularly interesting in final Hallstatt/Early La Tène. Princely graves die out before the fifth century (Pichlerova 1974), but it seems likely that an elite of chieftain rank are now picked out from their adoption of 'Scythian' features in burial, and doubtless in everyday display equipment. With the general tendency towards limiting actual Scythian penetration to the far south-east frontiers of Europe, the spread during the sixth and fifth centuries of Scythian cultural ideas into East-Central Europe is taken to signify a renewed interest in prestige borrowings from the Black Sea area. In the same way Slovakia is one of the regions of East Hallstatt where La Tène influences show an equal receptiveness of the elite to new cultural influences from the west.[36]

The Scythian 'factor', as noted earlier, is far more significant as a cultural influence than as a disturbing presence for East Hallstatt (Angeli 1980). It seems likely that the warlike prestige of the new Scythian/Kimmerian peoples was an attractive source of imitation amongst the late Hallstatt chiefs (horse equipment, burial rites, arrow and axe types), particularly after the remarkable success of the Scythians against the invading Persian imperial forces. The South East Hallstatt culture is also quick to adopt the Scythian accoutrements into its local cultural context, just as it likewise picks up what it finds attractive about the new western elite art style of Early La Tène. This culture continues with its traditional walled centres and princely mound burials through the Hallstatt D3 and Early La Tène phases of the fifth to early fourth century, during which time these new influences are absorbed (Gabrovec 1974, Knez 1974). Subsequently the marks of princely power cease by and large, although occupation at a reduced scale of complexity continues in the formerly defended sites, and ethnic continuity (and elite continuity) is argued throughout the La Tène, with the addition of a significant component of Celtic arrivals from the fourth century (Knez 1974, Gabrovec 1980). Whether the local political superstructure collapsed from internal reasons, or was broken down by the Celtic invasions, is unclear (Filip 1977, Gabrovec 1980), although the Scythian element is largely discounted as in any way contributory. But not suprisingly, the highly flourishing koine of the inner Adriatic breaks down too, and Slovenian culture becomes far more insular as the La Tène era develops.

Austria during this final Hallstatt to Early La Tène (A) phase (fifth to fourth centuries BC) provides further evidence that the main dislocation for East Hallstatt is not at the time when the West Hallstatt sphere flourishes (sixth century onwards) or when Early La Tène core culture arises in the west and spreads to the east (mid fifth century), but from the later fourth century onwards (Filip 1977, Pauli 1978). At tumulus cemeteries such as Hallein, local continuity of population is argued together with a rapid adoption of the new La Tène cultural repertoire (as seen for example in both male and female ornament and equipment) (Schwappach 1973, Pauli 1978). Cemetery decline and or relocation, and the shift to 'Celtic' burial in flat inhumation graves (or inserted into older barrows), is characteristic for the subsequent La Tène B (Ib-c) era in the region.[37]

THE WEST HALLSTATT SPHERE FROM HALLSTATT D, AND THE EARLY LA TENE CULTURE

We have earlier discussed the background in the West Hallstatt sphere (Burgundy in eastern France, southern Germany and Switzerland) of broad continuity of cultural development from the Late Bronze Age through Hallstatt C times, combined with a putative continuity of chiefdom structure throughout the region, sometimes centred on fortified foci, at other times arguably in more dispersed 'estate' foci. From the beginning of Hallstatt D (DI, early sixth century BC) once more these local elites emerge to view with the revival or elaboration of nucleated regional foci associated with prestige burials, the 'Fürstensitze' and 'Fürstengräber'. Yet in this phase the spacing of centres suggests large territories and even 'proto-state' structures, to be linked perhaps to the emergence of paramount chiefs or princes from an aristocratic stratum scattered through the region. The paramounts associated with the major putative centres and their particularly impressive prestige burials, seem to have dominated numerous district chiefs whose rich tumuli are found at various points around the suggested territory of each princedom (cf. Zürn 1974, Frankenstein and Rowlands 1978, Haerke 1979, 1982).

Developments in Settlement:

What little is known about the princely seat sites from settlement investigations, and the regional hierarchy of burials, suggests that large territories now centred upon the former sites (Fig. 4). However, very little is known of the form and nature of the subsidiary foci and the rural domestic sites.[38] What kind of centres and what kind of role are we likely to be dealing with? Almost all our information comes from one regional centre, the Heuneburg (Kimmig 1975a, b, Haerke 1979), and even this excellent excavation has only partially uncovered the interior of the defended area. It seems most likely that foci of different kinds of activity within the settlement

did not remain fixed in one sector of the site for each phase, and it is most plausible to envisage at all times: a part of the site devoted to craftwork at a specialist level; much of the site given over to domestic dwellings of a 'farm' type; and probably superior domestic accommodation and/or community structures occupied by the elite (this sector may be within the unexcavated area, although Kimmig draws attention to a 'notable building' of 30m. length, aisled, which Haerke ignores) (Kimmig 1975a, Haerke 1979, 1982). Exotic finds, chiefly from burials, also suggest that long-distance trade, especially from the Mediterranean, was concentrated in the hands of the central and district elites. The model of Frankenstein and Rowlands (1978), whereby the exotica are obtained via long-distance connections and then distributed to 'satellite', 'subordinate' chiefs, appears a promising line of research. It is further possible that some kind of redistributive, tithe system was operating to extract agricultural, labour and raw material surpluses from regional peasant populations to support these elites, their focal settlements and dependent specialists. Some of the craftwork at the centres seems indeed to have been of a luxury type destined only for elite consumption, but there is evidence to suggest that the division of labour at the main focus may have been paralleled by a similar if smaller-scale set-up at district chieftain foci[39] (see below). On the other hand, the production of display ornaments for the local aristocracy was probably a minor function of this focussing of craft activity, most craftwork being for items of wider circulation in metal, wood, bone and pot.[40] Arguably, concentrated production of the latter items at elite centres supplemented village production and was tied to distribution from the centres to surrounding rural settlements. However it is difficult to demonstrate any significant trade in such items between princedoms.[41] The larger nucleations themselves naturally provided an important market for such products, and economy of scale may have been a factor enabling competition with rural craftsmen. But it is certainly unrealistic to view the normal craft sector of later prehistoric European settlements, large and small, as elevated in centres such as the Heuneburg to a new phase of 'industrial centres'. Haerke strikes an appropriately deflating note when he comments: "Evidence of crafts, particularly metalworking, has been reported from a number of 'Fürstensitz' sites and also from some other hillforts. This may be more indicative of sedentary occupation of such sites rather than of a particular status and function within the settlement network because clear traces of metalworking have also been found in a humble, open lowland settlement of Hallstatt D date in the same geographical area" (1980).

As has already been pointed out, the establishment of the fortified regional 'princely centres' of Hallstatt D represents a revival and/or relocation of typical continental defended foci as had become widespread by the Late Bronze Age (wood box structure with earth fill and sometimes a stone façade). The underlying continuity of chieftain foci in Western Europe is partly concealed by the alternation between such nucleated communities and elite residence within villages or as 'estate'-like control points amid a dispersed settlement pattern. However, in some areas, it is possible to point to potential antecedent locations of the regional power structure, e.g. with the Heuneburg itself and the preceding Grosse Heuneburg, and similar examples (Haerke 1979). Even more striking is the evidence that suggests that the erection of 'princely' tumuli preceded the development of the nucleated regional centre (major examples include the Heuneburg, Mt. Lassois, the Hohenasperg and Breisach), demanding a contemporaray 'manor/estate' type focus for some generations of the princely power structure (Haerke 1979, 1982).[42] At the Heuneburg, the Talhau settlement may form part of such a pre-hillfort focus. The very early dating of the first princely tumuli in the Hallstatt D period makes the hypothesis of a revolutionary transformation of the region as a result of the founding of Massalia on the Provence coast c. 600 BC an implausibly overnight affair.[43]

Correlated with a higher level of complexity for West Hallstatt chiefdoms by Hallstatt D is the widespread adoption of the Eastern Hallstatt status behaviour in terms of prestige equipment and burial rites. These elements of aristocratic display had already begun to appear amongst Western chiefdoms in Hallstatt C, and include the typical four-wheeled waggon-hearse and horseman/archer 'steppe' equipment, under a great tumulus and with novel inhumation contrasted to non-elite cremation continuity. Particularly noteworthy is the precise copying of the East Hallstatt 'clan tumulus' variety of elite burial as recovered spectacularly at the Magdalenenberg (Spindler 1976), whilst other close parallel features can be found elsewhere. A similar act of pretension by emergent paramounts is the mimicry of a Greek colony fortification at the Heuneburg, when the initial traditional defencework is replaced by a mudbrick bastioned wall on a stone socle. This work is destroyed by fire and the rest of the rebuildings of the defences revert to traditional construction methods.[44]

In general, therefore, we have argued that the development of the Hallstatt D centres in the West merely reflects a phase of recurrence of nucleated foci in this part of Europe. Already-existing local elites concentrate with their dependent craftsmen and retainers into defended communities, perhaps consequent on a phase of more discrete 'estate' type foci, defended or open, which may have formed the residence of the 'princes' being buried in the early group of princely tumuli. The novel opportunities of the more productive Iron Age economy lead to the general rise of paramount, large-territory chiefdoms, as in many areas of temperate and Mediterranean Europe during this age, previously a rarer occurrence under Bronze Age economic conditions. Parallel or slightly out-of-phase developments of this kind over Europe encouraged an expansion and notable extension of long-distance exchanges, especially of items to emphasize the prestige of the new higher nobility. Internal redistribution is probably far more significant in these 'polities', both barbarian and Mediterranean, together with greater densities of essentially subsistence communities, than long-distance commercial exchanges.

The later florescence of Western Hallstatt, compared to the East, with only gradual development of comparable phenomena in some areas during Hallstatt C, then the full take-off of apparent 'princedoms' in Hallstatt D1, seems linked plausibly to the far greater degree of antecedent development of the East, with its vigorous high-culture of the Bronze Age. The arrival of the technological and other, agrarian changes, discussed earlier, helped to speed up the process of change in the West. Furthermore, as our chronological fixes accumulate, it seems likely that the rise of the West, though a widespread phenomenon through Hallstatt C and Hallstatt D, had also slightly differing rates of advance for major regions **within** the West Hallstatt sphere.[45]

Political Structure:

Within the sphere of the genuine territorial 'princedoms' of West Hallstatt, it seems reasonable to suggest the emergence of dynastic families, who should have created secure social, political and economic ties with what now become 'subordinate' foci within the polity; clearly from a cluster of originally comparable chieftain residences, one has now risen as pre-eminent, perhaps being relocated and enlarged to take account of its new increased function. Although it is extremely difficult to extract from Medi-

terranean historical accounts elements which might reflect the political structure of this part of the barbarian world at this era (much being only recorded later with strong risks of hearsay and legend), it may be inferred that an era dominated by 'kings' widely preceded the common aristocratic oligarchies recorded for the region in the final centuries BC (though in places kings survived). That some Classical references or at least the general inferences drawn from them for the pre-oligarchy period, suit the apparent archaeological picture of centralized princedoms, is clear, considering here in chronological terms the sixth to fifth centuries BC (and locally into the fourth century BC), and geographically the sphere of West Hallstatt and regions immediately to the north (i.e. that of the Hallstatt and Early La Tène princely graves) (Fischer 1973 p.448, Lessing and Kruta 1979 pp.42,70). The apparent breakdown of such centralization and supreme authority may likewise be studied in the context of the disappearance of such burials and centres during the mature La Tène period. Yet doubtless continuing on from the Bronze Age is the basic political structure of district chieftains, from whose midst one may reasonably conceive the paramounts of Hallstatt D and early La Tène to have emerged. This far more numerous, traditional and probably more stable structure seems to survive the apparent collapse of the princedoms, to form the nucleus of the oligarchies typical for the historic Celtic tribes. The parallel to the progressive displacement of kings by an aristocratic oligarchy in Italy and Greece deserves detailed further research, and one may note that the further stage of power displacement to the yeomen middle classes which occurred in many city-states in Greece ('the hoplite reform', cf. Snodgrass 1980), has even been suggested for parts of the Eastern Hallstatt world. But closer examination of the main evidence, the scenes of warfare in East Hallstatt art, argues that this world remained one dominated by a minority nobility, often riding to the scene of conflict then dismounting for heavy-armed clashes, as with the early Archaic Greek aristocratic armies, not proceeding on to be transformed into a genuine yeoman phalanx (Frey 1976, Gabrovec 1980). An **elite** infantry may arrive with La Tène.[33]

Exotic Imports and the Mediterranean Connection:

Especial attention is given to the new importance, primarily in these princely contexts of burials and centres during Hallstatt D, of Mediterranean imports, seemingly both from the Rhône corridor and ultimately the newly-established Greek colonies of Provence, and from the more familiar Hallstatt C connection with the peoples of northern Italy. Clearly emphasizing the special status of the West Hallstatt foci and associated elite burials, they have nonetheless also been used in extreme instances (most particularly by Frankenstein and Rowlands, 1978), as **explanations** for the rise and fall, and overall 'function' of the princes and their 'seats'.[46] Similar processes are considered to create the Early La Tène princedoms to the north, when creative impulses deliberately bypass the West Hallstatt in the fifth century BC, stifling the latter's raison d'être.

This 'prestige good economy/core-periphery/dependency' model deserves careful examination, especially because of the elegant analysis of the contents of princely tumuli it has given rise to, with supporting ethnographic interpretation, in the Frankenstein and Rowlands version. Initially it may be noted that we have already pointed to some significant difficulties with the model:

1) It is likely, despite the very sorry state of settlement archaeology in this overall region of Europe, that there was continuity from the Late Bronze Age of local chiefdom societies, based sometimes on nucleated, defended communities, or at other times on less obvious, dispersed

'estate' foci.[47] We must therefore avoid overstressing the significance of the rise of Hallstatt D proto-urban sites.

2)   Likewise, it would be a mistake to overestimate the meaning of the spread of Hallstatt D princely burial rites. We have to consider the existence of elite burials in parts of the region from the Late Bronze Age and Hallstatt C (including in the latter period the first examples of the normal Hallstatt D princely variety), and our belief that elites may display rank in other ways (as shown in the content of hoards). More acceptable is the inference that the regional political structure may now have developed from district chiefdoms into paramount kingdoms composed of a mosaic of the former under a central dynasty based on the new princely seat; quite possibly this development may have been under way, if not completed in some areas, during Hallstatt C. In drawing attention to their new status, these princely families adopted the regalia of their older counterparts of Eastern Hallstatt, as well as fripperies from the strange world of the Archaic Mediterranean states.

3)   Despite the excitement often generated (cf. Wells 1980a), by the appearance of nucleated settlement with evidence of numbers of craftsmen at work, much of this seems rather to a be a normal development for any community of the size of a large village or beyond in later prehistoric Europe, with the local needs for skilled work in metal, clay, wood, bone etc. Add to this the presence of district and regional elites, their retinues and economic capacity to maintain dependent specialists to cater for their special demands in prestige artifacts, then the admixture of master-craftsmen and more mundane artisans need generate no necessity for an external forcing role. Indeed parallel communities with similar specialization inferred in political and craft roles have been identified in most parts of Europe from mature Neolithic times onwards. The growing frequency and density of such settlements, as we have several times argued, is primarily to be related to positive feedback from the increasing density and agricultural efficiency of European population.

In addition to these points, we may cite further critical objections to the model. Particularly careful consideration must be given to the question of the precise role of the Mediterranean luxury items, especially when some remarkable aspects of this data set are given due emphasis. To begin with, we must underline the extreme scarcity of these Mediterranean imports, both in West Hallstatt and Early La Tène sites and burials. Not only are we made aware that only elite circles have access to these valuable exotica, but the absolute amounts represented are very small indeed.[48] The well-established confirmation of this state of affairs (which might perhaps have been accounted for as due to the poor recovery rate by archaeologists), is the actual condition of these imports when found. A considerable number of the known pieces show clear evidence, either from the chronology of importation and deposition, or in actual repairs and replacement work on the pieces, that these prestige items were being treasured for generations, (despite suffering damage), as heirlooms, before deposition into their current archaeological context.[49] This key evidence makes it extremely difficult, it seems to me, to erect any theory such as that of Frankenstein and Rowlands, whereby the Hallstatt princes rose to power by controlling the flow of such items to district chiefs as necessary status symbols; no-one seems to have had any kind of reliable flow of these imports, however powerful. The corollary is that the theory whereby the Greeks and north Italians were tapping West Hallstatt resources in return for, amongst other things, Mediterranean luxury products of this type, likewise falls into the same embarrassing poverty of such reciprocal goods.[50]

A closely related point concerns the implication of the 'heirloom' factor for the chronology of the West Hallstatt princedoms. Since the typical well-dated piece, such as a Black Figure vase fragment, points to a Mediterranean origin date of the sixth century, the end of the princely florescence is often set at c. 500 BC plus or minus some decades. The fifth century rise of the core Early La Tène tradition with its princely burials and chronologically later Mediterranean imports (especially Red-Figure ware), would therefore be a subsequent or even 'replacement' phenomenon. This Early La Tène core arises to the north of the West Hallstatt, primarily in the Middle Rhine and Champagne/Marne regions, and is conspicuous for a new elite community (from prestige burial evidence), who have modified their display repertoire to the two not four-wheeled chariot/hearse, and who import luxury pottery and metalwork with a much stronger Etruscan bias. On the traditional dating it would seem that the West Hallstatt sphere collapsed and Mediterranean trade routes shifted to a more northerly zone of emergent cultural florescence; or in terms of the 'prestige economy/dependency' model, the very shifting of Mediterranean exchange relations from the West Hallstatt towards the rising nobles of the north precipitated the collapse of the West Hallstatt princedoms, now deprived of their essential raison d'être (the 'Mediterranean connection').

The implications of the heirloom factor in creating depositional time-lags, taken together with rare dendrochronological fixes and the scanty but rapidly growing body of cultural and chronological information from West Hallstatt region rural settlements (especially surface finds), all suggest that the simple 'replacement' model is a gross oversimplification, and have opened up far broader interpretative perspectives for the decline of West Hallstatt and the rise of the La Tène Culture.[51]

The end of West Hallstatt and the rise of the La Tène Culture:

A provisional reinterpretation of developments in Western Europe during late Hallstatt D and Early La Tène times, based upon this important new information, might run as follows. A major elaboration of society, based upon wealth and status indicators, and probably intimately linked to demographic and economic expansion, appears to be taking place in those regions subsequently to form the La Tène heartlands (Middle Rhine and Champagne), in Late Hallstatt (D2-3) times, i.e. at a period contemporary to the florescence of the West Hallstatt 'princely' polities to their south (late sixth and first half of the fifth century BC). Around the latter point (c. 450 BC) the West Hallstatt sphere enters into a decline, but in the form of a gradual process of piecemeal abandonment of its central-places (which spans the remainder of the fifth century), and a much speedier process of cessation of princely burial (only one very fine example unambiguously occupies the late fifth century). At the same time as this decline of West Hallstatt commences, the new Early La Tène culture is born to its north, some of its Hallstatt chieftains are transformed into 'princes', and the pace of regional economic and demographic development in the north intensifies. But in the former West Hallstatt sphere imports from the Mediterranean are still being obtained at the diminishing number of major settlements, and a full participation in the novel La Tène A cultural format is observable both at surviving 'princely' seats and rural sites, and in both metalwork and pottery.

We have argued above that the presence of Mediterranean imports and prestigious burials in Hallstatt Europe is more indicative of the overall structure, and even 'health' of a complex socio-political system in any particular region than a key element in the latter's maintenance, and according to this model the La Tène A heartlands, together with major parts of the former East Hallstatt sphere, emerge as flourishing 'complex' in the later fifth century, whilst the West Hallstatt sphere in its La Tène A facies undergoes progressive socio-political devolution. If we reject the mercantile realignment model, the situation may perhaps be viewed as one of essentially unrelated processes, of internal socio-economic and socio-political breakdown in West Hallstatt, and vigorous demographic expansion and socio-political elaboration in the core La Tène regions of Champagne and Middle Rhine.

What is the relationship between the La Tène A core region and older Hallstatt developments? The Early La Tène core, centring on the Rhine and Champagne regions, with outliers, exhibits during La Tène A in the fifth century BC a notable emergence of princely burials and associated with them a new art style: this is created out of an indigenous amalgamation of Mediterranean, East European/steppe, Hallstatt Culture artistic influences together with an original creative transformation of these components into something quite unique - Celtic art. The princely burials show every sign of being an imitative series of those typical for Hallstatt elites. Although the new two-wheeled chariot is predominant there are plentiful links to the older tradition, including earlier and parallel use in rare cases of four-wheelers, together with other features taken over from the Hallstatt elite customs (Bretz-Mahler 1971, Harhoiu 1976, Stead 1979).[52] In fact, as regards the contribution that the Hallstatt Culture of Central Europe may have made to the repertoire of La Tène, it can be argued that whereas early La Tène metalwork bears a characteristic derivation from the westerly core regions, early La Tène pottery may represent a hybrid tradition emanating from Czechoslovakia (Collis, pers. comm.). Although the rich gifts include Mediterranean imports with a stronger Etruscan element than typical for Hallstatt, similar items are being imported into contemporary La Tène A sites in the former West and East Hallstatt regions, and there seems to be no discontinuity in the general, small scale flow of exotic luxury pieces from the Mediterranean into all three regions (Fischer 1973, Frey 1980, Lessing and Kruta 1979). Questions of access routes from different origin points and the varying prestige exchange networks involved, together with the decline in the number of West Hallstatt central places, seem to account for such regional differences as are observed. We do not require any more dramatic interpretation of trade route realignments being consciously carried out by the Mediterranean city-states, apart from the obvious fact that a new, more remote region was now emerging as a populous and more stratified society demanding status-enhancing customs and long-distance display pieces.[53] The new regions with princely graves continue the social tradition of Hallstatt, with a strong emphasis on a small, powerful elite; the new art style is confined to their milieu and does not extend to the rest of the population (Schwappach 1973, Neustupny and Neustupny 1961). The new style strongly influences the elite art of the former Hallstatt world, in both East and West, though a spectrum of receptivity can be observed. Hitherto curious is the absence of major nucleated foci for La Tène A in the west (Fischer 1973), but our earlier discussion of the variety of elite residences allows us to suggest that no major significance should be attached to the necessary alternative of smaller elite foci (Schindler 1974, Zürn 1974, Haerke 1979, 1982). During the fifth century, however, alongside this long-standing tradition of major and small scale elites with distinctive burials, there is emerging, both in the La Tène A of the West Hallstatt sphere and in the Early La Tène core, alongside such older rites, an increasingly popular inhumation rite in small mounds or flat graves, with the latter variant destined to become the norm for much of contin-

ental Europe from the fourth century or La Tène B (Ib-c) times (cf. above, and Champion, S. 1982). This important and poorly-understood transformation we have already entered into in the context of East Hallstatt, and will return to below, but in our emphasis here on the relative homogeneity of the fifth century 'princely' world of East Hallstatt, West Hallstatt and La Tène A, it is highly significant that these regional variants undergo profound changes between the fifth and fourth centuries, broadly contemporaneously, culminating in the general disappearance of this 'paramount' Hallstatt - La Tène A society and its replacement by one seemingly reflecting a different socio-political pattern across Europe (cf. Champion, S. 1982, Filip 1977).

As concerns the 'wave-effect' rise of these three regional florescences of princedoms, there are three major areas to explore in accounting for the sequence of developments as outlined, all having their current proponents:

1) Diffusion of the concept of 'princedom' amongst low-level chiefdom societies, plus the associated accoutrements (Kimmerian/Scythian, East Hallstatt, Mediterranean). It is extremely difficult to conceive how the simple 'idea' of conversion to a 'princedom' can produce a total socio-economic transformation, just as the Heuneburg can hardly be accounted for as a barbarian attempt to build an imitation Greek colony.

2) The growing colonization of, and interaction with, their barbarian hinterlands by the Mediterranean civilized city-states (Greek, Etruscan and those of other north Italian peoples), can be argued to have a strongly commercial aim, leading to progressive penetration and transformation of such barbarian societies in the hinterland of continental Europe - hence the later development of the more remote La Tène core territory compared to that of the more accessible West Hallstatt sphere.

This theory deserves much more serious consideration, and we shall begin with some obvious criticisms. Firstly, the initial florescence of East Hallstatt can hardly be ascribed to an early eighth-century metamorphosis inspired by Greek or Italian city-state interference, since neither group have the established organization or commercial pull at this stage for such an effect, nor is there any evidence to support such an argument in East Hallstatt developments. Even though the first Greek colonists in Provence are sixth-century in date, it is also hard to see how the contemporary rise of the Western princedoms can be ascribed to an immediate all-powerful level of interference from the contemporary fledgling Greek colonies, as if by spontaneous catalysis. As has been noted above, even arch-dependency theorists such as Rowlands will acknowledge that the complex political organization of the large princedoms of West Hallstatt must pre-date the flourishing of any proposed large-scale economic and political interactions with the Mediterranean states.

Secondly, the hypothesis of major commerce between the West Hallstatt princedoms and the Mediterranean lacks any supporting evidence. The recorded links are merely small quantities of luxury items for the local elite that may well be part of political gifts from individual Mediterranean communities (and subsequently circulating between local princely families and subordinate chiefs for similar purposes), to seal arrangements such as mutual respect of territorial power, non-aggression pacts, or peaceful low-level trade (that is sufficiently small scale to leave no obvious trace for us).[54] Here it must be remarked that a recurrent feature of the Greek colonial experience was hostility from barbarians in the hinterland zones. We have further to question the assumption that Greek colonies were primarily concerned with entrepôt roles. The general consensus on the phenomenon argues that their primary aim was to relieve population pressure by the search for new land, and that city foundations with strong commercial aims were very exceptional (cf. Bintliff 1982, with refs.).[55] To see the foundation of Massalia and other Western Greek colonies as a secure argument for wholesale, bulk, long-distance exchange between the Mediterranean and the West Hallstatt and La Tène A areas is therefore quite unjustified from the viewpoint of the Classical world, though it is of course reasonable to suggest that the merchants of these cities would have been interested in barbarian exports. Nonetheless such limited trade as may have flowed north and south in this fashion should have remained a poor second to the internal circulation of food, craft products, and raw materials within the city state territories themselves.

If one takes the most extreme example of an arguably anachronistic treatment of the barbarian and Mediterranean economies for this time-range, that of the studies by P.S. Wells (1979, 1980a, 1980b, 1981), we find some striking assumptions underlying his interpretation of historical processes that cannot be supported by the data of either side. Firstly, Wells accepts that the evidence of craft production and imports at the princely seats shows, without further discussion, the rise of new international commercial centres and major industrialisation, both a response to Mediterranean influence. The finding of a mould for a type of small ring at the rural West Hallstatt site of Hascherkeller is seized on as clear proof that even small rural sites are being transformed into nodes in this commercial/industrial revolution. A map of Western Europe centring on Hascherkeller is littered with trade arrows, including one for salt import to the area from Austria that defies the absence of any evidence from the site.[56] Let us recall Haerke's comments, cited earlier, commonsense observations that we enlarged on, that from the first Neolithic villages onwards people indulged in local craftwork and exchange, so that in later prehistoric Europe we may expect to find such activities in every corner of the countryside (just as in a traditional historic village in Europe until very recently). On a different but equally spurious plane, Wells erects from thin air a model of the economy of barbarian Europe wherein the demands of the Greek homeland for imports, especially grain, are channelled through their agents abroad, the colonies, to transform the native economies of the Hallstatt and La Tène world from locally orientated food production to commercial production for export.[57]

Related to this set of assumptions about commerce are other frequently-expressed but never closely-analyzed views about barbarian exports as stimuli to Hallstatt and early La Tène 'take-off'. Rowlands, for example (1980) informs us that the basis for the West Hallstatt polities was the activity of the princes as 'middlemen' in such commerce. A vague but popular link is made between the widespread occurrence of iron ore in the Middle Rhineland, the local rise of La Tène A princes, and the 'Mediterranean connection', (cf. Milisauskas 1978, with refs.) despite the particular transport problems such a bulky material poses, and the general availability of iron ore throughout the Mediterranean coastlands themselves (cf. Snodgrass 1980). The fact that the other Early La Tène core region, Champagne, has nothing but its excellent marl soils to recommend it, (cf. Collis 1977), is conveniently explained away by postulating a further 'middleman' role for it (an all-purpose argument that avoids the obvious by retreat into totally negative evidence; cf. Hodson and Rowlett 1974). The recent study by Freidin (1983) of Late Hallstatt, Early La Tène development in the Paris Basin (including the Marne), though impressively informed on the data base, is a disappoint-

ment on the theoretical level. It is admitted that no useful information is offered on population levels and local resources, yet the rise of this region is largely attributed to the "commercial power-base", for which no significant evidence is forthcoming (apart from the luxury imports that bear witness to the very degree of social elaboration that is to be accounted for).

Wells has interpreted the collapse of the West Hallstatt princedoms (1980a) as the result of the decline in the trading activities of Massalia and other colonial 'entrepôts' (cf. Hodson and Rowlett 1974), in the face of more accessible grain supplies from the Black Sea colonies. Apart from the arguments presented above on the improbability of such a scenario, recent research at Marseilles (Euzennat 1980) finds no support for a decline in the prosperity of the town during the fifth and fourth centuries BC.[58]

The alternative 'dependency' model offered by Frankenstein and Rowlands (1978) envisages a deliberate rerouting of trade lines away from West Hallstatt to the new La Tène core area to the north. We have already indicated our view that the small scale luxury import trickle that now expands to these latter areas is more a recognition of local, internal economic growth and socio-political elaboration, than a forced fruit of Mediterranean influence, and that Mediterranean trade is probably so minor a feature of West Hallstatt economics that such factors are hardly acceptable catalysts for regional developments. In any case, the recognition of significant continuity and survival of parts of the West Hallstatt central place network in La Tène A, undermines the whole 'rerouting' model. The disappearance of princely burials and centres in the latter part of the fifth century BC in the former West Hallstatt sphere, leads into major changes during the fourth century in large areas of the new La Tène A and former East Hallstatt spheres in burial tradition, and this has to have a deeper significance, just as the very origin and development of all three florescent zones require a more rounded model, incorporating local processual investigations, than the neo-diffusionist approach increasingly adopted at present.

3) Autonomous Regional Growth and 'Feudal' Models. We have already suggested that the background to the Hallstatt D princedoms in the West, and those of Hallstatt C-D in the East, as also those to arise briefly in the Early La Tène core lands, is the characteristic, long-lived chiefdom/paramount society of Bronze Age Europe. It has been pointed out that a wave of more elaborate 'princedoms' seems to spread across Europe from a source emergence in Hallstatt C of East Hallstatt, leading via West Hallstatt to the generally short-lived princely phase of La Tène A, before the transformation is completed to the mature La Tène chiefdom society expanding as a culture or ethnic diaspora over large areas of Central and Eastern Europe. Despite the borrowed finery and symbols of vigorous warriors on the Black Sea steppes and forest-steppe, and special but irregular imports of Mediterranean luxury display pieces for the table or the funeral procession, it has seemed more plausible to consider this pattern as reflecting the same injection of new productivity via iron technology into agriculture, and related changes in subsistence production, as was leading at precisely the same time to the transformation to a new level of complexity of Dark Age Greece and Villanovan north-central Italy. Rates of change would naturally vary, dependent on the relative development of the locally-antecedent socio-economic system, as well as other regional factors affecting the speed with which demographic and economic change moulded the local political structure. It is here claimed that the distribution of prestige goods and elite monuments reflects, indirectly, the regional achievement of the culmination of

this process, rather than in any significant way creating it. The territorial pattern of sizeable princedoms, as argued from the pattern of putative central foci, and central and satellite burials and foci, will have arisen and cohered via a process of integration of numerous chiefdoms under a paramount family or group of families, and as the precipitate of the novel potential in manpower and resources.

There is little doubt that with only the Heuneburg adequately excavated to modern standards (and even this only partially dug), the archaeological obsession with the rich tumuli with their sumptuous imports (cf. the classic Magdalenenberg tumulus with the 'prince' and numerous 'subject' satellite burials ranged appropriately around him), has denied us a serious look at Kimmig's original theory based on the agricultural support base for these princes, craftsmen and proto-urban populations. If we take Haerke's (1979) Thiessen polygon analysis of the major 'princely seats' and their inferrable territories, plotted against the main upland blocks, and then introduce a constant territorial module of a 40kms. radius circle (Fig. 4), it does appear that natural blocks of arable and grazing land are being linked into largish kingdoms (?) appropriate in size to the splendour of the associated princely burials (and significantly very much larger than the 5 and 10kms. radius territories discussed earlier in this chapter, cf. Figs. 1, 2, and 3). Whether we consider a medieval 'feudal' model (Kimmig 1975a, Zürn 1974) as an appropriate analogue, or something less formally structured, such as an elite superstructure riding the wave of indigenous economic growth and adapting to a more centralized, internally-differentiated hierarchy as a result - our emphasis will be on the control of resources. This is directly akin to the Marxist concern with the realities of power, of identifying the elite as those with power by virtue of their preferential rights to surplus resources of subsistence products, raw material and manpower (for a general discussion of this model with case studies, cf. Bintliff 1982).[59]

The rise and subsequent fall and/or radical transformation of such regional power systems, if we are to rule out dramatic changes in mental attitude (model one, above), or in Mediterranean patterns of interference (model two), needs to be sought in the 'health' of these regional systems themselves. With the current tendency to date the decline and collapse of the West Hallstatt sphere (La Tène A facies), and notable alterations in the cultural repertoire of the East Hallstatt sphere (La Tène A facies) **and** the Early La Tène heartlands, to the late fifth to fourth centuries BC, we are brought inevitably, as has been increasingly emphasized of late, into the striking circumstance that here indeed we have the much sought-after aid from the Mediterranean historical sources, an insight into remarkable developments at precisely this time within the barbarian world. These developments were noteworthy because they were directly affecting the Mediterranean states - the Celtic migrations. Clearest and most indisputable is the devastating colonization and related raiding of Italy by the 'Gauls', culminating (in tendentious hindsight) in the famous sack of Rome in 387/6 BC. A more important contemporary achievement was the loss to the Italian states and tribes of the far north of the country and the permanent weakening of the power of the Etruscan cities. Almost certainly around this time (fourth-century), 'Celtic' (mature La Tene, La Tène B/lb-c) culture begins its triumphant progress out of the core regions and through Central and Eastern Europe, commonly believed to involve the infiltration of West European bearers of this tradition amongst the East Hallstatt and neighbouring peoples; by the third century BC the Celtic expansion emerges again into history as the Celts erupt down the Balkans to pillage and colonize in Greece and Turkey. Classical tradition links the Italian

and Eastern European movements, and at least archaeologically the 'Celtization' of Central and Eastern Europe belongs to the same era as the occupation of Italy.

Of the varied historical explanations of this traumatic activity, provided by the threatened literate neighbours of the Celts, the clearest reported is that of over-population and land hunger. That the striking collapse of the central places and power structure of 'princes' is observed from the mid to late fifth century BC in the West Hallstatt sphere (D3 - La Tène A era), whilst major alterations in burial rite, settlement pattern and cultural repertoire occur also in the La Tène core and in the former East Hallstatt sphere, from this time and progressively through the fourth century and into the third (transformation from La Tène A to the La Tène B flat inhumation 'warrior' phase), could all reasonably be accounted for by postulating just such a breakdown in regional subsistence economies and demographic support structure in West Hallstatt and quite possibly in other areas of population growth in the Early Iron Age of continental Europe, with the resultant disintegration of the political leadership and extensive 'colonization' into neighbouring regions. Whether surplus population, swelling dense populations in Central and Eastern Europe, in this fashion, in turn gave rise to further colonial expansion as evidenced later in settlement attempts in south east Europe and beyond (e.g. the Celtic settlement of Galatia in Turkey), is a subject worthy of more processual explanation than the traditional study of the relevant battles has given scope for.[60] But we would once again seek to abolish the accepted distinction between the Mediterranean population expansion of the Early Iron Age (the Greek and Etruscan colonies), due to burgeoning land hunger, and the Celtic expansion into the Mediterranean and Eastern Europe, due to burgeoning land hunger. The Classical/barbarian dichotomy blinkers us from recognizing a common process of growth and external expansion at work, bound to bring these peoples into closer mutual contact. Such interaction can be at various levels, from the sporadic trade and treaty level (cf. the Hallstatt world), to more substantial trade (later La Tène), and ultimately military confrontation, when the expanding populations directly threaten each other's territory (e.g. the fourth to third century Celtic invasions of the Mediterranean, and the second century onwards advance of Rome into the European hinterland).

It seems to the present writer, that explanation '3' has most to recommend it, both in terms of the data and in terms of our current understanding of the ancient and late prehistoric economy. To what extent the genuine expansion of 'Celts' accounts for the spread of mature La Tène culture (La Tène B) in all parts of Western, Central and Eastern Europe is clearly a matter of dispute. It is quite possible that the chiefly elites of these regions as often before were highly receptive to new prestige sets, and certainly some were already in many areas employing early La Tène cultural forms and ideas. But some widespread disruption of the network of East Hallstatt (now 'La Tène') elites seems indicated, as in West Hallstatt, by the decline or abandonment of many central foci and of princely burial, during the time of the putative Celtic expansion to the east. There arise a remarkable number of examples throughout the old East Hallstatt region, as to the West, of a new and radically different kind of cemetery - flat inhumation graves, in which a low-level elite are detectable (with their richly-accompanied womenfolk) as 'warrior burials'. This pattern of course may represent a continuity of chieftain structure, surviving the loss of the paramounts, now decked with La Tène finery and prestige styles. But a new element is a contrast to the older princely burial symbolism of Hallstatt and Early La Tène, where the elaborate princes were poles apart from their subordinate population in grave style and contents. Now the analysis of grave wealth indicates a more smoothly flowing ladder of grave wealth from richest to poorest, all with similar burial form (though some chariots appear, but rarely, in the mature La Tène world). The significance of the general shift to inhumation for an increase in the quantity of gifts has been noted earlier, and it is a complex issue as to how far this rite-change in itself leads to a narrowing of the difference between commoner cremation and noble inhumation of former times, as opposed to the argument that such a change in disposal practices reflects a new attitude to the status of commoner vis-à-vis nobles. Overall, one may reasonably infer that statuses are now being blurred with the disappearance of the tumulus-inhumation versus flat-cremation dichotomy.[61]

Despite the plausibility of a model in which internal demographic-ecological problems led to the breakdown of West Hallstatt and perhaps other areas of contemporary Hallstatt-Early La Tène Europe, thus stimulating folk movements and/or Celtic infiltration, and reflected in the new burial symbolism of less complex political structure, it remains true that the apparent 'levelling' of social structure to a two-tier system ('warrior' chief families/peasants) from a three-tier one (Princes, chiefs, peasants), continues to dominate most of La Tène Europe up until the Roman conquest. However abundant Classical source evidence and alternative archaeological pointers prove the Late La Tène revival of a three-tier system (Celtic 'barons' at the core of dominant tribal oligarchies; chiefs; peasants/slaves). As with earlier phases of later prehistory, it must be suggested that elite display found ample scope in other directions - the clearest of which for archaeology are the mature and late products of Celtic art, which demonstrate the existence of a stratum of nobles with unparalleled access to luxury materials and true master-craftsmen. It may perhaps be truer of this later phase, than of La Tène B, when S. Champion writes (1982, p.71) of "the transformation of society from one essentially simple, if stratified, to one much more complex".

The Lausitz Culture

For comparison with these circum-Alpine developments, lest we be lured into the feeling that this is a purely 'Mediterranean contact-zone' phenomenon (as many would have us believe), let us turn to the far north of Europe. In a large area of Poland and East Germany, for several centuries spanning the Late Bronze Age and on through into the Early Iron Age, contemporary to the Hallstatt princely seats of the east and west Alpine regions, the Lausitz Culture produces a remarkable takeoff of dense rural populations focussing on urban centres, with much evidence for concentrated craft production and settlement planning. The build-up of very large populations prior to the appearance of the 'towns' or Burgwälle has been clearly documented, as has the integrated network of these latter district foci when they arise. The application of territorial analysis to one such region in Poland, including key sites such as Biskupin, reveals (Fig. 5) a remarkable density of population crowded into quite limited areas of land, in fact of the order of the small territories associated with early Iron Age hillforts in England. Clearly a very much more intensive agricultural production must be involved in the case of the Lausitz culture, quite possibly a dangerous over-exploitation, for some of these centres are considered to have contained thousands of people in addition to numerous rural satellite sites. By early La Tène times, just as in the West Hallstatt sphere, there is a remarkable collapse of this developed society, with general evidence for a dramatic shrinkage of the towns to mere hamlets or even abandonment. Not surprisingly, it is suggested by some scholars that the most important cause is land exhaustion. It is of

great importance that it is difficult to claim that this sequence of development is due to some external forcing role, from Mediterranean higher culture or anywhere else.[62]

Two further parallel case-studies may be introduced at this stage, to broaden the evidence to support our thesis of regular agrarian cycles in prehistoric Europe and their major effects upon socio-political structure. The first is an impressive study of a microregion in the neighbourhood of Berlin in East Germany (Wüstemann 1974; cf. Harding, this volume).[63]

Our second case-study is taken likewise from Northern Europe, again to provide an essential distancing from areas of the South where the neo-diffusionist arguments are still a reasonable counterpoise to local developmental processes. In a series of illuminating studies, Kristiansen has put together a highly persuasive correlation of site distribution maps, agricultural statistics and palaeo-ecological data, phase by phase, for the development of Denmark from the Late Neolithic to the La Tène Iron Age period (Kristiansen 1978, 1980, 1981, 1982). Supporting work by Randsborg reinforces the overall interpretation (1974a, b, c, 1982).[64]

EUROPE IN MATURE LA TENE TIMES

Characteristic of the middle period of the Iron Age (chiefly La Tène II/La Tène C third to second century BC), is a decline in hillfort usage, and a dominant emphasis in burials on the new social group between the traditional elite minority and the remaining peasantry: a warrior class. Some would maintain that an aristocracy, though broader in recruitment now, is still detectable, for example in the minority of burials with chariots in Western Europe, or by inference from the now mature products of the master-craftsmen of La Tène art. Population is still rising, and dense clusters of open settlement sites with closely adjacent foci of specialization may represent the undefended equivalent of the former hillfort nuclei (a settlement mode with possible parallels in the final pre-city phases of Archaic centres in the Mediterranean). One area well-documented in this respect is that of Clermont Ferrand in central France, where John Collis points to close Middle La Tène clusters of settlement, which during their life into Late La Tène times provide evidence for intensive craft specialization in a rural context (glasswork, metalwork and coin production) - the whole appropriate to 'rurally embedded' landed aristocrats who by the end of La Tène will move these populations en masse to the great adjacent hill of Gergovie to establish a major defended oppidum.[65]

The immediate parallels that spring to mind are similar 'archaic' pre- and proto-urban settlement patterns but in the Mediterranean. Compare the French picture and other landscapes discussed by Collis with similar features, to the pattern of dense hamlets marked by cemeteries illustrated by Anthony Snodgrass (1980) for the pre-city development of Athens, or to the pre-city hamlet clusters of the Etruscan cities illustrated by Tim Potter (1979).

At the inception of this period we have discussed the waves of migration (that had begun in La Tène I/La Tène A) out of Central; and later Northern, Europe into the far east, south, south-west and south-east of the subcontinent, with amongst other aims the intention, often realized of resettlement in a new homeland. We have seen these as the continental equivalent to the earlier and land-seeking explosion of Greek Mainland settlers abroad, or to the Etruscan colonization into northern Italy. On the other hand, it is characteristic in the ancient world for an expansion of the economy to consist of a denser infilling of land already occupied, or to be achieved by external territorial conquest; into marginal land, or fertile land belonging to someone else: "What passed for economic growth in antiquity was always achieved only by external expansion" (Finley 1978, pp.64-5). Perhaps, despite the great release of population pressure in early La Tène migrations, further temporary bottlenecks in the gradual increase in density and agricultural efficiency thoughout the middle Iron Age were to be linked with an external pressure valve (marked by the third to second century BC Celtic and Germanic migrations); certainly the decline or abandonment of most major defensive earthworks seems to indicate that growth could be sustained more normally within existing regional populations.

The final period of the pre-Roman Iron Age (Late La Tène, La Tène 3 or D, c. 120/100 BC to the Roman Conquest) represents a further stage in the evolution of more complex socio-economic structures in 'barbarian' Europe, with the appearance in a broad band through the centre of Europe, and eventually across into Britain, of 'oppida': despite their name, they are not, as too often stated, a sudden adoption of Mediterranean life by imitative groups of Celtic rustics after a visit to a Greek colony in Provence (or elsewhere).[66] There is probably a direct continuity of 'central-place' tradition from the Hallstatt nuclei through the early to mid La Tène undefined clusters of settlement and defended 'elite farms' into the erection of the great defences of the mature oppidum. Indeed the frequent use of a highly sophisticated wall construction on a quite remarkable scale around these giant oppidum enclosures, the 'murus gallicus', is demonstrably a combination of indigenous rampart traditions. One must also differentiate between the minority of oppida that seem to contain large resident populations as well as 'central place' functions, and those that were primarily for the latter and had large zones of refuge space, fields and grazing between scattered clusters of craft and residential quarters. It is possible that the more truly 'urban' centres represent nuclei for the larger, more truly centralized political groupings, and furthermore a significant degree of centralization of regional craftwork at the expense of rural production centres (e.g. Manching). The location of several oppida on or near major iron ore sources is clearly relevant to the central command over the source of much of the contemporary high productivity, and of the means whereby the gains of that productivity might be protected adequately and if possible improved at other communities' expense (weapons, the colossal amounts of iron incorporated in the murus gallicus ramparts); however it is highly unlikely that the macro-topographical location of the majority of oppida is a function of mineral resources or 'natural routes'. They should be considered primarily in terms of their central role to districts of notable fertility and dense population. In this respect we should pay far more attention to the signs of the importance of land and local agricultural products to these regional foci.[67]

From the Middle Iron Age on, we have scattered historical references to Celtic society, which can be supplemented with fuller accounts from the Late, oppida period, and with less confidence the tangled Irish and Welsh cycles of Laws and Legends preserved from the first millennium AD but believed to incorporate much earlier material. A general shift is hypothesized from numerous regional 'kings', towards an oligarchy (of a warrior aristocracy) over the Middle-Late La Tène period. If we can recognize an earlier stratum of dynasts, this would seem clearest in the Hallstatt, Early La Tène 'princely graves' and 'princely seats'. The rural nuclei of the Middle La Tène, with servicing functions apparently embedded in an open landscape of farms and fields, could perhaps represent some broadening of authority amongst a

much larger number of district notables, to be followed once again by a centralization of regional power within the defined limits of the later oppidum. The most highly developed region for such centralization of power and resource control would seem to have been central Gaul, with a number of tribal 'states' (Fig. 8) identified and analysed in a masterly study by Daphne Nash (cf. Nash 1975, 1978, 1981). Historical sources for the oppidum era suggest, at least for the most highly developed areas, that a council and rudimentary legislature, basing its activities in the most important oppidum of each region, was now wresting control of the use of force and the diversion of the regional surplus from district nobles into its own hands, (as a consensus of the overall elite, or more probably a select caucus of the aristocracy). In this respect it seems appropriate to see here the very process of state formation, and it is clear that the individual members of a 'tribe' were increasingly expected to recognize their common goals and contribute to the armed support and physical maintenance of the state's defences and 'treasury'. There is a shift from overlapping scatters of high value gold coins to more mutually-exclusive lower value silver and bronze coins centring on the key oppidum of each tribe. This has been interpreted as indicating the change from rival nobles minting gift coinage for their allies, to the 'state' controlling a more everyday medium of exchange with 'tribal' insignia.

Summarizing a very extensive body of research, Daphne Nash underlines what we consider to be the key internal processes that created increasingly larger political units within Celtic Europe (1981): "it is therefore likely that the late third and second centuries was a period during which a new pattern of territorial overlordship was imposed and consolidated in Gaul. I have argued elsewhere that the development of nucleated and defended settlements and the increase in luxury exchange with the Mediterranean during the late 2nd and 1st centuries must be seen as one outcome of the violent competition within the Celtic nobility for possession of territory, wealth, and armed retainers ... I therefore offer the suggestion that the early coinages were instituted at a time when the now firmly rooted nobilities moved into a new phase of political and economic growth, which this time took the form not of migratory expansion but a combination of intensified exploitation of existing territory, and attempts on the part of individual noble groupings to control increasingly large areas" (p.15).[68] Such political complexity would however seem to be unusual, and in most regions the oppida territories form a mosaic **within** each recorded 'tribe' and are still relatively autonomous; whether this latter pattern allows us to relate the 'tribe' back to the unpoliticized archaeological culture or a territorial grouping such as the Greek 'ethnos' is a question worth pursuing.[69]

Just as the Middle Iron Age saw a general decline in apparent settlement hierarchy over much of barbarian Europe and an equivalent reduction in burial differentiation, so the Late Iron Age (pre-Roman) provides a continued difficulty for social inferences in the frequent absence of notable status burials. It is clearly with some relief that archaeologists are able to link the rise of oppida and more centralized political groupings in southern Britain with the lavish gifts and special tumuli accompanying the supposed 'nobility' of the Aylesford-Swarling burial complex.[70] But although in the larger, more truly urban European oppida, there is evidence for rudimentary 'mansions' contrasted with 'humble' craftsmen's quarters, it would seem that the average 'aristocratic' household occupied a cluster of domestic houses, ancillary craft and storage structures, all within a common enclosure, either within the oppidum or amid the fields of that household (less commonly in a rural village). The variation in size of domestic structures is not great, although the number of enclosure structures and their composition has been seen to be significant for social differentiation. One is reminded of the absence of distinctive 'elite dwelling modes' at a notable remove from the remainder of the community, that seems characteristic for supposed chiefs' houses in settlements of the Neolithic to Bronze Age in Europe. The rural site of Gussage All Saints and the sophisticated analysis of the household units in Glastonbury Lake Village are eloquent in this respect.[71]

Despite the 'low key' of symbolic emphasis on rank in the **archaeology** of the later pre-Roman Iron Age, if we can accept the Classical authorities Celtic Europe had become increasingly a society of very sharp class divisions. Caesar puts it bluntly with his characterization of two classes: the free ruling warrior elite, and the dependent peasantry and slaves without political voice; between the two is a relationship either of subordinate clientage or mere ownership.[72] We are clearly very far removed from social forms entertained for earlier periods, with communal leadership stemming from kinship pyramids or 'achieved status' from specific service to the community. However, the origins of this state of affairs is unresolved. The most favoured view is to consider that the role of the elite in approved 'management' of communal surpluses in food, minerals and labour (including captive slave labour), was until the oppidum period played out within traditional kinship contexts and consensus leadership roles. With the great takeoff in trade with the Mediterranean world, the possibility of converting such surplus into the personal, private 'capital' of the elite (in the form of gold coinage, increased quantities of imported luxury goods, etc.) led to a breakdown of such structures and a re-alignment towards a dependence of the masses on individual aristocrats, regardless of kinship or ascribed role, in terms of their provision of capital.[73]

What is left unclear is how the average dependent peasant is brought into the power of the elite class, from whom must flow the essential agricultural surplus and labour force to support that elite and its regional and international exchange systems. Not for him the wine amphorae and luxury tableware, although many scholars argue that the redistribution of such desirable items and the additional handouts of booty and slaves from war parties, (both controlled by leading aristocrats), could be sufficient to secure a retinue of lesser 'nobles'. Caesar specifically mentions indebtedness for the servile status of the peasantry, and there are other references that seem to imply very considerable private estates manned by large workforces. In the light of the persuasive arguments of Professor Finley and his school concerning the 'Ancient Economy', with the emphasis firmly on private land-holding for elite dominance in the Classical world, one might consider the possibility that social differentiation in the Celtic (and Germanic) world had now become firmly established via gross variations in private land ownership (cf. Bintliff 1982). Such a suggestion provides a complementary and possibly alternative approach to the source of power and wealth of leading aristocrats and earlier 'kings' and 'princes', in the pre-Roman Iron Age. We cannot however be at all sure whether the desire for prestigious imports encouraged competing nobles to increase their estate size and yields (an analogous situation has been analysed by Mike Rowlands (1979) in West Africa, and is a possibility he raises for the European Iron Age), **or** whether the rise of a 'landed aristocracy' concentrated a larger surplus into fewer hands and stimulated more intense exchange (a view with much to recommend it in terms of the most appropriate functional model for pre-Industrial economies in Europe).[74]

I have elsewhere (Bintliff 1982) offered a re-analysis of the development of Mycenaean civilization in Mainland Greece during the Middle and Late Bronze Age, exploring the potential of this 'differentiation of landholding' model for the metamorphosis of village headmen, 'big men' and lineage heads into a class of privileged nobles and princes residing in mansions and palaces. A pattern that appears highly significant in this process is a dramatic rise in population and remarkable intake of cultivated land, leading to the equally rapid rise of a settlement hierarchy culminating in large controlling centres with palaces and an administrative bureaucracy. I suggested that initial minor economic distinctions, prevalent due to ascribed and achieved status in the early period villages, became grossly exaggerated with the great land intake, during which those colonizing the wasteland become dependent on the wealthier members of the community in a patron-client relationship. As we have seen, phases of land intake on a large scale are characteristic features of recurrent agrarian cycles in prehistoric Europe, due to novel technologies, ecological adaptation, or recovery from previous phases of over-exploitation, depopulation and cultivated-area decline. As the model develops, district and then regional hierarchies of landowning elites are erected by alliance and intermarriage. A recent re-interpretation of the Mycenaean archives has led its most authoritative commentator, John Chadwick, to postulate a 'feudal society' in which power and privilege are a function of landed wealth.

The model has further applications, e.g. Archaic Greece, Republican Italy, perhaps late Dark Age to Medieval Europe. The fit to the data is suggestive, and the implications are that we must always consider the regional basis to Medieval and earlier society and economy in Europe (cf. Bintliff 1981). Rather than stress the essential dependence on each other of these regions, as they are drawn into early states and empires, we should consider an alternative wherein each incorporated region remains for the most part an introverted economy, most of its surplus being consumed internally by its superstructure (even if that is imposed or introduced from without) leaving a small fraction to be milked for external consumption (tax, exchange). The crucial corollary for social structure is that both before and after state/empire formation, the emergence and maintenance of elite strata is for the most part to be sought in their control over the means of production in their region. Although this can include mineral resources (metal, salt, etc, and very rarely such an association can be shown in the European Bronze and Iron Ages), in almost all instances this must have been control over land and agricultural labour.[75] How far back beyond the hypothesized examples cited above, this preferential access can be envisaged in terms of private and hereditary control, is quite unknown, until it yields to preferential access at the ascribed chief, lineage head or achieved 'big man' level.

One can, moreover, point to more dramatic implications of this suggested social pattern. If elite status is associated with landed estates, the pressure to achieve higher rank or secure sizeable holdings for one's descendants is a natural spur to a continual pushing back of the limits of cultivation and grazing, and to more intensive use of traditional areas of exploitation. At the same time, we have already argued that inadequate population control amongst farming populations in Pre-Industrial Europe is responsible for a recurrent pattern of demographic climax and collapse, as over-exploitation produces rapidly diminishing returns at the essential subsistence level. We have suggested that demographic climax is also intimately linked with cultural climax and moves towards or the achievement of, proto- or full urbanism and a complex division of labour. Finally, although each cycle has a certain inevitability, regardless of technological and agricultural innovation, one can underline the way in which such innovations alter the parameters of climax growth. As a result, averaged out on a long time span, the suspected population of Europe appears as a logarithmic curve from Palaeolithic to immediately pre-Industrial times. Yet looked at in detail, the smooth curve is seen to consist of a regular pattern of quite drastic upswings and downcurves; although the highpoints tend to be higher each time, the nadir points can frequently fall well below earlier peaks and even earlier lowpoints. These cycles of growth and decline are, it can be argued, primarily a reflection of expansion and contraction of the extent and productivity of regional food production. They appear to contradict the oft-cited thesis of Boserup (1965), that when population rises to a dangerous level, appropriate changes in technology and economy will arise to allow the crisis to pass, though at the expense of increased energy input per head. Instead they are more in keeping with the gloomy thesis of Malthus (First Essay on Population, 1798), in which population moves relentlessly towards over-exploitation, to a stage of famine, disease, strife - which latter combine brutally to shift densities to a more reasonable level.

The recurrent cultural collapses, settlement hiatuses of later prehistoric and ancient Europe may fruitfully be studied with this neo-Malthusian model in mind, and it is surely of particular interest that medieval historians such as Leroy Ladurie (1978), Hilton (1978) and Postan (1975, Hatcher and Postan 1978), have recently used just such a model for the severe decline in late Medieval Europe (the 'Crisis of Feudalism'); hat Robert McAdams (1978) and Karl Butzer (1980) have employed an identical model for drastic fluctuations in Mesopotamian and Egyptian culture over several millennia of development; and that R.W. Adams (1977) has recently found such a model to conform most satisfactorily with the detailed data now available for the rise and collapse of the classic Maya civilization in Mesoamerica.

Moreover, in all these cases, as in my own recent study (1982), there is a remarkable agreement on the place of social elites in the cycle: they develop to far greater prominence on the crest of the wave of demographic and agricultural florescence (due to factors already discussed); their maintenance of power rests on personal, preferential access to agricultural products and labour, generally assured by the proliferation of estates or hereditary rights to peasant surpluses; they fail, as a group, to adopt any efficient 'management policy' towards regional exploitation rates, preferring to 'milk' a deliberately inflated surplus product from an increasingly over-exploited and often marginal resource base (such surpluses being invested in prestigious monument constructions, ceremonial centres, palaces, castles, luxury goods, and socially-approved warfare - for example, Crusades); the inherent tendency for expansion to yield to decline and collapse is exacerbated by such associated managerial incompetence, which hastens the ensuing Dark Age and deepens its impact on population and cultural complexity.[76]

Colin Renfrew (1973a) and Grahame Clark (1979) have placed on a plinth the chieftains, princes and aristocracies that seem so general a phenomenon of European society from the later Neolithic to Feudal times. This stratum we are told, was the essential catalyst for any kind of growth of the economy or development of useful innovations, the leading sector that pushed Europe to ever greater complexity and sophistication.[77] Returning to our simplified model of the growth of European population, with its background accumulation of innovation and socio-economic elaboration, there is perhaps an

important partial truth to be assimilated here (spiritual sustenance from the past for practitioners of Conservative archaeology?). Moving on to our more detailed inspection of that curve, with its recurrent deep oscillations, one is tempted to ponder what comfort it might have been to increasingly undernourished peasants, in the shadow of imposing•elite monuments, to know that institutionalized inequality was an essential requisite for some dimly-perceived welfare-state of the remote future (after a few more demographic 'hiccups' of course), (spiritual comfort to practitioners of Social Democrat archaeology?). I am not even sure that any of the important innovations that raised the parameters of each growth cycle owe their original discovery and widespread implementation to the elite sector (with current understanding of early bronze metallurgy in Eastern Europe, or the takeoff of everyday iron tools, for example); with the erosion of their role as wet-nurse and financier of economic and technological progress, the 'privileged' of the past become increasingly exposed to charges of exploitation and parasitism (spiritual comfort to practitioners of Socialist archaeology?).

ACKNOWLEDGEMENTS

I am particularly grateful to Dr John Collis of the Prehistory Department, Sheffield University, who has read and commented on the text of this chapter. A number of errors and weakness were thus revealed. Sarah Champion of Southampton University provided invaluable advice on the controversy surrounding late Hallstatt and Early La Tène chronology.

NOTES

Note 1
Cf. notes 63, 65 and 66 in my Neolithic chapter (this volume), for a brief discussion of Bronze Age settlement and social hierarchies, and in general cf. the sound, deflationary analysis of Coles and Harding (1979).

Note 2
Cf. notes 59 and 63 in my Neolithic chapter (this volume) for the background to the well-evidenced general increase in the size and distribution of occupation traces in Bronze Age Europe compared to the Neolithic period. Also cf. Coles and Harding (1979), Fowler (1978), Wailes (1970), and innumerable regional studies such as Higham (1968), Manby (1980).

Note 3
Cf. notes 27, 28, 43, 57, and 63, in my Neolithic chapter (this volume), for Neolithic and Copper Age examples of putative 'agrarian cycles' and the accompanying theories. It is there argued that the continual lack of urban and civilizational take-off in barbarian Europe beyond the Aegean and Iberia during the Bronze Age bears witness to the further operation of the same limiting factors in human ecology. For specific Bronze Age case-studies of this phenomenon, see below.

Note 4
The cases of Denmark and the Lausitz sphere will be treated later in this chapter, where ecological overkill can be argued in Bronze Age and Bronze-Early Iron Age contexts. We might here, however, briefly mention the well-known major discontinuity in the occupation of major, long-lived settlements in Eastern Europe, that characterizes the Middle Bronze Age. Often ascribed to

massive invasions from a variety of directions (cf. Gimbutas 1965, Hänsel 1968) or a dramatic shift from mixed farming to nomadic pastoralism, these implausible interpretations (on grounds of our current views of the scale of the societies involved, the realities of primitive agriculture, and the realities of the archaeological data), should probably yield to the testing of the proposition that the previous, long-lasting balance between settlement patterns and densities and the local environment had broken down and required a radical (Danubian 2 or Post-Copper Age type, cf. Neolithic chapter) relocation of settlement and reorganization of agricultural strategies. Such an explanation makes reasonable sense of the remarkable changes in the nature of the archaeological record, suggesting as it does, very large populations continuing in the general area of the settlement abandonments (from cemeteries and hoards primarily), with strong continuity of regional cultural assemblages. This model, which rejects the unsupported and improbable nomads and imperial armies recently prevalent in the literature, is also the research direction that Coles and Harding point to in their treatment of the problem (1979).

The elaborate Wessex Culture of Early Bronze Age southern Britain, and its dramatic disappearance and replacement by an apparently less complex society in the Later Bronze Age, has similarly recently been interpreted as a response to ecological overkill: "It is interesting that the greatest change in the whole of British prehistory occurs immediately after the greatest display of ritual and hierarchical symbolism ... Rather than involving climate deterioration, it seems more satisfactory to lay the main emphasis on social disruption arising from those changes in the natural environment that were precipitated by human misuse. The great displays and ritual monuments" of the Early Bronze Age Wessex Culture "were part of the strain building up within the existing framework of society. The existing social and hierarchical relations could no longer be supported by their economic underpinnings" (Bradley and Hodder 1979, pp.98-9). Furthermore, recent research on the Neolithic and Bronze Age settlement of the Shetlands by Alisdair Whittle has led to a similar model of an agrarian cycle, commencing with Neolithic settlement c. 3000 BC onwards and a dense exploitation of the landscape, proceeding through cumulative land overuse linked to climate deterioration, and culminating in an environmental and cultural collapse by 1000 BC: "the establishment, growth, maintenance and decline of an early agricultural settlement" (Whittle 1980, pp.52, 36).

Note 5

The accumulation of very detailed regional evidence for the British Isles has encouraged these remarkably high population estimates for the late pre-Roman Iron Age (Fowler 1978, Cunliffe 1978b; Burgess 1980, Ch. 4). In particular, the link-up now being explored between the environmental archaeologist and the field archaeologist has allowed one to see the vast scale of Iron Age clearance and enclosure undertaken for more intensive exploitation (Smith 1978, Champion 1979, Bradley 1981). Moreover, it is very noticeable that old cultivated zones that had perhaps been relegated to a less intensive use by the later Bronze Age, such as the southern chalklands, are once again taken into more intensive use.

In Denmark, also recovering from possible over-exploitation in Neolithic and Bronze Age times (as discussed later), the Iron Age witnesses a remarkable rise in population and renewed expansion (from a phase of retraction), into marginal land that is only to be reached again by reclamation in the nineteenth century (Kristiansen 1980). Likewise in Sweden there is evidence for later Iron Age agrarian expansion and conversion of extensive systems of land use into intensive ones

(Lindquist 1974). In France there is similar evidence on a regional level for an Iron Age population boom, e.g. in the Champagne area (Bretz-Mahler 1971). In West Germany and Switzerland, dense Iron Age populations exhibit the British phenomenon of a renewed intensive intake of core areas for mixed farming, that had been neglected, arguably from overuse, during the Bronze Age (Balkwill 1976). In Czechoslovakia, archaeological and historical sources suggest a great increase of population in Iron Age times (Kruta 1975, Preidel 1979, Koutecky and Venclova 1979). The Polish cemetery evidence for the Late Bronze Age and Early Iron Age Lausitz Culture is even more remarkable (cf. Harding this volume, and further, below).

Parallel to this crucially significant population boom and new aspect to the European landscape north of the Alps, is a contemporary Iron Age population take-off in Italy (Potter 1979) and Greece (Snodgrass 1980). It is more helpful, and positively enlightening (see below) to consider these contemporary developments as stemming from similar processes at work over the whole of Europe during this time.

Note 6

Cf. notes 59, 63 in my Neolithic chapter (this volume) for the Bronze Age background. Apart from the very important role of the iron ploughshare in increasing farming efficiency (cf. below), it has also been suggested that a far more efficient type of plough came into use during the Iron Age. If the Bronze Age may have improved on the simple Neolithic ard by the diffusion of the heavy, twisting ard, Iron Age farmers would seem to have been equipped in areas of heavy soil with an ard plough provided with iron coulter and share (Wailes 1970, Zimmermann 1978, Lantier 1973). There is also considerable evidence for a further broadening of the range and quality of cultivated plants during the Iron Age beyond the Bronze Age spectrum (Knörzer 1979, Willerding 1979, Renfrew J. 1973, Hillman 1978). In particular the widespread cultivation of rye and oats would have enhanced crop production in the wetter, more acid soils of northern and parts of north-western Europe, especially in the new, less favourable climate mode of the Subatlantic era whose inception broadly coincides with the beginning of the Iron Age. The widespread adoption of spelt wheat and hulled barley, autumn sown cereals, would have improved arable productivity (Cunliffe 1978a, p.178, Bradley and Hodder 1979 p.101). Crop samples throughout Western Europe show a far greater number of cultivated varieties of crops in use, which must be intimately linked to the much wider range of soils now under intensive use and the evidence for site economic specialization (Martin Jones, pers. comm.).

Major use of plants presently considered as weeds, despite their nutritious properties, is also especially notable in Iron Age domestic contexts (Liversage 1977). Less clearly documented are other important examples of inventive improvements in farming and food processing during the Iron Age, such as the Gallic harvesting machines, advanced querns and technically sophisticated cart tyres (all areas where the 'barbarians' may have been more advanced than the Mediterranean civilizations - cf. Rowlett 1968).

Note 7

Cf. note 63, Neolithic chapter. It is quite debatable whether the average peasant farmer had access to regular kits of high tin-bronze artefacts, and indeed only such good quality metal tools would have been worth acquiring as functional improvements on stone and bone equivalents. It is exceptional to find scholars querying the real significance of 'Bronze Age' innovations in technology this way (such as Vigneron, 1981), although Milisauskas boldly states: "The production of bronze artifacts was never on

176

a scale large enough to provide readily available goods to all the people. Only high-ranking individuals could obtain bronze tools, ornaments, and weapons; most people had to continue to use stone, bone, and wooden implements ... The flowering of bronze technology may be related to the increased use of bronze artifacts in the social and ideological subsystems of these cultures as symbols of rank and status, and as objects in rituals" (Milisauskas 1978, pp.208-9). And more obliquely, Phillips (1980, p.199) comments: "Many European archaeologists have pointed out that the total volume of Early and Middle Bronze Age metalwork could not possibly reflect full-time working of a large number of bronzesmiths".

Of course, it is essential to point out that the valuable metal was being regularly broken up as it wore out or snapped, and recast to serve future generations. Just how many lives a bronze artifact possessed in later prehistoric Europe is a worthy subject for research modelling, but the work of metal analysis has shown that as the Bronze Age progressed the average object becomes increasingly more difficult to assign to ore source due to secondary melting down and pooling of scrap pieces. On the other hand, intelligent comparative study of series of artifacts of the same type in Denmark by Kristiansen (1978) suggests that many pieces were treasured for generations, becoming visibly worn down in the process. The amount of new metal to be supplied from the south east to metal-less Denmark, to replace that lost from the system of metal circulation in the form of hoards and burials, would appear to have been very small on a yearly basis. A rather intriguing snippet of evidence from Late Bronze Age Greece might offer a parallel, although the special context and problems of interpretation need stressing. The palace archives of the Mycenaean state of Pylos in the south-west Peloponnese, in the last year of the palace, record what seems to be a centrally-organized collection of bronze from all over the realm; yet the quantities involved are probably very small indeed (Chadwick 1976, p.139ff). Although it is generally suggested that a possible hostile threat to the realm was stimulating pooling of all metal, however sacred or cherished, for armaments, an attractive alternative would be to suggest that bronze was usually treated in this fashion in prehistoric Greece, a land that by this time was probably relying entirely on long-distance trade for fresh (un-recycled) supplies of both tin and copper.

Certainly a sample of statistics of bronze finds from different parts of Europe enhances one's impression of the extraordinarily low absolute quantities recovered to represent large regions and lengthy periods of time (cf. for example, on the well-published Czech evidence, Neustupny and Neustupny 1961, Novotna 1970, and Furmanek 1973; for Wales and the Welsh Borders, Leese 1979). A recent study by Flanagan (1982) of the Irish Earlier Bronze Age metal industry illustrates the situation very neatly: "The production-capacity of the Irish Earlier Bronze Age industry has often been described in glowing terms ... the actual volume of production ... suggest (s) ... that statements such as these ... fall far short of reality" (p.93). Plotting axe finds over time, the surviving corpus represents a mere two or three axes a year, or a total consumption over 350 years of 725kgs. of metal. Including halberds and daggers merely raises the total weight to 809kgs. "These levels of consumption seem insignificant beside the postulated capacity of Irish Bronze Age mines of some 732 tonnes" (p.93), yet to argue that we have lost that proportion of metal objects required to make up the shortfall of known over potential consumption is beyond belief, as 700 tonnes would account for two million axes (p.90). In a comparative study of bronze finds from Iberia and Austria very similar conclusions are drawn (pp.94-5).

If bronze was indeed for much of the Bronze Age a material unavailable for most domestic tasks, what was the peasant largely relying on? Apart from wood and bone implements, hardstone and flint may well have continued as staple raw materials. Recent surface work around Stonehenge has led to the conclusion: "An understanding of excavated flint assemblages suggests that (in areas where it occurs freely) large quantites of such material may be expected as late as the Middle Bronze Age at least" (Richard 1982, p.100). A similar observation has been made for Greece (C. Runnels, pers. comm.)

Despite the strong degree of uncertainty thus revealed, it seems more than likely that further research into improvements in food production, both in the range and productivity of crops and domestic animals, and in the gradual advances made in the capability of the ard plough, may cause us in future to relegate bronze tools to a secondary role in the expansion of population and cultivated area that is observable through the Bronze Age (cf. above and Wailes 1970).

Note 8
The regional importance of the inception of widespread iron-working, in terms of the new availability en masse to every farmer of a tough set of tools, enabling more efficient woodland and scrub clearance and cultivation of heavier or otherwise marginal land, has frequently been pointed out (cf. Wailes 1970). In Denmark, for example, the postulated retraction of settlement and cultivated area of the Bronze Age is reversed with the local Iron Age (here parallel to the mature, not early Iron Age of Southern and Western Europe), in which agriculture revives and old heathland and previously neglected heavy clay soils are put to the plough (Kristiansen 1980, 1978). In Sweden one can see an even later population explosion and expansion of cultivated and cleared land, argued to be due to the very late introduction of general iron-working in this area (Welinder 1975). In Britain, a study of several regions within England demonstrates a significant population expansion into areas of heavy soils during the Iron Age (Marshall 1977). But the key appearance of the iron ploughshare would have been making its presence felt already in the early stages of iron-using in each region, and finds of this implement indeed appear in such contexts (cf. Schwab 1976). Bouzek (1978) makes an important distinction between the increasing frequency of specialized iron usage during the Late Bronze Age of Central and Eastern Europe, and the full Iron Age from 700 BC where much of Europe began to adopt the general use of large iron tools in everyday life.

Probably significantly, the amount of iron in circulation and the range of iron tools, grow throughout the Iron Age, and already in the early 1960s the revolutionary implications of the wide array of iron agricultural and craft tools of the late Early Iron Age were being stressed by the Neustupnys (1961 -ploughshares, sickles, spades, scythes etc.). Metallurgical specialists remind us, nonetheless, that steel was achieved in only a minority of these iron objects and that many if not most of them were less 'hard' than top quality bronze. Yet for working purposes, iron possessed, even unsteeled, a crucial advantage over bronze: cast tin bronzes are not ductile enough to survive a forceful blow without breaking, whereas iron will bend and can be straightened (Tylecote 1976, Pleiner 1980). This gain over the brittleness and working problems of bronze, and related improvements in the flexibility of the new metal, combined in a crucial way with the ready access in almost every area of Europe to local sources of iron: "iron rapidly became the most important material and its use and technology influenced the development of organized social systems" (Pleiner 1980, p.375). Pleiner goes on (p.384) to stress the wave effect of iron-using, with an early widespread use in Southern Europe (the Mediterranean world of the nascent Greek and Etruscan civilizations, and the neighbouring Hallstatt Culture north and east of the Alps), reaching Scandinavia (cf. above) centuries later.

Note 9
Cf. my Neolithic chapter (this volume), note 63, and earlier references covering Copper and Neolithic Age 'centres'.

Note 10
In thus putting the dominant stress on ecological and demographic factors in the development of Iron Age Europe, we are continuing the fundamental approach adopted in my Neolithic chapter of this volume, and one that reflects many of the important and challenging insights of the late Eric Higgs (1972, 1975). Such an approach is also that advocated in several stimulating studies by S. Welinder, who states: "War, trade, religion, social organization, etc. certainly are of importance when trying to understand a society that is restricted in time and space, but in a perspective of thousands of years they will disappear or at least stand out as less important than the slow but irreversible ecological and demographic changes and the fundamental agricultural food production" (Welinder 1975, p.25).

As far as I am aware, most scholars hitherto have tended to treat the remarkable takeoff of Italy, Greece and Hallstatt Europe, as evidenced in terms of increased population density, the proliferation of district centres (often or increasingly fortified), the elaboration of an associated high culture or civilization, and a highly-emphasized dominant aristocratic elite (Potter, Snodgrass, op. cit,; Die Hallstatt Kultur, 1980) in **independent** explanations, failing to break the traditional barrier of Classics/Prehistory by positing a unitary model accounting for these largely concurrent phenomena. However, the common factor of a clear increase in agricultural productivity, to support this new level of dense population, must rest upon the vital effect of iron to the peasant economy and improvements suggested in crop practices (cf. above). In this model, the three adjacent regions rise towards high culture or civilization in parallel, increasingly interacting together in terms of population overspill and exchange systems, until the Italian core area finally succeeds in incorporating its neighbours into an imperial system.

Note 11
A well-documented example can be seen in Cunliffe's (1976) study of the development of the hillfort landscape around Danebury, Hampshire, where in the earlier Iron Age we can see a mosaic of small hillfort territories, each controlling or acting as a focus for an area of around 5kms. radius (Fig. 1). By the later pre-Roman Iron Age almost all the regional hillforts seem to go out of use, except for Danebury itself, which seems to grow proportionately in importance and complexity, perhaps now acting as a focus for the much larger area formerly split into smaller territories. The first phase of the process at Danebury seems to be seventh to sixth centuries bc, and from this time there is an enormous boom of hillfort construction in the British Isles, paralleling a wider European trend, and resulting in some thousands of such territorial monuments dotting the countryside as community 'focal points' (Cunliffe 1976, 1980, 1981a).

The role of the focal settlement, including early hillforts, had indeed been passed on from examples during the later Bronze Age. This is clearly indicated by recent research into British Later Bronze Age 'central places' in southern England, which have important similarities to early hill-forts in the same region (Bradley 1981). One can also find good continental parallels from the Bronze Age for the new Iron Age and Archaic Mediterranean district foci. To illustrate the comparison one might set side-by-side, a Thiessen polygon analysis of Late Bronze Age hillfort territories in Bohemia (Fig. 2), with a similar mosaic created out of the Archaic-Classical city state pattern in Boeotia (Fig. 3), central Greece. Both sets of data, and an Early Bronze Age network of central places in Czecho-slovakia (Neolithic chapter, Fig. 1), produce small 'polities' centring on defended sites and of approximately 10kms. radius. Such continuity or similarity is indeed to be expected from our model of the **enhancement** of earlier trends, rather than discontinuities or dissimilarity, for each successive phase of later European prehistory. Thus we can contrast the small numbers of major foci in total, in Britain and on the continent, belonging to the Bronze Age as compared to the Early Iron Age, and generally the degree of elaboration of the sites concerned increases markedly in the later era. There is clearly a likely functional comparability between the Bohemian hillforts and the earlier Czech central places and the early historic Greek 'mini states' brought into conjunction above: these networks reflect a primitive level of district centralized co-ordination, with access thresholds (time/-distance) a plausible limiting factor. Yet the human population serviced by these three networks will almost certainly be on entirely different scales, likewise the range and sophistication of the services available from the three kinds of focus on our present knowledge will be significantly contrasted. A bridge between the later two levels of 'central place' development can reasonably be formed by introducing the more developed Early Iron Age hillfort centres of temperate Europe (e.g. the Western Hallstatt 'princely seats' discussed below).

Note 12
The process by which small district centres are replaced by regional foci on an ever larger operative scale, as in the Cunliffe model, has been illuminated by Colin Renfrew's coinage of the ESM or Early State Module (1975), in which he has argued that early states tend to arise by the peaceful or forceful coalescence of a mosaic of small political units. Likewise, in Cunliffe's longer perspective of British Iron Age political development (1976), the plethora of tiny hillfort territories of the early centuries of the Iron Age yields by elimination to fewer, territorially more powerful hillforts during the Middle pre-Roman Iron Age; then in some areas to a smaller number of lowland oppida, and finally an even smaller number of territorial oppida, during the Late pre-Roman Iron Age, with the final giant blocks in south-eastern England approximating to primitive states of the ESM variety and on a similar scale (Celtic kingdoms) (Fig. 7). Paralleling this diachronic unfolding of a hierarchy of 'central places' it is generally assumed that there existed controlling elite groups associated with each focus, whilst the smaller hillforts represented the sphere of "petty chieftains" (cf. Piggott 1982 p.67).

Note 13
The current tendency, to which the writer would suscribe, suggests a major feedback of the new high regional densities into enhanced centralization and political development. Bradley and Cunliffe have both considered the rise of hillforts and larger, more effective political units during the Iron Age as responses to population pressure (cf. Cunliffe 1971, 1978; Bradley 1971, 1981). "Strains ... are clearly seen in the increasing construction of defended sites. These hillforts gradually increased in size and number during the Iron Age. At the same time the economic evidence suggests intensification and expansion ... A steady increase in known sites implies substantial population growth ... Thus, during the Iron Age there is evidence of increasing pressure on the environment and of

agricultural intensification ... These factors underlie the continued crystallization of regional cultural units and of clearer hierarchical differences" (Bradley and Hodder 1979 pp.101-2). Fowler, concentrating on the late pre-Roman Iron Age when the population and productivity was particularly striking in comparison to earlier areas, puts the case bluntly and provocatively (1978, p.7): "Rather should we perhaps see a more rapid population increase in the last century BC than there had ever been before, producing absolute numbers of Domesday order by the Roman Conquest and certainly of a different order from anything the Lowland landscape had had to cope with earlier. The landscape implications of this, in terms of settlement patterns and types, of territorial arrangements, of food production, and of culture contact ... have not received the attention they deserve .... Indeed, much of the archaeology of our pre-Roman Iron Age may well be explicable in terms of this completely new phenomenon in Lowland history, a magnitude of and rapidity of change in population numbers not previously experienced".

Note 14
"in the Middle and Late Bronze Ages in much of Europe rather homogeneous cremation burials replace the earlier inhumations which contained variable grave goods. Given the inferred presence of a ranked society in the Early Bronze Age and given the continuity of much of the archaeological record from Early to Late Bronze Age, it is unlikely that these homogeneous burials reflect the introduction of an egalitarian social organization in the Late Bronze Age. But for further tests of the hypothesis of ranked Bronze Age societies, we need to identify material remains other than mortuary remains that may reflect ranking within Late Bronze Age social organization" i.e. hoard bronze finds (Levy, op. cit: pp.49-50)

Note 15
In Hallstatt Culture times, the continuance of urnfield burial for the majority of the population exhibits a striking contrast in gift poverty to the revived tumulus burial for the elite with varying amounts of wealth in the chamber. More real space, and more symbolic space are involved in this reversal of the Middle to Late Bronze Age trend (cf., e.g. on Czech burials Filip 1977, Koutecky 1968).

Note 16
The characteristic elite markers of the Hallstatt Culture (armour, swords and tumuli), despite stylistic transformations from the Black Sea region, are essentially developed out of the local Late Bronze Age traditions in central Europe (Angeli 1980).

Note 17
In a study of the Late Bronze Age hillforts of Hallstatt B Bohemia (Nynice Culture), V. Saldova (1977) sees them as the likely core from which later Hallstatt 'princedoms' of the area developed. There is actually little trace of internal differentiation in buildings, and one would point to the Bohemian metal finds for clearer indications and the wealthy burials of the region, (and perhaps the very organization of manpower to construct these sites), for the existence of central people for these proto-central places. Nonetheless with that reservation noted we can otherwise fully agree with Saldova's conclusions, a very notable set in contrast to the exaggerated role assumed for similar sites of the Western Hallstatt Culture: "Die spätbronzezeitlichen Burgwälle in Westböhmen waren also weder vorübergehende Zufluchtsorte, noch militärische Festungen zu Verteidigungszwecken, noch Herrensitze, sondern dauernde besiedelte befestigte Höhensiedlungen von überwiegend agrarischen Charakter, verbunden mit Heimerzeugung - Töpferei, Spinnerei, Weberei. Als wahrscheinliche Wirtschafts -, Handels-, Gesellschafts-und vielleicht auch Religionszentren, die Keime einer politisch - admin-

istrativen Funktion in sich trugen, errichtet in einer Zeit von Stabilisierung und Entfältung der Gesellschaft, bilden Sie einen der ausdrucksvollsten Belege fur die in der Spätbronzezeit eingetretenen Veränderungen in der gesellschaftlich-ökonomischen Entwicklung, aus denen die Hallstattkultur 'fürstlichen' Charakters hervorwächst" (p.161).

Note 18
No exception is the gigantic hill fort of Závist near Prague, in Bohemia. Its vast, 170ha. extent, revealed Late Bronze Age (Knoviz Culture) material everywhere, and on the highest plateau ('acropolis') a palisade enclosed a putative ritual area. Around 50ha. of the site were fortified at this time. The site will be further elaborated as a regional centre in early La Tène times. Continuity of chiefdom organization and use of defended centres is found at other sites of the region in Hallstatt C (Motykova 1977, 1978).

Note 19
Alexander (1980) rightly summarizes the Central European Urnfield era as a time of expansion and crystallization, with hillforts and warrior burials showing a pattern of social and political organization that will characterize 'Barbarian' Europe in the Iron Age.

Note 20
"Die oft relativ kurze Belegungsdauer der Befestigungen selbst ... könnte ein Hinweis auf noch nicht festgefügte Machtverhältnisse sein. Es ist offensichtlich noch nicht zu einer institutionalisierten Herrschaft von 'Adels-Dynastien' gekommen. Diese Entwicklung ist erst in der frühkeltischen Späthallstattkultur festzustellen, der sich der gesellschaftliche Abstand zwischen Herrschern und Beherrschten weiter vergrösserte, womit letztlich die Grundlagen des keltischen Königtums geschaffen wurden" (p.59). Likewise, Dusek (1973) sees the Urnfield princely burials of the Slovak Velatice and Caka groups as "Kometenhaft" chiefs, but yet the foundation of Hallstatt Iron Age princedoms here. Tim Champion (1982) suggests that problems with over-exploited land in the earlier Bronze Age led to a reorganization of society by Urnfield times, with enhanced stress on property rights and control over rights to land. The organizing elite are identifiable from rich graves amid cremation cemeteries, and in late Urnfield times from fortified hill-sites with evidence for craft specialization and access to luxury goods. In Hallstatt C rich burials continue to be found but most of the 'central places' go out of use.

Note 21
An even clearer example is in Moravia, where defended centres (Burgwälle) are found in the late Urnfield period. Stary Zavek for example is occupied in Hallstatt B, but goes out of use in early Hallstatt Culture times (Hallstatt C) to be resettled as a princely seat in Hallstatt D. However, in the gap in occupation, a Hallstatt C princely burial is erected at the site! (Podborsky 1974). Curiously, although arguing absolutely for the Western Hallstatt (Hallstatt D) florescence as the outcome of the interference of the civilized Mediterranean peoples, Rowlands (1980) is willing to admit that earlier phases of elite burials and organization can be identified in the future Hallstatt zone - such as Bz D/Hallstatt A1 and Hallstatt B2-3. Naturally, an internal explanation would weaken the Hallstatt case, so we are offered a vague causation from the external world, in mysterious (and highly dubious!) "continental-wide pulsations". Nonetheless, in what seems to be a major shift in the 'revolutionary change' position of Frankenstein and Rowlands (1978), Rowlands concedes for the final West Hallstatt princedoms that: "this type of political structure could not have been generated through external contacts, but these conditions allowed the further development of tendencies

towards increased hierarchization that already existed in their Hallstatt B/C antecedents" (p.29).

Note 22

Study of the eastern French Hallstatt Culture, with major 'princely graves' and putative 'residences' of Hallstatt D date, shows a significant development cycle originating in the local Late Bronze Age (Wamser 1975). In late Urnfield times, tumulus burial is revived and even some inhumation burials appear, and wealthy burials reappear with such graves, contrasted to the continuing poor cremation tradition. In Hallstatt C this trend continues with rich tumulus inhumations for men and women, setting the scene for the Hallstatt D florescence of 'princedoms' in the region.

Note 23

As noted above, the revived tumulus chamber is the setting for far more lavish status gift offerings than was usual in Urnfield times, offering greater scope for elite display in what seems to be a new era of more enhanced distinctions both between the elite and the peasantry, and between grades of elite.

As for warfare, the new emphasis on horse equipment and occasional Hallstatt scenes of armed warriors on horseback, probably do not imply regular cavalry formations or set battles on horseback. The huge, heavy slashing sword and the absence of spurs suggests that, as in Homeric warfare, the horse or waggon/chariot acted as a tactical 'taxi' to ferry the elite to and from, and from one part to another of, the battlefield. A formal, prolonged combat would take place between heavily-armed warriors on foot, and in loose formation to judge from the space required to operate the Hallstatt sword to its best advantage.

Note 24

Firstly, recent research tends to suggest that the peoples around the Black Sea, both in prehistoric and historic times, combined sedentary or semi-sedentary farming of the highly fertile Black Earth soils with short-range and long-range (or 'nomadic') pastoralism. Those groups sharing cultural features termed 'Thraco-Kimmerian' from this period seem to be local farmer-herder folk in the European USSR, that adopted by diffusion from Central Asia their typical warrior prestige equipment and a tendency towards a greater emphasis on long-range pastoralism (Terenozkin 1980). Secondly, there is now wide agreement that the spread of Thraco-Kimmerian elite equipment and burial rites into the Eastern Hallstatt sphere is a matter of influences diffusing into a continuing, indigenous context, and of the adoption by local European chieftains of a new social symbolism to mark out status individuals. The new cultural items remain foreign in local traditions, just as with previous Black Sea influences (Angeli 1980, Gabrovec 1980).

Note 25

However as mentioned earlier, the Mediterranean influence of this time is merely the latest in a long history of mutual cultural exchanges, with especial emphasis on elite prestige items and styles, going well back into the Bronze Age and in which the people north of the Alps were generally the more influential.

Note 26

In the south east Hallstatt sphere for example, notables are buried as 'knights', whereas in other areas of East Hallstatt and in Western Hallstatt, the aristocrat's 'charger' is represented by appropriate equipment alongside the four-wheeled hearse (Gabrovec 1980). The trend towards inhumation is also more pronounced in some regions than others, being typical for Hallstatt elite burials in the south eastern Alps, but from Austria through Bohemia/-Moravia and into Western Hallstatt frequently found alongside prestige burials still employing cremation. In Slovakia cremation remains dominant for even the most princely burials (Gabrovec 1974, Neustupny and Neustupny 1961, Pichlerova 1974).

Note 27

These burial features owe perhaps more to local Balkan tumulus burial traditions than to Black Sea influences, and it is of prime importance that close parallels to these mounds are now being discovered amongst the late Hallstatt 'princely graves' and 'nobles' graves' of Western Hallstatt, such as Hirschlanden and, most spectacularly, at Magdalenenberg (Gabrovec 1974).

On the edge of the eastern Alps, in the Sopron mountains of Hungary, a network of defended hillforts with associated tumulus cemeteries arises in Hallstatt Iron Age times, contrasted to the contemporary flat grave cemeteries found with smaller unfortified sites. A direct parallel has been made to the contemporary transformation of Slovenian society (Patek 1982).

Note 28

Kromer (1958) identified in the Hallstatt cemetery three distinct 'classes': warrior protectors, the heavy labour miners, and a technical commercial group. An imbalance in the sexes and age groups was also claimed, to argue against the cemetery representing a natural community rather than selected portions of a population living elsewhere. However, recent discussions and analyses of the burial data from Hallstatt and from the poorly-known Hallein cemetery groups suggest a very different interpretation (Kilian-Dirlmeier 1969, 1971, Maier 1974, Hodson 1977, Pauli 1978, Hodson 1980). The Hallstatt cemetery is generally argued to have been set out from the first as a burial zone, within which discrete foci of burial were used throughout the life of the cemetery. However the most recent research on the cemetery (Hodson 1980, and pers. comm.) has revised this model in favour of a straightforward horizontal displacement across the cemetery area over time. At any stage of the cemetery's use, however, it still seems that contemporary burials are deliberately arranged in clusters comprising a broad spectrum of wealth, age and sex appropriate to a social group representing a cross-section of the total community. In Hallein such sub-groups are actually spatially distinct, and it is argued that as population in the associated community rose over time, so the Hallein cemetery expanded outwards as well as continuing to see its original clusters added to by infilling (Pauli 1978 p.369, Zeller 1980a p.163). Separate groupings of settlement traces are claimed to accompany the discrete burial zones at Hallein (Pauli 1978 p.507). Each 'cluster' comprises burials of the minority, wealthy 'warrior' type, as well as those formerly attributed to Kromer's other classes of role. In fact no obvious 'miners' graves' exist, merely gift distinctions reflecting status, from giftless graves, through ranked, to a smaller number of notably rich burials (especially warrior's, but females are included in this class). It is further argued that a reasonable spectrum of adult, child, male and female burials exists for the different clusters. The remote, non-agricultural location of the Hallstatt cemetery, and to a lesser extent the low potential of the Hallein plateau for quality subsistence production, surely indicate that the population buried there reflect salt-mining communities. The variable gift wealth would therefore reflect status within these settlements, most plausibly mirroring both rank within the kinship system (e.g. clan heads, extended family eldest males) and achieved status ('big men'). Given the need for role differentiation within the salt industry, it is plausible to argue for the wealthiest graves as belonging to those with a supervisory/organizational capacity, the basic labour being carried out by 'lower status' people. The clear burial clusters would seem to represent subdivisions within the industrial community, possibly, as Kromer suggested, reflecting discrete residential groups (hamlets, or small villages). If all roles and statuses and a real 'community' appear within each cluster, they probably represent independent 'teams' each working all or part of a particular mine area. At Hallein, for example, some eight to nine burial clusters are recognized, and it has been suggested by Schauberger that five major mine areas each employed around 10-12 man teams, giving a total workforce of around 50 plus. Such a workforce would be equivalent to around 250 people (one adult male to a family of five), to which we must add organizational and practical tasks away from the actual active face being carried out by other individuals (though female and child labour is likely to be involved here). The far larger known expanse of the Hallstatt cemetery might suggest a total live population of some 90 families (c. 450 people). The burial clusters are likely, then, to indicate a hamlet-sized social group (probably less than a dozen families) and the 'elite' wealthier graves are therefore of the correct frequency for 'big men' or clan elders. This conclusion is close to that reached by Pauli in his penetrating analysis of Hallein society as indicated by its cemetery (1978 pp.505, 516).

It is important to note, however, again following Pauli (1978 p.394), that the limited areas so far excavated and carefully recorded of the Hallein cemetery probably represent a skewed sample of the cemetery 'population'. Male warrior burials are far commoner than in the much better known Hallstatt cemetery. Pauli accepts that the figures of 26% from Hallstatt - closely comparable to the frequency of warrior to other adult male graves in Celtic Europe generally -will probably be the final proportion at Hallein when far more of the burial areas are uncovered. Richer graves are not noticeably given preferential, more conspicuous sites within the cemetery area. It is likely that both upland locations were inhabited by men, women and children during the temperate half of the year, although known settlement remains are continuously used only at Hallein. Where occupation areas have been revealed, it is argued that they represent seasonal occupation from communities resident the rest of the year in more favourable agricultural zones. Given the suspected small size of the populations working both mine sites, one might naturally expect that these migratory communities were otherwise resident in the immediate region. This plausible hypothesis seems fully borne out by Pauli's investigations on the cultural affinities of the domestic assemblage at Hallein (1978 pp.417, 499). The less spectacular and 'international' aspects of the Hallein artefacts all point to a limited and local geographical catchment for the seasonal workers at the salt mines in both Hallstatt and La Tène times.

A final point of interest concerning Hallstatt and Hallein is that of their inter-relationship. At present the archaeological finds suggest that Hallstatt is already flourishing in Hallstatt C, Hallein not till Hallstatt D. There are reasons to think that Hallein may have been a daughter foundation of Hallstatt. On the other hand, C14 measurements seem to point to mining at Hallein in Hallstatt C times, and a great deal is still to be uncovered of the total cemetery area (the recent Eislfeld excavation radically altered our perception of the site, for example; cf. Pauli 1978, pp.367, 483,487).

Note 29
The famous Athenian industry in fine painted pottery, with a distribution throughout the Mediterranean and Black Sea shores and beyond into their hinterlands (including the late Hallstatt and Early La Tène chieftains' tables), was run from a great number of totally independent small workshops in Attica, whose total specialist workforce is estimated to be little more than 500

(compare this to the suggested population of the state of Athens at some 200,000). Moreover, the distribution of Attic pottery was almost entirely by carriers of other states, alongside other kinds of products, and the Athenian state had no interest in the organization of this commerce (Snodgrass 1980).

Note 30
In Slovakia for example, there is plentiful evidence for the organization of Hallstatt society, from distinctive princely tumuli, high quality prestige art products (both local and long-distance exchange pieces), and settlement foci (the fortified hilltop sites or 'Burgwälle' with special features) (Dusek 1973). Particularly interesting is the 'princely seat' of Molpir near Smolenice, a large and heavily defended community with indications of a regional role in craft and trade and the suggestion of social distinctions in internal residences (Dusek 1974). Similar evidence comes from neighbouring Moravia and Bohemia (Podborsky 1974, Saldova 1974, Neustupny and Neustupny 1961).

Note 31
As often in the past, northern Italy and West-Central Europe offer an alternative exchange sphere to the East-West continental nexus, and already in the limited Mediterranean imports of the seventh century the role of contacts to Etruria and the north-east Italian peoples is clear.

Note 32
Even as recently as 1982, S. Champion remarks that we are sadly 'unclear what is happening' in much of West Germany during Hallstatt C, when elite burials go on from Hallstatt B but the obvious hilltop foci regularly go out of use till a revival in Hallstatt D.

Note 33
It is perhaps rather jejeune to try to associate the burial changes with changing concepts of the passage to the afterlife, especially as we have no obvious way to test this suggestion. Yet possibly the interment of the unaltered body may imply a belief in transference of the spirit in the form it was buried in; here the revived attention to dress and status ornaments, together with gifts and offerings for use in the passage to, and in, the afterlife 'in the spirit world', would form a natural accompaniment.

The change of sword type from the heavy, slashing and stabbing weapon of Hallstatt to the stabbing La Tène variety may perhaps be linked to the appearance of tactical formations of infantry, with less room for swinging weapons. Since this type of formation is characteristic for the 'citizen/hoplite' armies of contemporary Greek and Italian states, there may be some wider significance to these military rearrangements. If cemetery contents suggest a broadening of status symbols and far less emphasis on the very powerful and their subordinates, contrasting Hallstatt custom to La Tène, then maybe the ubiquitous 'warrior grave' of the latter era represents the new importance of the hamlet chief/'big man' in warfare and economic and political influence? (But **not** the peasantry, cf. infra).

Note 34
After remaining flourishing in the Hallstatt tradition in Hallstatt D (Filip 1977, 1978), Bohemia is very receptive to the new elite art style of Western La Tène, and in its contemporary princely graves such as Chlum shows very close links to the early burial assemblages of the core La Tène region, as well as a vigorous new phase of Hallstatt Geometric art to be found elsewhere in the Hallstatt D3/Early La Tène princely graves of East Hallstatt (Schwappach 1973). The new two-wheeled chariot burial-

rite for nobility, characteristic for the core La Tène regions in the west, arrives in the area (Stead 1979), and at the same time a small quantity of the now popular Etruscan imports typical for western exotica filters through into Bohemia (Saldova 1974).

Note 35
Apart from the traditional failure to take the achievements of barbarian Europe seriously, a hangover from diffusionist days, the only other factor is the discovery not far away of possible fragments of Etruscan imports from lost princely burials (Motykova 1977). To believe that the organizers of the Zavist acropolis monuments, whatever they were planned to be, had the ability to obtain small quantities of luxury goods from a lengthy series of exchanges, is one thing; to suggest that they had any real awareness of the nature of Mediterranean architecture and religion is pure speculation. We might be better employed comparing this activity to the prestige monuments of Mesoamerica, or Neolithic Britain, with their anthropological inferences, than playing an unwarranted neo-diffusionist game. Far too much is made of the slightest Mediterranean influence in Central Europe, such as part of an Attic vessel from Kadan in Bohemia of transitional La Tène age, and limited Etruscan-style imports from the fifth century BC onwards (Nemeskalova 1978).

Note 36
But it is clear that both streams of influence continue the earlier pattern of adoption by the local leadership of new and attractive forms of display, as the novelties are clearly being absorbed into the local context with strong continuity (Pauli 1980b, Neustupny and Neustupny 1961). In the detailed analysis of the Chotin cemeteries, Dusek, though arguing for ethnic change, nonetheless reveals much evidence that supports the more accepted view of local ethnic continuity and Scythian diffusion (1977). These technically 'late Hallstatt' sites (fifth - fourth centuries BC) show the gradual transformation of local, Hallstatt tradition, cremation rites into assemblages coloured by Scythian style horse equipment and horse burials and other associated gear, together with the gradual adoption of wheel-turned pottery (likewise diffused from the Black Sea). Inhumation takes over piecemeal from cremation over time. But the same classes of dead appear, progressively shifting in cultural markers: poor, average, very rich.

Note 37
The Hallein settlement for the salt mining community appears to grow continually till the fifth century BC (final Hallstatt D3). Then in the period La Tène A, parallel to Early La Tène in the west (pace Pauli 1978), a notable rise in complexity seems indicated (Maier 1974) by a great expansion in the domestic settlement and burial zones and the accompanying development on the Ramsaukopf of a fortified hillfort, suggested to be an elite residence ("Herrensitz") from the contemporary presence in the cemetery of two of the new chariot burials, (one of which is described as 'princely' and has important close links to the rich finds from contemporary Early La Tène princely graves in the Middle Rhine and further west). It should be pointed out, however, that Pauli considers the chariot burials especially the very rich 44/2 example, as in reality likely to represent statuses well below the putative West Hallstatt and Middle Rhine La Tène A 'princes'. He argues that the peculiar wealth of the two salt-mining communities raised the average level of display wealth for all ranks in society, and that the smallish communities concerned could at most produce village chiefs or 'big men' (1978, pp.515-16). Beyond the enlarged settlement the contemporary tumulus graves contain rich imports reflecting the important Italian connection and wider influences north of the Alps.

As will be discussed in detail below, much play has been made of shifting trade routes in accounting for concentrations of wealth and status in Celtic (and Germanic) Europe. In particular the decline of the West Hallstatt sphere and the rise of the La Tène core lands is linked to a redirection of commercial contacts emanating from Italy. It is therefore noteworthy that the rapid acceptance in some areas of Central and Eastern Europe, formerly of East Hallstatt tradition, of Early La Tène styles, combines knowledge of new developments in the core regions of La Tène with an **independent** set of exchange systems across the eastern Alps to the Mediterranean (Pauli 1978 p.467).

Note 38
The kind of research desperately needed is such as that reported from western Switzerland by Schwab (1976). Very extensive research in the Freiburg area in the putative territory of the Châtillon-sur-Glâne princely seat has identified dense regional rural settlement and some 50 isolated tumuli and 17 tumuli fields considered as 'upper class'.

Note 39
The recent excavation of a new princely tumulus at Hochdorf is illuminating in this respect. It probably represents a 'provincial' chieftain within the wider territory of the Hohenasperg centre. Many of the luxury items seem to have been made at the burial site itself (bronze, iron, gold-work) (Biel 1981).

Note 40
Iron-working, bronze-working, probably also glassworking and that in coral, amber, lignite, bone and antler, have been demonstrated or argued for the Heuneburg craft sector (Kimmig 1975a, b, Frey 1980).

Note 41
Thus, for instance, scientific analysis of the fineware from the Heuneburg and Châtillon-sur-Glâne (Switzerland) shows distinctly separate, local production groups (Maggetti and Galetti 1980).

Note 42
The necessity of urban or even 'proto-urban' centres for developed settlement systems of proto-state or even state type, has been disproven by research into the 'hamlet-cluster' form of early state foci in Archaic Greece and Italy (cf. Potter 1979, Snodgrass 1980). The same sources remove the necessity of major defences, too.

Note 43
Though clearly supporting such a 'revolutionary change' scenario, Haerke nonetheless underlines the already-existing background of focal centres in Hallstatt C: "the emergence of a settlement hierarchy in south-west Germany took place before Mediterranean influences made themselves felt on a large scale in central Europe" (1980; cf. Haerke 1982 p.204). Rowlands is also concerned by the extreme difficulty of a short-term diffusionist metamorphosis of the political and settlement structure of Western Hallstatt, and in discussing the centre-province model of paramount and district dependent chiefs for Hallstatt D, he is even prepared to confess: "this type of political structure could not have been generated through external contacts, but these conditions" i.e. the new Mediterranean contacts "allowed the further development of tendencies towards increased hierarchization that already existed in their Hallstatt B/C antecedents" (1980 p.29).

Note 44
It is fair to say that the mudbrick wall was primarily an act of prestigious display, rather than an attempt at imitative functional improvements based on an awareness

of Greek military architecture. A major mudbrick construction is unsuited to the moist, temperate south German climate, and could only have been protected from the inevitable rainwater dissolution by a substantial roof structure. The latter, wooden affair would have been an easy target for enemy incendiarism. Not surprisingly, the end of the mudbrick wall shows fragments of fallen, burnt wooden plank roofing material, followed by a return to tried and tested defences (Frey 1980). (In opposition to this view, J. Collis has reminded me (pers. comm.) that the mudbrick wall actually lasted longer than the local wall type at the site).

Note 45

Thus Haerke (1979, 1982) distinguishes already for Hallstatt C the key area wherein Hallstatt D princely seats will emerge, with its smaller, internally structured district foci, from the parallel zone to the north, where more traditional, large and less sophisticated hillfort foci are found. Likewise, as noted, Hallstatt C waggon graves, the first sign of more elaborate power hierarchy perhaps, are very confined in the West. During Hallstatt D, the number of more sophisticated foci rises dramatically, and is a far more widespread phenomenon, tied frequently to the geographical expansion of the elite burial sites. To the north of West Hallstatt, although princely seats do not emerge in Hallstatt D, fortified foci multiply during this period, and in Early La Tène there are signs in this northern swathe of a notable rise in rural settlements, linked to the emergence in several regions of princely burials (though seemingly without subsequent development of princely seat proto-urban foci) (Haerke 1979, 1982). Despite this time-lag from south to north, it must be emphasized that within parts of the core West Hallstatt sphere the climax princely florescence can be almost as late as, and even contemporary with the north. In eastern France, for example, although a clear local evolution of elite burials can be traced back to the end of the Bronze Age, the most striking finds of this kind belong to the 'Vix Horizon', now placed in the fifth century very shortly before the rise of La Tène A north of West Hallstatt, Mediterranean finds are also rare in the region until this period (Wamser 1975; cf. below).

Note 46

In the cited version of this model, local, low-level leaders heading kinship-pyramids (cf. Fried 1967) become aware of an external outlet (here the Greek colonies, and the Italic communities secondarily), for local surpluses that were formerly redistributed amongst the general populace. They redirect these surpluses abroad in return for an assured flow of luxury prestige items, by the possession of which they distance themselves from their previously embedded social role. They now form a new distinct class of entrepreneurs, displacing traditional sources of authority and status by preferential access to prestige display items and more tangible accumulation of privileged rights over supplies of food, labour and raw materials. However, the fickle Mediterranean traders shift their supply routes, leaving the West Hallstatt princes stranded without the luxury status-creating items they had utilized to bind district chiefs to their regional paramountcy. The entire superstructure collapses back to its antecedent level of district chiefs, though in the new contact zone to the north a network of princes is created by Mediterranean commercial interference (the Early La Tène sphere). But while the flow of status symbols and more tangible trade goods concentrates on the West Hallstatt, it gives rise to proto-urban centres for the collection and distribution of imports and exports; here the newly created wealth is displayed, and imitative industrial and commercial developments to those of Mediterranean cities arise; the chief beneficaries, the elevated paramount families, establish their princely seats, well-defended from envious neighbours, and impress their peasantry with the form and content of dynastic princely tumuli.

Note 47

The great Heuneburg site was itself an important district site in the Bronze Age, and it is likely that in Hallstatt C the local elite were based in a nearby focus at the Grosse Heuneburg. There is then an intermediate phase in which it may have resided at an 'estate' focus such as the Talhau (to be associated with the first of the princely tumuli nearby), before the subsequent erection of a revived Heuneburg nucleated focus that dominated the rest of Hallstatt D. Indeed, many further examples of small elite power centres must be accepted for Early La Tène groups to the north of West Hallstatt, where princely burials are known without comparable nucleations (cf. Collis 1981a).

Note 48

For the eastern France area for example, despite a continuous tradition of increasingly elaborate elite burials from the Late Bronze Age into genuine 'princely' levels by Hallstatt D, Mediterranean imports are rare indeed until the fifth century BC, Hallstatt D3 'Vixien' phase (Wamser 1975). The Marne Culture, a key core region for Early La Tène culture, exhibits only occasional Mediterranean pieces from its prolific cemeteries (Bretz-Mahler 1971). Local imitations of genuine imports have confused the real situation in some cases, especially for Early La Tène, when most 'Mediterranean-style' pieces seem to be locally manufactured (Frey 1980).

Note 49

At the Heuneburg it has often been observed as a curious feature that almost all the Greek fineware fragments stem from the final phase of occupation - yet occasional fragments occur from the earliest levels - are the latter out of context? More likely it appears now that they represent crucial evidence that the bulk of the scanty, treasured import pieces were conserved until the final decline and destruction of the site. Published figures are remarkably low, e.g. around 50 fragments of Black-Figure ware, and around 15 wine amphorae. Almost all of the Black-Figure pieces are from the top of the Hallstatt stratigraphy (I), with but a few from levels IV, III and II (see further, below).

Note 50

To argue that most exchanges were of perishable items, archaeologically-speaking, (food, salt, slaves, etc.) does not explain the inadequacies of that portion of the commerce that is preserved (and which after all initiated the commerce theory), nor can such a theory be considered seriously until independent positive confirmation appears. There are other reasons to be highly sceptical of this neatly unprovable hypothesis. Here we must emphasize the difficulty of using the very limited and partial data from West Hallstatt sites far general explanations of the processes at work in this period. Fischer (1973) rightly criticizes much of the past theorizing on West Hallstatt developments as "impressions not analyses", and Rowlands has recently (1980) admitted that he can see no current alternative to setting up models for this and other data sets that though internally consistent are not susceptible to disproof.

Note 51

The traditional chronology places the Hallstatt C/D transition c600 BC, running the final Hallstatt phase (Hallstatt D3) to c. 500 BC which is also the approximate date for the birth of La Tène culture (La Tène A/Ia) to the north. Such a chronology permits with ease a unifying model of contemporary collapse and rise phenomena, and 'wave' effects, matched in the Frankenstein and Rowlands interpretation (1978) to regional displacements in commercial networks to the Mediterranean. On the other hand, the apparent poverty of La Tène A material in the West Hallstatt sphere, till La Tène B times, has encouraged German scholars (Zürn, Kimmig, Pauli) to erect a very different chronological and cultural historical scheme, in which Hallstatt D coexisted as an archaic cultural format in the West Hallstatt sphere contemporary to La Tène A in the northerly origin zones of the La Tène Culture (Champagne and Middle Rhine). Evidence adduced in favour of this latter model includes 'mixed deposits' (of a 'Mischkultur' supposedly), occasional artifactual cross-links between the two 'cultures' and dating evidence which points to a fifth century BC existence for Hallstatt D3 (cf. Kimmig 1975a, b, Pauli 1978, Haerke 1979).

The real difficulty lies in:
a)   the scarcity of absolute dates at appropriate resolution for clarifying the relationship between Hallstatt D1-2/Hallstatt D3/La Tène A;

b)   the over-emphasis on princely burials which are inadequately tied to the few excavated major settlements;

c)   an almost total ignorance till very recently concerning the chronology and cultural contents of non-princely rural settlements;

d)   the 'heirloom' character of much if not all Mediterranean imports whose date of manufacture is the main chronological evidence for West Hallstatt and Early La Tène findspots. For general references to the heirloom aspects of Mediterranean imports cf. Fischer (1973), Kimmig (1975a, b), Haerke (1979) Champion S. (1982). The evidence from the Heuneburg has been mentioned above (note 49). For the adjacent Hohenasperg territory and its putative district foci, the presence of fifth century Red-Figure ware at Klein Aspergle had already alerted scholars to the possible late use of the Hohenasperg centre from that associated princely burial, but this mid-fifth century date material could have been kept for a further one or two generations, to judge from the breaks on the pottery concealed by gold sheet (Kimmig 1975b, Frey 1980). The Grafenbühl burial from the same territory with imports of around 600 BC manufacture but Hallstatt D2 fibulae, shows a very long heirloom use for the Mediterranean exotica (Zürn 1975), and the recent Hochdorf tumulus discovery revealed an imported Greek cauldron with local additions to it (Biel 1981). The eastern France West Hallstatt culture shows a climax development in Hallstatt D3 (Wamser 1975), with heirloom deposits such as at Vix (Kimmig 1975b, Hodson and Rowlett 1974), and also obvious fifth century imports belonging to a Hallstatt D3 **and/or** local La Tène A ultimate phase of the regional central places of princely character (such as at Château-sur-Salins, cf. Hodson and Rowlett 1974). Switzerland provides a similar picture to eastern France (Haerke 1979).

However it does seem possible that resolution may be approaching the hitherto polarized positions described above, of contemporaneity or succession, that have split German-speaking and other scholars of Early Iron Age Europe (especially British specialists). This compromise solution might be outlined and explained as follows:

1)   The central fact that indicates the correct interpretation is the existence in the Champagne area, specifically at Les Jogasses, of distinctive Hallstatt D3 and La Tène A assemblages, and the same situation at the cemetery of Dürrnberg-Hallein in Austria. Regrettably (cf. Pauli 1978 p.469) the Champagne evidence is urgently in need of up-to-date reappraisal and the case for 'succession' is not unambiguously proven, allowing Pauli to imply that the two assemblages might have conceivably

co-existed as subcultural variants (the argument he puts forward for supposed inter-penetration or Mischkultur of D3 and La Tène A in parts of West Hallstatt). At Hallein however the evidence is quite clear, and Pauli himself in his masterly summary volume of the site publication (Dürrnberg-Hallein III, 1978), pointedly indicates the chronological succession from D3 to La Tène A as separate phases at the site. The characteristics of these finds from Hallein are so clearcut that it is more than special pleading to suggest that the La Tène A here is a much later facies than La Tène A elsewhere. In fact Pauli's contorted time-lag hypothesis seems to run counter to all the evidence and is forced on him by an a priori position of contemporaneity based on his researches in south western Germany.

That south western German data from Baden-Württemberg are also now in need of revision, very much as a result of recently published information on rural settlement sites in the region. It seems clear that there are a large number of hitherto poorly-researched rural sites which include a significant proportion dated to La Tène A (the period whose supposed virtual absence had stimulated the model that local D3=La Tène A elsewhere). Moreover, sites now exist, at no great distance from each other, with quite distinctive separate assemblages in both metalwork and pottery, typical for Hallstatt D2-3 and La Tène A respectively. The hiatus in population and settlement no longer exists in the traditional sequence to encourage a lengthening of D3 towards the local La Tène B threshold (S. Champion, pers. comm.). The existence of Mischkultur sites need not in fact imply total or even predominant contemporaneity of Hallstatt D3 and La Tène A, as transitional sites must be expected. In any case the use of the D3 and La Tène A labels by German scholars frequently rests not on a total assemblage, but on the presence/absence of individual artifact types that need not each one have an exact currency terminating or commencing with the D3/La Tène A boundary.

In general therefore the present data base seems to confirm the traditional model that the so-called D3 facies is antecedent to La Tène A in both the former West Hallstatt sphere, in East Hallstatt contexts where La Tène A makes an early appearance, and in the core western regions of Early La Tène.

2)   On the other hand, the current state of play as regards chronology appears to confirm the German view that Hallstatt D in its final D3 facies occupied a major part of the fifth century BC, even though this is not inconsistent with a minimal overlap to La Tène A, which is now in turn increasingly taken by many authorities to occupy the latter half of the same century and the early fourth century BC.

Dendrochronology of the West Hallstatt Magdalenenberg tumulus suggests a date for the transition Hallstatt C/D c. 570 BC, which plainly makes the compression of Hallstatt D1, 2 and 3 into the remainder of the sixth century problematic. The late Hallstatt D context at Befort in Luxembourg provides confirmation with dendro-dates of 468 and 457/6 BC (Haerke 1979 p.13; Pauli 1978 p.429). According to Pauli (1978 p.426) the Hallstatt D3 classic princely burial of Vix, associated with the West Hallstatt culture centre at Mont Lassois in eastern France, not only contains a decorated Greek dish of 530-520 BC manufacture but an undecorated Attic dish import recently dated to c. 480 BC. Mont Lassois itself has produced Hallstatt D2/3 but no La Tène A traces (Haerke 1979 p.99). The situation at the Heuneburg is highly controversial. The final level is described by the excavators as 'La Tène A' though no precise La Tène features are indicated and the absence of Red-Figure imports and appropriate fibulae are contrary to such a designation. A casting-mould for an Etruscan flagon, suggesting a 480-460 BC date would merely fit into a final pre-La Tène A, early fifth century era of Hallstatt D3 (cf. Haerke 1979, pp.96, 150, 157, and above discussion). The great currency in fibulae of D3 type in Italy is also significantly in the fifth century (Pauli 1978 p.429).

For La Tène A beginnings, imports span the early and late fifth century BC in terms of manufacturing date in the Mediterranean, but in no case demand a commencement at c. 500 BC. They could all probably be reconciled with a general spread of La Tène A styles from mid-century onwards (cf. Pauli 1978 p.434). Thus the Hallein chariot grave with particular wealth contains an Attic dish manufactured around the second quarter of the fifth century, and that of Somme-Bionne in Champagne an Attic dish c. 430-420 BC (Pauli op. cit. p.434). A down-dating of the La Tène A/B transition on the basis of a revaluation of the Waldalgesheim Style has been proposed, offering compensatory time in the fourth century for La Tène A developments (Pauli op. cit. p.419).

3) To come full circle, the German position of a survival of the former West Hallstatt communities through the La Tène A period, parallel to the rise of wealthy burials and population increase in the new core Early La Tène florescent regions of the Champagne and Middle Rhine, seems to be receiving widespread confirmation from the available (but still poorly-researched data).

First and foremost is the case of the Hohenasperg princely seat and its accompanying princely burials. There is undeniable continuity of tradition and presumably of political structure arguable from the Klein Aspergle tumulus, whose riches conform to a clear La Tène A format and include Greek imports manufactured c. 460-450 BC but almost certainly much later in final deposition (cf. above on repairs) (Frey 1980 p.76). The Hohenasperg itself is very poorly-known but has yielded La Tène A sherds (Haerke 1979 p.97). In eastern France the Château-Sur-Salins princely seat demonstrates even clearer the degree of continuity, with the La Tène A layer 5 producing considerable quantities of Attic Red-Figure ware (Haerke 1979 p.149). In Switzerland, the Châtillon-Sur-Glâne princely seat is argued to continue into La Tène A on stylistic and import considerations (Haerke 1979 p.149). Other major sites usually assigned to 'central place' roles in the West Hallstatt sphere and where evidence of La Tène A occupation is claimed, include Ipf, Britzgyberg, Uetliberg, Breisach and Marienberg (Haerke 1979, pp.97, 150).

The widespread evidence now being published and analyzed for extensive rural La Tène A settlement in the overall Baden-Württemberg region (cf. above) is clearly complementary to the continuance of occupation at many defended centres. On the other hand, there are also numerous cases in the West Hallstatt sphere where no La Tène A finds or associations can be documented and it is likely that the centres concerned did not survive the transition period. Haerke summarises the situation as follows: widespread discontinuity can be found in site occupation, especially in eastern France but also in north west Switzerland and south western Germany, but in the latter regions "apparently continuity was the rule" (Haerke 1979 p.173). The new era is one of 'deterioration' and 'stagnation' (p.242). In particular, with the exception of Klein Aspergle, princely burials disappear at this time, even if defended foci continue in use, **yet** nonetheless the resident elites at surviving centres are still able to obtain Greek and Italian imports.

4) We must further emphasize that a dramatic contrast between a sudden, cataclysmic collapse of society in West Hallstatt, and a contemporary spectacular emergence of wealth and status in the La Tène core regions, is not only unlikely from the above discussion, but is also at odds with the situation during Hallstatt D in the Champagne and Middle Rhine. The little-known Hallstatt D of the Champagne demonstrates in its metalwork and waggon burial rite both wealth and status, as does the early series of 'burials of nobility' with similar furnishings in the Middle Rhine (the Hundheim-Bell group) (cf. Haerke 1979 p.20) associated probably with 'chieftains' seats' (Haerke op. cit. p.143). Occasional finds of two-wheeled chariots typical of La Tène A prestige burials can be documented already during late Hallstatt D in the core West Hallstatt sphere (e.g. eastern France), as well as in both core regions for La Tène A (Pauli 1978 p.432, Stead 1979).

5) In conclusion, the **rise** of the future La Tène A core zone, in terms of population, wealth and status distinctions, must be seen as contemporary to the late florescence of the West Hallstatt sphere, between the latter sixth and first half of the fifth century BC. Around the latter point the West Hallstatt sphere enters into decline, but in the form of a gradual process of piecemeal abandonment of central places (which spans the remainder of the century), and a much speedier process of the cessation of rich graves. At the same time as this West Hallstatt deterioration commences, La Tène A is born to its north, and there population appears to take a rapid jump and political statuses are further elaborated. In the former West Hallstatt sphere, imports are still arriving at the diminishing number of centres, yet full participation in the novel La Tène cultural format can be observed at both major and minor sites, in metalwork and pottery.

We have already argued (cf. above) that the presence of Mediterranean imports and prestige burials is more indicative of the overall structure and even 'health' of the complex socio-political system than key elements in the latter's maintenance. Following this interpretation the La Tène A core lands emerge, together with major areas of the former East Hallstatt sphere (now stylistically La Tène A) as flourishingly 'complex', whilst the West Hallstatt sphere proceeds through a progression of apparent socio-political devolution. Some putative centres of the former West Hallstatt sphere cease to receive imports and erect prestige burial monuments (e.g. the Heuneburg), others (e.g. the Hohenasperg) continue apparently much as before. No simple model with the north rising upon the ruin of the south seems appropriate, especially as regards a supposed withdrawal of commercial contacts from the Mediterranean to the West Hallstatt region. The situation may be more in keeping with an essentially unrelated process of internal socio-economic and/or socio-political breakdown in West Hallstatt and vigorous demographic expansion and socio-political elaboration in the core La Tène A regions. The latter may be seen from the seemingly sharp rise in evidence for settlement and burial in the early La Tène Champagne in comparison to the Hallstatt era (cf. Bretz-Mahler 1971) and from the less spectacular infilling of the landscape in the Rhineland Hunsrück-Eifel culture (cf. Haerke 1979), but as noted above, in both regions the start of these important regional florescences is increasingly traceable to Hallstatt D.

Note 52
Further continuity is demonstrated by the appearance of occasional two-wheeled chariot burials in Hallstatt D in both West Hallstatt and the future La Tène core regions (cf. note 51, above).

Note 53
On this key point, S. Champion (1982) surely makes the correct warning to simple 'dependency' assumptions, when she writes: "the regional shift from southern Germany to

the Middle Rhine in the fifth century and the contemporary development in Switzerland of new patterns of life and death suggest internal changes in European society that may have affected the relationship with the Mediterranean just as much as those events in the Mediterranean, underlined by Frankenstein and Rowlands, which may have caused a lessening of interest in Europe north of the Alps" (p.71).

Note 54

Already in Hallstatt C individual notables in the West Hallstatt sphere and beyond were receiving such Mediterranean luxury items, the flow merely increasing during Hallstatt D/La Tène A times - but the same emphasis on exotic display pieces is found, especially tableware in pot or metal. It is not even necessary to assume that these vessels accompanied a 'wine trade' as the quantities of amphorae over this period are both very low, and in distribution over time and space not comparable to that of the imported vessels and cups. The overall effect is far from suggesting 'trade' and has led to most authorities investigating a diplomatic role for these preserved items (Fischer 1973, Lessing and Kruta 1979, Frey 1980).

An interesting parallel may be sought in the highlighting of indigenous tribal princes in Free Germany during the Roman era by luxury imports from the Roman world. Todd suggests (1977, pp.41-2) that elites founded on agricultural expansion and agricultural wealth were receiving such imports by long distance exchange for use as status symbols, and in some cases the exotica were diplomatic gifts from the Empire.

Note 55

Not surprisingly the links between the colony and its mother state were therefore often tenuous (with the majority of new settlers frequently from numerous other states), and examples are common of colonies siding against their official founder state in subsequent interstate wars. A regular organized entrepôt role for the colony to supply its home city, or other specific trading partners, as a keystone of such a foundation, is unusual and in general contrary to the spirit and practice of the 'ancient economy' (Finley 1973). It would be extremely difficult to supply a colony that was not mainly self-sufficient in subsistence production from its own territory, given the absence of formal commercial organizations within the Greek state or between its citizens, and the very low role of trade and industry in the budget of most Archaic states. The overall implications of the research of the 'Finley school' of ancient economic historians are that the trade and industry activities of the Greek colonies would have been of far less account in their productivity and wealth than their own intra-regional food production.

Although one can make a far better case for Phoenician sites in the Western Mediterranean as including a high proportion of trading posts, as opposed to locally rooted, self-sufficient farming communities with strong exchange interests, it is the writer's unorthodox view that the normal description of Phoenician civilization as fundamentally centring on industry and commerce will likewise, in time, yield to a more balanced conception. In this revision we may identify core areas of Phoenician settlement where the prime activity was sophisticated mixed farming and industry for local needs, and peripheral contact zones where activity was far more orientated towards an entrepreneurial role. Within the core zones we may include the Phoenician homeland in the Levant, where the network of major city-states forms a neatly defined mosaic of approximately equal territorial cells, comparable to Renfrew's (1975) 'early state module' for Etruscan states, and provides each Phoenician city with a significant hinterland of fertile arable and grazing land

(author's unpublished research); also, and remarkably neglected in the literature, the vast hinterland territory of the great North African city of Carthage, known to extend some 150kms. from the city into the fertile Tunisian countryside, and defined formally by a great demarcation ditch - a region that soon became populous with towns and farms, thriving on the unusually fertile soil and climate of this zone of North Africa (cf. Potter 1980); western Sicily should also be included in the core, internalized areas. For the peripheral zones, several of the Spanish sites with Phoenician activity well evidenced might be representative, although one may fairly doubt that locally based farming settlements did not develop within the very wide area of Phoenician influence, considering the long period of that influence in the Iberian peninsula. This controversial rethink of Phoenician settlement and economy in the East Mediterranean homeland and abroad is very much at odds with the commercial/industrial dominance assumed in the recent study by Frankenstein (1979). It is worth noting, however, that her view was already challenged in a most penetrating critique by R. Mc. Adams (1979).

Note 56

In Wells (1980b) we are told of Hascherkeller, that "the principal result of the first two seasons" is to "have revealed that this prehistoric community was very much involved in the general growth of commerce and industry during the early phase of the Early Iron Age" . . . "very active in production and trade" . . . "actively involved in a variety of manufacturing and trade activities" (p.328). The evidence presented for this grandiose scenario falls far short of these claims. Thus, "evidence for metalworking " is "abundant" (p.326), - this turns out to concentrate on the discovery of two pin fragments, a lump of bronze seen as casting debris and a mould for bronze finger-rings. On this basis we are told to rethink our West Hallstatt model of metalworking "at a small number of specialized industrial centres" (p.326 - an astonishing description for the princely seats!) to allow for a broader Industrial Revolution. Graphite found at the site could be local or exotic in origin - naturally the latter is assumed likely. Even bone-working and weaving activities are blandly assigned to this new 'industrial' environment, supposedly quite distinct from the economy of traditional, indigenous type before the Mediterranean metamorphosis.

With relief one may turn to the sober realism of Biel and Joachim (1979), who describe very similar evidence from the Hallstatt D site of Feilbach, such as bronzeworking, the production of fibulae - but merely in terms of smallscale craft production by a rural community to meet local needs.

Note 57

"Much of the colonisation by Greek cities was done primarily to establish new sources of wheat for the mother cities as well as for new colonial populations" (Wells and Bonfante 1979, p.21). The Fürstensitze show "Intensive trade relations" and "abundant Mediterranean luxury products" (p.18). In another study (Wells 1980a) these are described as "commercial centres" marking the transformation of the whole of Central Europe from self-sufficiency to international commercial production. The insurmountable difficulties of which no mention is made, of shifting such an implied series of food mountains from this vast region, the great majority of which is well off any navigable river to the Mediterranean, with no known maintained heavy transport land routes, must make this suggestion beyond probabilitiy (cf. Finley 1973), even without re-introducing our previous conclusions concerning the limited scale of any exchange systems from the Mediterranean at this time. Grain shipments by sea from the coastal cities of Sicily, or the Black Sea Greek colonies, are a very different matter, but these fundamental constraints on ancient trade are relevant through to the Late Roman Imperial period.

Note 58
In response to these new data, Wells is forced to rethink (Wells and Bonfante 1979), but merely offloads the problem into historic limbo by introducing eastern Mediterranean 'events' as at work moulding the fate of the West Hallstatt barbarians! One is here approaching the diffusionist-revival, impressionistic analysis of local sequences that sometimes pervades M. Rowlands' interpretations (viz. the "continental-wide pulsations" of his 1980 paper). In a similar simplistic vein, Wells writes that the barbarian Celts, (their appetites for fine tableware doubtless sharpened to fever-pitch as a result of their slavish dependency on Mediterranean trade), determine to invade Italy, abandoning their homelands in pursuit of the usual rape, pillage, etc., "lured by the attractions of Mediterranean life" (1980a, p.6; possibly founder-fathers of the Club Méditerranée?) - hence the fourth century Celtic settlement.

Note 59
Interestingly, Rowlands has recently discussed the process of differentiation within Celtic society in a way that is remarkably similar to the author's own model, at least as far as the stages we quote from here (Rowlands 1980). We begin with the important analytical focus on district surplus control: "consistent relationships exist between kinship form, patterns of marriage alliance (and the kinds of dependency and ranking these promote) and the size of the minimum political units on which the accumulation of socially significant wealth must depend". With more implied relevance to later pre-Roman Celtic society, though we see its equal validity to Hallstatt times, he continues: "The development of a dual or tripartite class structure in late Celtic society, as usually understood, would have had to have occurred at the expense of kinship and to have resulted from the elaboration of various cross-cutting mechanisms of status differentiation and clientage based on non-kinship principles" - "Inequalities between households and within households are reinforced by the same processes of unequal productive capacity, and by the monopolisation and manipulation of marriage alliances and attendant political processes. A more absolute stratification between 'nobles' and 'commoners' can develop as a result of the intensification of these processes" - "Poorer households lose their social identity and are re-invested with the only one available to them, as dependents or clients of richer and more powerful households within the clan. This process of 'sloughing off' poorer households and their reduction to client status leads to the emergence of elite and commoner strata within the same clan or phratry which will cross-cut all clans within a given territorial unit. An aristocratic elite tends to emerge, defined essentially by its relations to land, wealth, dynastic alliance, genealogical ordering and ritual knowledge, and differentiated from a commoner substratum that retains a reduced and politically insignificant kinship ordering". Thus far (op. cit. pp.6-16), we are in full agreement, but then, quite gratuitously, and for a priori reasons of preference, the whole structure hitherto erected is deprived of its own energy to live and develop, by the introduction into the argument of the external 'handle' of Mediterranean manipulation; to our view, the tail wagging the dog. And curiously, it is subsequently admitted that the Hallstatt political structure "could not have been generated through external contacts" (p.29).

Note 60
The Celtic Migrations. On the remarkable coincidence of events c. 400 BC, we may recall the reasons discussed earlier for the dismemberment of complex society from

450-400 BC in the West Hallstatt sphere (Early La Tène facies), directly linked by Kimmig (1975b) and others to the Celtic migrations. In a recent chronology (Pauli 1980c) the end of the Heuneburg and Mont Lassois is placed as late as 390-370 BC, directly parallel to the Italian invasions. As seen, there is no reason for supporting such a late date for either site, but after the abandonment and/or destruction of the princely seats and cemeteries, there is the evidence for relocation of settlement in new areas of the landscape, and the associated takeover of the flat cemetery/inhumation rite, in West Hallstatt (cf. Wamser 1975). These changes and similar settlement and burial alterations in the core La Tène and East Hallstatt spheres are frequently directly linked to the Celtic migrations (Zürn 1974, Frey 1980, Pauli 1980a, S. Champion 1982). The discovery of archaeological traces of the historic early fourth century settlement of Celts in Italy is often seen as most appropriately tied to the region suffering the greatest discontinuity - the former West Hallstatt sphere, and it is possible to analyse the Roman traditions as indicating a major origin zone for the invaders between Rhône and Rhine, i.e. West Hallstatt (Pauli 1980b). Scholars place the main Celtic settlement in northern Italy between the late fifth century and the Rome sack 387/6 BC (Nemeskalova 1978, Frey 1980). For the parallel spread of Celts eastwards, both Classical traditions and archaeological research agree on a contemporary and related movement to that shown for the Italian invasion. The early fourth century is the generally accepted date both for the historic eastern migrations, and for the appearance in a vast region running through Central into Eastern Europe (the former East Hallstatt sphere and neighbouring lands to the north) of the flat inhumation 'warrior' cemeteries associated with La Tène B(Ib-c) styles and generally identified with the process of 'Celtization' (cf. Filip 1977, Hodson and Rowlett 1974, Lessing and Kruta 1979, Nandris 1976, Pauli 1980b). However, the possible minority genuine immigrant population demonstrable from the analysis of later historic sources, and commonsense inferences on the level of indigenous settlement, finds a confirmation in the strong local context into which La Tène objects and styles become embedded (cf. Wozniak 1976). Nonetheless, by the third century BC, when the 'Celts' irrupt into the Hellenistic world of the East Mediterranean, they clearly intend to settle in large numbers, as the Balkan kingdom of Tylis and Turkish Galatia demonstrate (Lessing and Kruta 1979, pp.71 ff.). And a Celtic 'dominance' over much of the north Balkans by 290 BC is accepted (Alexander 1980, p.225). A parallel Celtic migration wave to Iberia is much more problematical, and scholars have looked at influences there from as early as the Late Bronze Age for the traces of Celtic arrivals, who at least by 250 BC should have occupied or dominated much of the peninsula (Alexander 1980, p.225).

The logical conclusions to be drawn from the great process of colonization are amply confirmed by the Classical traditions regarding the Celtic migrations both to Italy and to Eastern and South-Eastern Europe. The emphasis on over-population and land hunger explains the clear attempts to settle by whole populations, rather than hit and run raids by marauding bands (Zürn 1974). That the push to Italy and to Eastern Europe were both linked events, reflecting West European population and land problems, is interestingly expressly recorded in traditions preserved in Livy and Pompeius Trogus. Unfortunately, the variety of tribal groups named for these movements, and the difficulty of locating their homelands at this era, constrains a more exact use of the sources for matching regional archaeological discontinuities in barbarian lands (for a general discussion of the sources and archaeology, cf. Lessing and Kruta 1979; also cf. Pauli 1980b, Zeller 1980).

Note 61

It is difficult to isolate one area within which the major transformation to the typical mature La Tène B(Ib-c) flat inhumation rite originated. This may in any case be a less significant question than the reasons why much of Europe north of the Alps converted to the rite, and indeed it seems likely that several discrete areas had either retained inhumation through the Hallstatt/La Tène A phase or moved together towards the new format from cremation and/or tumulus forms. Certainly it must be noteworthy, however, that a leading area for the development of cultural styles in La Tène A, the Marne region, has a prominent early place in the rite transformation. Already in the Jogassien late Hallstatt graves here we see flat inhumation as a normal burial form, including 'warrior' burial, trends merely continued in the numerically far greater series of La Tène A graves (Collis 1977). Elsewhere in Champagne and other parts of France inhumation had continued to be common alongside cremation during the time range of the Hallstatt Culture (Bretz-Mahler 1971, Hodson and Rowlett 1974, Freidin 1983). Already in Hallstatt C, eastern France also participates in the popular East Hallstatt subculture of tumulus inhumation associated with characteristic weaponry and horse gear (Freidin 1983). In Jogassien and La Tène A there continues this distinctive element of separate princely burials that links the Marne to the wider Hallstatt traditions (including four-wheeled cart burial -cf. Freidin 1983). Also in the fifth century, the West Hallstatt region witnesses individual examples of flat inhumation graves or even cemeteries, alongside the final flowering of the tumulus inhumation/cremation complex, and increasingly the 'warrior' sector appears in these new burials. Switzerland is particularly notable in its early adoption of the characteristic flat cemetery of warrior aspect, and with a smooth curve of wealth (Filip 1977, Hodson and Rowlett 1974, S. Champion 1982, Stead 1979). But in general, it is the fourth century, after the collapse of the 'old order' that sees the universal rise of La Tène B (Ib-c) style flat inhumation cemeteries in former West Hallstatt (Zürn 1974, Wamser 1975, Hodson and Rowlett 1974). In non-West Hallstatt France beyond the Marne, the takeover of inhumation proceeds gradually from the fifth century onwards. If the princely tradition disappears in the West Hallstatt region and Marne by the fourth century, in favour of the new rite alone, in the Middle Rhine the princes survive as far as burial records suggest into the fourth century, but then yield to the prevailing pattern elsewhere (Filip 1977, Collis 1977, Stead 1979).

However the unusual popularity of chariot burials in the Marne area (c. 140 can be listed - Stead n.d.) during La Tène A and B (La Tène I, fifth to fourth centuries BC), and their gift associations, seems to argue that the traditional Hallstatt high-level elite symbol, the wheeled hearse, has now become a symbol open to what must be the equivalent of district chieftains; possibly further evidence of a process of social levelling in burial symbolism typical for La Tène Europe. In the cultural or even ethnic offshoot of the Marne Early La Tène culture, the east Yorkshire Arras Culture of England, the evidence of chariots seems to reflect a similar devaluation of the emblem of rank.

In the East Hallstatt sphere, some areas had always continued with inhumation as a major or minor rite, even for princely burials, throughout Hallstatt times (cf. supra). However, it is the fourth century again that witnesses the wholesale conversion of Central and Eastern Europe to the norm of flat inhumation cemeteries with a warrior sector and with a smoothly graded wealth pattern. Although as elsewhere, outstandingly rich burials have all but ceased at this time, occasional chariot graves or burials with unusual wealth continue to occur, but as clear exceptions to the general socio-political trend. The

emphasis on the lower level elite, the district chieftains and 'big men', throughout this great new La Tène B (Ib-c) world of West, Central and Eastern Europe, fits the high frequency of 'warrior' burials, and the small size of the communities represented by the typical flat cemetery (and increasingly being identified on the ground as settlements in the vicinity of the cemetery). Likewise, the spread 'downwards' at this time of the La Tène art style, from its La Tène A (Ia) confinement to the princes, seems to underline the changed social structure (Filip 1977, Lessing and Kruta 1979, Stead 1979).

On the other hand, as noted earlier, the changed symbolism may be illuminating for us, in a socially-significant way, a new importance to the already-existing lower-level elite of Hallstatt and La Tène A times. In the Polish province of Silesia, for example, when the dominant cremation rite with poor gifts of Hallstatt and La Tène A times yields to the La Tène B adoption of birite customs (in which the important inhumation sector includes warrior graves and a richer average gift complement), we need not follow the traditional line that here we see the living-together of incoming western Celtic elites and their subordinate local Lausitz peasantry (Gedl 1978). It could well be that statuses obscured for us in the earlier rite (a highly plausible inference as we shall see in our investigation of the Lausitz culture, below), are now underlined with the adoption of western burial symbolism. The presence in such cemeteries of genuine Celtic immigrants, as opposed to Celtized local elites, is an open question, even if we have accepted the general thesis of Celtic migration into Eastern Europe.

Professor F.R. Hodson (1979) has reminded us, illustrating his paper from recent cemetery excavations, of the possibility that 'Celtic society' may have been far less standardized in its class structure than we imagine. For West-Central Europe his review of diverse cemetery 'societies' of Hallstatt and Early La Tène data concludes: "Even such interpretations as these make it difficult to believe that any standard form of social organisation existed ... in this area at this time" (1979 p.29).

Whilst we have been concerned with pointing out a distinction in later European prehistory between the universally prevalent district elite structure of 'big men' or 'chieftains', and the rarer occurrences of more powerful territorial leaders - 'paramounts', 'princes', the variety of cemetery patterns for so-called 'Celtic communities' need not be irreconcilable with such a generalization. High status families may be buried in separate cemeteries, and most rural community cemeteries could be expected to lack regional notables. A broad class distinction such as the above between high-level elites, low-level elites, and commoners, still leaves ample room for local divergences in burial symbolism and treatment for emphasizing other distinctions (sex, age, family or clan structure, non-kin sodalities, etc.) Finally, it might be argued that variation from cemetery to cemetery in burial symbolism informs us about local differences in the cultural expression of status and role which may well be obscuring more fundamental similarities in actual social structure.

Note 62

The Lausitz Culture is a regional phenomenon of remarkable extent in both the temporal and spatial dimension. Characteristic features of the typical assemblage begin to be widespread c. 1400 bc and then dominate Poland, East Germany and major parts of Czechoslovakia (Moravia and Slovakia) for some 1000 years, till the fifth century BC (Coblenz 1971, Gedl 1977, Milisauskas 1978). Studies of the evolution of the culture emphasize two fundamental points: firstly that it arose from indigenous local roots in each area of its distribution, as a result of a great surge of population and land intake during the Late Bronze Age and Early Iron Age (often into more marginal lands than hitherto). Secondly, that the florescence of its network of proto-urban foci and associated satellite rural settlements is time-transgressive, as is the dramatic decline of the culture and its 'towns'. It is therefore with good reason argued that each area moved at its own pace towards a more elaborate society, and that the inherent instability of Lausitz socio-economic structure led to an inevitable dissolution of that specific form of society at varying time-intervals across its vast area of distribution.

A major part of this zone of north-central Europe is composed of glacial and periglacial soils of very varied composition, but frequently less favourable sandy and clayey groups that had been under-exploited by earlier populations. One can observe an increasing exploitation as the Neolithic progresses in this zone (cf. Bogucki 1979, Kruk 1980) but, as elsewhere in Europe, it is particularly during the Bronze Age that intensive settlement activity occupies the whole region. Pressure on older lands and increasing adaptation to new econiches are factors often associated with this process, as well as more specific aspects such as the development of major cultivation of rye and oats, hardy plants well-suited to the ecology of this zone of Europe (Ostoja-Zagorski 1974, Alexander 1978). Other features of the Lausitz adaptation that underlay this notable expansion of mixed farming communities, as evidenced by archaeological finds, includes a wide range of cultigens (cereals, pulses - but also intentional recovery of nutritious 'weeds'), major effort on a strong stock-breeding component, and significant hunting of wild game (Coblenz 1971, Ostoja-Zagorski 1974). These broad-spectrum adaptations, in combination, must account for the long-life of this very populous culture, its remarkable spread through a landscape of very varying quality in subsistence terms, and notable colonizing achievement (Lausitz settlement is well represented up to 250m. above sea level and findspots occur as high as 7-800m. in the uplands of the border country between Germany, south Poland and Czechoslovakia) (Coblenz 1971, Milisauskas 1978).

A whole series of regional studies (cf. Coblenz 1971, Bukowski 1971, 1974, Gedl 1976, 1977, Breddin 1975, Rajewski 1974), enable one to compare rates of change towards the classic 'Burgen' or 'fortified town' phase. In Silesia and Great Poland, e.g., a dense level of settlement during the pre-town period of Middle Bronze Age and early Late Bronze Age is represented by scattered, small and short-lived sites in the vicinity of much longer-lived cemetery fixed points in the landscape. These cemeteries also form the continuity locally into the phase of development of district settlement foci, from the later Late Bronze Age into the Hallstatt Iron Age era (Hallstatt B on into Hallstatt C/D). In a detailed survey of developments within the Liswarta Basin (Gedl 1976), once again it is the Middle Bronze Age 'Vorlausitz' (Pre-Lausitz) phase that shows the commencement of the settlement expansion, followed by a very striking takeoff of population density in the Late Bronze Age true Lausitz Culture emergence period, producing a visible wave-like infilling of the landscape. Here also, at a detailed level, cemeteries in core areas provide clear continuity across these developments. In some areas the climax density may already be achieved in Late Bronze Age times (especially Hallstatt A 2), e.g. Brandenburg (Breddin 1975), and be on the decline when elsewhere the culture is still on the demographic ascendant. The fortified nuclei or 'Burgen' begin in many areas during the Late Bronze Age, especially Hallstatt B, though they are more frequent by Hallstatt C/D times (Rajewski 1974); a broad generalization puts them earlier in the west, later in the east, of the Lausitz sphere (Galuszka 1963, Coblenz 1971). Where the Burgen are late in arising there are associated indications of delayed overall settlement climax, e.g. in Great

Poland with major forest clearance horizons in the pollen record from Hallstatt C on (Bukowski 1974). But the total picture offered by both local and general studies of the Lausitz settlement development is one of a great series of individual micro-regions (Siedlungskammern), conditioned largely by geography, within which the indigenous communities enter into a pronounced demographic expansion in Late Bronze Age and Hallstatt times, frequently (but not always), crystallizing out into regional settlement patterns composed of numerous 'cells' - Fig. 5 (landscapes comprising a fortified 'town' and dispersed rural satellite sites) (cf. Coblenz 1971, Bukowski 1974, Gedl 1977). The 'Burgen' often develop on or near a smaller open site from the preceding settlement build-up phase. The peak of the Burgen occurs in Hallstatt C-D times, when the Lusatian Culture enters the full Iron Age, and as elsewhere we may attribute accelerated development to the introduction of iron tools in all aspects of everyday life (cf. Pleiner 1980).

The particular interest for European prehistoric development in the Lausitz Culture lies in the outstanding fortified centres, which seem to form nodes for discrete districts of dense rural settlement (Coblenz 1971). Although one may expect that variations in land quality and topography over the vast area of the culture will be reflected in variable 'cell' size for these 'polities', some overall regional regularities have been observed. The range of inferred territories runs from 100-800sq. kms., with the western Lausitz generally at the lower end, the eastern at the upper end of the spectrum. If the cells were to be truly centred on their foci, such territories would encompass land from 7-15kms. radius out from the 'town'. In actual fact, available maps with relevant details of soil distributions etc., suggest that more irregular territories exist matched to the discontinuous distribution of more fertile land and lake/river networks. The general distance between nearest neighbouring centres is recorded as 15-25kms., consistent with the above estimates of total cell boundary distance. (Cf. Bukowski 1971, 1974, Coblenz 1971, 1974, Ostoja-Zagorski 1974, Milisauskas 1978, Galuszka 1963, Henneberg and Ostoja-Zagorski unpubl.).

As for the relationship between the nucleated foci and smaller rural sites, most studies consider them intimately linked as an inter-dependent system (cf. Galuszka 1963, Coblenz 1971, Ostoja-Zagorski 1974); however, whilst some suggest that the Burgen act as regional service centres for a dispersed peasantry, others maintain that the population of each cell normally resides in the focus and uses the rural locations for temporary purposes (seasonal cultivation, hunting, raw material extraction, etc.; cf. Rajewski 1974, Bukowski 1974). This important distinction deserves closer comment. Firstly, some areas of Lausitz Culture reach typical high rural density without establishing central foci, e.g. the far east of the distributional sphere (Bukowski 1974, Rajewski 1974). In others, larger settlements and smaller exist, without the pronounced fortified 'town' focus emerging (Gedl 1976). In general, Burgen arise out of previous agglomerations of rural settlement. Indeed the focus may represent an upgrading of an older rural site of smaller size, or a relocation of such (Bukowski 1974). If the rise of the centre requires a population pooling, there is evidence from some detailed local analyses of a process akin to 'synoecism', the concentration of people from the land immediately around the focus into its enclosed habitation area (Piontek and Kolodziejski 1981, Bukowski 1971). As for the rural sites, a major difficulty lies in the scant attention hitherto paid to them by archaeologists, in contrast to the considerable number of excavated Lausitz cemeteries and the partial excavation of many Burgen (Milisauskas 1978). There is little doubt that the known rural settlements must represent a very small proportion of their original density, if we bear in mind not only their scantier vestiges but more importantly, the truly phenomenal number of Lausitz cemeteries scattered across the landscape (cf. Harding, this volume; Milisauskas (1978) quotes 2830 for Poland alone). The cemeteries are increasingly being tied in to adjacent rural settlements, and taken together with the rare excavations of rural sites, that reveal substantial house structures and evidence for normal domestic activities including metalworking, the evidence seems to point convincingly to the model of 'urban' plus 'rural' populations living independently (Bukowski 1974, Milisauskas 1978). The rural sites do seem to be shorter-lived than the centres, which suggests farms or hamlets shifting around, perhaps in order to rotate the infield around the cultivated area; the cemeteries, however, are often much more stable in location, limiting any interpretation of true 'shifting agriculture' (cf. Piontek and Kolodziejski 1981, Coblenz 1971, Bukowski 1974).

As for the 'urban' sites, their surface area varies from one to ten hectares, occasionally more, but knowledge of their interiors is often vague and perhaps too much emphasis is placed on a small group of Polish sites with reasonably good data. At Biskupin, for example, a fairly full picture of the internal plan was obtained by excavation, leading to house estimates of over 100 contemporary structures. On an extended family module of some 10-12 occupants, a total population of 1000-1250 is arrived at (Rajewski 1974). The Sobiejuchy centre in the same region is given a projected 2500 inhabitants (Ostoja-Zagorski 1974). Although trial excavations confirm that many other foci have a similar plan of regular, close-packed domestic units (Rajewski 1974), the Biskupin model is certainly not typical for the foci as a whole. Other investigations show that large areas enclosed elsewhere are probably given over to craft quarters, communal food preparation and stock/arable plots (Coblenz 1971); at Wicina e.g. only 30% of the site is described as domestic quarters (Piontek and Kolodziejski 1981). The concentrated dwellings of the smallish Biskupin enclosure (2ha.) imply in any case a substantial extramural activity zone, if only to accommodate stock. It may also be questioned whether the known dwellings are indeed occupied by one or several families, and recalculations using Naroll's formula for Biskupin reduce its population to 700-750 (Milisauskas 1978).

Taking focal and satellite sites together and allowing for under-representation of the latter, most estimates of total 'cell' territory population are in the range of one to several thousand people (cf. Ostoja-Zagorski 1974, Henneberg and Ostoja-Zagorski unpubl.). The degree of organization and integration suggested by such central foci is underlined by the archaeological evidence for communal construction work: an estimate of the labour involved in building one such centre is 900,000 man-hours (Henneberg and Ostoja-Zagorski unpubl.) whilst the effort and raw material involved in great breakwaters, bridges (120m. long example at Biskupin), and wooden streets is matched by the equivalent requirements involved in the great circuit defences in box rampart form incorporating earth, wood and stone (Coblenz 1971, Milisauskas 1978). The buildings are often in a uniform style and plan, and their regimented rows are divided by regular streets that may converge on open squares (Rajewski 1974). Craft and small scale industrial activity are well-evidenced in these foci, as well as frequent finds of luxury items, including gold (Coblenz 1971, Bukowski 1974). Occasional pieces of the latter class seem to be imports, from the Middle Danube/East Hallstatt sphere and north Italy. On the other hand, metalworking is well-evidenced from rural open sites, and bronze, which seems to have been generally a scarce commodity in the Lausitz culture, is mainly recovered from rural hoards (Bukowski 1974).

Considering the unambiguous evidence of complex organization within these 'polities', running parallel as they do to the flourishing chiefdom and paramount systems of later Bronze Age Central Europe, and then to the princedoms of the Hallstatt sphere, the question naturally arises as to the precise political structure of the Lausitz Culture. In traditional terms, the archaeological evidence is universally agreed to betray little hint of chieftains, let alone princes. Often a focus will contain one building notably larger than the norm (Coblenz 1971) which, as we have noted earlier, is no more or less than the equivalent feature optimistically identified for the clearer-attested chieftains elsewhere as their 'residence'. As for burials, the urned cremations of the frequently very extensive Lausitz cemeteries are almost exclusively akin in their gift poverty and simple grave practice (Bukowski 1971, Caplovic 1974, Rajewski 1974). However, occasional examples are known of individual graves or even groups within cemeteries, where 'rich' burials appear in clear contrast to the norm (Coblenz 1971, Rajewski 1974, Bukowski 1974). These can be flat cremations, but in many cases the wealthier burials have the inhumation rite. At this point a connection may be made to an earlier discussion of the effect of the Urnfield rite upon grave wealth. In most of the Lausitz sphere, Early to Middle Bronze Age burials are inhumation, often under a tumulus, and cemeteries exhibit the 'normal' broad spectrum of wealth and inferred rank. From the Late Bronze Age and generally through to the end of Lausitz around the transition to the La Tène era, burial customs rapidly change towards the urn-cremation, generally in flat graves. Associated with this shift is a decline or disappearance of gifts to the dead, and the apparent disappearance of 'rank' (Gedl 1977). Yet throughout the life of the culture, inhumation remains as a minority custom; at the cemetery at Opatow for example the inhumation burials of Hallstatt C times include wealthy graves (Gedl 1976). When in the great expansion of the revived inhumation rite to Eastern Europe, that is associated with the 'Celtic' flat inhumation cemeteries of La Tène B, inhumation burial arrives or returns to popularity, in the Lausitz world, it seems reasonable enough to question the assumption (Gedl 1978) that the wealthy and powerful Celtic elite are being buried alongside their new subjects (the still cremating, impoverished Lausitz peasants). Equally plausible is the interpretation that links the return of inhumation and provision of a range of gifts with the dead, with a revival locally (if under foreign inspiration) of a burial symbolism which seeks to emphasize rather than obscure the range of statuses in society, just as that symbolism had been extinguished through the many centuries of Lausitz burial uniformity. It is, therefore, the present writer's thesis that the pre-Lausitz ranking was not abolished at the very period when organizational complexity grows to a remarkable climax in north-central Europe, rather that the Lausitz elite generally found other means to **display** their status than burial pomp, which apart from the monumental co-operative building projects at the foci, are perhaps to be sought in future analysis of the role of hoards and prestige objects (cf. Levy 1978).

The uniform view on the role of the Lausitz nucleated foci or Burgen, is that they functioned as regional central places, in terms of the provision of administration, justice and exchange, on the model of an historic market town, and with the strong defences offering protection for the surrounding population (Galuszka 1963, Coblenz 1971, Bukowski 1974). It is agreed that such a function is far more likely than any origin in distant commerce or the control of valuable raw materials (Coblenz 1971). The emphasis on defences is no longer reasonably to be ascribed to a mythical confrontation between Bronze Age 'empires' of continental Europe (Lausitz being one! - cf. Gimbutas 1965, and contra, Coles and Harding 1979); "supra-regional political events were not the reason for their construction, but the tension that arose between individual groups in the process of societal evolution" (Coblenz 1971). Behind the central place emergence is demographic pressure creating the need and scope for higher organizational levels of people and settlements. Further proof of the indigenous and localized roots of the Lausitz phenomenon is the oft-cited empirical observation of the varying times of emergence and submergence of the population climax and florescence of Burgen (cf. Coblenz 1974, Bukowski 1974).

Despite this seemingly self-sufficient explanation of the development of Lausitz, the sheer impressiveness of the defended foci has caused local archaeologists to wobble at the knees at the work of mere barbarians, so remote from the Mediterranean civilizations. While recognizing the dominant indigenous forces behind the expansion of settlement and rise of regional foci, some scholars clearly cannot accept that the local populations were capable of such highly-organized proto-urban layouts, and have recourse to a civilizing influence from the Mediterranean. The planned cities of the Etruscans are taken as the model, transported hither in some vague way along with the occasional tangible long-distance import (Ostoja-Zagorski 1974). One authority, however, feels emboldened enough to state: "on suggère même la possibilité d'un séjour de petits groupes d'Etrusques en Poméranie et en Grande Pologne" (Niesiolowska-Wedzka 1976). Apart from the quite incidental nature of Mediterranean imports into Northern Europe throughout this period, the pressing need to seek diffusionist explanations for monumental activity in prehistoric Europe has been effectively demolished (Renfrew 1973).

The human ecology of the Lausitz Culture is a subject of great importance, but regrettably, the challenging and promising models that are published tend to lack precise data to test them. One model demonstrates a match of foci to the best soils, whilst another claims that soil quality is no determinant of their location (Galuszka 1963, Bukowski 1971, Ostoja-Zagorski 1974, Bukowski 1974). Some interpretations seem to take the present landscape for purposes of locational analysis, others argue that much change has occurred in soil conditions since the first millennium BC (Ostoja-Zagorski 1976). The view that overuse of arable and grazing land precipitated the collapse of Lausitz has to be set alongside calculations that known population densities could have been nourished from a fraction of the established polity territory (Ostoja-Zagorski 1976, Henneberg and Ostoja-Zagorski unpubl., Piontek and Kolodziejski 1981). If one can attempt to thread one's way through these contradictions and describe some general features of the environment and subsistence, one may note that the major sites (foci) and satellites are particularly associated with the lakeside and valley soils and with the more fertile medium to light soils of the surrounding land. Further out there are often extensive areas of poorer soils. It is generally argued that garden culture or at least intensive farming/gathering/lush grazing was carried out on the immediately accessible lake/valley soils, with dry farming of cereals on the better parts of the surrounding land. Woodland, or open grazing, characterized the extensive poorer and more distant land ascribed to the 'cell' (and hunting and gathering), though it seems that satellites well away from the focus would tend to be associated with localized areas of more fertile land (Bukowski 1974, Ostoja-Zagorski 1974, 1976). The impression of potential overuse of land comes from the study of the core area of each cell, the land immediately around the focus, which may also contain a number of satellite sites within a few kilometres' radius or less. The converse viewpoint, stressing the

great extent of the cell in comparison to the area of land required to support the estimated contemporary population, rests instead on the low number of known rural sites to exploit the extensive lands beyond the immediate focus hinterland. It is possible to reconcile these contrary impressions, if we argue that archaeological recovery of small rural sites has been at a very low level due to their scanty traces; the phenomenal number of cemeteries, which should represent a considerable extramural population, supports this suggestion. (For comparison, we might cite a statistic from our own field-by-field, intensive survey in Greece, where the density of **visible** surface sites representing small farms of the first millennium BC is some 30 times that recorded by modern extensive surface surveys, and we estimate that only three fifths of the original number of such farms has survived as a surface feature.) The inhabitants of the central focus would have concentrated their own subsistence activity within an area up to 5kms. out from their base (Vita-Finzi and Higgs, 1970), an area where there is frequently evidence of rural habitation sites and cemeteries (Ostoja-Zagorski 1974, Bukowski 1974). A population seeking to feed itself well below carrying capacity within such a radius, and of the order of 1,000 or more, might well be considered as pushing environmental constraints, with soils of such varied quality and 'resilience' (cf. Ostoja-Zagorski 1976, Henneberg and Ostoja-Zagorski unpubl.) If one were to suggest that the major part of the 'cell' attached to each focus, that land too distant from the focus to be considered easily exploitable from it, was filled with rural farms and hamlets at a far denser level than hitherto recovered, though consistent with the hints of rural cemeteries and the remarkable packing of the Burg settlement, then one might return to the hypothesis that a reasonable argument for land pressure in the Burg micro-region could be extended provisionally to the remainder of the cell centring on this focus (cf. Piontek and Kolodziejski 1981 for supporting data). Such an argument would fit in with the evidence for colonization of the more striking marginal lands of this part of Europe by the Lausitz (especially the uplands), and with the very wide range of resources being tackled (Gedl 1976, Coblenz 1971, Ostoja-Zagorski 1974).

Considerations such as these lead one to take seriously the frequent suggestion that the striking collapse of the Lausitz Culture phenomenon is not to be ascribed to external attack, but to a fundamental breakdown in the human ecology of these communities. The parallels to contemporary and earlier examples of cultural disjunction, where an ecological factor may be considered a strong possibility (cf. earlier this chapter, and my Neolithic chapter, this volume), reinforce the significance of Tringham's general model for European prehistoric development (cf, Neolithic chapter), and my own (1982) model along similar lines for agrarian cycles in Aegean prehistory and history. In addition to the elements noted above for the Lausitz, one may also observe that many features of the Lausitz distribution are closely paralleled by local Roman period and Medieval settlement patterns, considered to be very intense exploitation phases, the latter indeed over-extended as in much of Europe (Ostoja-Zagorski 1974). Ostoja-Zagorski (1974, pp.139-40) argues that the potential for over-exploitation is strongly suggested by the data available, especially if internecine warfare weakened the strength of the subsistence economy (many foci are 'destroyed' more than once before final abandonment or depopulation, and the effort of defences presupposes a consistent security threat): "the demographic density of the Lusatian culture tribes, noticeable especially at the decline of the Bronze Age and the Hallstatt period, was probably disproportionate to their technical abilities concerning the management of crops during fertile and poor harvests as well as the ability to prevent various epidemic diseases. It seems, that when the concentration of Lusatians in fortified settlements exceeded a certain permissible level there occurred a sudden catastrophe which resulted in a significant decrease in the population number, or even in a complete depopulation of certain regions".

The evidence for the actual collapse of the Lausitz Culture is clear cut. All the major Burgen are either totally abandoned or reduced to small open settlements; very frequently there is an associated destruction level (Bukowski 1971, Ostoja-Zagorski 1974). Although other small sites go on into the succeeding period, in some areas virtually all traces of settlement vanish at this time. This rather undermines one detail of the model of Henneberg and Ostoja-Zagorski (unpubl.) where over-exploitation of the land round the Burgen causes the mere dispersal of the inhabitants into the surrounding landscape, allowing equal numbers of people to exist in a more evenly balanced pressure on available land. Pollen also suggests depopulation (Gedl 1976). The Lausitz cultural assemblage gradually becomes transformed into the unimpressive Pomeranian Culture, without centres, or the intrusive cultural repertoire of La Tène B (Coblenz 1974, Ostoja-Zagorski 1976). However, as stressed earlier (cf. Rajewski 1974) both the rise and fall of the Burgen, and of their associated dense rural populations, happen at different times in different regions of the vast Lausitz sphere. Most of the Burgen fall out of use after Hallstatt C, c. 600 BC, or on the threshold to La Tène, in the fifth century BC (Rajewski 1974, Coblenz 1974, Gedl 1978).

Apart from the ecological factor and/or internal debilitating warfare between the individual foci, an additional element often cited is raiding by the Scythians from their foothold in south-east Europe (Rajewski 1974). We have already had reason to restrict the scope of the Scythians in the case of East Hallstatt, and most Lausitz authorities consider the potential role of Scythian incursions to be either absent/minimal, or merely contributory to a more fundamental internal breakdown of the Lausitz system (Bukowski 1971, 1974, Ostoja-Zagorski 1974, 1976, Coblenz 1974, Rajewski 1974).

In conclusion, we may consider the development of a centralized settlement system and inferred socio-political elaboration, within the Late Bronze Age and Early Iron Age of North-Central Europe (Lausitz sphere), as an independent manifestation of the internally evolved complex society, to set in parallel to similar processes behind the florescence of Hallstatt society and other regional developments in later prehistoric Europe (e.g. at Zavist). Small 'polities' arise as a result of a dramatic rise of population, acting as centres of servicing and control; the life support system for remarkably dense settlement rests on an arguably over-extended wide-based economy (cf. the Nandris (1976a, 1980) 'Climax Economy'), whose long-term weakness may well have led to the collapse of the complex superstructure of 'towns' and an inferred managerial elite. Finally, the territorial scale of these 'polities' deserves comment (Fig. 5). They fall between the major hillfort territories of the Late Bronze and Early Iron Age (ten kilometres radius or so; Figs. 1, 2), the territories of archaic city states (e.g. those of Boeotia, of a similar scale; Fig. 3), and the large princedoms of West Hallstatt (some tens of kilometres radius, average 40kms.; Fig. 4). In concentration of population within the focus, they may well surpass all these parallels, although the larger West Hallstatt 'cells' probably included more than one population centre in their considerable territory. It is here argued that the broad similarity between these developments reflects the independent operation of similar processes, with the emphasis firmly on population growth, changing patterns of land use, and adaptive and opportunistic managerial developments in the socio-economic sphere.

Note 63
This area was densely settled during the Late Bronze Age and Hallstatt Culture era (1100-500 bc), and forms in many respects a naturally bounded settlement unit or 'Siedlungskammer' (girdled by sand zones and major river depressions). Appropriately its cultural content at this time shows strong internal homogeneity and distinctiveness from neighbouring regions; this justifies the recognition of a unique 'Seddin Culture', so-named after a strikingly rich 'King's Grave' at a central point of the region. But there is in fact a whole series of unusually rich and elaborate burials at separate locations within the settlement unit. As for settlements, those about which details are available include farms and small villages (e.g. Perleberg). The majority of burials would seem to conform to contemporary European-wide urnfield, flat grave, practice, but there is a significant minority of other burial forms which are associated with almost all the indications for wealth and status individuals. But since all belong to the same overall culture and there is a general continuity throughout the region over time, and all burial variants inter-penetrate geographically, it is most likely that the different forms of burial mark status distinctions between members of the same society.

The lowest status group in this Seddin society is argued to be those buried in the flat graves; metal objects are rare and are small pieces that were probably the end-product of much recycling. Within these cemeteries there appear small numbers of Bell Graves and Stone Cist Graves; they are more elaborate affairs, and generally have a more generous gift assemblage. It is suggested that they may represent a low-level of authority ('big man', clan head, headman of a small district?). The true governing elite are identified with the tumulus cremation burials. These appear to be concentrated into three separate clusters within the Seddin micro-region, and are set apart from the flat grave cemeteries. Since they are basically contemporary in use, and share a common burial format, it is suggested that we have here three distinct territorial centres each with its own elite core group. The tumulus clusters contain variable gifts, from low or absent offerings through reasonably wealthy to mounds whose form and contents place them alongside some of the most impressive burials of Bronze Age Europe. Allowing for the reasonableness of the argument that tumulus burial in itself within this cultural context may represent a higher status than wealthy burials within the other types of burial, it may be claimed that the ranking within the class of tumuli reflects status amongst the regional elite. In any case, with tumuli containing offerings, the gifts found place their occupants in a very different social sphere from other types of grave. Metal objects are far commoner and tend to be larger and more complex artifacts; there is also a symbolic aspect, with weapons featuring prominently. In Hallstatt C, the wealthiest graves introduce the exotic Hallstatt Culture prestige kit of horse harness. This latter, richest group of graves also sees the most elaborate burial chambers. The Seddin King's Grave e.g. had a stone corbelled vault, and walls that were carefully plastered and decorated in multi-colour paint. Unusual types of pottery vessel, made locally, and imports of pottery and metal, are found in these tumuli, contrasted to the offerings in flat graves, which are household artifacts of local manufacture, generally showing signs of wear.

In summary, Wüstemann (1974) considers that within the Seddin microregion a warrior aristocracy arose in the Late Bronze Age and persisted until a dramatic collapse at the threshold to the La Tène era. The contemporary social structure of at least three major status/power levels, and lesser subdivisions, is demonstrated from the burial evidence, and geographical factors point to three contemporary aristocratic foci within the Seddin region.

At this stage he reminds us of Sprockhoff's interpretation of the same data. He saw the Seddin King's Grave as the burial of the ruler of the whole Siedlungskammer, who rose to such eminence because he "controlled passes" ... "he gained economic and political power, for which the surrounding land offered otherwise no basis". Wüstemann rightly finds such a sweeping hypothesis without foundation and quite anachronistic in its assumptions, and reminds us that it is a characteristic of the Central European Bronze Age to witness the sporadic appearance in time and place of enhanced social stratification. Such phenomena underline the fundamental importance of local factors, even though internal and external elements naturally interweave as the elites extend their contacts beyond their region of origin. Although, therefore, the Seddin Culture sees its leaders deploying exotic finery "the outer forces on Seddin social development can only have been secondary - and primary would have been the local economy and the possibility of wealth accumulation on an enlarged surplus". The military role can also be over-estimated, as there is little beyond the burial symbolism to point to regular hostilities affecting the Seddin population.

It is possible to add some comments on the rise and fall of the Seddin Culture, from additional examination of the data presented by Wüstemann. The number of flat cemeteries and rich tumuli rise to a peak from the early to the late phase of the Late Bronze Age, and this peak is largely sustained through the Hallstatt Culture era; by the full Early Iron Age of La Tène times (fifth century BC), the tumuli and flat cremation cemeteries have disappeared or seriously declined in number, indicating a clear breakdown of the Seddin socio-political tradition. In Wüstemann's analysis, the internal driving force would have been disrupted, and he mentions the changeover to iron and possible climatic shifts as relevant to this breakdown. The region is not a very fertile one for prehistoric agriculture, and one may well wonder whether the rise and fall of cemetery evidence at all levels may not reflect a broader fluctuation in population and settlement density, which would introduce the question of a cycle of extensive-intensive-extensive agriculture spanning the rise and fall of the Seddin Culture and its elite superstructure. But whether we consider human ecology as a promising explanation, or other causes, the basic thesis of Wüstemann seems supported by the available data, i.e. that this small scale florescence is internal in its origin and development. A soil decline and/or climatic change explanation for the collapse of this cultural phenomenon would also be internal, but the spread of iron-using to replace bronze is more complex. One of Wüstemann's suggestions is that the local elites, who had risen to power by controlling local surpluses of food and labour, were able to control population with bronze weapons and their special access to precious bronze for tools; with iron-using arriving on a large scale, local resources would make metal accessible to all, with far-reaching consequences in terms of warfare and trade dependence - hence perhaps the loss of power by the Seddin elites. The difficulty here is that supplies of bronze to the vast bulk of the population appear to have been so meagre that it is hard to imagine they had any vital effect on local agriculture; the suggested population rise of the Late Bronze Age may well have had more to do with crop and cultivation improvements of this era. In most other areas of Europe the arrival of iron tended to have the reverse effect, of stimulating socio-political development to even greater elaboration (as with the Hallstatt sphere or Lausitz, as analyzed earlier). Obviously the definitive answer demands far more research on the settlement sites of the culture, and ecological investigations, but we might suggest that the rise and fall of the Seddin phenomenon provides a further example of the temporary achievement of a higher level of political structure in later prehistoric

Europe, failing to be sustained due to local 'managemental failure' (over people and resources).

Note 64
Denmark is divided into five basic regions on eco-geographic grounds, and the data base comprises the massive total of prehistoric burial mounds recorded by parish for the country (and in particular, the great numbers from Periods 2 -6 of the Bronze Age, c. 1500-500 bc). It is closely argued that the density and distribution of burials is a function of the relative fertility of each major region, and of each individual parish within it. But since burial sites for Period 1 are artificially low this period is generally ignored, and likewise Periods 5 and 6 are amalgamated to boost sample size; finally we are left with c. 1000 graves per unit in order to compare the distributional features of Periods 2, 3, 4, and 5/6.

From all surviving evidence, including burials, it is clear that from the transition Middle/Late Neolithic, there is a marked expansion of settlement numbers and distributional area, both in Denmark as over much of North West Europe. Palaeoecological studies suggest that very considerable areas of the landscape, including now much marginal land, were quite clear of woodland and were given over to arable/grazing. Particularly striking is the great colonization during the Corded Ware phase of the poorer sandy soils of western Jutland, associated with major clearance in the pollen and palaeosol record. This is at a time when the more fertile east of Jutland had already largely become a heavily cultivated/grazed, open landscape, and the evidence should reflect population pressure (neatly parallel to Late Neolithic expansion onto marginal land elsewhere e.g. in Britain). Initially the great overall increase of population and the easing of pressure on older cultivated lands may have nourished a short-lived era of surplus production and the rise of more complex social systems of chiefdom type; surpluses for exchange and the prestige needs of an emergent elite stimulated a thriving import of bronze from the south and precious metals. This period of general florescence broadly lasts till the end of Period 3 (c. 1100 bc, or early in the traditional Late Bronze Age), when settlement retraction becomes the dominant trend. "The economic growth in western Denmark was seen to have been accompanied by political and commercial expansion, including south western Norway and north Germany, and this might have been on the point of transforming the system into a more centralized direction. This was blocked, first of all by the constraints imposed by the economy, but perhaps also by political counteraction" (Kristiansen 1978, p.177). The economic constraints were inherent in the short-term advantage but long-term disadvantage of the massive intake of poorer soils that characterizes the earlier Bronze Age of Denmark. Already not long after clearance, these sandy soils, deprived of protective woodland, began to be transformed from semi or full brown earths to acid soils, and the process of creating the typical present day heathlands of west Jutland had begun. As the Bronze Age progresses, the deterioration of these marginal lands becomes so severe that they are largely abandoned, settlement pulling out completely or nucleating into those districts best able to continue to provide a reliable subsistence base. The physical decline of the soil and the disappearance of cultivation or maintained pasture indicators can be closely followed from palaeoecological investigations. In contrast to the retraction and abandonment of settled land in west and central Jutland, the richer more resilient soils of east Jutland and the Islands permit much greater stability of settlement and subsistence, although even here, over the Bronze Age, continued over-reliance on land first opened up in early Neolithic times leads to a noticeable encroachment of impoverished heathland and similar signs of ecological crisis for local mixed farming populations.

"Thus we can observe that by the end of the Bronze Age the whole of western Denmark was experiencing a growing economic crisis, characterized by deteriorating ecological conditions of reproduction resulting in diminished yields, denser populations" due to population contraction into the best land "and restricted possibilities of geographical expansion. As this is paralleled by decreasing consumption of bronze and increasing isolation we are inclined to believe that local economic development was crucial for establishing those exchange networks through which bronze flowed. When expansion and economic growth was blocked by the constraints of the system (which were altered during that process) the exchange network fell apart and the flow of bronze was reduced proportionately" (op. cit. pp.177-8). As for the more fertile zones of south and east Denmark, despite serious pressure on them: "Due to their higher PP (productive potential) these zones were able to maintain a stable economy without significant changes throughout the Late Bronze Age", and therefore continue to show wealth concentrations and princely graves (op. cit. p.178). In general, Kristiansen suggests that in the fluctuations of settlement and the finds of bronze "local economic changes may have played a decisive role" (p.169). The cycle identified (which will be repeated in the Iron Age with renewed expansion into the marginal zones, he refers to as one of 'evolution' and 'devolution': "As evolutionary we term a development towards centralisation and wealth accumulation whose primary base was a significant increase of absolute surplus probably implying a growing dominance of vertical relations" (i.e. social hierarchy)." As devolutionary we term a process where the functioning of a social system leads to a degradation of the conditions of production resulting in diminishing returns, a blocking of political and geographical expansion which ultimately may alter social and political relations" (pp.178-9).

During the local 'Later Bronze Age' (c. 1100-500 bc and equal to the latter part of the traditional Late Bronze Age and the Hallstatt Culture era), the general decline of bronze imported from the south is accompanied by a great change in deposition away from burial display and towards deposition in hoards. This has generally been interpreted as reflecting a breakdown in elite display behaviour towards more communal ritual deposition (cf. also Levy 1978) as a result of the collapse of the economic power base of the Bronze Age chieftains. It is a phenomenon naturally most clearly marked in west Jutland, but is also widely evidenced in the less noticeably weakened economies of the east of Denmark.

Overall, both Kristiansen and Randsborg (1974a, b, c; 1982) demonstrate that the phase of expansion gives rise to more elaborate political structure in Denmark, marked by increased signs of social stratification in burial and a steady import of exotic metals (which are concentrated in elite burials and commonly represent elite equipment). The ecological miscalculation, probably stimulated by demographic pressure in the old settled lands, that encouraged colonization en masse of marginal zones, led eventually to a forced abandonment or severe contraction of settlement into the more resilient lands. Kristiansen argues that no great change in population size occurred, rather that the settlers were forced to retreat into narrow patches of better land in the west and their origin lands in the east. This poses some difficulties. Firstly one would like to know how the compressed populations managed to improve local productivity to cope with far higher densities, especially when even the best lands of the east are being eaten into by heathland. Secondly, do the population data support a constant overall figure for Denmark for each phase? The answer to the first point is that no evidence has been forthcoming for improved land use. To the second one may question whether the burial data may not indicate a significant population fluctuation.

This latter point is, however, bedevilled by the range of dates given for the duration of the individual Bronze Age periods to which the burials are assigned. However, if we adopt the chronology of Coles and Harding (1979), we find that the c. 1000 graves per Periods 2-4, and the same for 5/6 together, may actually correspond to time periods of unequal length (i.e. 300, 100, 200 and 400 years respectively). Converted to graves per century, we find that the inferred population ratios would run as follows: 4:12:6:3. It does seem rather striking that this suggestion of a dramatic rise and fall of population should correspond exactly to the great expansion and retraction of settlement in Denmark. One may, therefore, with the chronological doubts hindering closer definition, put forward the alternative view that the forced retraction of settlement led to a real decline in overall population in Demark, and only thus could the surviving fertile lands sustain their general level of population throughout the centuries of pressure.

Not unexpectedly, the traditional lure of the 'Mediterranean Connection' proves irresistible, despite the extreme remoteness of any cultural linkage. Rumblings from the East Mediterranean and the Mycenaeans make a curious appearance in the midst of Kristiansen's otherwise well-argued analysis of what is clearly a locally confined sequence. The collapse of the Mycenaeans is seen as in some oceanic wave effect to have its repercussions on the Baltic coasts, furthering the stress on end-second millennium bc societies in Denmark. Likewise, the stress is kept up when a revived Greece puts out West Mediterranean colonies which divert Hallstatt Europe's attention from the bronze needs of their former Nordic trade partners. Needless to say, it does not seem required of us from the local data to resuscitate Montelian fantasies to account for the development cycles of Scandinavia, where accumulating research is providing us with far clearer processes at work on a regional level.

The inception of the full Iron Age in Denmark provides a new motor to drive the cycle into motion again, the widely available metal powering a renewed land intake especially into heavier clay lands in eastern Jutland. Additional agricultural improvements are argued to be linked to major landscape enclosure, and manuring and grazing control within the new, carefully-run field units. Pollen evidence shows widespread clearance, including reclamation of heathland. The impoverished west Jutland is resettled. However, in the late second century BC, the rising imperial power of Rome is seriously threatened by a major migration of Cimbri and Teutons, of whom at least a major part have been argued to have originated in Jutland. Allowing for the customary exaggeration of the size of the migrating tribes, their full community status (warriors and families) and intention to conquer and settle are well attested, and seem to point to a remarkable population surplus, if not renewed land shortage by this time. Kristiansen (1978, p.182) notes that the Iron Age population expansion, especially into the poorer land of west and north Denmark, reached the level of nineteenth-century reclamation, and was clearly an impossible long-term strategy: "This reflects a severe population problem, accelerated by the impossibility of expansion, which ultimately had to release a migration ... the Teutonic and Cimbric people". However, either by this colonial experiment, or further improvements in agricultural productivity and social reorganization of production, the period from the first century BC to the fourth century AD is characterized by strong evidence for elite wealth concentration (based on land control), with putative chiefly residences in villages, and rich burials (Kristiansen's 'Fürstengrabgesellschaft' or princely grave society). Randsborg includes a warmer climate in the factors favouring a regional florescence during Roman Iron Age times.

194

Kristiansen includes north Germany in his Late Iron Age revival and upward movement in the demographic-agrarian cycle. The eventual dramatic decline of this region of Northern Europe after this new false dawn of expansion, has been superbly analyzed in the settlement history of the island of Sylt, off the west coast of Jutland (Kossack et.al. 1974), where the roots of the Dark Age are exposed.

In a more recent discussion of the period (1982), concentrating on social change, Kristiansen continues to demonstrate the primary role of agricultural surpluses and ecological crises in the Danish sequence from Early Neolithic to Late Pre-Roman Iron Age. Neolithic chieftains are evidenced in megalithic and earthen barrows which "gradually developed from single chiefly burials of big chiefs to local territorial cult places for ancestor worship and burial places of chiefly lineages" (p.258) "The economic basis of these territorial chiefdoms lay in the high productive potential of the former forest soils" (p.259). As settlement expands in the later Neolithic and Early Bronze Age onto poorer lands, a new kind of chiefdom is supported - theocratic chiefs tied to a monopoly over long-distance exchange networks, and inhabiting sizeable longhouses. Despite this seeming allegiance to the prestige-good model, we are then told: "However, population density and the distribution of wealth generally reflect the productive potential of larger areas" (p.265). It is indeed the agricultural collapse and crisis of the Later Bronze Age that creates, and is symbolized by (rather than caused by) the disruption of external exchange networks, a state of affairs that Kristiansen has to admit in his hedging commentary: "Although economic constraints imposed by the transformation of the environment quite evidently created barriers to the functioning of the social system, and thus seem to have determined both the decline of Early Neolithic territorial chiefdoms and Bronze Age theocratic chiefdoms, it is worth reflecting on the fact that culmination periods ... correspond to periods of international exchange" (p.268).

Note 65
After the great Early Iron Age (Hallstatt/Early La Tène) florescence of fortified centres in continental Europe (princely seats or less complex hillforts), there is a marked trend towards the abandonment of most of these sites in favour of smaller undefended settlements or small defended sites with easy access to their rural supportive landscape. Already the core Early La Tène area with its traditional princely burials is accompanied by the latter types of settlement (with the Champagne area marked by small open sites, the Rhineland by small defended sites; cf. Bretz-Mahler 1971, Schindler 1974). The Middle La Tène era forms over wider areas a striking interval before the Late La Tène era when the landscape once more begins to be controlled from major fortified foci (cf. Nash 1978). Not surprisingly the widespread disappearance of the very numerous hillforts of the early Iron Age centuries, or their replacement in some areas (e.g. Britain) by isolated foci with larger territorial interests (cf. above, note 12) can create the illusion of depopulation, as over much of Europe field survey is in its infancy and generally the well-known sites are hillforts. A period characterized by smaller sites - open villages, hamlets and farms - may well remain poorly known unless more intensive survey or complementary evidence becomes available. We would therefore revise traditional interpretations of apparent settlement hiatuses recorded between Early and Late La Tène in the Mosel, Saar and Reichenhalle regions (Menke 1971, 1972), and elsewhere. Fortunately, the typical mature La Tène flat inhumation cemeteries of Central and Eastern Europe are increasingly being linked to closely adjacent settlement sites. The prevalence of small communities is underlined by this pairing, as almost all Celtic cemeteries analyzed appear to represent a mere two to three families in the contem-

porary community. The distance between cemetery and settlement, also on a predictably small scale, is of the order of a few hundred metres. The individual communities lie densely across the landscape at intervals of a few kilometres. Similar evidence comes from the French La Tène cemeteries and settlements (cf. in general Lessing and Kruta 1979).

Despite this evidence for a dense population carpeting continental Europe at a farm-hamlet level, the existence of low-level ranking in the cemeteries and rarer but consistent finds of higher ranking burials, point towards the continuing existence of district headmen/chiefs, and in some areas, more notable families or individuals. Where hillforts continue, but with a reduced presence, one may suggest the activity of such co-ordinating elites, but elsewhere one must look much closer at the patterning and nature of the rural communities for signs of rank and specialization. John Collis in particular is constantly reminding us that local foci do not have to be based on hillforts, and we have already seen in the work of Haerke and others that elites may reside in rural 'estate' sites not much larger or more notable than the farms and hamlets of the peasantry - even more indistinguishable before excavation. We shall look in more detail at putative elite 'proto-villae' later, but examples that may belong to this class can be assigned to the Middle La Tène age. More interesting perhaps is Collis's model of proto-urban agglomerations consisting of several closely spaced rural sites, each in itself seemingly no different from the typical hamlet/village of the flat cemetery diaspora, at least until excavation. At Aulnat, in south-central France, a cluster of rural sites seems to combine a primary mixed farming role in their fertile lowland environment with a very broad range of industrial and craft activities. Increasingly, exotic imports appear, and eventually by Late La Tène the scale of this specialization and finds of coin moulds seem to indicate both the presence of elite individuals and a regional service role for this partially dispersed, rurally-embedded focus. In other words, many of the functions of a town may have been exercised, though on a smaller scale of production and for a smaller dependent region, by such Middle La Tène foci: "These villages would seem to be primarily agricultural, but also partly industrial, as though industry had not yet been centralized at this period" (Collis 1980, p.46). Craft specialisation includes working in bronze and iron, precious metals (gold and silver), glass, coral, bone and possibly pottery (Collis 1982). Collis describes a number of further examples of possible Middle La Tène (La Tène B/C) rural agglomerations that seem to act as similar foci, some of which are transformed or transferred into genuine nucleated enclosed sites or 'oppida' in the revival of fortified foci in Late La Tène (e.g. Breisach, Basel in the Upper Rhine, Macon and other sites in the Saône region, and Levroux near the Massif Central). The imposing true 'town' of Late La Tène Manching in Bavaria has some similarities to this group, in that it commences with two Middle La Tène cemeteries close to each other and commanding a fertile plateau. By the transition to Late La Tène the settlement has been transformed from two putative hamlets to a large nucleated community, which during the final pre-Roman La Tène era reaches truly urban proportions (though still apparently reserving major parts of the enormous defended plateau for subsistence production) (cf. Collis 1973b, Krämer 1975).

Our earlier recognition of the continuing co-existence of putative, scaled-down elite residences **and** more socially-embedded, elite plus peasant, rural agglomerations finds especial relevance in Collis's most recent views on developments in the Aulnat region. It seems possible that **parallel** to the role provided by the Aulnat cluster, there exists a potential hilltop elite site at Corent in the same area (Collis 1982). Defended 'proto villa' rural sites of the local elite may indeed be hypothesized to form a major feature of continuity from the Bronze Age chiefdom society into that of the historic Celts with their landed wealth and clients inhabiting numerous rural estates.

It will be argued below that the native pattern of defended 'estate centres' and proto-urban dispersed foci may well be the most important and widespread form that La Tène central places take (even where the latter become enclosed within a giant defensive system as 'oppida'). The image of a genuine densely packed Celtic 'town' plan occupying the major part of a great enclosure may be an illusory conflation of quite exceptional instances (most notably Manching) and Celtic towns that post-date the Roman conquest and are inextricably tied to Imperial development and resettlement schemes. The synoecism of Aulnat and other small communities into the Gergovie oppidum, for example, now seems to belong to the latter category of urban creation (Collis 1982). Yet Collis still makes the case that within the mature La Tène development from the fourth to second centuries BC, the dispersed foci seem to grow in number and in their range of functions, often in overall size too, in many separate areas of the La Tène world. And parallel to the later group of more complex dispersed foci there begin to rise the first true Oppida, e.g. at Manching and in Czechoslovakia.

Note 66

Though we will argue that Iron Age foci were in general neither urban nor Mediterranean inspired, it is on the other hand undeniable that the immediate 'barbarian' hinterland of the Greek colonies in Provence was significantly influenced by colonial forms and habits of urbanization in its own development of a settlement hierarchy. Yet even here, the Greco-Roman trappings seem to decorate foci whose rise and function combines Mediterranean influence and a purely local dynamism akin to wider La Tène processes (Benoît 1975, Hatt 1976, Février 1975).

Note 67
OPPIDA AND LATE PRE-ROMAN IRON AGE URBANIZATION.
Particular attention has for long been focussed in Iron Age studies on the evidence for a major process of transformation of Celtic society during the final pre-Roman centuries, most clearly marked by the erection of impressive and extensive defence works around what are arguably regional 'central places' with political, economic and ritual functions that anticipate or fulfil 'tribal town' expectations. These sites or 'oppida' arise chiefly from the late second century BC onwards, in La Tène 3, with some late Middle Iron Age 'early starters' earlier in that century (Collis 1975, Lessing and Kruta 1979, Nash 1978). Links between this visible centralization and the development of more coherent tribal polities with a central government (as witnessed by Classical sources for this period), have been explored in the search for the processes that may give rise to primitive states, based on the belief that at least some regions of Late La Tène Europe were emergent states (cf. Nash 1975, 1978). We shall discuss this most important development in terms of a number of individual aspects fundamental to the rise and function of oppida within Celtic society.

1   Oppida Origins: Formal Consideration

We have already introduced the 'Aulnat Model' of Collis, where a cluster of minor rural sites includes a potential for regional servicing within the context of a primarily rural and agrarian-centred settlement pattern and economy (cf. above and Collis, 1979a). An alternative but related development is the minor rural site that grows at variable rates into a proto-urban community. One is here mindful of the question of scale and function, as the

assignment of very large defended areas to a class of 'densely occupied proto-towns' is very controversial and not well-supported by archaeological evidence (see below). Nonetheless, the Late La Tène era 'foci' of oppida type, whatever their true demographic status, can in several cases be shown to stem from an in situ or locally transferred process of settlement enlargement (of population and range of functions) (cf. Collis 1975, 1980, 1982 and supra). That most obviously 'urban' of oppida, Manching in Bavaria, represents an extreme example of this enlargement model, but Collis rightly warns us against using Manching (particularly because of its usefulness as a rare example of a recently dug oppidum) as any kind of model to aid us with less well known oppida: "too anomalous for a general model" (pers. comm.). With its very low-profile Middle La Tène village beginnings we are totally unprepared for the logarithmic growth that the settled area undergoes between 150 and 50 BC, and its internal layout is quite different from what details we have available from other pre-Roman foci (ignoring oppida layouts that are essentially post-Conquest, cf. note 65). A further model is provided by the continuity between Bronze Age and Hallstatt defended foci represented in the hillforts and putative elite rural foci (defended and undefended) of Early to Middle La Tène times. Although almost universally in La Tène Europe where chronology is precise, there is an apparent hiatus in hillfort usage in Middle La Tène times, (cf. above, and Collis and Ralston 1976), there are exceptional regions e.g. central Germany, Provence and Britain, where they continue, even if reduced in number. Less conspicuous noble 'manors' (cf. above) almost certainly provide an even more significant element of continuity in the Continental landscape for specialized foci of regional importance, despite their far less imposing appearance. They are likely to be a characteristic feature of the La Tène world from the Early phase, and may provide the basic building block of the layout, and function, of the oppida. From the hillfort and defended 'manor' traditions can be derived the complex stone, earth and timber defenceworks of the oppida (Collis 1975).

2   The Role of the Oppida

Nash succinctly summarizes the various functions for which there is good or substantial evidence (1978) : defended refuges in a bellicose society; the site of tribal (civitas) and local administration; market centres for regional and long-distance exchange (note concentrations of Mediterranean luxury goods, and locations often on major rivers); production centres for regional and long-distance distribution (note artisans' quarters and industrial debris, products specific to particular oppida, locations often near iron ores); residence of a tribal nobility. So far so good; but such an approach fails to tell us of the relative importance of these varied activities to the occupants of the oppidum and surrounding populations. We should for example be suspicious of a type of enclosed site, supposedly uniform in function, that can range from some tens of hectares in size up to Stradonice at 80ha., Manching at 380ha. and Kelheim at 600ha.! The Heuneburg supposedly fulfilled most of these roles at a mere 4.5ha., and its suspected 'territory' is certainly equal to that assignable to most oppida. Jan Filip exhorts us to be far more critical: the mind model of oppida is culled from a melange of hints from Caesar - he describes a number of Gallic foci under rather specific if not peculiar political and military conditions. From this scholars derive a picture of communities more or less urban, with dense populations, developed craft production and an emphasis on local raw materials. However, such a model is hardly to be generalized from (Filip 1978). Rather, considering the oppida over a longer time range, and as a Europe-wide phenomenon: "As a rule the oppida are found where there was a high density of population, well-developed production and changes in the socio-economic structure, and from this point of view they are sometimes compared to urban forms. **This is not generally valid"** (Filip, 1977, p.227; final emphasis the present writer's). To clarify Filip's rejection of urbanism and the Caesarian mind-model, specific functions attributed to oppida need to be carefully examined in turn.

Oppida as 'Towns': In various papers Collis has claimed that the oppida conform to broad expectations for Pre-Industrial towns, with marked class divisions in internal layout (the elite in courtyard houses, the proletariat in trading accommodation along street fronts). However, apart from 'exceptional' Manching, and some features of Czech sites, much of our evidence for such urban features is derived from post-Conquest layouts in France (Preidel 1978) and the wider-attested and probably more reliable examples of internal planning are very different from any historic town plan (cf. below), even if there are indeed status distinctions in style of accommodation. Collis also emphasizes craft production for the region. Once again, Manching (graphite ware) provides the best example, with a very widespread specialist distribution in Western Europe. Even here, though, Collis reminds us that trade in graphite wares is already important in Early La Tène times and it would be false to see the oppida as fundamental to such specialist activity (Collis 1973b). If one tries to link other oppida to long-distance or even major regional industrial or craft production and marketing, very few offer tangible evidence. Filip (1978) considers that Manching has only one possible parallel amongst the Czech oppida, Stradonice, as a significant production centre, the rest being quite different, and elsewhere he finds only Bibracte a further possible parallel (which is basically post-Conquest in this context). Additional support for urban industry is often sought from the frequent association of oppida with iron ore sources. This is after all the late Iron Age, and objective commentators remind us that iron ore is so widespread and plentiful in Europe and so fundamental to everyday life by this stage, that in every part of Europe now they expect all largish communities (i.e. from the village upwards) to be actively manufacturing their own tools (cf. Pleiner 1977). One really needs to ask whether iron ore in any particular region is so scarce that it needs 'protecting', or would control the location of the regional centre in preference to any other considerations. The logic of such assumptions is not apparent, and at one of the oft-cited examples, Kelheim, with ore sources actually within the great enclosed area, makes no serious sense (see below). Certainly the anachronistic approach exemplified in a recent paper on the Titelberg in Luxembourg (Thomas 1975), where the usual traces of craftwork and local iron ore are blandly and uncritically converted into a claim to have identified: "One of the first industrial towns to be established north or the Alps", cannot be taken seriously. Apart from the failure to demonstrate at any single oppidum that the normal source of 'income' came from 'industry', or 'commerce', (in fact our evidence tends to a very different conclusion,) we may merely remind ourselves that even in the Classical Mediterranean world, ancient historians regularly underline the vast gulf between the Industrial and Pre-Industrial city. Finley and others find the current evidence totally consonant with Hume's penetrating insight that "I do not remember a passage in any ancient author, where the growth of a city is ascribed to the establishment of a manufacture" (Finley 1973, p.22). Here and elsewhere (Finley 1977) the very limited role of industry and long-range commerce for the economic foundation of ancient towns is clearly exposed, in favour of a general model stressing regional administration, the residence of an elite subculture (whose income is derived from rural estates) and a broadly parasitic role on the region. Even the growth of urban trades and specializations is largely a phenomenon servic-

ing the urban populations themselves, paid for from rural incomes rather than any wealth generated by the town itself.

Another much-cited example of an 'industrial town' or even 'industrial state', is the Magdalensberg oppidum in the Austrian Alps near Villach, believed to be the centre of the kingdom of Noricum. Here there is good evidence for a Roman trading community in residence and intense local exploitation of a very high grade iron ore which was exchanged across the Western Mediterranean (Alexander 1980, Moosleitner 1980). But as Finley points out, such partial information about the Norican economy does not begin to justify Alföldy's model for Noricum: "the economic life depended on agricultural production, pastoralism, mining, industry - above all iron-smelting and metal-working - and trade" (Finley 1977, p.327).

Even at Manching, whose status as an urban site with strong commercial activity is the strongest, if isolated, those who promote its irrelevance to local agriculture avoid discussion of what use the major part of the vast enclosed area was put to, in the absence of settlement evidence. Of 380 ha enclosed, the core 'built up area' could be as small as a mere 80ha., although the excavators suggest a much larger proportion. But in any case, on all speculative reconstructions considerable empty space is discernible (Krämer 1975). Let us recall that the site began as a fertile lowland plateau, seemingly under cultivation from at least two smallish rural communities: they appear to amalgamate into a village central to the plateau, which grows into a true agglomeration of town proportions. Yet apparently much, if not most, of the defended area remained as mixed farmland exploited by our assumed 'industrialists and merchants'. If it be claimed that the defences merely follow the lie of the land, it much be answered that a similar pattern of farmland incorporation appears increasingly typical of lowland oppida, almost all of which have far smaller core occupation areas than Manching. Furthermore, the land is completely flat and the site layout **led** to stream diversion. Recently, John Collis appears to be moving away from earlier models where, for example, the developed Medieval town is classed as analogous to the oppidum. He admits that the evidence is growing that large tracts within oppida were open, unsettled land. Moreover, the commerce and industry centred on the oppida is no 'market trade' capitalist activity, but a strictly controlled sector of a broader centralized administration of each region by a dominant elite - 'administered trade', which is also centred on putative 'ports of trade' such as Hengistbury Head on the English Channel coast (Collis 1979a). Although this may seem a nuance of economic history, it is a far more fundamental step taking Collis into the 'Substantivist' fold of Weber, Polanyi and Finley. Rather than stressing the oppidum as a regional node of commercial exchange of imports and exports, marketing of cash crops locally etc., an abode of 'merchants' and 'craftsmen', the new emphasis concentrates on the centres as residences of a ruling elite, where they carry out a range of roles **including** the manipulation of local and long-distance exchanges. Might we not suspect that the true source of the economic wealth and political power of these elites, as in the Classical city, may lie more in the relationship of the oppidum and its nobles to the agricultural wealth and dispersed raw material sources of the large territory associated with the oppidum, than in the craft products made in, or trading shipments arriving in that defended focus?

Oppida as Regional Refuge Centres:

The visible strength of Late La Tène fortifications for lowland and hillfort oppida underlines the perceived aggressive atmosphere of the period over much of continental Europe. Moreover, the great extent of circuit typical for a large proportion of examples - together with the virtual absence (cf. above) of a truly 'urban' build-up of the defended interior, suggests that surrounding populations would probably have taken refuge within. This role is clearest with the giant oppida such as several south German examples in the hundreds of hectares range (Filip 1977). The fallibility of the 'defended iron ore' model is clearly shown in a recent study of the enormous oppida of Kelheim, a 600ha. enclosure beside the Upper Danube (Herrmann 1975). Firstly it is abundantly clear that no 'town' population ever occupied this rugged rock, on the surface indications. Secondly, there can be no logic in erecting a defencework that required a vast non-resident population to man, merely in order to defend iron ore veins or their miners, whilst the suggestion of a river-control point is likewise difficult to take seriously on this scale. By far the most reasonable role for the giant enclosed area is as a regional refuge and 'tribal' assembly point. That is not of course to deny the possibility of a permanent or semi-permanent small community within the enclosed area, perhaps of elite or general regional servicing status, and indeed evidence for such a settlement has been identified, **but** from an artificial extension of the line of defences into an adjacent tract of valley land (doubtless for easier access to farmland, the river and neighbouring communities).

Certainly if one looks carefully at the Classical references to Celtic foci described as 'oppidum', 'urbs', in context, they are very variable in their meaning, and analysis of Caesar's usage suggests that in a large number of cases a defended area with stores is being used by local regional populations as a temporary refuge centre, creating for us an apparent series of towns during the Gallic Wars (Preidel 1978). Even the recent claims of Stanford (1980) to have evidence for remarkably dense 'town like' build up of domestic structures within some Welsh Marches hill-forts, is seen by Collis as both exaggerating the scale of the archaeological traces and more likely to represent tiny shelters for military purposes (perhaps even 'age-set' exercises; Collis 1981a). The refuge factor is often raised as a prime mover in the setting up of a number of Late La Tène oppida in southern Bohemia, particularly as a response to the known threat to Celtic communities from the advancing Germanic groups (Filip 1977, 1978). One factor that is considered to point to an abnormal siting is the general absence of typical flat cemeteries in the hinterland of these oppida, as if they were often removed from natural concentrations of rural settlement for strategic reasons. However it has to be remembered that this form of burial, typical as it is for Middle La Tène times in much of Europe, virtually disappears in Late La Tène times in favour of shallow cremation burials that are far more difficult to spot and locate. But where findspots of the latter, new and far less impressive mode of disposal have been recovered, it is much more in agreement with the Late La Tène settlement pattern of Central Europe (Benadik 1977). The great oppidum of Zavist near Prague must also be mentioned, as it is in fact on the edge of a territory dense with burial sites of typical flat inhumation style. In general the role of the Czech oppida is likely to have been more than a mere 'bolthole', and regional servicing in terms of administration, elite residences and specialist concentration must be functions that not only require future testing but are suggested by the limited data already available (Collis 1976, Preidel 1978, Filip 1978).

Oppida as political 'central places':

As the list of major defended Late La Tène sites grows in number and the map of their distribution over continental Europe (cf. Cunliffe 1979, fig. p.64) resembles an almost uninterrupted network of points, it becomes increasingly

difficult to attribute those of any particular region as a specific historical response to events or factors of unique local relevance (e.g. the threat of Germanic invasions, the influence of Provence towns, or feedback from the settlement of Celts in the Po Valley alongside Mediterranean towns). These are merely secondary phenomena "welche die gleichzeitige Entwicklung der oppida und ihres Wirtschaftssystems in den westlichen und mittelöstlichen Gebieten nicht erklären können" (Lessing and Kruta 1979, p.84). The same infill of the map, seen on a regional level, is tending to produce networks of such foci at similar intervals across the landscape, seeming to form regular territorial cells or minor 'polities'. Despite the great stress put on the long-distance connections of Manching, it still fits confortably into the evenly-spaced pattern of oppida in southern Germany (Zürn 1977) (Fig. 6). Zürn's study of the Finsterlohr focus within this series successfully relates that centre to a dense rural settlement in the surrounding countryside, and points to an associated coin distribution that emphasizes the same link up between central focus and hinterland. Regular spacing recognizable between oppida elsewhere in Europe points to an identical process of crystallization out of a mosaic of smallish tribal/sub-tribal centralized 'polities' (cf. Motykova 1978 for Czech examples, Nash 1978 for central Gaul, Cunliffe 1976 for southern Britain). One looks forward to detailed analyses of the territorial network in other regions of Europe, such as, for example, Yugoslavia, where the well-established and flourishing settlement pattern of the Scordisci evidence a very dense population and a whole series of central, fortified sites of La Tène 3 date (Jovanovic 1981). It should no longer seem curious to record that the Scordisci are apparently little involved in Greco-Roman trade at this time.

Apart from these encouraging signs of a growing interest in the formation of centralized political units at a similar scale over La Tène Europe, one now expects the development of greater research interest into the dependent nature of these foci on well-populated and well-cultivated territories. Marshall's (1977) analysis of English La Tène 2-3 hillforts in the Cotswolds (including complex multivallate examples up to 49ha. in area) illustrates the potential of such work. The fertility of associated land proved to be correlated significantly with the scale of the fortified enclosure: "This relationship could reflect the interdependence of population distribution and agricultural potential of surrounding areas" (op. cit. p.352). Although the upper end of Marshall's hillforts is comparable in scale to many of the smaller European oppida, we consider that present evidence does **not** support any essential threshold between the large and giant oppida and the smaller foci that are still often referred to as hillforts for this period. One may indeed note that Suetonius refers to the 20 large and medium size hillforts of south western England that Vespasian had to reduce one by one, as oppida, and there seems no good reason not to view these sites, or a planned hillfort of medium size such as Danebury, as non-urban central places with a regional service and administrative role (Burnham 1979) - a model that suggests they are merely smaller-scale centres for 'polities' of smaller scale than the large 'oppida' of south eastern England and the continent (Fig. 1). In many respects it is these lesser foci that provide continuity with the less frequent manifestations of centralization and hierarchy we have observed in the Bronze and Copper Ages of Europe.

Two further points of importance develop from these last considerations. Firstly, if oppida arise to service population concentrations, why is their distribution not entirely regular across the landscape, like market-towns in some geographical model? We may begin to answer this point by recalling that regular networks of oppida **are** actually beginning to be recognized in several separate regions of

La Tène Europe. But it still seems clear, allowing for the continual increase in known oppida sites, that just as with the central places of Hallstatt Europe, there exist substantial regions where few if any major defended foci are to be recognized. A well-documented example is the clear dichotomy between south eastern Britain with a neatly patterned mosaic of oppida and the north and west where oppida are rare and even major hillforts are present in very variable density (cf. Cunliffe 1976, 1978; and Fig. 7). This contrast has encouraged the interpretation of oppida as the result of close cross-Channel influence on the south east, or even of waves of immigrants (despite the gross discrepancies between the archaeology and relevant historical sources). Peter Fowler brings a refreshingly different perspective to the problem (1978) by pointing out that south east Britain as a whole, or lowland Britain, due to its pre-eminent agricultural fertility, has formed the most developed and densely settled zone of Britain from as far back as Neolithic and Bronze Age times, and it is precisely here that we would expect to find a natural breeding ground for a new and higher level of central place and polity by the Late pre-Roman Iron Age. Whether the concept of the great, defended lowland oppidum was borrowed from across the Channel, or developed in parallel to the continent, is of little consequence, as it is the function of these foci and the regional socio-economic structure that they arose to serve that opens up our understanding of the phenomenon.

The second discussion point concerns the scale of the territory attached to an individual central place. As we have seen (Fig. 1), the rash of Early Iron Age hillforts frequently indicates smallish service areas that may be encompassed within some 5-10kms. radius from the focus. Obviously such distances and land area would not normally be intensively exploited from the site or vicinity of the focus itself, arguing for a series of satellite farms and hamlets (on this scale, based e.g. on the Danebury region (Cunliffe 1976), the equivalent of some four small villages in total for each hillfort cell). The hillfort would nonetheless be accessible in a mere one or two hours from the most outlying farm, allowing a day return with ease. A very large number of Greek city states existed on the same simple central place scale e.g. the cluster on Lesbos (cf. Fig. 3). Even in the final centuries BC and the first century AD, the smaller oppida and hillforts that appear in less centralized regions, or as subsidiary centres below a genuine great oppidum (cf. Nash 1978), will have operated on a similar scale. The overall population of focus inhabitants at such minor centres will not have produced such an intolerable burden on the immediate subsistence catchment of the focus that complex arrangements will have been necessary for food imports for the very survival of the focus. But when we move into the league of greater oppida, which seem to control very extensive territory or at least act as a key focus for such a region, and where permanently or temporarily a more populous community may exist, it is necessary to ask whether a steady flow of supplies would have been coming, often some distance and over very slow tracks. Nandris puts the case succinctly: "It is possible to argue that the Neolithic village is not a fundamental break between site and resource zone. It is related to the resource zonations of the surrounding environment in a way very similar to hunter/fisher sites. Oppidan/urban settlement does constitute such a fundamental break, in that in the town a greater population and a wider range of complex activities, specialisations and exotic materials, are being supported than could be done by any direct subsistence exploitation of the accessible surrounding resource zones" (1976, p.724). While acknowledging the validity of this model for certain oppidum sites, we must ask ourselves whether indeed the typical oppidum or larger hillfort was sufficiently populated that its subsistence needs could

only have been drawn from its extended territory. The answer at present would seem to be a firm 'no'. Firstly, as argued above, almost all known foci appear to stand out more in the range of activities than in the great size of their population. Exceptions such as Manching provide the only cases where the resources of districts well beyond the 'Danebury' day-return supply zone may have become essential for the day to day existence of the site. Let us remember that estimates of Medieval towns' external food support requirements call for the agricultural surplus of some ten villages, representing arguably a far smaller zone of surrounding settlement than many of the great oppida possess. If the oppidum territory is correlated to oppidum scale without the direct causative link of food needs, what is the essential connection between the total territory and the focus?

At this point one introduces what an eminent authority has argued to have been the role of the Mediterranean Classical town (Finley 1973, 1977): as the centre of elite residence and 'culture'; of corporate elite decision-making; of the craft workshops (that operate as much for elite prestige purposes as for regional everyday artifact production); of trade in and out of the territory (again as much for elite exotica as for more everyday items and materials). To this we must add, as we have seen, the function of a regional refuge point. For the development of Iron Age centres, therefore, as the links between district elites tighten, by treaties and inter-marriage for example, and tribal elites cohere into recognizable classes with common interests transcending local concerns, so the scope for the central focus grows in step with its expanding sphere of servicing. The scale of the centre and the size of its territory are indeed intimately related, but through the medium of those rural elites who in ever increasing numbers are identifying themselves with centralizing activity and a new subcultural life in such a distant focus. The process of amalgamation of innumerable district political units into a much larger mosaic of polities (cf. Renfrew's (1975) ESM model) as outlined here (and cf. Bintliff 1982) is in turn, and fundamentally, the result of pressures brought on by the new demographic and agrarian conditions of the Iron Age itself, as has been argued in detail at the beginning of this paper.

Oppida as residences of a landed nobility:

In the preceding sections we have suggested that the average oppidum can scarcely be considered as an industrial or merchant town, or any kind of urban nucleation in simple population terms. With few known exceptions (and most of these are doubtful), the picture that may be emerging is one of a network of regional defended central places, offering refuge and a rallying point to surrounding rural inhabitants, as well as a focus for regional political activity. Foreign trade seems to be especially concentrated at and perhaps controlled from these points, although this is likely to represent the greater wealth and exotic tastes of those permanently or temporarily resident there rather than a genuine 'disembedded' commercial free-for-all for the oppidum hinterland. The fundamental element in the rise and functioning of oppida could be the attraction to district elites of a focus for political aspirations and 'class interests', as well as a subcultural environment with international connections and an elite-dependent establishment of specialist craftsmen. We shall shortly turn to the overall reasons for locating the power and wealth of La Tène elites in land, but the very character of the archaeological traces within oppida leads us to an identical emphasis. The first aspect to stress is the basic model from which it seems likely most oppida developed: the Aulnat type of rural site or site-complex where the rise of specialist craftwork and long-distance trade grew out of firm roots in a mixed farming economy. Many oppida consist of vast expanses of lowland enclosed by complex defences, beyond which they dominate considerable resources of arable and grazing (we will be considering some outstanding examples in Britain). The very limited domestic traces, together with the elite associations of the finds, point us to the inference that the minority occupying the oppida would have been very much concerned with the surpluses available from surrounding and adjacent fields and pastures. Preidel (1978) comments on the evidence from a number of oppida for a domestic occupation sector comprising what appear to be large farm establishments of a wealthy class (e.g. Stare Hradisko, Hrazany), whose regional political power is reflected in their association with coin minting, and whose economic power is reflected in adjacent establishments of specialist craftsmen. It is at their command that great regional corvées of rural peasants have been drafted in to fill years of off-season work on the enormous and elaborate oppidum defence works. The great Zavist oppidum may likewise contain within its final La Tène ramparts a number of separate small settlements of a strongly farming nature linked by stone-paved roads. Aside from the usual evidence for craftsmen and minting, the household complexes have all the appearance of fenced off, sizeable farm establishments - appropriately distinct from non-oppidum parallels in their rich house fittings (Motykova 1978). Rather than mislead ourselves with clearly unsatisfactory analogues in Medieval towns (cf. Clark and Piggott 1965, Fig. 94) we would be better to follow Preidel in his parallel to Medieval manors. In general then, we are suggesting that the oppida represent either the relocation of elite estates into a more concentrated form on a defended hilltop, or even more clearly betraying the landed interest, a rural landscape which is merely 'enclosed' by giant ramparts and ditches but retains its embedded, country character.

Such a controversial interpretation nonetheless removes the necessity of a dramatic arrival of 'towns' in La Tène 3 Europe, and makes it less difficult to comprehend why there are large areas of Celtic Europe where characteristic oppida are less numerous or absent (cf. Filip, 1978 for Eastern Europe and Cunliffe, 1978 for the very uneven distribution throughout the British Isles). In these instances, there may well have existed a dense network of elite foci of the Aulnat type, or of the discrete defended estate unit type (cf. earlier discussion). These regions would appear to be lacking a single common centre for their inhabitants, or at least our putative elite foci lack the giant defenceworks that should distinguish one as preeminent for us. We may reasonably hypothesize that such regional communities are less far along the road to centralized polities.

Despite the suggestion of a strong interest in the immediate arable and pasture resources of the district surrounding or even partly enclosed by the oppidum, the scale of most oppida territories reflects the interaction of the oppidum and elites whose estates would be well beyond regular access from the regional focus. The south German network (Fig. 6) which includes the sparsely inhabited oppidum of Finsterlohr (Zürn 1977) offers a good example, and we may imagine that as oppida develop in size and range/scale of functions they are offering an alternative residence to an increasingly larger number of nobles.

At this point we can introduce the remarkable evidence from the British oppida (Fig. 7). Colchester/Camulodunum is by far the most impressive both in archaeological terms and in the hints of Classical sources: "In its heyday ... probably the most influential settlement in the country" (Crummy 1980c, p.43). With 15 miles of earthwork enclosing some 15 square miles of land (c. 4000ha.), the site provides a powerful clue to the degree of centralization and organisation amongst the south eastern

English tribe of Trinovantes for whom it provided a focus in the immediate pre-Conquest era. It has been known for some time that within this vast area of lowland landscape there were at least two areas of intensive occupation. Firstly a sector of domestic residence at Gosbecks, and then down by the river Colne with easy marine access, the Sheepen sector, seemingly more of an 'industrial' area with evidence of metalworking, potting, brick and tile manufacture and debris of a Celtic mint, as well as clear potential for reception and despatch of trade goods. The Gosbecks sector was poorly known, but had the intriguing honour of being the site of an extensive Roman sanctuary after the Conquest when the new Colonia town of the region was established nearby. But the details of the vast enclosed landscape were otherwise a mystery, apart from associated highly prestigious burials, allowing continued speculation about pre-Roman town life. However during the 1970s careful study of cropmarks, particularly under the unusual drought conditions, revealed at Gosbecks what appears to be a large defended homestead from which led a complex system of trackways and field boundaries; this agricultural landscape stretches across most of the southern half of the oppidum along the fertile land to the north of the valley of the Roman river. Taken with the evidence that even the Sheepen specialist community did not seem to be at all dense, the emerging picture of the site is of clusters of households dispersed amid a 'rural landscape' but all under the protective umbrella of the great dyke system (Crummy 1980a). "The convergence of the trackways and dyke systems suggests that the native farmstead was the site of the royal household or, put another way, that the oppidum was in pre-Roman days a royal estate, Gosbecks being its agricultural base set out on the fertile soil just north of the valley of the Roman river and Sheepen being its industrial and commercial centre based on water-borne transport via the river Colne. This is a major point which has wide implications generally ... However, if correct, the importance of the Gosbecks sanctuary is easy to understand since it would seem to have been based on a site not only sacred since pre-Roman times but also with dynastic associations for the Trinovantes" (Crummy 1980b, p.264). "This latest interpretation of Gosbecks ... prompts a radical reinterpretation of Camulodunum itself, namely that the entire settlement was in reality a huge private estate under royal ownership" (Crummy 1980c, p.45). The suggestion of an imposed defence system developed around a pre-existing 'manorial' estate agrees with the internal structures, which have clear parallels to open settlements elsewhere: "Only its size sets Camoludunum apart from other sites but not its various components". As for the dyke system: "There is no elegant plan here ... but rather a motley collection of earthworks each built to answer an immediate need and not much else" (Crummy, pers. comm. 1980).

A second major oppidum lies adjacent to the Roman town of St. Albans/Verulamium, at Prae Wood, forming the tribal focus for the Catuvellauni, western neighbours of the Trinovantes. Recent research (Hunn 1980) has identified an integrated dyke system at the site enclosing an area of over 140ha. Within this zone the layout seems to represent at least three homestead enclosures tied to field boundaries. One homestead in particular appears to be an early feature around which the total network developed, and has a double-dyke defensive perimeter. Nearby this sector of the site the evidence for a mint has been identified (Cunliffe 1978). The formal similarities to Colchester are clear, with the suggestion of an enclosed estate landscape with elite/tribal focus associations. Our knowledge of the oppida at Chichester and Silchester (cf. Cunliffe 1978) is tantalizingly scanty, but it is highly unlikely at either site that the dyke systems considered to be pre-Roman enclosed nucleated 'urban' foci. Chichester in particular, with a very extensive area of lowland landscape sealed off behind barrier dykes inland, and hints of a commercial shore sector at the coast, together with what looks very much like a series of internal land divisions, may form an especially close parallel to Camulodunum.

It is surely symptomatic of our changed conception of the tribal focus and the agricultural ties of Celtic elites even of the highest level, that a recently-discovered rural enclosure in East Anglia, north of the Colchester region, has been suggested as one of several sub-tribal focal centres for the first century AD Iceni tribe. The enclosure at Gallows Hill, Thetford, is not very large (4.5ha.), but impressively defended for its size. The triple rampart of the final phase, and a long 'ceremonial way' into massive gates, contributed to many miles of palisade fencing. Three domestic houses of the middle phase are of typical Iron Age farmhouse plan but are considerably larger in scale and detail. The overall impression is of the estate centre of a major elite community, yet conceived of as a greatly-elaborated version of a typical wealthy farm. The Iceni are known to have formed sub-tribal units or 'pagi' and it is suggested that Thetford and another recently discovered focus at Stonea Camp represent political centres for these districts (Selkirk 1981; T. Gregory, T. Potter, unpubl. research). Further evidence for dispersed elite foci is discussed in note 71, below.

Note 68

Nash's view, of the centralization into larger political units as a kind of resolution of internal pressures over resources and power, is echoed by Lessing and Kruta: "Zu Beginn des 2. Jahrhunderts verfügt die keltische Welt also über kein einziges ausreichendes Mittel mehr, um den Bevölkerungsüberschuss, die Ursache der Spannungen, abzubauen. Daraus entsteht ein je nach Region mehr oder weniger ausgeprägtes Ungleichgewicht, das der Durchführung des Strukturwandels der keltischen Gesellschaft einen besonders günstigen Boden bereitet. Ihr deutlichstes Zeichen ist das Auftauchen einer städtischen Formation einfächster Art, die gewöhnlich mit dem lateinischen Ausdruck oppidum bezeichnet wird" (1979, p.82). Here the internal tensions cannot be broken by external release as in the era of Celtic migrations, since neighbouring lands have now reached sufficient political and military development so that such predatory expansion is yielding to a reverse pressure from the expanding populations of Italy, and from the Germans and Dacians.

Although it has been customary to discuss Late La Tène coinage as the evidence for a Mediterranean-inspired shift towards a genuine 'market economy' in both the narrow and most general sense, the current consensus is very much removed from this position. Coins begin to be minted in the Celtic world in several major regions between Gaul and the Middle Danube around 200 BC and their role seems to have been to replace the use of gold in varied forms with a new form imitating the precious coin used to pay Celtic mercenaries in the Mediterranean. Yet the Celtic gold coins continued to act in the same context as is known for these Hellenistic mercenaries and as inferred for pre-coin Celtic gold circulation: to pay armed retinues and cement alliances.

We have most information about the development of native coinage in Gaul. Here the early series of the final third and of the second century BC are high value, precious coins, with very loose distributions for each type and usually inter-penetrating and overlapping distributional spheres. This pattern is seen as reflecting a very large number of rival district chiefs and the absence of regionally dominant authorities. Power is decentralized, and diffuse foci of authority are each represented by a 'trademarked' minor production of wealth items that are spread in irregular radii as gifts and payments for services, to allies and 'clients'. This interpretation (Nash 1978, 1981) is closely matched by the evidence we have discussed for pre-oppidum settlement patterns: "in the early phases of La Tène political and military authority was distributed over a multitude of petty chieftains" (Nash 1978, p.460). Tracing these 'petty chief' distributions to Middle and early Late La Tène rural foci has been increasingly successful (Collis 1981b).

During the La Tène 3 era, the rise of oppida as putative central places for larger and more centralized political units of tribal or sub-tribal groups, is accompanied by a corresponding shift in many regions to the production of only one or two types of precious coin within each area; issues of these more restricted types are larger in quantity, their distributions are well-defined and rarely overlap. Some of these coin zones can be related to the general area occupied by specific Gallo-Roman tribal territories or 'civitates'. It is suggested that coin production is moving increasingly towards central control from the key oppidum/oppida of each tribe, under the direct authority of an oligarchy of the higher nobility (or in some cases where the institution survived - the tribal king). The precious high value issues in gold and silver continue, and are seen as marking gifts and payments to rural elites for military and administrative services, as well as providing a common wealth medium for regional tax collection amongst the better-off. But there now develops a lower value silver currency and then a small coin bronze currency. These, however, tend to be confined in distribution to the oppida themselves. It is argued that the low value coins are a kind of 'town' currency made there and used there, to pay for 'state services' such as military service, craft production by resident specialists and oppidum building forces. Essentially the state coinage is issued to cover the living costs of 'servants' of the state who are prevented from labouring or overseeing their own food (and wealth) production (Nash 1978, 1981). Such a limited degree of coin mobility within the special subcultural environment of the oppidum rules out any genuine town-rural hinterland coin exchange in market transactions: "whatever 'low value' coins were produced for, it was not to facilitate market exchange which is a secondary factor, and this is true for Roman and Medieval Europe as it is for pre-Roman. Such a coinage was normally made for official payments to state workers, soldiers, jurors, and so forth" (Collis 1981c, p.122). Collis goes on to distinguish between the wide tribal dispersal of high value coin in the countryside, associated with the distribution of bronze vessels and imported wine amphorae etc., mirroring the distribution of a high social class across a political territory, and on the other hand, the concentration of coins of low value at major sites, representing the limited circulation of more regular and numerous coin payments amongst the oppidum elite and attendant specialist workforces. Allen (1976) places the same emphasis on coinage as 'socially-embedded' rather than acting as a free medium of everyday exchange; rich Celts, as in historic references to Gallic nobles, would have been wealthy in land, cattle and slaves, not money.
In the oppida-dominated landscape of southern Britain it seems likely that there remained an uneasy balance between district nobles and the central oppidum authorities, as in contrast to much of Gaul, coin issues of the first centuries BC and AD show the persistence of 'rival chief' coinage alongside issues purporting to be a central 'state' issue (Cunliffe 1981c).

If this contemporary viewpoint of the significance of Celtic coinage runs directly counter to the previously widespread dogma that it marks the emergence of a free 'market' or even 'Market' economy, it is very much a reflection of a revision of our ideas about the role of coinage in the civilized Mediterranean world. To give an extreme example, Rome did not produce its own coinage till the third century BC (Reece 1981). The role of any free market is also limited in Collis' (1979a) general application of Polanyi's concept of 'administered trade' for the oppida-centred long-distance exchange systems. In this model, considered typical for Archaic (primitive) states, it is argued that a monopoly on trade is invested in the central authority of the state, hence it is confined in scope and scale and in no sense 'commercial', and its effects on the overall socio-economy of the population of the state are appropriately restricted due to such preferential, confined channels of access and the absence of the possibility of a widespread transformation of rural economies from outside. Even Haselgrove (1979) - an exponent of neo-diffusionist models for Mediterranean manipulation of the Celtic economy, sees the bronze coinage as still 'embedded' in non-market relations.

Note 69

Instances where one particular oppidum seems obviously pre-eminent for a particular tribe (such as Manching, or the southern British centres), are far rarer than tribal areas where several oppida are equally impressive, even if one of their number may have acted as primus inter pares. It is generally suggested that the degree of apparent hierarchical complexity of the settlement pattern may betray the most highly centralized from the commoner, semi-integrated power networks. In central Gaul, e.g., (Fig. 8) the individual tribes by La Tène 3 were operating with fairly clear borders and an internal set of sub-tribal political divisions - the pagi and sub-pagi units. Even in this series of relatively well-centralized tribes, the districts continued to exercise a degree of independence. For the Bituriges there are some four to five major oppida which would seem to mark discrete pagus foci, and a further 20 or so sizeable defended sites. Together they recall Caesar's reference to 20 'urbes' of the Bituriges, with the majority probably acting as sub-pagus centres with some district administrative and economic role (Nash 1978).

The existence of tribal formations that precede political integration at a single focus raises the interesting and important question (briefly mentioned in my Neolithic chapter, this volume), of ethnic groupings in later prehistoric Europe, their origin and wider role in everyday life. Although most Iron Age tribes are located and circumscribed from Classical references and geographical inferences, it has been possible to isolate cultural spheres in terms of distinctive archaeological distributions that are known to be, or are suggestive of, ethnic groupings. Perhaps the best-known example relates to the Germanic tribes and the work of Egger (cf. Todd 1975, Fig. 5), but research by Holste and Bergmann has identified comparable regional 'cultural spheres' going back into the Bronze Age (cf. Bergmann 1967). The preference of the Greek term 'ethnos' to 'state' for Iron Age tribes with but semi-integrated administration (Nash 1978), brings into play the parallel within Greece itself between the highly focussed city states and the more widespread political form of the ethnos (with a recognizable cultural uniformity but multiple centres of authority) (Snodgrass 1980). It is argued that Greek ethnos units may have maintained a distinctiveness via shared cults and a tradition of common ancestry, reinforced by common dialect.

Note 70

It has frequently been commented on that the Late La Tène era furnishes a curious contrast between the dramatic elaboration of social structure, art and monuments, and a contemporary neglect of elaboration in burial tradition. Of Central Europe, Filip reports (1978, p.431): "At the end of the second and beginning of the last century BC, the era of the flat Celtic cemeteries in Central Europe came to and end" and elsewhere, (Filip 1977, p.223): "So far no burial grounds have been found in

relation to the oppida; whether this reflects a profound religious and cult transformation connected with the general change in the Celtic social structure, or whether it was the outcome of the historical situation which hastened the phase of strongly fortified oppida, one cannot as yet determine". As hinted at here, one possible element is the breakdown of Celtic dominance in Central Europe during this general time period in the face of the historically-attested attacks and colonization by Germanic groups from the north and Dacian groups from the east. Indeed the aggressive movements of more northerly tribes such as the Cimbri, and the beginning of the Dacian westward expansion from Eastern Europe towards Central Europe, can be dated to this final second, early first century BC (Benadik 1977).

However, this local, historical explanation is inadequate because the trend away from an easily recognizable burial tradition is general throughout the Celtic world at this time, and beyond. From the late Middle La Tène age, cremations become increasingly popular, (indeed in some areas the Early La Tène flat cemeteries are cremations, providing a tangible continuity to older traditions), and in the Late La Tène of the last century BC and later they are standard over most of Celtic Europe. Accompanying this change in custom, as we have noted in previous epochs, went a severe reduction in gifts for the deceased, and those that continue to be left may be the victims of cremation too (even chariot graves that probably mark a local notable can contain mere fragments of the prestige vehicle). The ashes in this cremation custom appear most frequently to have been scattered in shallow depressions in the ground, less commonly put in an urn with a similar context (Lessing and Kruta 1979, Lorenz 1980, Rieckhoff-Pauli S. 1980). Not surprisingly it is extremely hard to detect and record such burials, and over wide areas of France, Switzerland, Germany and Austria, as well as Czechoslovakia, formal burials are remarkably rare in the archaeological record (cf. Collis 1977). In the Marne region it is well-recognized that the nineteenth-century excavators were adept at picking out the characteristic dark, Early La Tène inhumation graves against the chalky soil (12,000 La Tène burials were found between the 1860s and World War I), but the La Tène cremations of the region are hardly represented at all (Stead n.d., p.15). Caesar's claim (Gallic Wars vi. 19. 4) "it is only a short time since the slaves and clients who were known to have been loved by the dead man were cremated along with him when the funeral was properly carried out" - might imply that a most prestigious rite to contemporaries (human sacrifice) could leave the most impoverished traces to the excavator. In Britain the poverty of formal burial has been a problem from the later Bronze Age and this merely continues through to the Roman Conquest in all but a few special regions, although 'careless' inhumation may be the most common disposal practice (Whimster 1977). In Scandinavia the Iron Age is generally a period of gift poverty with cremations, as elsewhere, and but rare exceptions of 'chiefly graves'. Indeed Todd (1977) considers cremation burials to be the norm in Northern Europe from the Middle Bronze Age until the end of the first millenium BC, with inhumation being general only in the era of the Later Roman Empire.

It would, therefore, seem more plausible to account for the rite change in terms of Filip's other factor, the socio-ideological explanation, which is as far from our real comprehension as it is for the similar rite transformation that occurred in the European Late Bronze Age. The undisputed disruption in Central and Eastern Europe caused by the mixing of peoples and cultures (Celts, Germans and Dacians) would appear to be an unsatisfactory explanation. Indeed, it is noteworthy that in areas where Germanic groups became dominant, the Celtic warrior-grave rite can reappear (Werner 1977).

Less difficult to account for are regions where formal burial in a more noticeable rite continues through Late La Tène. The Scordisci in the Danube-Belgrade area for example have large burial grounds for this period, and there are rich Celtic cemeteries in northern Italy such as at Bellinzona (Filip 1977). In the region occupied by the Treveri tribe, formal burial with plentiful gifts carries on into the Roman era (Haffner 1977). In Britain, the tradition of the continental Early-Middle La Tène cemeteries with chariot burials appears anomalously in the limited region of east Yorkshire with the 'Arras Culture', often considered to mark a genuine colonization from the Champagne area of France, or at least very close cultural links across the North Sea (Stead 1979). The tradition is at its most flourishing in England **after** the main period of the Champagne cemeteries, and there does seem to be a tendency for areas peripheral to the main distribution of Hallstatt and La Tène cultures to continue with archaic practices, (although the 'princely' symbolism seems to have moved to a lower social context in Yorkshire as arguably in the original Early La Tène Marne group - cf note 61). In Free Germany princely graves are a notable feature of Late La Tène times (Fischer 1973), and four-wheeled waggon burials are still found here during this era (Joachim 1973). In south eastern England, the Late La Tène with its spectacular lowland oppida and other indications of complex proto-state organization exhibits a compromise in its burial tradition (Collis 1977, Cunliffe 1978). In line with other evidence for strong influences from across the Channel, which probably includes a limited amount of colonization/emigration from Belgic tribal country into the area south of the river Thames, and much subsequent influence on native dynasties north of the Thames, the cremation rite is adopted, generally in urns of continental inspiration. But these cremations are found not carelessly scattered around the area of occupation but in formal cemeteries and, moreover, the pattern of gifts and layout of graves betrays very clearly that strongly hierarchical social structure that we know existed throughout the sphere of the contemporary continental Celts but is usually not exhibited there in burial rites. Most of the south eastern English cemeteries of this tradition (the largest group being that of Aylesford-Swarling) have gifts, and there are obvious gradations of wealth that are underlined by the placing of wealthy grave groups within special enclosures inside these cemeteries, around which less wealthy satellite graves are laid out. Although generally flat graves, a number of tumulus burials which include what are clearly elite burials belong within this general tradition (the Welwyn Group).

Note 71
Clarke's (1972) brilliant analysis of a village community of the later Iron Age at Glastonbury in Somerset, using sophisticated correlations of structures and artifacts, together with the application of later Celtic sources for analogies, reveals the dominance of a module within the village of a co-residential group of male relations plus wives, associated workshop and storage facilities, and finally of some kind of overall leadership for the whole community. This is very much the kind of lower level ranking that emerges, for example, from the frequency of richer individuals amid the flat grave cemeteries that typify mature La Tène times.

One can directly compare such embedded, intra-village leadership with nucleated communities known beyond the Celtic sphere, in Germanic north west Europe. In north western Germany for example, during the final pre-Roman and Roman era Iron Age, discrete districts of cultivable and grazing land (Siedlungskammern) are associated both with dispersed farms and some larger, nucleated communities. A well-investigated example of the latter is Feddersen Wierde, where for several centuries the village was composed of a number of farms, amongst

which a special farm stands out within its own enclosure; amongst its unique features is a higher than average stall area for stock and evidence for craft specialization and trade. Eventually this chieftain's farm is converted to an even more distinctive three-aisled hall (Schmid 1978). In west Jutland, at Hodde, around the final century BC and the first century AD, another village, here estimated at some 2-300 people, includes a notable chieftain's farm enclosure throughout; it had twice the normal stall capacity and a concentration of fineware pottery. The excavator links the class to which the Hodde 'lord' may have belonged to the few recorded Iron Age elite burials in Denmark, such as Kraghede and Langa, where as in other regions peripheral to the original spheres of Hallstatt and La Tène culture, chariot burials survive late on in the Iron Age (Hvass 1975).

Even more interesting is the accumulating evidence for discrete elite foci in a purely rural environment, particularly in the light of our earlier discussion of such sites in the context of Western Hallstatt and Early La Tène society. Daphne Nash (1975) points out that the historical sources, artefactual and coin evidence available for Celtic society indicate a basic structure of nobility and peasantry from as early as the beginning of the third century BC, whereas oppida become widespread only from the late second century BC. Except where hillforts continue through the Middle Iron Age, it is obvious that elite residences must have been dispersed across the countryside, either within dependent nucleated communities as exemplified above for Celtic and Germanic society, or as free-standing rural estate centres. The concentration of gold torques, a well-attested elite symbol, away from defended centres in England (Collis 1981a), and the coin moulds commonly being recovered from minor rural sites on the Continent (Neustupny and Neustupny 1961, Collis 1981b), has generally underlined this poorly-researched sector of aristocratic residences set amongst their immediate source of wealth and power, the land.

In Holland, the absence of hillforts and the poor contexts and low quantities of prestigious artwork have hitherto led scholars to envisage a society with no visible leadership structures to compare with more 'complex' developments elsewhere. Waterbolk (1977), however, argues that society had probably two levels of integrative leadership (in the period c. 350 BC to AD 100). The first he detects as one of the village chiefdoms, marked by a regular pattern of defended foci, inside of which the main features are food storage structures. Clusters of these chiefdoms may, he hints, have centred on regional centres.

Interestingly, the Dutch enclosures are reminiscent of the Thetford 'aristocratic' estate centre mentioned earlier from the other side of the North Sea. It has been argued by a number of British Iron Age specialists (Bowen, Wainwright, Jones) that one can detect, in general, within known British La Tène settlements, a class of rural site of a different scale and importance from the ordinary run of smallish peasant establishments. This class, typically represented by Little Woodbury and Gussage All Saints, is one of large farm layouts, often with imposing entrance avenues of antennae form (here we may note the very pretentious approach to the Thetford site), and perhaps accommodating as many as 30-60 people (Wainwright 1979). These are considered to be estate centres of a chiefly elite and it is particularly appropriate that excavation of Gussage revealed significant specialist craftwork at the site, including the manufacture of chariot-fittings. Collis (1977) notes with insight of the rich burials in a large swathe of Late La Tène north western Europe (his 'North Gallic Culture' of the Rhineland-north France-south eastern England): "Generally these rich burials are not associated with the oppida and other major settlements, Lexden (Colchester) and ... Kelheim being the exceptions. Unfortunately we know little of the settlements to which the rich burials belonged, but generally they seem to be small, of the size of farms or small hamlets. In south eastern England they are all within a radius of about 70-80kms. from Colchester, along with a series of less rich burials which produce items such as shale beads, bronze mirrors, and silver brooches ... The 70-80kms. radius is possibly the zone where the use of gold coinage from Colchester is most concentrated" (1977 p.6 - cf. note 68, this chapter, for the significance of the coinage distributional sphere).

Finally we may cite an important contribution to this topic from study of the settlement pattern of the Treveri tribe (spanning the country either side of the border between West Germany and the Low Countries). Haffner (1977) reports that continuing research has revealed a clear three-tier settlement hierarchy for the Late Iron Age (Fig. 9). At the top are oppida such as the Titelberg, at the bottom a whole series of small, undefended rural sites. The middle tier comprises substantial rural defended enclosures of an impressive character, identified as estate residences of the noble class, probably the 'Castella' referred to by Caesar. Associated with one of these sites is evidence for rich burials. The best-known example of these proto-villae is the Altburg bei Bundenbach, a well-fortified 1.5ha. enclosure that is provided with an inner defended 'sanctum' interpreted as the chief's residential quarter. As with the Dutch enclosures, considerable storage facilities are accompanied by domestic features for only a select number of inhabitants, an indication perhaps of the chief's redistributive role (Schindler 1975, 1977).

Note 72

Caesar, Gallic Wars (1, 1). "Political authority rested solely with the nobility at all periods, whose position was ensured by their maintenance of retinues and agricultural clients" (Nash 1978, p.467; cf. also Preidel 1979). This power base was still operative under Roman rule and in AD 21, Julius Florus "could muster clients and debtors like his ancestors for a revolt against Roman authority" (op. cit. p.468). Furthermore, there were "no popular assemblies, and although the Celts had chattel slaves (mostly captives of war) the population of any state was divided among a range of dependent statuses from a semi-servile labourer or debt-bondsman who was virtually a slave, to members of the nobility" (op. cit. p.469). The existence of such a social system can be argued for Celtic society from Early La Tène times, with the support of the limited historical references for the pre-Conquest era (Nash 1975). The one element of change was the gradual replacement of a formal and probably very limited tribal kingship by an inner caucus of nobles in most of Celtic Europe. The importance of institutional religion, in the form of the Druids, must not obscure the fact that the latter formed an alternative source of power and prestige to young nobles from that offered by warfare and the accumulation of land and clients (Lessing and Kruta 1979, pp.87 ff., Rieckhoff-Pauli S. 1980). The very close parallel between this socio-economic system and that typical for Greco-Roman society in the Mediterranean needs no special pleading (cf. Finley 1973, Bintliff 1982). A less obvious parallel, but no less valid and illuminating, is that drawn with early Medieval Europe and its estate and dependent serf society (Bintliff 1982, Rieckhoff-Pauli S. 1980). Julius Caesar knew all too well the political realities not only of his own, but of Gallic tribal society, when he gave short shrift to the Bellovaci who had complained that the 'ignorant rabble' had forced the tribe into war. The rabble, he replied, does nothing unless the leading men of the tribe put them up to it (Lessing and Kruta 1979, p.40). Even allowing for traditional exaggeration in Classical accounts of the Celts, the scale of

Celtic 'power serfdom' must be indicated by the story of the great aristocrat Orgetorix, of the Helvetii tribe (Gallic Wars, 2.1). When due to be arraigned in chains for high treason before the tribe, he escaped immediate prosecution by summoning 10,000 slaves from his estates, together with numerous retainers and debt-bondsmen. Caesar also reports a Gallic tradition where the cremation of notable personages was accompanied by the sacrifice of "slaves and clients who were known to have been loved by the dead man ... when the funeral was properly carried out" (Gallic Wars v. 19. 4, quoted by Stead n.d. p.40). Whether this happened with any real frequency (or at all!) is unclear, but such a statement, however apocryphal, is a powerful reflection of the accepted relative status of aristocratic and client/slave rights and privileges in Celtic society.

Despite this apparent polarization of Celtic society, there remains a rather grey area left open for those who wish to find a primitive democracy amongst the Celtic and Germanic tribes of the Iron Age (Filip 1977, Randsborg 1982; cf. Preidel 1977, 1979). The scope for some kind of politically-effective, yeoman middle class is claimed from the references to assemblies of the tribal levy, or of those of the arms-bearing class, suggesting to some a military democracy with at least some political counterpoise to the inner clique of the aristocrats. Such an elaboration of the political system is, however, difficult to reconcile with our sources, especially when they are carefully scrutinized and analyzed as a whole. Although many scholars have enthused about the potentially 'open' and even entrepreneurial nature of Old German society, where chiefs held sway by organizing useful functions and services for surrounding peasants (e.g. Randsborg 1982), and with the elite having to persuade the populace at special assemblies towards certain courses of action, there are strong objections to such a reconstruction (Preidel 1977, 1979). Firstly, the totality of historical sources for Celtic and Germanic society underlines the Caesarian polarity between the all-powerful elite (with or without a king) and the dependent multitude (however many sub-statuses we care to recognize within the latter class). A recent review of Germanic burial practices from the archaeological record (Todd 1977) provides separate confirmation. The pattern suggested above, of local elites associated with a retinue of clients may be detected in numerous cemeteries of the earlier Roman Iron Age in the Elbe region. Here male cemeteries are separate from female and the former consist of a high proportion of graves without goods and a minority with burial wealth and warrior equipment (including imports). Todd emphasizes the contrast to any pattern we might expect if kinship were a major organizational element. Above the level of local chiefs and 'big men' are a series of widespread but not very numerous 'princely burials' distinguished by unusual wealth concentrations and a preference for inhumation over traditional and otherwise customary cremation rites (e.g. the Lübsow group, the Elbe-Saale group) - these may in part be identified with the persistence of tribal kingship amongst the Germans. Despite current tendencies to tie these regional elite manifestations to the prestige-good model (cf. Hedeager 1980) on account of the inclusion of Roman import pieces in these luxury burials, Todd strikes the appropriate note in his stress on the symbolic role of these exotica to mark locally-achieved status, rather than their potential role as creators of status. These distinctive and widespread 'paramount' burials reflect: "shared customs in the upper realms of Germanic society, fostered no doubt by diplomatic contact and by intermarriage between the leading families of different tribes ... Wheeler wrote of the Lübsow group 'It was as though now, with a advent of new resources under the Early Empire, the 'new rich' were reviving the magnificence of their own past ... An intertribal fashion, based upon an access of wealth, had swept across Central Europe in front of the organised and masterful approach of the culture of the Mediterranean'. We might now add that the 'new rich' were not all that new and that they owed their 'access of wealth' to the opening up to agriculture of rich tracts of land in northern and central Germania" (Todd 1977 p.41; cf. this chapter notes 5 and 64).

Secondly, the reality of a peasant-army parliament is seriously in doubt. For the Marcomanni, a Germanic group who formed a dominant elite in Bohemia by Imperial times, Preidel argues that the probable total armed levy of the non-slave population (of the order of 90,000) is totally out of scale with any realistic assembly, where no more than a few thousand might reasonably be expected to have been in a position to participate in audible debate. Such a proportion of free-men as the latter would fit very neatly with estimates of the aristocratic sector in these societies, of the order of a mere three to eight per cent. One may indeed make a strong case for a distinction between the elite warrior force (in both Celtic and Germanic ethnic groupings), perhaps permanently in readiness for war or raiding, and the emergency tribal levy of every free-man (cf. Zeller 1980). The quality of the latter force, in training and equipment, is likely to have been in no way proportional to its size. Again making allowance for exaggeration, the effectiveness of small Roman armies against far larger tribal levies is unsurprising. At the siege of Alesia, when clearly an emergency levy (but not total) was in operation, Caesar reports enemy forces of 250,000 footsoldiers and 8,000 aristocrats (Gallic Wars 7,5). However much we suspect his figures, we might have more confidence in the ratio between the two classes. When the migrating Celts had swept through the Balkans and founded the long-lasting realm of Galatia in Turkey, we once more have some opportunity to study the effective scale of government, from contemporary and later descriptions (Lessing and Kruta 1979, pp.73 ff). Some 20,000 Celts, three tribes, are put as the total migrating population; of these naturally but a few thousand would have been adult, free warriors; yet the ruling assembly of the resultant tribal confederacy numbered but some 300. Preidel comments reasonably: "Diese Organisation ist aller Wahrscheinlichkeit noch keltisches Erbe" (p.73). Thirdly, even if one were to dispute the case being made for the exclusive nature of those attending tribal assemblies, our cumulative evidence on the degree of dependence of all inferior classes upon the all-dominant chiefly elite would argue that decisions would be made on the basis of aristocratic 'block votes', whether in the presence or absence of other classes: "Es gab zwar bei besonderen Anlässen auch 'Volksversammlungen' zu denen alle waffentragenden Männer kommen müssten. Aber da 'die meisten' entweder als Soldaten oder Leibwächter (ambacti) ihren Herren gehörten, bzw. als Bauern oder Hirten durch Pachtverthältnisse zu Gehorsam und Gefolgschaft verpflichtet waren (clientes), lag die Entscheidung letzlich doch bei dem Adel" (Rieckhoff-Pauli, S. 1980, p.42).

These tentative suggestions of the scale of the controlling minority might hypothetically be fed back into a settlement context. A core, professional warrior elite of under 10% of the free population might represent one elite individual for a nucleated or dispersed community of some dozen or so free families, i.e. the equivalent of a hamlet chief. This plausible context for our references puts us firmly back into that great underlying continuum of later prehistoric society, the network of minor and major chiefdoms across Europe. It also undermines those who attempt to introduce only at a late stage (the Late La Tène for Rowlands (1980); for Randsborg (1982), the late Viking era), such a system of class polarity based on land, tenants, clients and slaves. (Cf. also on this point, Todd 1977).

An additional insight is achieved if one were to accept this general reconstruction of Celto-German society, when regarding the apparently confusing succession of migrating peoples in Central and East-Central Europe. If, for example, the Celts sweep into regions occupied by local populations, both then being overrun by Dacians or Germans, where does one conceive the 'swamped' populations fitting in within the context of the new, dominant tribal organization? Only rarely can we invoke a genuine emigration by the defeated, in most cases we must assume that 'Celtic' or 'Germanic' tribes were in reality composed of diverse ethnic and cultural groups. Moreover, if we accept the probability of a dense occupation of continental Europe from mature La Tène times, 'ethnic replacement' in areas such as Central Europe is more likely to have been a case of the arrival of a more effective elite warrior force, demoting or more probably merging with the established aristocracy. For the vast majority of the population, the 'free' and unfree, it would be little more than a change in, or minor modification of, their landlords or protectors; the structure of society, and their subordinate role, would remain unchanged (De Laet 1976, Preidel 1977, 1979, Pauli 1980; cf. Kolnik 1977).

A final element in this discussion is the brief report given by Caesar of the customs of the Germans (Gallic Wars 1, 2). Caesar's authority here is generally considered to be far less reliable than in his numerous first hand accounts of Gallic society, as his unintentionally humorous account of the fauna serves to remind us (Riekhoff-Pauli, S. 1980). The claims for a lack of agricultural activity are, of course, flatly contradicted by archaeological evidence, and the socio-political hints are very much at odds with much fuller, later sources and the archaeological data. Nonetheless, it is possible to suggest that behind the seemingly very garbled account of Caesar there lies an interesting reflection, about which he was misinformed, of elite life amongst the Germans. The description of a population devoting its life to hunting and warfare, uninvolved in agriculture, may be inaccurate for the population as a whole, but could well have been a report of the lifestyle of the people 'who mattered' amongst the Germans, the elite. With the land cultivated by slaves, clients, tenants, serfs, it would certainly have been natural for the elite to have maintained a characteristic lifestyle of this nature (Preidel 1977, 1979). Caesar's mention of regular redistribution of land, and even a kind of shifting agriculture, though to some extent paralleled in the probably more reliable account of Tacitus (Germania), is also very hard to reconcile with our current knowledge of settlement patterns, unless the discussion is really concerned with fallow rotation on a large scale. Caesar's oblique hint of 'discretionary allocation' becomes clearer in Tacitus, where we are told that land is allotted according to rank. If there was indeed an established custom of regular land redistribution, the power and support base for the elite may have been fixed as much to dependent manpower as to particular plots of land, exacting agricultural and labour surpluses from wherever the annual crop was being produced.

Note 73
Thus Nash, despite an excellent insight into the role of local economic control in Celtic elite power, falls victim to the seductive 'deus ex machina' role of the Mediterranean interference model. She argues that external events such as the decline of mercenary service by Celts for Hellenistic kingdoms, and the rise of Roman demands for slaves in return for luxuries, stimulated intense internal competition within the Celtic world for more status goods. Chiefs aimed at a steady flow of captives out, in hopes of a monopoly in local redistribution of Mediterranean imports. The rival chiefs somehow amalgamated into steeper power hierarchies, from which a centralized administrative structure for each tribe arose (cf. Nash 1975,

1978). In the much less sophisticated study of Crumley (1974) on this phase of Celtic society, despite once more the recognition that the lower orders of society were in a client relationship towards the aristocracy and that there could have been a system of land tenure deriving from the top echelons of society, we are nonetheless led to believe that Celtic society moved from inherited to achieved status activated by the wealth of the Classical world (cf. Phillips 1980, p.257). Haselgrove, imitating the Frankenstein and Rowlands (1978) treatment of Hallstatt political elaboration with a neo-diffusionist model, applies it to the pre-Roman Iron Age of southern Britain (Haselgrove 1979, 1982). He stresses the link between the shift to a centralized coinage, the issuing of a small-change bronze coinage, the striking of personal names on such coins, and the construction of the Welwyn type burials in the Home Counties (with strong import display): "control of Roman imports may have enabled the promotion of such individuals in the hierarchy" (1979, p.203). Yet such a model fails to explain why an intensive, early first century BC trade between the continent and 'ports of trade' on the English south coast at Hengistbury Head and Mount Batten "had little lasting effect on the socio-economic structure of the Iron Age communities of southern Britain" (Cunliffe 1981, p.31). Neither does it explain why the post-Caesar intensive trade into the 'Belgic' and 'para-Belgic' developed tribes of south eastern England (Aylesford-Swarling zone) concentrates on Essex and all but ignores Kent (Cunliffe op. cit.).

Note 74

The general arguments and theory involved in this most important debate have already been rehearsed earlier in this chapter when we considered the socio-economic development of Hallstatt Europe. We have also begun to accumulate evidence in favour of a similar explanation of Late La Tène socio-political structure, with the emphasis on regional control over the means of production (land, agricultural labour) rather than industrial and mercantile entrepreneurship. In one of his last published papers, D. Allen (1976) expressed some telling insights into Celtic society, much in accordance with the approach adopted by the present writer: "No Celtic land ever became a granary of Greece or Rome. We often hear of the dense populations of Celtic lands; we also hear of frequent movements in search of new agricultural land ... Despite the popularity in Rome of Gaulish hams and geese, there is no reason to think that there were any large agricultural surpluses from which money was earned. In iron, but not in other metals, the European Celts were broadly self-sufficient. The exports from which they could earn were largely ores, hides and pre-eminently slaves. But there is every reason to think that the proceeds of this traffic were spent up to the hilt on the sought-for imports from the Mediterranean world. These included luxury goods ... but more especially ... wine. It was no coincidence that the value of a slave and of an amphora of wine were equal" (Allen, op. cit. p.20). Allen goes on to suggest that the Roman trader in Gaul was often a speculator in land, rather than in commodities, and underlines the generally-recognized point that Celtic coinage of this era was not an indication of free market activity on a Mediterranean model, but firmly 'embedded' into a taut internal social hierarchy. Rich Gauls will be so on the basis of land, cattle and slaves, not money, and the references to debt should be placed firmly in the former sector of power over the subsistence sector and manpower. Preidel (1978) on behalf of the Central European evidence, offers a similar damaging critique of the 'world economy' approach: "Überhaupt ist man grundsätzlich geneigt, den vor - und frühgeschichtlichen Handel zu überschätzen" (p.72). The evidence of long-distance trade is primarily concerned with the subcultural interests of a small elite. Ian Hodder (1979) has also recently challenged the prevailing orthodoxy and criticized anachronistic assumptions about the Late La Tène economy of Britain. An 'embedded' and non-market economy is posited, and we are reminded that even the now classic study by Peacock of the Iron Age pottery trade in south western Britain is as likely to be a socially-controlled distribution as the commercial 'market' proposed by Peacock (1968, 1969). The much-cited Classical references for the first century AD trade of Britain with the Continent are suggested as reflecting merely the elitist 'conspicuous consumption' sector of the Celtic economy in which diplomacy may have ranked highly (with prestige imports being deposited in Welwyn type burials and found at elite residences such as oppida).

Overall, the model in which elite imports feature prominently as a prime causative factor in the elaboration of Celtic socio-political structure is very difficult to support, and the value of such trade is rather in its reflecting the status quo of rank, and the achievement of centralized polities that the Mediterranean powers considered it worthwhile to come to official terms with (both for reasons of strategic policy and in recognition of the usefulness of organized, barbarian supplies of slaves). The scale of Celtic socio-political pyramids, and the absolute dependency ties, that our sources agree on, argue for a far more fundamental system of class control than the sprinkling of elite gew-gaws can possibly account for. The ability of an Orgetorix to assemble thousands of men from his estates and clients, is far from isolated, and we might cite a further example to add to that of Florus to illustrate that such powers continued into better-documented Roman times. In the rising against Nero, Julius Vindex, a Roman senator but more importantly a Gaulish 'baron', was able to attract his fellow territorial dynasts to his cause; they came with their host of clients, a hundred thousand (Syme 1977).

The dependency of the ordinary peasant can be convincingly explained from his reduction to tenant or client status within a universal system of elite support for subsistence agriculture. The attachment of minor elite members to the household of prominent aristocrats, seemingly a second fundamental feature of Celto-Germanic social hierarchy, is known to be a product of the ability of leading nobles to offer them a lavish level of 'hospitality' (i.e. a 'living') and the prospect of a share in the slaves and portable wealth that accrued from endemic inter- and intra-tribal warfare (Nash 1975, 1978, 1981). The parallels to the retinue of Medieval feudal lords are clear-cut. Even when totally-different models are offered for earlier eras, it is noteworthy that by the late pre-Roman Iron Age in many parts of Europe numerous scholars postulate a land-based political and social hierarchy (cf. Rowlands (1980) for Celtic Western Europe, Kristiansen (1980) and Lindquist (1974) for Scandinavia).

Putting this debate into a wider perspective, the Marxist scholar Klejn provides an essential element in a modern evaluation of the workings of the prehistoric and early historic economy (Klejn 1972). He points out that archaeologists have moved away from the original, early nineteenth-century theory of periods of the past based on technology, towards a developmental scheme combining economy and technology (i.e. from the Three Age scheme and its subsequent subdivisions towards 'revolutionary' transformations such as farming, urbanism, etc.). This shift, from the attitude of Thomsen and his followers, to that of Childe, has been given formal status in the theorizing of Braidwood. Yet Braidwood is to be criticized as typically 'bourgeois' in failing to see that mere changes in economy are by themselves minor in significance compared to the associated shifts in the vital relationships of production. One thus finds the curious situation that prehistoric and proto-historic societies are analyzed from a techno-economic standpoint, whereas historic societies receive a treatment in which social relationships are seen as fundamental to economic processes. Klejn here quotes Avdusin: "Mit dem Auftreten der schriftlichen Quellen hört diese Periodisierung nach dem Material der Arbeitsgeräte auf, die wichtigsten historischen Veränderungen widerzuspiegeln, und im weiteren wird die Darlegung des historischen Materials zur Geschichte der Klassengesellschaften nach sozialökonomischen Formulationen (Sklavenhalter-und Feudalgesellschaft) durchgeführt" (Avdusin 1967, p.5, quoted in Klejn, op. cit. p.23). Clearly scholars of the late '70s and of the 1980's are far more concerned than those of previous decades to establish the nature of past social systems; yet Klejn's critique still holds bite in that most of this contemporary 'social archaeology' isolates discrete elements in a socioeconomic system (often because these are easiest to analyze and best preserved) and fails to construct a model of the over-riding systems of economic production. Antonio Gilman (1981) offers a very similar attack upon the established views concerning the rise of complex social hierarchies, in this case in the context of Bronze Age Europe: Childe had stressed the self-interest of nonproducers in getting surpluses under their control, and in the Near East McAdams has characterized early trade as serving more the interests of the agents of exchange than fulfilling broad social needs. Earle has brought to light the fallacy of seeing complex chiefdoms such as those in the Pacific, as socially desirable for communal benefit, rather than systems of elite exploitation. Harris, though opting for the 'social services' theory for elite dominance, expresses strong unease at such a functionalist explanation: "What were the rewards of those who were cut off from the two-million year old heritage of free access to resources? ... Why was control of soil, water, and even the air yielded up into the hands of a relatively small group of people?" (Harris 1971, p.393, quoted in Gilman, op. cit.). Gilman concludes of these elites "That their actions do not serve common interests" (op. cit. p.4).

To abolish, once more, the barriers between 'barbarian' and 'civilized' socio-economic systems, we may fruitfully compare the relationship of the Celtic and Germanic chief or 'big man' to his slaves, tenants and clients, with that of the Greco-Roman citizen to his agricultural and domestic slaves and tenants. Of the latter culture, but with a far wider relevance, De Ste. Croix comments: "The essential problem of production in every civilised society is how to extract a sufficient surplus from the primary producers in order to give at least some people enough leisure for government, the arts and sciences, and the other necessities and luxuries of civilised life. The technological level of the Greco-Roman world was a good deal lower than is generally realized ... In such a society, unless nearly everyone is to have to work nearly all the time, and have virtually no leisure, some means has to be found of screwing a substantial surplus out of the lowest class. The Greeks and Romans, among other means, employed slaves for this purpose: that is to say, they forcibly imported men and women whom they deprived of virtually all rights and compelled to labour for their masters, and they probably did this to a greater degree than any earlier society" (De Ste. Croix 1957, p.57). Perhaps ironically, even those scholars who ultimately lean towards explanations based on commercial wealth recognize, but fail to give adequate treatment to, these fundamental relationships of exploitation within proto-and early historic societies. Thus Nash on the Gauls (1978) acknowledges that coercion was required in Celtic society to ensure the provision of an adequate surplus to keep "a non-producing warrior nobility but also ... a juridical, religious and artisan class patronised by them, which was likewise freed from direct agricultural production" (p.470).

Note 75
We have hitherto presented a case, briefly summarized by

Gilman as follows: "while the commodity-exchange theory of elite origins may be useful in other settings, in later prehistoric Europe it founders on the apparent self-sufficiency of local communities. Trade was mostly confined to luxuries" (1981, p.5).

It is of great interest to examine the relationship between this model of regional economic and social differentiation and the process of engulfment of small geographical regions by imperial systems. Most scholars concerned with the development of empires appear to agree that complex societies have denser populations, deploy more powerful productive forces and, once established, tend to expand at the expense of less populous and hierarchical neighbours (following Carneiro's (1978) 'Principle of Competitive Exclusion'). We have already had cause to quote the great historian of antiquity, Finley, on the nature of ancient empires: "What passed for economic growth in antiquity was always achieved only by external expansion" (1978, pp.64-5). A similar view is expressed for early civilizations in the Near East by Larsen (1979, pp.92-3): "The three basic political structures in the Mesopotamian traditions, city state, territorial state ('country') and empire, are related to each other in a dynamic system where the operative element is territorial expansion. It is typical of the Mesopotamian world that major territorial units and empires are named after a city, an observation which by itself indicates the fundamental role played by the city-state. Mesopotamian history cannot be understood in terms of a unilinear development, but seen against a background of recurrent breakdowns we do seem to find a clear trend towards more complex organization. With regard to the empires this growing complexity is accompanied by a move towards larger units and a stronger centralization so that more extensive areas come under direct rule". From the third to the first millennium BC this process culminates in imperial systems dominating almost all the land area of the Near East.

Larsen's analysis is to be found in an important volume (1979), under his editorship (Power and Propaganda) that examines the nature of early imperial systems, particularly those of the ancient Near East. Especially relevant to the point of view we are presenting here, is the visible confrontation between the Formalist, neo-diffusionist analysis of these civilizations, presented by Larsen, Eckholm and Friedman, and Frankenstein, and contrasting papers more aligned with Substantivist, regionally-based sympathies. The reactive challenge is most powerful in a masterly review paper for the volume, by R. McAdams (1979), who brings out a number of significant points of much wider relevance. A principal objection he raises is to the Formalist assumption that an expanding empire acts to concentrate 'capital' at its centre (or as Larsen puts it for a prime case-study - the Assyrian Empire was a giant vacuum cleaner): "What is much less certain ... is the extent to which the early deployment of capital in the production process became a self-generating force for change, with more than a fairly slight resemblance to the Industrial Revolution that introduced our own era. And equally debatable is the extent to which" Eckholm and Friedman "are accurate in regarding ancient empires as centre-periphery systems in which the centre 'accumulates wealth based on the production of a wider area' " (McAdams 1979, p.394). Adams moves on to consider the distinction necessary between light freight of special value, and bulk movement of heavy raw materials and foodstuffs. Like Finley on the Ancient Economy of Greece and Rome (1973), Adams sees this distinction ignored at the cost of a genuine understanding of the real nature of the economies involved. As both writers remind us, the high bulk goods are very expensive to move any distance on land, yet such material, including subsistence surpluses, would have been the major product of every province of empire and the vast majority of imperial subjects: "Merely to introduce this elementary consideration is to expose a weakness of the approach taken by the symposium as a whole, for technical and logistic factors of this kind received little or no attention from any of us" (Adams, op.cit. p.397). When, for example, the Assyrians conquered Babylonia "it is of interest that the goods removed were luxuries rather than raw materials, reaffirming the importance of the heavy transport costs that was indicated earlier" (p.399). For Egypt, the growth of imperialism seems often to have reflected internal power struggles rather than any conceivable import-export balance: "neither the composition nor the absolute scale of plunder and tribute exacted from conquered lands may be as important as whether the benefits of empire accrued to reinforce the position of elites who were strategically located to press for further conquests" (p.400). And when too much is made of the pretensions of the Akkadian imperial experiment, it is essential to be reminded that possession of the great manpower and food production of the Mesopotamian heartland of Sumer was its real strength: "it was the Akkadians' relatively more durable dominance over the Sumerian south that supports this status rather than their very wide ranging but apparently ephemeral conquests outside of the Mesopotamian alluvium" (p.402).

Proceeding from this critique to an alternative formulation of core-periphery relations between an imperial central zone and its provinces, Adams is worth quoting at length: Lattimore (1962) has pointed out "that traditional empires were structured by radii of military action, civil administration and economic integration that in this order were of characteristically decreasing length. The calculus of pre-industrial transport costs and delays once more enters as a vital element ... What this gave importance to, in any empire, was a limited number of densely populated, highly productive regions, that could be depended upon for revenue as well as for military forces out of all proportion to the real differences in their preexisting economic status, or even to their loyalty. Herein lies the possibility of a reformulated core-periphery dichotomy that transcends its metaphorical status and provides us with a strong working hypothesis" (op. cit. p.401). The following summary from Skinner (1977) of the situation in traditional China is also particularly apposite, and is then introduced by Adams: "In the absence of mechanized transport, a dispersed population places severe limitations on feasible levels of commercialization and revenue extraction. By increasing the cost of delivering administrative and economic services, population dispersion depresses both administrative and economic central functions. Great distances relative to the total magnitude of productivity discourage a real specialization and the division of labour. By contrast, a dense population concentrates demand for products to the point where it pays to extract them efficiently. Large accessible markets make possible good returns for investment in land, encourage cash-cropping and foster a real specialization. It goes without saying that population density is itself a function of productive potential in relation to prevailing technology" (Skinner 1977, p.232). Combining these several insights into an overall conclusion, Adams states: "This analysis" of Skinner "is directed toward a traditional empire ... but its general relevance is apparent. Implied in it is the highly significant suggestion that imperial centres need not necessarily be thought of as well defined, antecedent homelands of conquering peoples. To varying degrees instead, they were themselves generated by the process of imperial expansion and consolidation, even if the involuntary transfer of resources from the peripheries may have played no determinative part in this process. As thus reformulated, the hypothesis encourages us to look for a richly diversified set of features that differentiated cores from peripheral regions, rather than merely the forms and degrees of political subordination and economic exploitation" (Adams, op. cit. pp.401-2).

The present writer has developed a comparable model based upon the development of the historic imperial state of ancient Sparta (cf. Bintliff 1977a, b). In brief, the mosaic of regions surrounding an expansive state has each its varied potential, within a given level of technology; some may already have achieved that potential with a complex high culture or civilization, others are below potential for reasons of late colonization or previous over-exploitation. The achievement of imperial incorporation of this mosaic is not to attempt the impossible (in antiquity) of converting regional surplus to central 'capital', but for the central community to expand logarithmically those landscapes within which it reproduces itself on the basis of abundant estates, sources of raw materials and dependent manpower (cf. Bintliff 1981). 'Lebensraum' for the dominant imperial nation, but usually with effective integration for local indigenous elite communities, is the simple solution to the constraints of distance and liquidation of local assets. Moses Finley comments, challengingly: "It is one of the most remarkable facts in the history of Roman imperialism that, once conquest of a territory was complete, Roman administrators and Roman soldiers were so scarce as to be hardly visible. Day-to-day administration was left largely to the local communities and their officials; the bulk of the Roman army was stationed in the frontier provinces, aimed against the outside world, not against the subjects within ... The incorporation of provincial aristocrats, oligarchs, and landed magnates into the Roman ruling class inexorably led, by the third century, to the replacement of Roman rule over subject peoples by a single territorial state, ruled by an emperor and his associates drawn from all parts and peoples of the territory" (Finley, 1978, pp.67-8). The flavour of economic regional realities also permeates a striking paper by Fulford (1978) which aims at quantifying the role of external trade in the overall economy of the province of Roman Britain. After the pre- and early-Conquest period of imbalance in which Imperial imports are prominent, the typical product of Romanization is observed: a dramatic decline in such items as indigenous production takes over.

However, the new 'management' stimulates production of products and raw material that other provinces require, so the mature imperial era would maintain earlier levels of trade or exceed them. Yet a well-argued parallel investigation into the archaeological correlates of Medieval trade prompts the major conclusion: "These figures may give the impression that trade in the medieval period (and hence the late Roman period) played an important part in the economy. The opposite is probably nearer the truth ... Thus for the fourteenth century it is extremely unlikely that exported goods would have accounted for even 5% of gross national product which, as has been suggested, might be comparable to the late Roman situation" (op. cit. p.68). Not surprisingly the development of provincial towns cannot reflect nodes of concentration of manufactured products and other surpluses, dependent on an international market economy, but the ancient equivalent of county towns for primarily agricultural populations, 'consumer' 'parasite' towns (Finley 1973, 1977; cf. R.F. Jones, this volume).

Note 76
For a similar view of elite exploitation cf. Gilman (1981). Timothy Gregory (this volume) has this to say from the standpoint of the Byzantine Empire: "We have, I think, come a long way from a simplistic study of empires only 'from the top' and generally realize that they are frequently only shadows and ephemeral structures that take advantage of serendipity events to siphon off economic and political profit while leaving the underlying social fabric reasonably unaffected".

208

Note 77

"Hierarchy and social inequality were not merely the invariable accompaniment but the formative factor in the emergence of higher cultures. And by high cultures I mean those whose upper classes observed, or failed to observe, canons of behaviour furthest removed from those of the lower animals ... Whereas the peaks of cultural achievements, the finest products of human craft, were exclusively associated with and indeed helped to define and signal the highest levels in hierarchical societies, the objects and structures used by the mass of the population ... were often comparable with those of their prehistoric forebears. The conclusion is surely inescapable that without a hierarchical structure, without a marked degree of inequality in consumption, the astonishing diversity and perfection of ... civilisation could hardly have been achieved ... Archaeology tells us that the finest artefacts made by man, the most superb and diverse embodiments of his humanity, were made to celebrate social systems founded on hierarchy and inequality" (Grahame Clark, 1979, pp.19-21).

BIBLIOGRAPHY

ADAMS, R.E. 1977 - "Apocalyptic visions: the Maya collapse and Mediaeval Europe", Archaeology 1977, pp.292-301.

ADAMS, R.McC. 1978 - "Strategies of maximization, stability, and resilience in Mesopotamian society, settlement, and agriculture", Procs. of the American Philosophical Soc., vol. 122, pp.329-35.

ADAMS, R.McC. 1979 - "Common concerns but different standpoints : a commentary", pp.393-404 in M.T. Larsen (Ed.) Power and Propaganda. Akademisk Forlag, Copenhagen.

ALEXANDER, J.A. 1978 - "Frontier studies and the earliest farmers in Europe", pp.13-29 in D.Green, C. Haselgrove, M. Spriggs (Eds.) Social Organization and Settlement. British Archaeological Reports, Int. Ser. 47, Oxford.

ALEXANDER. J.A. 1979 - "Islam in Africa: the archaeological recognition of religion", pp.215-28 in B.C. Burnham and J. Kingsbury (Eds.) Space, Hierarchy and Society. British Archaeological Reports, Int. Ser. 59, Oxford.

ALEXANDER, J.A. 1980 - "First-millennium Europe before the Romans", pp.222-26 in A. Sherratt (Ed.) The Cambridge Encyclopedia of Archaeology. Cambridge University Press, Cambridge.

ALLEN, D.F. 1976 - "Wealth, money and coinage in a Celtic society", pp.200-208 in J.V.S. Megaw (Ed.) To Illustrate the Monuments. Thames and Hudson, London.

ANGELI, W. 1980 - "Die Hallstattkultur", pp.11-19 in Die Hallstatt Kultur.

AUSGRABUNGEN IN DEUTSCHLAND Teil I, 1975 - Röm.-Germ. Zentralmuseum, Mainz.

AVDUSIN, D.A. 1967 - Archeologija SSR. Moscow.

BALKWILL, C.J. 1976 - "The evidence of cemeteries for later prehistoric development in the Upper Rhine valley", Procs. of the Prehistoric Soc. Vol. 42, pp.187-213.

BARTH, F.E. 1980 - "Das prähistorische Hallstatt", pp.67-79 in Die Hallstatt Kultur.

BEITRAGE ZUM RANDBEREICH DER LATENKULTUR, 1978 -Zeszyty Naukowe Uniwersytetu Jagiellonskiego CCCCLXXXV, Prace Archeologiczne Z. 26. Warsaw and Cracow.

BENADIK, B. 1977 - "Zur Datierung des jüngsten Horizontes der keltischen Flachgräberfelder im Mittleren Donaugebeit", pp.15-31 in B. Chropovsky (Ed.) Ausklang der Latène-Zivilisation.

BENOIT, F. 1975 - "The Celtic oppidum of Entremont, Provence", pp.227-59 in R. Bruce-Mitford (Ed.) Recent Archaeological Excavations in Europe. Routledge and Kegan Paul, London.

BERGMANN, J. 1967 - "Ethnosoziologische Untersuchungen an Grab- und Hortfundgruppen der älteren Bronzezeit in Nordwestdeutschland", Germania Vol. 45, pp.224-40.

BIEL, J. 1981 - "The late Hallstatt chieftain's grave at Hochdorf", Antiquity Vol. 55, pp.16-18.

BIEL, J. and JOACHIM, W. 1979 - "Vorgeschichtliche Siedlungsreste mit Gusstiegeln bei Fellbach-Schmiden, Rems-Murr-Kreis", Fundberichte aus Baden-Württemberg, Vol. 4, pp.29-53.

BINTLIFF, J.L. 1977a - Natural Environment and Human settlement in Prehistoric Greece. British Archaeological Reports, Suppl. Series 28, 2 Vols., Oxford.

BINTLIFF, J.L. 1977b - "New approaches to human geography. Prehistoric Greece: a case-study." pp.59-114 in F.W. Carter (Ed.) An Historical Geography of the Balkans, Academic Press, London.

BINTLIFF, J.L. 1981 - "Theory and reality in Palaeoeconomy: some words of encouragement to the archaeologist", pp.35-50, in Economic Archaeology, edited by A. Sheridan and G. Bailey, British Archaeological Reports, Int. Series 96, Oxford.

BINTLIFF, J.L. 1982 - "Settlement patterns, land tenure and social structure: a diachronic model", pp.106-11 in Ranking, Resource and Exchange, edited by C. Renfrew and S. Shennan, Cambridge University Press, Cambridge.

BOGUCKI, P.I. 1979 - "Tactical and strategic settlements in the Early Neolithic of Lowland Poland", J. of Anthropological Research Vol. 35, pp.238-46.

BOSERUP, E. 1965 - The Conditions for Agricultural Growth. Allen and Unwin, London.

BOUZEK, J. 1978 - "Zu den Anfängen der Eisenzeit in Mitteleuropa", Zeitschrift für Archäologie, Vol. 12, pp.9-14.

BRADLEY, R. 1971 - "Economic change in the growth of early hill-forts", pp.71-83 in M. Jesson and D. Hill (Eds.) The Iron Age and its Hillforts. University of Southampton.

BRADLEY, R. 1981 - "From ritual to romance: ceremonial enclosures and hill-forts", pp.20-7 in G. Guilbert (Ed.) Hill-fort Studies: essays for A.H.A. Hogg. Leicester University Press, Leicester.

BRADLEY, R. and HODDER, I. 1979 - "British Prehistory: An Integrated View", Man, Vol. 14, pp.93-104.

BREDDIN, R. 1975 - "Die bronzezeitliche Besiedlung zwischen Tornow und Zinnitz, Kr. Calau, auf Grund der Ausgrabungsergebnisse", pp.153-59 in Symbolae Praehistoricae.

BRETZ-MAHLER, D. 1971 - La Civilisation de la Tène I en Champagne: le facies marnien. Gallia, Suppl. 23. Editions du CNRS. Paris.

BUKOWSKI, Z. 1971 - "The character of settlement of the Lusation Culture in the phase of fortified settlements in Silesia and 'Great Poland'", Wiadomosci Archeologiczne, Vol. 36, pp.155-77.

BUKOWSKI, Z 1974 - "Besiedlungscharakter der Lausitzer Kultur in der Hallstattzeit am Beispiel Schlesiens und Grosspolens", pp.15-40 in B. Chropovsky et al. (Eds.) Symposium zu Problemen.

BURGESS, C. 1980 - The Age of Stonehenge. J.M. Dent and Sons, London.

BURNHAM, B.C. 1979 - "Pre-Roman and Romano-British Urbanism? Problems and Possibilities". pp.255-72 in B.C. Burnham and H.B. Johnson (Eds.) Invasion and Response: the case of Roman Britain. British Archaeological Reports, 73, Oxford.

BUTZER, K.W. 1980 - "Civilisations: organisms or sytems?". American Scientist, Vol. 68, pp.517-23.

CAPLOVIC, P. 1974 - "Junghallstattzeitliche Funde im Orava-Gebiet", pp.41-59 in B. Chropovsky et al. (Eds.) Symposium zu Problemen.

CARNEIRO, R.L. 1978 - "Political expansion as an expression of the principle of competitive exclusion", pp.205-33 in R. Cohen and E.R. Service (Eds.) Origins of the State. Institute for the Study of Human Issues, Philadelphia.

CHADWICK, J. 1976 - The Mycenaean World. Cambridge University Press, Cambridge.

CHAMPION, S. 1982 - "Exchange and ranking: the case of coral", pp.67-72 in C. Renfrew and S. Shennan (Eds.) Ranking, Resource and Exchange. Cambridge University Press, Cambridge.

CHAMPION, T.C. 1979 - "The Iron Age: Southern Britian and Ireland", pp.344-432 in J.V.S. Megaw and D.D.A.Simpson (Eds.) Introduction to British Prehistory. Leicester University Press, Leicester.

CHAMPION, T.C. 1982 - "Fortification, ranking and subsistence", pp.61-6 in C. Renfrew and S. Shennan (Eds.) Ranking, Resource and Exchange. Cambridge University Press, Cambridge.

CHROPOVSKY, B., DUSEK, M. and PODBORSKY, V. 1974 -(Eds.) Symposium zu Problemen der. Jüngeren Hallstattzeit in Mitteleuropa. Verlag der Slowakischen Akademie der Wiss., Bratislava.

CHROPOVSKY, B. 1977 - (Ed.) Ausklang der Latène-Zivilisation und Anfänge der Germanischen Besiedlung im Mittleren Donaugebiet. Verlag der Slowakischen Akademie der Wissenschaften, Bratislava.

CLARK, G. 1979 - "Primitive man as hunter, fisher, forager, and farmer", pp.1-21 in P.R.S. Moorey (Ed.) The Origins of Civilisation. Oxford University Press, Oxford.

CLARK, G. and PIGGOTT, S. 1965 - Prehistoric Societies. Hutchinson, London.

CLARKE, D.L. 1972 - "A provisional model of an Iron Age society and its settlement", pp.801-70 in D.L. Clarke (Ed.) Models in Archaeology. Methuen, London.

COBLENZ, W. 1971 - "Die Lausitzer Kultur der Bronze- und frühen Eisenzeit Ostmitteleuropas als Forschungsproblem", Ethnogr. -Archäol. Z. Vol. 12, pp.425-38.

COBLENZ, W. 1974 - "Die Burgwälle und das Ausklingen der westlichen Lausitzer Kultur", pp.85-99 in B. Chropovsky et al. (Eds.) Symposium zu Problemen.

COLES, J.M. and HARDING, A.F. 1979 - The Bronze Age in Europe. Methuen. London.

COLLIS, J.R. 1973a - "Burial with weapons in Iron Age Britain", Germania Vol. 51, pp.121-33.

COLLIS, J.R. 1973b - "Manching reviewed", Antiquity Vol. 47, pp.280-83.

COLLIS, J.R. 1975 - "Excavations at Aulnat, Clermont Ferrand", Archaeological J. , Vol. 132, pp.1-15.

COLLIS, J.R. 1976 - "Town and market in Iron Age Europe", pp.3-23 in B. Cunliffe and R. Rowley (Eds.) Oppida in Barbarian Europe. British Archaeological Reports, Int. Ser. 11, Oxford.

COLLIS, J.R. 1977 - "Pre-Roman burial rites in north-western Europe", pp.1-12 in R. Reece (Ed.) Burial in the Roman World. CBA Res. Rep. 22.

COLLIS, J.R. 1979 - "City and State in pre-Roman Britain", pp.231-40 in B.C. Burnham and H.B. Johnson (Eds.) Invasion and Response: the case of Roman Britain. British Archaeological Reports, 73, Oxford.

COLLIS, J.R. 1980 - "Aulnat and Urbanization in France: a second interim report", Archaeol.J. Vol. 137, pp.40-9.

COLLIS, J.R. 1981a - "A theoretical study of hill-forts", pp.66-76 in G. Guilbert (Ed.) Hill-fort Studies: essays for A.H. Hogg. Leicester University Press, Leicester.

COLLIS, J.R. 1981b - "Coinage, oppida and the rise of Belgic power: a reply" pp.53-5, in Cunliffe, B. (Ed.) Coinage and Society.

COLLIS, J.R. 1981c - "A typology of coin distributions", World Archaeology Vol. 13, pp.122-28.

COLLIS, J.R. 1982 - "Gradual growth and sudden change - urbanisation in temperate Europe", pp.73-78 in C.Renfrew and S. Shennan (Eds.) Ranking, Resource and Exchange. Cambridge University Press, Cambridge.

COLLIS, J.R. and RALSTON, I.B.M. 1976 - "Late La Tène Defences", Germania, Vol. 54, pp.135-46.

CRUMLEY, C.L. 1974 - Celtic social structure: the generation of archaeologically testable hypotheses from literary evidence. The University of Michigan Press, Ann Arbor.

CRUMMY, P. 1980a - "Camulodunum", Current Archaeology, no. 72, pp.6-10.

CRUMMY, P. 1980b - "The temples of Roman Colchester", pp.243-83 in W. Rodwell (Ed.) Temples, Churches and Religion: Recent Research in Roman Britain, British Archaeological Reports 77, Oxford.

CRUMMY, P. 1980c - "Camulodunum", Popular Archaeology, December 1980, pp.43-5.

CUNLIFFE, B. 1971 - "Some aspects of hill-forts and their cultural environments", pp.53-69 in M. Jesson and D. Hill

(Eds.) <u>The Iron Age and its Hillforts</u>. University of Southampton.

CUNLIFFE, B. 1976 - "Hill-forts and oppida in Britain", pp.343-58 in G. Sieveking et al. (Eds.) <u>Problems in Economic and Social Archaeology</u>.

CUNLIFFE, B. 1978a - <u>Iron Age Communities in Britain</u>. 2nd Edition. Routledge and Kegan Paul, London.

CUNLIFFE, B. 1978b - "Settlement and population in the British Iron Age: some facts, figures and fantasies", pp.3-24 in B. Cunliffe and T. Rowley (Eds.) <u>Lowland Iron Age Communities in Europe</u>. British Archaeological Reports, Int. Ser. 48, Oxford.

CUNLIFFE, B. 1979 - <u>The Celtic World</u>. Bodley Head, London.

CUNLIFFE, B. 1980 - "Danebury", <u>Popular Archaeology</u>, December 1980, pp.7-12.

CUNLIFFE, B. 1981a - "Danebury, Hampshire. Third Interim Report on the Excavations 1976-1980", <u>Antiquaries J.</u>, Vol. 61(2), p.238-54

CUNLIFFE, B. 1981b - (Ed.) <u>Coinage and Society in Britain and Gaul</u>, CBA Res. Rep. 38.

CUNLIFFE, B. 1981c - "Money and Society in pre-Roman Britain", pp.29-39 in B. Cunliffe (Ed.) <u>Coinage and Society</u>.

DE LAET, S.J. 1976 - "Native and Celt in the Iron Age of the Low Countries", pp.191-98 in J.V.S. Megaw (Ed.) <u>To Illustrate the Monuments</u>. Thames and Hudson, London.

DE STE. CROIX, 1975 - Review of Westermann, W.L. 'The Slave Systems of Greek and Roman Antiquity'. <u>The Classical Review</u>, Vol. 7 (N.S.) pp. 54-9.

DIE HALLSTATT KULTUR 1980 - Frühform europäischer Einheit. Ausstellungskatalog. Land Oberösterreich, Abteilung Kultur, Linz.

DIE KELTEN IN MITTELEUROPA 1980 -Ausstellungskatalog, Keltenmuseum Hallein, Österreich, 1 May - 30 Sept. 1980, Salzburg.

DUSEK, M. 1974 - "Der junghallstattzeitliche Fürstensitz auf dem Molpir bei Smolenice", pp.137-50 in B. Chropovsky et al. (Eds.) <u>Symposium zu Problemen</u>.

DUSEK, S. 1973 - "Zur Frage der militärischen Demokratie in der urgeschichtlichen Entwicklung der Slowakei", <u>Slovenska Archaeolgia</u>, Vol. 21 (2), pp.409-22.

DUSEK, S. 1977 - "Zur chronologischen und soziologischen Auswertung der Hallstattzeitlichen Gräberfelder von Chotin", <u>Slovenska Archaeologia</u>, Vol. 25 (1), pp.13-46.

EUZENNAT, M. 1980 - "Ancient Marseille in the light of recent excavations", <u>American Journal of Archaeology</u> Vol. 84, pp.133-40.

FEVRIER, P. -A. 1975 (1977) - "L'Habitat dans la Gaule Méridionale", <u>Cahiers Ligures de Préhistoire et d'Archéologie</u>, Vol. 24, pp.7-25.

FILIP, J. 1977 - <u>Celtic civilization and its heritage</u>. Collet's Academia, Wellingborough/Prague.

FILIP, J. 1978 - "Celtic strongholds as an indicator and a reflection of the evolution and the structure of Celtic society", <u>Archaologicke Rozhledy</u> Vol. 30, pp.420-32.

FINLEY, M.I. 1973 - <u>The Ancient Economy</u>. Chatto and Windus, London.

FINLEY, M.I. 1977 - "The Ancient City: From Fustel de Coulanges to Max Weber and Beyond", <u>Comp. Studies in Society and History</u>, vol. 19,pp.305-27.

FINLEY, M.I. 1978 - "Empire in the Graeco-Roman world", <u>Review II (1)</u>, pp.55-68.

FISCHER, F. 1973 - "Keimelia: Bemerkungen zur kulturgeschichtlichen Interpretation des sogenannten Südimports in der späten Hallstatt-und frühen Latène-Kultur der westlichen Mittleuropa", <u>Germania</u> Vol. 51, pp.436-59.

FLANAGAN, L.N.W. 1982 - "The Irish Earlier Bronze Age Industry in Perspective", <u>JRSAI</u>, Vol. 112, pp.93-100.

FOWLER, P.J. 1978 - "Lowland landscapes: culture, time, and personality", pp.1-12 in S. Limbrey and J.G. Evans (Ed.) <u>The effect of man on the landscape: the Lowland Zone</u>. CBA Research Report no. 21.

FRANKENSTEIN, S. 1979 - "The Phoenicians in the far west: a function of Assyrian imperialism", pp.263-94 in M.T. Larsen (Ed.) <u>Power and Propaganda</u>. Akademisk Forlag, Copenhagen.

FRANKENSTEIN, S. and ROWLANDS, M.J. 1978 - "The internal structure and regional context of early iron age society in south-western Germany", <u>Bull. of the Institute of Archaeology, University of London</u>, Vol. 15, pp.73-112.

FREIDIN, N. 1983 - "The Early Iron Age in the Paris Basin: A Study in Culture Change", <u>Oxford Journal of Archaeology</u>, Vol. 2, pp.69-91.

FREY, O. -H. 1976 - "The chariot tomb from Adria: some notes on Celtic horsemanship and chariotry", pp.171-79 in J.V.S. Megaw (Ed.) <u>To Illustrate the Monuments</u>. Thames and Hudson, London.

FREY, O. -H. 1980 - "Der Westhallstattkreis im 6. Jahrhundert v.Chr.", pp.80-116 in <u>Die Hallstatt Kultur</u>.

FRIED, M.H. 1967 - <u>The Evolution of Political Society</u>. Random House, New York.

FULFORD, M. 1978 - "The interpretation of Britain's late Roman trade: the scope of medieval historical and archaeological analogy", pp.59-69 in <u>Roman Shipping and Trade</u>, edited by J. du Plat Taylor and H. Cleere, CBA Res. Rep. 24.

FURMANEK, V. 1973 - "Zu einiger sozial-ökonomischen Problemen der Bronzezeit", <u>Slovenska Archeologia</u>, Vol. 21, pp.401-08.

GABROVEC, S. 1974 - "Die Ausgrabungen in Sticna und ihre Bedeutung für die südostalpine Hallstattkultur", pp.163-87 in B. Chropovsky et al. (Eds.) <u>Symposium zu Problemen</u>.

GABROVEC, S. 1980 - "Der Beginn der Hallstattkultur und der Osten", pp.30-53 in <u>Die Hallstatt Kultur</u>.

GALUSZKA, A. 1963 - "Die Frage von Genese und Funktion der Burgwälle der Lausitzer Kultur in Niederschlesien", <u>Arbeits - und Forschungsberichte zur Sächsischen Bodendenkmalpflege</u>, Vol. 11/12, pp.511-17.

GEDL, M 1976 - "Studies on settlement of the River Liswarta Basin in the Bronze and Early Iron Age", <u>Archaeologia Polona</u> Vol. 17, pp.211-30.

GEDL, M. 1977 - "Bemerkungen zur Vorlausitzer Kultur", Zeits. f. Archäologie Vol. 11, pp.49-66.

GEDL, M. 1978 - "Gräber der Laténkultur in Kietrz, Bezirk Opole", pp.9-72 in Beiträge zum Randbereich.

GILMAN, A. 1981 - "The development of social stratification in Bronze Age Europe", Current Anthropology, Vol. 22, no. 1, pp.1-23.

GIMBUTAS, M. 1965 - Bronze Age Cultures in Central and Eastern Europe. Mouton, the Hague.

HAERKE, H. 1979 - Settlement Types and Settlement Patterns in the West Hallstatt Province. British Archaeological Reports, Int. Ser. 57, Oxford.

HAERKE, H. 1980 - "Early Iron Age Hill Settlement", unpubl. paper given to the conference, Hillforts in Britain and Europe. Oxford University Extramural Dept., January 1980.

HAERKE, H. 1982 - "Early Iron Age Hill Settlement in West Central Europe: Patterns and Developments", Oxford Journal of Archaeology, Vol. 1, pp.187-211.

HAFFNER, A. 1977 - "Neue Forschungen zur Archäologie der Treverer", pp.95-105 in B. Chropovsky (Ed.) Ausklang der Latène-Zivilisation.

HANSEL, B. 1978 - Beiträge zur Chronologie der mittleren Bronzezeit im Karpatenbecken. Rudolf Habelt Verlag, Bonn.

HARHOIU, R. 1976 - "Sittentypen in den Späthallstattzeitlichen und Frühlatènezeitlichen Fürstengräbern aus Westdeutschland und Ostfrankreich", Studii si Cercetari de Istorie Veche si Arheologie, Vol. 27 (2), pp.181-202.

HARRIS, M. 1971 - Culture, Man, and Nature. Crowell, New York.

HASELGROVE, C. 1979 - "The significance of coinage in pre-Conquest Britain", pp.197-209, in B. C. Burnham and H.B. Johnson (Eds.) Invasion and Response: the case of Roman Britain. British Archaeological Reports, 73, Oxford.

HASELGROVE, C. 1982 - "Wealth, prestige and power: the dynamics of late iron age political centralisation in south-east England", pp.79-88 in C. Renfrew and S. Shennan (Eds.) Ranking, Resource and Exchange. Cambridge University Press, Cambridge.

HATCHER, J. and POSTAN, M.M., 1978 - "Agrarian class structure and economic development in Pre-Industrial Europe. Population and class relations in Feudal Society", Past and Present, Vol. 78, pp.24-37.

HATT, J. -J. 1976 - "Le Pègue et l'histoire de la Gaule", Archéologia, Vol. 98, pp.46-60.

HEDEAGER, L. 1980 - "Besiedlung, soziale Struktur und politische Organisation in der älteren und jüngeren römischen Kaiserzeit Ostdänemarks", Praeh. Zeits. Vol. 55, pp.38-109.

HENCKEN, H. 1968 - Tarquinia, Villanovans and Early Etruscans. Cambridge, Mass.

HENNEBERG, M. and OSTOJA-ZAGORSKI, J. (Unpubl.) - "Use of a general ecological model for reconstitution of prehistoric economy: the Hallstatt period culture of Northwest Poland".

HERRMAN, F.-R. 1975 - "Grabungen im Oppidum von Kelheim 1964 bis 1972", pp.298-311 in Ausgrabungen in Deutschland.

HIGGS, E.S. 1972 - (Ed.) Papers in Economic Prehistory. Cambridge University Press, Cambridge.

HIGGS, E.S. 1975 - (Ed.) Palaeoeconomy. Cambridge University Press, Cambridge.

HIGHAM, C.W. 1968 - "Patterns of prehistoric economic exploitation on the Alpine Foreland", Vierteljahreshefte Naturf. Ges. Zürich, Vol. 113, pp.41-92.

HILLMAN, G. 1978 - "On the orgins of domestic rye - Secale Cereale", Anatolian Studies, Vol. 28, pp.157-74.

HILTON, R.H. 1978 - "Agrarian class structure and economic development in Pre-Industrial Europe: a crisis of Feudalism", Past and Present, Vol. 80, pp.3-19.

HODDER, I.R. 1979 - "Pre-Roman and Romano-British tribal economies", pp.189-196 in B.C. Burnham and H.B. Johnson (Eds.) Invasion and Response: the case of Roman Britain. British Archaeological Reports, 73, Oxford.

HODSON, F.R. 1977 - "Quantifying Hallstatt: some initial results", American Antiquity Vol. 42, pp.394-412.

HODSON, F.R. 1979 - "Inferring status from burials in Iron Age Europe; some recent attempts", pp.23-30 in B.C. Burnham and J. Kingsbury (Eds.) Space, Hierarchy and Society. British Archaeological Reps. Int. Ser. 59, Oxford.

HODSON, F.R. 1980 - "Ramsauer und Hallstatt: Eine Zwischenbalanz", MAG Wien, Vol. 110. pp.53-9.

HODSON, F.R. and ROWLETT, R.M. 1974 - "From 600 BC to the Roman Conquest", pp.157-91 in S. Piggott, G. Daniel and C. McBurney (Eds.) France Before the Romans. Thames and Hudson, London.

HUNN, J.R. 1980 - "The earthworks of Prae Wood: an interim account", Britannia Vol. 11, pp.21-30.

HVASS, S. 1975 - "Das eisenzeitliche Dorf bei Hodde, Westjütland", Acta Archaeologia Vol. 46, pp.142-58.

JOACHIM, H. -E 1973 - "Ein reich ausgestattetes Wagengrab der Spätlatènzeit aus Neuwied, Stadtteil Heimbach-Weis", Bonner Jahrbücher Vol. 173, pp.1-43.

JOCKENHÖVEL, A. 1974 - "Zu befestigten Siedlungen der Urnenfelderzeit aus Süddeutschland", Fundberichte aus Hessen, Vol. 14, pp.19-62.

JOVANOVIC, B. 1981 - "Les guerres et l'economie des Celts orientaux dans la vallée du Danube", pp.207-29 in Abstracts, 10th Congress of the Union of Pre- and Protohistoric Sciences, Mexico, Oct. 19-24, 1981 (Miscelanea, Sect.8).

KILIAN-DIRLMEIER, I. 1969 - "Studien zur Ornamentik auf Bronzeblechgürteln und Gürtelblechen der Hallstattzeit aus Hallstatt und Bayern", Ber. Röm. -Germ. Komm. vol. 50, pp.97-189.

KILIAN-DIRLMEIER, I. 1971 - "Betrachtungen zur Struktur des Gräberfeldes von Hallstatt", Mitteilungen der Österreichischen Arbeitsgemeinschaft für Ur- und Frühgeschichte Vol. 22, pp.71 ff.

KIMMIG, W. 1975a - "Early Celts on the upper Danube: the excavations at the Heuneburg", pp.32-64 in R. Bruce-

Mitford (Ed.) Recent Archaeological Excavations in Europe. Routledge and Kegan Paul, London.

KIMMIG, W. 1975b - "Die Heuneburg an der oberen Donau", pp.192-211 in Ausgrabungen in Deutschland.

KLEJN, L.D. 1972 - "Die Konzeption des 'Neolithikums', 'Aneolithikums' und der 'Bronzezeit' in der archäologischen Wissenschaft der Gegenwart", Neolithische Studien I, pp.7-29.

KNEZ, T. 1974 - "Hallstattzeitliche Hügelgräber in Novo Mesto", pp.243-52 in B. Chropovsky et.al. (Eds.) Symposium zu Problemen

KNORZER, K.-H. 1979 - "Über den Wandel der angebauten Körnerfruchte und ihrer Unkrautvegetation auf einer niederrheinischen Lössfläche seit dem Frühneolithikum", pp.147-63 in Festschrift Maria Hopf, edited by U. Körber-Grohne. Rudolf Habelt Verlag, Bonn.

KOLNIK, T. 1977 - "Anfänge der Germanischen Besiedlung in der Sudwestslowakei und das Regnum Vannianum", pp.143 ff. in B. Chropovsky (Ed.) Ausklang der Latène-Zivilisation.

KOSSACK, G. et.al. 1974 - "Zehn Jahre Siedlungsforschung in Archsum auf Sylt", Ber.Röm. -Germ. Komm., Vol. 55, pp.261-427.

KOUTECKY, D. 1968 - "Grossgräber, ihre Konstruktion, Grabritus und soziale Struktur der Bevölkerung der Bylaner Kultur", Pamatky Archeologicke Vol. 59 (2), pp.400-87.

KOUTECKY, D. and VENCLOVA, N. 1979 - "Zur Problematik der Besiedlung des Nordwestlichen Böhmens in der Latènezeit und Römischen Kaiserzeit. Die Siedlung Pocerady I and II", Pamatky Archeologicke, Vol. 70, pp.42-112.

KRAMER, W. 1975 - "Zwanzig Jahre Ausgrabungen in Manching, 1955 bis 1974", pp.287-297 in Ausgrabungen in Deutschland.

KRISTIANSEN, K. 1978 - "The consumption of wealth in Bronze Age Denmark. A study in the dynamics of economic processes in tribal societies", pp.158-90 in K. Kristiansen and C.Paludan-Müller (Eds.) New Directions in Scandinavian Archaeology. The National Museum of Denmark, Copenhagen.

KRISTIANSEN, K. 1980 - "Besiedlung, Wirtschaftsstrategie und Bodennutzung in der Bronzezeit Dänemarks", Praehistorische Zeits., Vol. 55 (1), pp.1-37.

KRISTIANSEN, K. 1981 - "Economic models for Bronze Age Scandinavia - towards an integrated approach", pp.239-303 in A. Sheridan and G. Bailey (Eds.) Economic Archaeology. British Archaeological Reports, Int. Ser. 96, Oxford.

KRISTIANSEN, K. 1982 - "The Formation of Tribal Systems in Later European Prehistory: Northern Europe, 4000 - 500 BC", pp.241-80 in C. Renfrew, M.J. Rowlands and B.A. Segraves (Eds.) Theory and Explanation in Archaeology. Academic Press, New York.

KROMER, K. 1958 - "Gedanken über sozialen Aufbau der Bevölkerung auf dem Salzberg bei Hallstatt, Oberösterreich", Archiv für ur- und frühgeschichtliche Bergbauforschung, Mitt. No. 13, pp.39-58.

KRUK, J. 1980 - The Neolithic Settlement of Southern Poland. (Edited by J.M. Howell and N.J. Starling). British Archaeological Reports, Int. Ser. 93, Oxford.

KRUTA, V. 1975 - "Les habitats et nécropoles laténiens en Bohême", pp.95-102 in P. -M. Duval and V. Kruta (Eds.) L'Habitat et la Nécropole a l'Age du Fer en Europe Occidentale et Centrale. Librairie Honoré, Paris.

LANTIER, R. 1973 - "La Campagne Gauloise", pp.319-22 in Estudios Dedicados al Profesor Dr. Luis Pericot. Instituto de Arqueologia y Prehistoria, Universidad de Barcelona.

LARSEN, M.T. 1979 - "The tradition of Empire in Mesopotamia", pp.75-103 in M.T. Larsen (Ed.) Power and Propaganda. Akademisk Forlag, Copenhagen.

LATTIMORE, O. 1962 - "The Frontier in history", pp.469-91 in O. Lattimore, Studies in Frontier History. Oxford University Press, Oxford.

LEESE, M.N. 1979 - "A statistical study of Welsh Bronze Age metal artifacts", Abstracts, Procs. of the Annual Conference at the Computer Centre, Birmingham, 'Computer Applications in Archaeology'.

LE ROY LADURIE, E, 1978 - "Agrarian class structure and economic development in Pre-Industrial Europe. A reply to Professor Brenner", Past and Present, Vol. 79, pp.55-59.

LESSING, E. and KRUTA, V. 1979 - Die Kelten. Herder Freiburg, Basel - Wien.

LEVY, J. 1978 - "Evidence of social stratification in Bronze Age Denmark", J. of Field Archaeology, Vol. 5, pp.49-56.

LINDQUIST, S. -O. 1974 - "Landscape on Gotland during the Early Iron Age", Norwegian Archaeological Review, Vol. 7, pp.6-32.

LIVERSAGE, D. 1977 - "Kulturlage in Dänemark um die Zeitwende, beleuchtet durch neuere Funde", pp.209-21 in B. Chropovsky (Ed.) Ausklang der Latène-Zivilisation.

LORENZ, H. 1980 - "Bemerkungen zum Totenbrauchtum", pp.138-48 in Die Kelten in Mitteleuropa.

MAGGETTI, M. and GALETTI, G. 1980 - "Composition of Iron Age fine ceramics from Châtillon-s-Glâne (Kt. Fribourg, Switzerland) and the Heuneburg (Kr. Sigmaringen, West Germany)", J. of Archaeological Science, Vol. 7, pp.87-91.

MAIER, F. 1974 - "Gedanken zur Entstehung der industriellen Grosssiedlung der Hallstatt- und Latènezeit auf dem Dürrnberg bei Hallein", Germania Vol. 52, pp.326-47.

MANBY, T.G. 1980 - "Bronze Age settlement in Eastern Yorkshire", pp.307-70 in J. Barrett and R. Bradley (Eds.) The British Later Bronze Age. British Archaeological Reports, 83, Oxford.

MARSHALL, A.J. 1977 - "Environment and agriculture during the Iron Age: statistical analysis of changing settlement ecology", World Archaeology Vol. 9, pp.347-56.

MENKE, M. 1971 - "Zur Vor- und Frühgeschichtlichen Besiedlung im Reichenhaller Becken", Archäologisches Korrespondenzblatt Vol. 1, pp.113-16.

MENKE, M. 1972 - Review of R. Schindler, 'Studien zum vorgeschichtlichen Siedlungs- und Befestigungswesen des Saarlands", Praehistorische Zeitschrift, Vol. 47, pp.122-31.

MILISAUSKAS, S. 1978 - European Prehistory, Academic Press, New York.

MOOSLEITNER, F. 1980 - "Handel und Handwerk", pp.93-100 in Die Kelten in Mitteleuropa.

MOTYKOVA, K., DRDA, P. and RYBOVA, A. 1977 - "The position of Zavist in the Early La Tène period in Bohemia", Pamatky Archeologicke Vol. 68, pp.255-316.

MOTYKOVA, K., DRDA, P. and RYBOVA, A. 1978 - "Metal, glass and amber objects from the Acropolis of Zavist", Pamatky Archeologicke, Vol. 69, pp.259-343.

MÜLLER-KARPE, H. 1959 - Beiträge zur Chronologie der Urnenfelderzeit nordlich und südlich der Alpen. Römisch-Germanische Forschungen 22, de Gruyter, Berlin.

NANDRIS, J. 1976a - "Changing premisses of exploitation in r-and K- societies during the Early Neothermal Period in South-East Europe (c. 10,000 - 3000 BC)", Unpubl. lecture (cyclostyled) to the Brit. Assoc. for Advancement of Science at Lancaster, Sept. 1-18, 1976.

NANDRIS, J. 1976b - "The Dacian Iron Age: a comment in a European context", pp.723-36 in Festschrift für Richard Pittioni I. Archaeologia Austriaca, Beiheft 13, Wien.

NANDRIS, J. 1978 - "Some features of Neolithic Climax Societies", Studia Praehistorica, Sofia, 1978, 1-2, pp.198-211.

NASH, D. 1975 - The Celts of Central Gaul - some aspects of social and economic development as background to the Roman Conquest in the light of numismatic and archaeological evidence. D. Phil. thesis, Oxford University.

NASH, D. 1978 - "Territory and state formation in central Gaul", pp.455-75 in D. Green, C. Haselgrove and M. Spriggs (Eds.) Social Organization and Settlement. British Archaeological Reports, Int. Ser. 47, Oxford.

NASH, D. 1981 - "Coinage and state development in central Gaul", pp.10-17 in B.Cunliffe (Ed.) Coinage and Society.

NEMESKALOVA-JIROUDKOVA, Z. 1978 - "Der Einfluss der Antiken Welt auf die keltische Münzprägung in Böhmen und Mähren", Eirene, Vol. 16, pp.71-9.

NEUSTUPNY, E. and J. 1961 - Czechoslavakia Before the Slavs. Thames and Hudson, London.

NIESIOLOWSKA-WEDZKA, A. 1976 - "Recherches sur la genèse et la fonction des castra du type 'Biskupin' à la lumière des civilisations méridionales", Slavia Antiqua Vol. 23, pp.17-38.

NOVOTNA, M. 1970 - Die Axte und Beile in der Slowakei. Praehistorische Bronzefunde IX, 3. Beck Verlag, München.

OSTOJA-ZAGORSKI, J. 1974 - "From studies on the economic structure at the decline of the Bronze Age and the Hallstatt period in the North and West Zone of the Orda and Vistula Basins", Przeglad Archeologiczny, Vol. 22, pp.127-50.

OSTOJA-ZAGORSKI, J. 1976 - "Recherches sur le problème du déclin des castra de civilisation Lusacienne", Slavia Antiqua, Vol. 23, pp.39-73.

PATEK, E. 1982 - "Recent excavations at the Hallstatt and La Tène Hill-Fort of Sopron-Varhely (Burgstall), and the Predecessors of the Hallstatt Culture in Hungary", pp.1-56 in D. Gabler, E. Patek and I. Voros, Studies in the Iron Age of Hungary. British Archaeological Reports, Int. Ser. 144. Oxford.

PAULI, L. 1978 - (Ed.) Der Dürrnberg bei Hallein III. Beck Verlag, Munich.

PAULI, L. 1980a - "Die Herkunft der Kelten", pp.16-24 in Die Kelten in Mitteleuropa.

PAULI, L. 1980b - "Das keltische Mitteleuropa vom 6. bis 2. Jahrhundert v. Chr.", pp.25-36 in die Kelten in Mitteleuropa.

PAULI, L. 1980c - Die Welt der Kelten. Salzburger Landesausstellung, Wallchart. Keltenmuseum, Hallein.

PEACOCK, D.P.S. 1968 - "A petrological study of certain Iron Age pottery from Western England", Proceedings of the Prehistoric Soc., Vol. 34, pp.414-27.

PEACOCK, D.P.S. 1969 - "A contribution to the study of Glastonbury Ware from South-Western Britain", Antiquaries J., Vol. 49, pp.41-61.

PHILLIPS, P. 1980 - The Prehistory of Europe. Allen Lane, London.

PICHLEROVA, M. 1974 - "Zum hallstattzeitlichen Hügelgräberhorizont in der Südwestslowakei", pp.363-70 in B. Chropovsky et al. (Eds.) Symposium zu Problemen.

PIGGOTT, S. 1965 - Ancient Europe. Edinburgh University Press.

PIGGOTT, S. 1982 - Scotland Before History. Edinburgh Unversity Press.

PIONTEK,J. and KOLODZIEJSKI, A. 1981 - "Excavations at Wicina, Poland", Current Anthropology, vol. 22, pp.73-74.

PLEINER, R. 1977 - "Extensive Eisenverhuttungsgebiete im Freien Germanien", pp. 297 ff. in B. Chropovsky (Ed.) Ausklang der Latène-Zivilisation.

PLEINER, R. 1980 - "Early iron metallurgy in Europe", pp. 375-415 in T.A. Wertime and J.D. Muhly (Eds.) The Coming of the Age of Iron. Yale University Press.

PODBORSKY, V. 1974 - "Die Stellung der südmährischen Horakov-Kultur im Rahmen des Danubischen Hallstatt", pp. 371-426 in B. Chropovsky et.al. (Eds.) Symposium zu Problemen.

POSTAN, M.M. 1975 - The Medieval Economy and Society. Penguin Books, London.

POTTER, T.W. 1979 - The Changing Landscape of South Etruria. Elek, London.

POTTER, T.W. 1980 - "The western Mediterranean and the origins of Rome", Ch. 34, pp.227-31 in A. Sherratt (Ed.) The Cambridge Encyclopedia of Archaeology. Cambridge University Press, Cambridge.

PREIDEL, H. 1977 - "Handel und Verkehr zwischen Mittleren Donau und Ostsee in den ersten Jahrhunderten n. Chr.", Bohemia vol. 18, pp.9-34.

PREIDEL, H. 1978 - "Die keltischen Oppida", Bohemia vol. 19, pp.65-84.

PREIDEL, H. 1979 - "Die Bevölkerungsverhältnisse in Böhmen und Mähren in den Jahrhunderten um Christi Geburt", Bohemia vol. 20, pp.13-36.

RAJEWSKI, Z. 1974 - "Was Wehrsiedlung-Burgen sowie deren Überbauung an wirtschaftlich-gesellschaftlichem

214

Wert bergen", pp.427-33 in B. Choropovsky et.al. (Eds.) Symposium zu Problemen.

RANDSBORG, K. 1974a - "Social stratification in Early Bronze Age Denmark: a study in the regulation of cultural systems", Praehistorische Zeits. Vol. 49, pp.38-61.

RANDSBORG, K. 1974b - "Population and social variation in Early Bronze Age Denmark", Kuml 1973/4, pp.197-208.

RANDSBORG, K. 1974c - "Prehistoric populations and social regulation: the case of Early Bronze Age Denmark", Homo Vol. 25, pp.59-67.

RANDSBORG, K. 1982 - "Rank, rights and resources - an archaeological perspective from Denmark", pp.132-39 in Renfrew and Shennan (Eds.) Ranking, Resource and Exchange.

REECE, R. 1981 - "Roman monetary impact on the Celtic world - thoughts and problems", pp.24-28 in B.Cunliffe (Eds.) Coinage and society.

RENFREW, C. 1973 - Before Civilization. Jonathan Cape, London.

RENFREW, C. 1975 - "Trade as action at a distance: questions of integration and communication", pp.3-59 in Ancient Civilization and Trade, edited by J.A. Sabloff and C.C. Lamberg-Karlovsky. University of New Mexico Press, Albuquerque.

RENFREW, C. 1979 - "Systems collapse as social transformation: catastrophe and anastrophe in early state societies", pp.481-506 in C. Renfrew and K.L. Cooke (Eds.) Transformations: Mathematical Approaches to Culture Change. Academic Press, New York.

RENFREW, C. and SHENNAN, S. 1982 - (Eds.) Ranking, Resource and Exchange. Cambridge University Press, Cambridge.

RENFREW, J.M. 1973 - Palaeoethnobotany: the prehistoric food plants of the Near East and Europe. Methuen.

RICHARDS, J. 1982 - "The Stonehenge environs project - the story so far", Scot. Arch. Review, Vol. 1, pp.98-104.

RIECKHOFF-PAULI, S. 1980 - "Des Ende der keltischen Welt: Kelten - Römer - Germanen", pp.37-47 in Die Kelten in Mitteleuropa.

ROWLANDS, M.J. 1979 - "Local and long distance trade and incipient state formation on the Bamenda Plateau in the late 19th century", Paideuma, Vol. 25, pp. 1-19.

ROWLANDS, M.J. 1980 - "Kinship, alliance and exchange in the European bronze age", pp. 15-55 in J.Barrett and R. Bradley (Eds.) The British Later Bronze Age. British Archaeological Reports, 83, Oxford.

ROWLETT, R.M. 1968 - "The Iron Age north of the Alps", Science vol. 161, pp. 123-134.

SALDOVA, V. 1971 - "Die Westböhmischen Späthallstattzeitlichen Flachgräber und ihre Beziehung zu den zeitgleichen Westböhmischen Hügelgräbern", Pamatky Archeologicke vol. 62 (1), pp. 1-134.

SALDOVA, V. 1974 - "Östliche Elemente in der westböhmischen hallstattzeitlichen Hügelgräberkultur", pp. 447-68 in B. Choropovsky et al. (Eds.) Symposium zu Problemen.

SALDOVA, V. 1977 - "Die sozial-ökonomischen Bedingungen der Enstehung und Funktion der Spätbronzezeitlichen Höhensiedlungen in Westböhmen", Pamatky Archeologicke, vol. 68, pp. 117-163.

SAXE, A.A. 1970 - Social Dimensions of Mortuary Practices. Ph. D. Dissertation, University of Michigan (Unpubl.).

SCHINDLER, R. 1974 - "Hallstättische Höhenburgen im Saar-und Moselraum", pp. 435-446 in B. Chropovsky et.al. (Eds.) Symposium zu Problemen.

SCHINDLER, R. 1975 - "Die Altburg von Bundenbach und andere spätkeltische Befestigungen im Trevererland", pp. 273-286 in Ausgrabungen in Deutschland.

SCHINDLER, R. 1977 - Die Altburg bei Bundenbach. Phillip von Zabern, Mainz.

SCHMID, P. 1978 - "New archaeological results of settlement structures (Roman Iron Age) in the north-west-German Coastal area", pp.123-45 in B. Cunliffe and T. Rowley (Eds.) Lowland Iron Age Communities in Europe. British Archaeological Reports, Int. Ser. 48, Oxford.

SCHWAB, H. 1976 - "Erforschung hallstattzeitlicher Grabhügel im Kanton Freiburg", Mitteilungsblatt Schweiz. Ges. f. Ur- und F.- Geschichte 7 (25/26), pp. 14-33.

SCHWAPPACH, F. 1973 - "Frühkeltisches Ornament zwischen Marne, Rhein und Moldau", Bonner Jahrbücher vol. 173, pp. 53-97.

SCHWIDETZKY, I. 1978 - "Anthropologie der Dürrnberger Bevölkerung", Beitrag, pp. 541-581, in Pauli 1978.

SELKIRK, A. 1981 - "Thetford", Current Archaeology, no. 81, pp. 294-297.

SIEVEKING, G. de G., LONGWORTH, I.H. and WILSON, K.E. 1976 - (Eds.) Problems in Economic and Social Archaeology, Duckworth, London.

SKINNER, G.W. 1977 - (Ed.) The City in Late Imperial China Stanford University Press, Stanford.

SMITH, C. 1978 - "The landscape and natural history of Iron Age settlement on the Trent gravels", pp. 91-101 in B. Cunliffe and T. Rowley (Eds.) Lowland Iron Age Communities in Europe. British Archaeological Reports, Int. Ser. 48, Oxford.

SNODGRASS, A. 1980 - Archaic Greece: the Age of Experiment. Dent, London.

SPINDLER, K. 1976 - Der Magdalenenberg bei Villingen. Führer zu vor- und frühgeschichtlichen Denkmälern in Baden-Württemberg, 5. Stuttgart.

STANFORD, S.C. 1980 - "Hillforts of the Welsh Marches", Popular Archaeology December, 1980, pp. 16-20.

STEAD, I.M. 1979 - The Arras Culture. Yorkshire Philosophical Society, York.

STEAD, I. n.d. - The Gauls. Celtic Antiquities from France. British Museum Publications.

SYME, R. 1977 - "Helvetian Aristocrats", Museum Helveticum, vol. 34, pp. 129-140.

TERENOZKIN, A.I. 1980 - "Die Kimmerier und ihre Kultur", pp. 20-29 in Die Hallstatt Kultur.

THOMAS, H.L. et.al. 1975 - "The Titelberg: A hill fort of Celtic and Roman times", Archaeology vol. 28, pp. 55-57.

TODD. M. 1975 - The Northern Barbarians, 100 BC - AD 300. Hutchinson University Library, London.

TODD, M. 1977 - "Germanic burials in the Roman Iron Age ", pp. 39-43 in R. Reece (Ed.) Burial in the Roman World. CBA Res. Rep. 22.

TYLECOTE, R.F. 1976 - A History of Metallurgy. Metals Society, London.

VIGNERON, E. 1981 - "Contribution de l'analyse des données a l'étude des débuts de la metallurgie dans le Midi mediterranéen français", pp. 10-33 in Abstracts, 10th Congress of the Union of Pre- and Protohistoric Sciences, Mexico Oct. 19-24, 1981 (El Origen de la Metalurgica Sect.).

VITA-FINZI, C. and **HIGGS, E.S.** 1970 - "Prehistoric economy in the Mt. Carmel area of Palestine: site catchment analysis", Procs. Prehistoric Soc. vol. 36., pp. 1-37.

WAILES, B 1970 - "Plow and population in Temperate Europe", 154-179 in B. Spooner (Ed.) Population, Resources, and Technology Cambridge, Mass.

WAINWRIGHT, G.J. 1979 - Gussage All Saints. An Iron Age Settlement in Dorset. Dept. of the Environment Archaeological Reps. No. 10, London, H.M.S.O.

WAMSER, G. 1975 - "Zur Hallstattkultur in Ostfrankreich", Ber. Röm.-Germ. Komm. 56, pp. 1-178.

WATERBOLK, H.T. 1977 - "Walled enclosures of the Iron Age in the north of the Netherlands", Palaeohistoria vol. 19, pp. 98-172.

WELINDER, S. 1975 - Prehistoric Agriculture in Eastern Middle Sweden. Acta Archaeologica Lundensia series in 8⁰ Minore No. 4, Lund.

WELLS, P.S. 1980a - "Contact and change: an example on the fringes of the Classical world", World Archaeology vol. 12, pp. 1-10.

WELLS, P.S. 1980b - "The Early Iron Age settlement of Hascherkeller in Bavaria: preliminary report on the 1979 excavations", J. of Field Archaeology vol. 7, pp. 313 -328.

WELLS, P.S. and BONFANTE, L. 1979 - "West-Central Europe and the Mediterranean", Expedition, vol. 21(4), pp. 18-24.

WELLS, P.S., BENEFIT, B., QUILLIAN, C.C. and STUBBS, J.D. 1981 - "Excavations at Hascherkeller in Bavaria: Field Research into the Economy of a Late Bronze/Early Iron Age Village", J. of Field Archaeology, vol. 8, pp. 289-302.

WERNER, J. 1977 - "Schlusswort", pp. 403-413 in B. Chropovsky (Ed.) Ausklang der Latène-Zivilisaion.

WHIMSTER, R. 1977 - "Iron Age burial in Southern Britain", Proceedings of the Prehistoric Soc., vol. 43, pp. 317-327.

WHITTLE, A. 1980 - "Scord of Brouster and early settlement in Shetland", Arch. Atlantica, vol.3, pp. 35-55.

WILLERDING, U. 1979 - "Zum Ackerbau in der jüngeren vorrömischen Eisenzeit", pp. 309-330 in Festschrift Maria Hopf, edited by U. Körber-Grohne. Rudolf Habelt Verlag, Bonn.

WOZNIAK, Z. 1976 - "Die östliche Randzone der Latènekultur", Germania, vol. 54, pp. 382-402.

WÜSTEMANN, H. 1974 - "Zur Sozialstruktur im Seddiner Kulturgebiet", Zeits. für Archäologie, vol. 8, pp. 67-107.

ZELLER, K.W. 1980 - "Kriegwesen und Bewaffnung der Kelten", pp. 111-132 in Die Kelten in Mitteleuropa.

ZELLER, K.W. 1980a - "Die neuen Grabungen auf dem Dürrnberg - Techniken und Ergebnisse", pp. 159-181 in Die Kelten in Mitteleuropa.

ZIMMERMANN, W.H. 1978 - "Economy of the Roman Iron Age settlement Flogeln, Lower Saxony - husbandry, cattle farming and manufacturing", pp. 147-165 in B. Cunliffe and T. Rowley (Eds.) Lowland Iron Age Communities in Europe. British Archaeological Reports, Int. Ser. 48, Oxford.

ZÜRN, H. 1972 - "Zur Chronologie de südwestdeutschen Späthallstattzeit und die Datierung der Fürstengräber", pp. 487-500 in B. Chropovosky et al. (Eds.) Symposium zu Problemen.

ZÜRN, H. 1975 - "Der 'Grafenbühl', ein späthallstattzeitlicher Fürstengrabhugel bei Asperg", pp.216-20 in Ausgrabungen in Deutschland I.

ZÜRN, H. 1977 - "Grabungen im Oppidum von Finsterlohr", Fundberichte aus Baden-Württemberg, vol. 3, pp. 231-264.

216

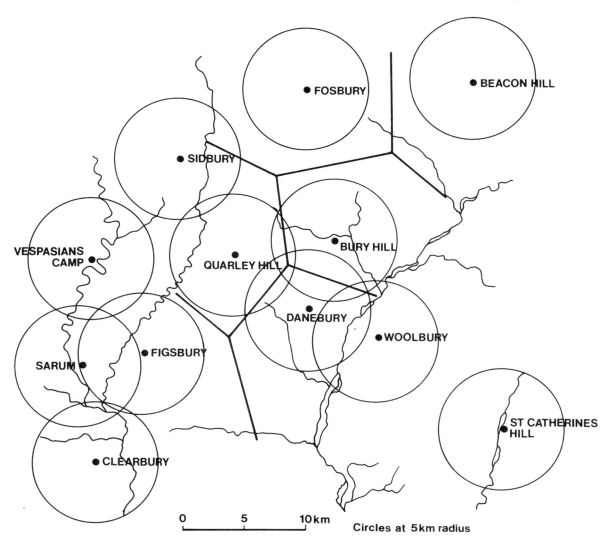

Fig Ia

Early Iron Age hillforts in the area west of Winchester, southern England. Data and partial Thiessen polygon network after Cunliffe 1976, Fig. 4. On a farming catchment of 1 hour or 5kms. radius (circles) from each defended focus, the sites are poorly spaced for rational non-competitive teritorial exploitation. This assumes that land use was tied to a home base in or beside the hillfort.

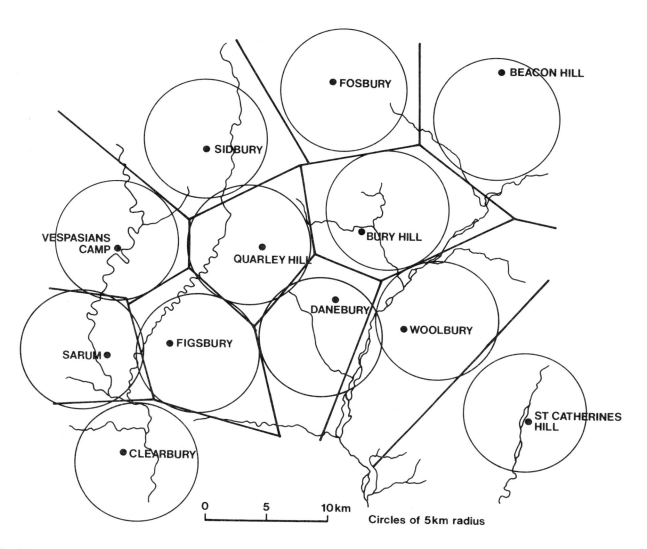

Fig Ib

The same data base re-analysed. The Thiessen polygon network is redrawn and completed. It is here assumed that most farmers dwelt in farms and hamlets outside of the hillfort and scattered about the Thiessen-defined territory of each focus. The relevant catchment statistic is therefore the ease of access from the territory into the 'central place' for varied 'services' and these cells allow access within 1-3 hours for the most outlying sectors (giving a day-return potential that forms a characteristic threshold lilmiting the catchment of simple 'service centre' systems). Circles of 5kms. radius are fitted into each cell regardless of the symmetry to the hillfort locus, to emphasize that the land area (and therefore perhaps population module?) of these territories is generally very regular.

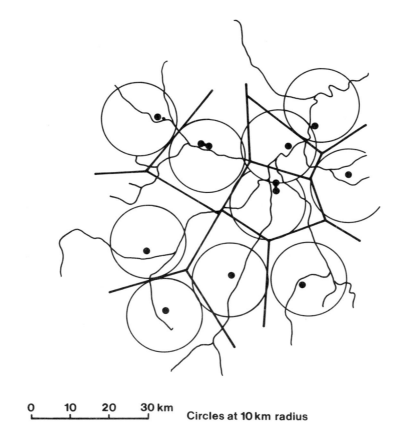

0   10   20   30 km
Circles at 10 km radius

Fig 2

Territorial analysis of late Bronze Age hillforts in West Bohemia, Czechoslovakia (data from Saldova 1977, Fig. 31). Earthwork sites that are spatially very close are assumed to be alternative foci, or chronologically successive, for the same territorial community. As in Fig 1b, the putative political units are outlined using Thiessen polygons, and an heuristic module (of 10kms. radius in this case) fitted regardless of centre into these cells. The circles indicate a significant degree of comparability in the partitioning of the landscape. Access potential to the 'focus' for servicing rural satellite communities would be available for almost all the landscape within a day-return.

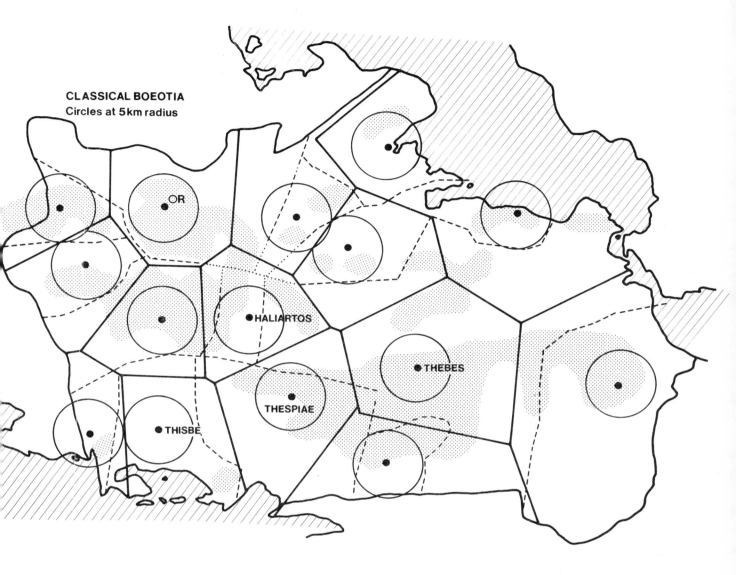

CLASSICAL BOEOTIA
Circles at 5km radius

OR

HALIARTOS

THEBES

THESPIAE

THISBE

Fig 3

City-state territories of Archaic to Classical Boeotia, Central Greece. The 15 states were all independent early in the period and the Thiessen polygon cells suggest that a broad degree of territorial parity may have existed at this time (Tanagra, the furthest east, being a notable exception). Fitting of 5kms. radius circles concentric around each city locus gives a scale that allows the detection of servicing potential. Clearly almost all districts in Boeotia were within a day-return of such a service focus (2-3 hours travel each way, c. 10-15kms.). As population rose dramatically through this period, secondary service centres arose in the interstices between the political foci, satellite market towns. Current research by the Cambridge/Bradford Boeotia Project suggests that day-return servicing continued for particular functions to the city itself but lower-level servicing of rural populations now focussed on their satellites at around 1 hour access time. The concentric 5kms. circles demonstrate the probable secondary catchment for each city, and point to sufficient remaining territory for 1-3 satellite service centres per cell.

These suggestions from geographical theory and field survey of the archaeology can fortunately be compared to actual state boundaries derived from written sources (dashed lines). Although a number of states have actual territories broadly similar to Thiessen prediction, almost all deviations elsewhere document the historically-attested, aggressive expropriation of their neighbours' lands by the major powers of Thebes and Orchomenus (OR). The comparison of Thiessen boundaries and the actual boundaries as recorded by Classical times illustrates the process by which this early state mosaic is moving towards a much larger ethnic polity, Boeotia, under one or other of the two leading states (in the event, Thebes).

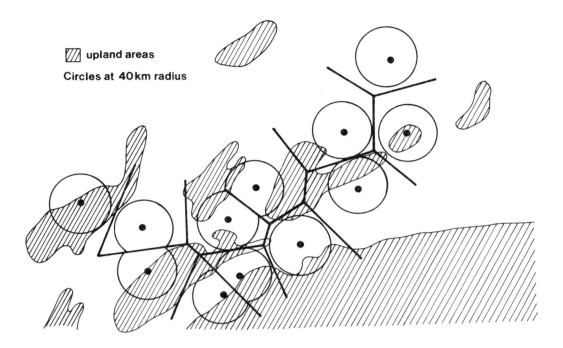

Fig 4

Putative territories for the Western Hallstatt 'princely' polities of the Hallstatt D era. Thiessen analysis, modified, from Haerke 1979, Fig. 54. The addition of a very large, 40kms. radius circle, reveals the considerable size of these territories, and the impossibillity of a standard day-return access role for much of the rural population. This poses interesting questions about the precise function of the focus and the probability of numerous secondary foci within each cell awaiting future study. The major upland areas plotted on the map suggest strongly that the polity frontier zones may frequently co-incide (marginal land?) and that although in many Thiessen cells the unshaded lowland component (main farming area, main population concentration?) exists with the key site at its centre, in many other cases the key site is located on the edge of the most fertile land (as the proportion of upland in each concentric circle demonstrates). For a more realistic comparison of mixed farming territory per polity the 40kms. circles could be located without reference to the key site but within each cell so as to cover as much lowland as possible.

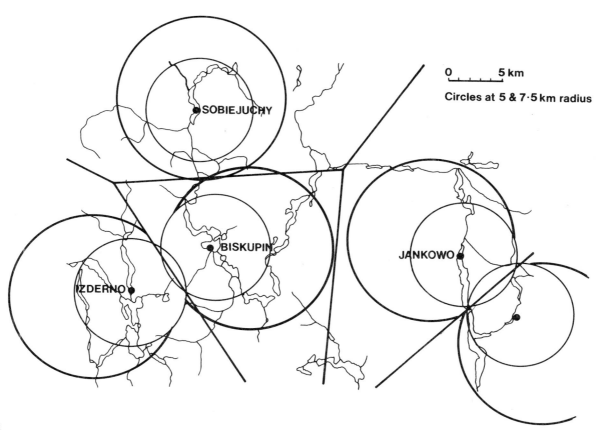

Fig 5

A sector of the fortified 'town' network of the Lausitz Culture in Poland, between the rivers Oder and Vistula (after Ostoja-Zagorski 1974, Fig. 7). Given the high density of population inferred or proven for the major settlements themselves, the 5kms. radius circle represents the approximate farming catchment out from the site. The 7.5kms. radius circles on the other hand are placed without regard to the site as centre but fitted into the Thiessen territorial cells constructed around each fortified centre. Although a rather coarse heuristic device, the larger circles suggest that cell territories may be of similar order of size, and also demonstrate that all sectors of each cell are within a day-return of the focus for servicing purposes (satellite rural sites are probably a major feature of the settled landscape). Finally the importance of lakes, rivers and their associated soils is highlighted by the inner catchment circle.

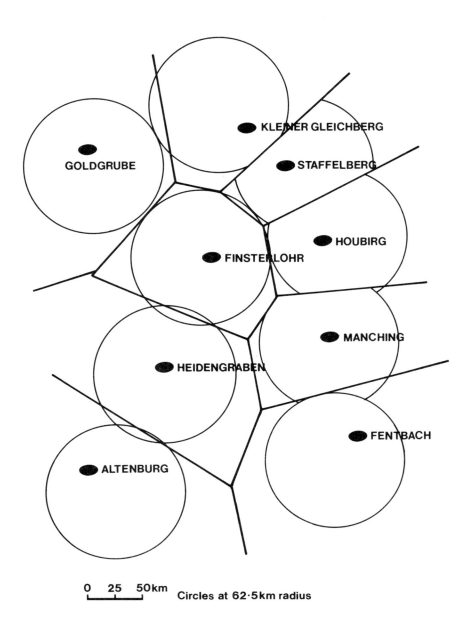

0   25   50km
Circles at 62·5km radius

Fig 6

Territorial network of late La Tène oppida in South Germany (data after Zürn 1977, Fig. 31). Putative 'polity' cells for each oppidum are created by Thiessen polygon analysis. Given the very large size of these teritorial units, servicing access on a day-return basis and the farming catchment immediately around each site are on too small a scale to affect the size of the polity mosaic. The best-fit heuristic circle for comparison of oppidum territories is 62.5kms. These 'polities' are clearly operating on a more advanced integrative level than that of simple servicing networks, but the broad similarity in scale of territory, and the interdependent packing of oppidum territories point to a balanced process of political expansion from numerous foci that maintain broadly equivalent territorial status.

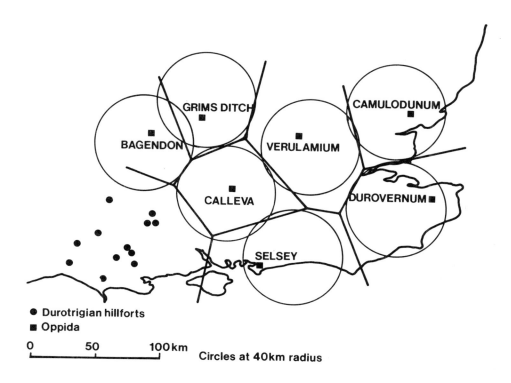

Fig 7

Major lowland oppida in Southern Britain, 0-40 AD, and to the south-west a zone of uncentralized tribalism focussing on a swarm of hillforts (data base and Thiessen analysis from Cunliffe 1976, Fig. 11). These large polities are too large to represent simple market/servicing catchments on a day-return threshold basis, as the heuristic circles of 40kms. radius demonstrate. These are located asymmetrically to the oppidum loci and merely fitted to the Thiessen cells to allow comparison of territory scale. In general the oppidum cells are significantly similar in size and should reflect a comparable process of mutual political expansion and centralization to that shown in Fig. 6.

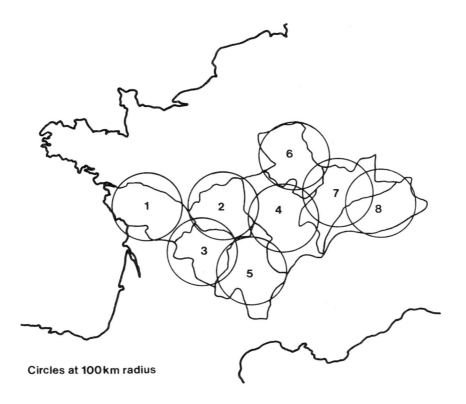

Circles at 100km radius

Fig 8

Late La Tène tribal states (civitates) of Central Gaul (first-century BC), after Nash 1978, Fig. 1. The best fit heuristic circle for territorial comparison is 100kms. radius, and this module demonstrates a closely comparable polity size. The great dimensions of these units represent an integrative process well beyond the simple servicing systems shown on earlier figures, and a process of mutual political expansion from numerous foci in balanced territorial growth.

   Key: 1 – Pictones; 2 – Bituriges; 3 – Lemovices; 4 – Aedui; 5 – Arverni; 6 – Lingones; 7 – Sequani; 8 – Helvetii.

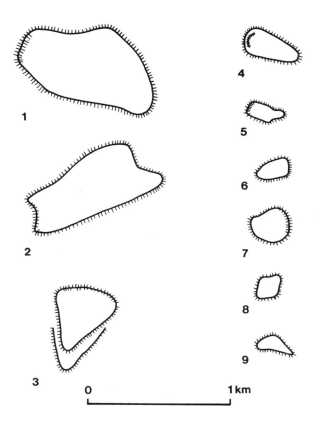

Fig 9

Oppida and 'Castella' in the western sector of the territory of the Treveri tribe (Western Germany/Benelux region; after Haffner 1977, Fig. 5). Major political foci, oppida: 1 - Titelburg; 2 - Kastel; 3 - Otzenhausen. Minor foci, 'castella', putative residences of local nobility : 4 - Kordel-Burgberg; 5 - Bundenbach-Altburg; 6 - Limbach; 7 - Trier-Ehrang; 8 - Landscheid; 9 - Hoppstädten-Weiersbach.

8

THE ANCIENT GREEK WORLD

Anthony Snodgrass

Even firm believers in social evolution do not often pursue their quarry into the field of Ancient Greece. It was no co-incidence that Gordon Childe's Social Evolution, although dealing extensively with the Aegean, stopped when it got to Homer (and only included him because Childe, in keeping with his generation, regarded him as a primary source for the Late Bronze Age Aegean world). There is a feeling that the wealth of evidence available for Classical Greece not only fails to illuminate the processes of social evolution, but somehow actually obscures them. This feeling, I think, boils down to a belief that the Classical Greek experience was unique and inexplicable, or at least too extraordinary to be covered by any general evolutionary laws. I reject this belief and would argue instead that there are a number of archaeological approaches, some of them well tried in other fields, others by definition only applicable to literate and advanced cultures like that of Greece, which can be and are already being fruitfully applied to the world of Classical Greece; and that the benefits are seen not only in the better understanding of that world, but also in the better understanding of the archaeological approaches themselves. In other words I think, as a few non-Classical archaeologists like the late David Clarke also thought, that historically-documented cultures are a potentially invaluable testing-ground for theories and models developed elsewhere - if only they can be brought to bear. This view is closely linked to another doctrine, rather less of a minority one this time, to which I also subscribe: that the distinctive characteristics of Classical Greece were in fact formed in an earlier period, the dark age and the ensuing Archaic age, when our dependence on archaeological evidence is rather heavy; so that we need not be embarrassed by the presence of a mass of historical documentation.

What are these archaeological approaches to which I refer and how can they illuminate social evolution? I would single out a handful of the most valuable ones, all of them familiar by now in one context or another but some of them relatively untried in this particular area. There is first of all settlement archaeology: at its best, this involves the careful excavation and observation of some sizeable sample of a settlement site, preferably over a sequence of periods. I introduce the word 'sample' here because of the first of our local difficulties that arise in the Greek world: most Greek settlements are simply too big, at least by the full Classical period, to be excavated in toto, quite apart from the fact that a high proportion of them have remained major centres of population ever since, and so are buried now under supermarkets or were destroyed long ago in the laying of gas mains. This helps to explain why there are so few well-excavated Classical settlements. Secondly, there is grave

archaeology: the full excavation and publication of cemeteries - again the bigger the better - complete with extended cluster-analyses, statistics of associations and so on. Third, and even more obviously under-exploited, there is cult or sanctuary archaeology. One has only to think for a moment to realise the huge potential importance of this for Classical Greece. Think of the first five Classical Greek sites that enter your head, and I will wager that at least three and quite likely all five of them are sanctuaries: they probably include the Athenian Acropolis, Delphi, Olympia and, perhaps, Delos or Epidauros. All of these and many other sanctuary sites have been prodigiously rich in finds; yet how much do we know of the working of a Classical sanctuary? Surprisingly little. There is, needless to say, an excuse or alibi once again: this time it is the fact that Greek sanctuaries operated in a way which produced relatively little stratification. I have noted that the chapter titles in a newly-issued American work, Advances in Archaeological Method and Theory edited by Michael Schiffer, include one that is called 'Cult archaeology and unscientific method and theory'; a better title one could not imagine for the study of Greek sanctuary-sites, though unfortunately on past trends it is a fair bet that the paper will prove not to make extended reference to Classical Greece. This is a hint that the shortcomings I have referred to are not confined to Greece.

Next, I would point to distribution studies: a central preoccupation of archaeologists everywhere now, but again one especially suited to a culture as prodigal of artifacts as Classical Greece: particularly of painted pottery, but also of coins and metalwork of equally distinctive types. Here again there is a contrast between the wealth of potential evidence and the limited use to which it has been put. It has been estimated that the world's museums hold some 40,000 Attic Red Figure vases alone and most of them have a known provenance. Sixteen thousand of them were catalogued by Beazley and attributed between about 500 painters, thus making them quite closely datable. Yet only the most primitive kind of work has been done on their distribution; as with all Greek fine pottery, their dispersal overseas has mainly been harnessed to an undifferentiated conception of 'trade' and recorded on distribution maps which seldom give any indication of quantity and never answer the most important question of all, namely in what kind of archaeological **context** they were found. But think of their potential statistical value!

This brings me to the fifth suggested approach, what might be called applied art history. Here we have something which is largely peculiar to the archaeology of advanced cultures. By 'applied' I refer to the kind of work which consists, not of the evaluation, dating and attribution of artistic products, but of moving on from that to use the results archaeologically; I shall give examples presently, but clearly there are some works of art which, by their nature, have considerable social significance. Finally, the sixth approach which I would mention is that of demographic studies. The raw material for these is essentially the same as that for the first two techniques that I listed, settlement archaeology and grave archaeology; but here the same evidence is used for a different and narrower purpose. Once again, the sheer quantity of evidence is one of the great advantages that Classical Greece has to offer: hundreds and hundreds of fairly closely dated burials, in particular.

It is time to ask what are the main questions and problems to which such approaches can be directed. In terms of social evolution, the Greek world offers a whole series of partly contemporaneous developments; if some of them are largely peculiar to Classical Greece **in their day**, they are none the worse for that, since in many cases a fairly similar course of events was ultimately to unroll itself, centuries or even millennia later, in other parts of the world. I place first the process which began and ended first chronologically: the transition from tribesman to citizen. By putting it thus baldly, I am simplifying; but it remains true that, by a date no later that 600 BC, most of the free adult male population of Greece has the status of membership of a community - not always a city-state, sometimes a looser federation of some kind - and that the clearest, hardest division across Greek Society was henceforward that between citizen and non-citizen. It is almost equally certain that this state of affairs had not existed for very long before about 600 BC. Those who argue (like Baechler 1980) that there was continuity of the Greek state or the Greek city from the Bronze Age down to Classical times seem to me to fly in the face of all the evidence except a very loose resemblance between the two eras of urbanization. Therefore the concept of citizenship must have an origin and period of growth in the generations before 600 BC and there are few more important processes in the social evolution of Greece than this one for us to try to chart. Somehow we have got to detect the form of society that prevailed in Greece before the rise of the city-state, and observe how it transformed itself into the phenomenon with which we are all more or less familiar. I still incline (pace Roussel 1976) to envisage this as a form of tribalism, simple rather than complex: that is, without the elaborate subdivisions of phratry and genos, our evidence for which is relatively late (if indeed it falls within the pre-state period at all) and which may even, with the eye of faith, be detected in some burial groupings of the eighth century BC in Attica, Thessaly, Argos, Achaea and the islands (cf. Snodgrass 1971, pp.195-6 and 387-8).

Then there is a second process which is sometimes confused with the first, namely the transition from an economy entirely agriculturally- or pastorally-based to a partially urbanized one. The clearest proof that these were two separate processes is the fact that there was a substantial time-lag between them: the city-state arrived long before real urbanization took place, and was indeed founded throughout its existence on a peasant system of land-holding; at first, it seems, it was impossible to become a citizen without also being a landowner. Political and material developments, however obviously related, could take place independently of each other. A third process which, yet again, is often allowed to shade into the preceding one, but which should nevertheless be distinguished as a quite separate development, is the growth of chattel-slavery in Greece. As long as the picture of Greek slavery as an essentially industrial phenomenon prevailed, it was reasonable enough to see it as merely an aspect of the growth of urban society. But today, especially since the recent work of Jameson (1977/8), Greek slavery has assumed a position too extensive and too important for that. Rather, it must be seen as the underpinning for the whole economic system of the advanced city-state, including the component whereby rural smallholders were enabled to take an active part in city politics through having agrarian slave labour at their disposal.

A further development, though primarily political, has such obvious social implications that it must be included in any account of social evolution: I mean the development in forms of government. It is a fact that some Greek states, within a space of about 300 years, progressed from a form of tribal monarchy, through a period of more or less absolute aristocratic rule, then one of what might be called constitutional aristocracy, then one of more or less popular dictatorship (the tyrannies) to moderate democracy and finally to radical democracy. All of this was not of course accomplished without social change, and to a certain extent it was even motivated by social forces. Fifth and different yet again, is another process which must be classed as political: the changes in the importance of the role of the state. Some time after it first came into being (typically in the eighth century BC), the Greek state embarked on a long power-struggle against its strongest rival, that is its own richest and most influential citizens. From being merely a useful and increasingly effective counter in the board-games of Greek aristocratic politics, the state gradually advanced until by the fifth and fourth centuries, especially in the democratic regimes, it became a ferocious and at times ungrateful-seeming taskmaster, cutting even its greatest servants down to size at every opportunity. Then in the Hellenistic period, mainly it seems under the stress of economic weakness, it sinks back somewhat into dependence on the wealth and patronage of its leading men: the relationship which specialists call 'evergetism'.

There are other processes which, in the context of Classical Greece, seem to me scarcely less important than those already mentioned, but about which I shall have less to say: the growth of literacy, which through the medium of the alphabet attained a greater range of social diffusion than the world had previously seen; the economic advance from the prestige-oriented system of gift-exchange which Homer portrays, to a genuine though partial mercantilism (I should however stress that I am firmly of the camp of those who confine this 'mercantilism' to a very limited significance and to a very late period - that is, later Classical and Hellenistic - with land-ownership playing a far greater role - cf. Finley 1973); and finally that cultural process of assimilation whose result can be summed up in the word koine - that is, the gradual merging of a host of local and regional characteristics into a more or less uniform, pan-Hellenic norm. The clearest example of it is perhaps a linguistic one: the destruction of the ancient regional dialects of Greek and their absorption into a new common language, throughout much of the Greek world, in the years after c. 400 BC.

Altogether I have now listed eight major processes; I would claim only that they are among the most important media of social evolution in Classical Greece, not that they are the eight most important. Before that, I gave a list of six archaeological approaches by which one might investigate these processes. Six by eight: that gives a theoretical matrix of 48 fields of study of Greek social evolution through archaeology. But of course they do not all work: some of the approaches I have named, such as demographic study, are by their nature restricted in scope and cannot be use to tackle such questions as the growth of literacy. Some of the problems I have posed - in particular, that of the political progress from monarchy to democracy - are inherently difficult to 'get at' through archaeological means. But I want to devote the rest of my chapter to giving examples, sometimes of the successful application of one of these approaches to one or more of the problems, more often merely of signposts for future work that should be possible.

One could reasonably argue that it is the first of the approaches, settlement archaeology, which is potentially the richest and most direct source for knowledge of social evolution. An initial point to be made is that many Greek archaeologists have begun to feel that the excavation of town-sites, traditionally the prime form of settlement archaeology, has some severe limitations. By excavating part of an ancient town, you can certainly build up some form of picture of the changes in density and extent of housing and in the material standards of living. But to base your picture exclusively on this is to rest on the false assumption that Greek civilization was entirely town-based.[1] To answer the equally important questions of **why** these changes in an ancient town took place, or **where** the new people might have come from or the missing ones gone to, one can only make limited progress from the evidence of the town itself - from the occupation debris within the houses, for example. To extend and deepen the investigation, it is really essential to include the town's rural hinterland as well as the main settlement itself; and for this, excavation as traditionally conceived is poorly adapted, at least in Greek conditions. The small number of excavations of farms and village-sites so far undertaken in Greece have, it is true, been encouraging in the amount of knowledge that they have yielded, but this is largely a measure of our previous ignorance. A number of archaeologists in Greece are turning their eyes to more productive and cost-effective methods, such as aerial photography and, above all, area surveys. Survey has been late in coming to Greece, but energetic efforts are now being made to catch up. The great undertaking of the 1960s, the University of Minnesota Messenia Expedition, has been brought a step nearer to total fulfilment recently by the partial publication of the excavations at its control site of Nichoria. Among other things, this has somewhat broadened the original chronological emphasis of the survey, which came in for some criticism for being concentrated on one period only, the Bronze Age. The general tendency of surveys in the 1970s and 1980s is certainly towards covering all periods. This extension of thematic and chronological range has to be paid for by a compensatory narrowing of the geographical range: I hope that the admission of a regional or local emphasis will soon become a matter of pride rather than shame. There was in fact already a strong but hidden bias in the conclusions derived from traditional urban excavations, but it was usually overlaid by the excavators' claims for the importance of their sites for Greek culture as a whole.

I am not going to give a list of all the survey projects, ranging from one-man research projects to major team undertakings like the Stanford/Indiana Argolid Exploration Project, which are currently going on in Greece. It will be years before we can really assess their contribution, even though we can already see that it is going to be very great. Instead let me pick out, much more selectively, one or two examples of more traditional settlement excavations which seem to me to have made an unusually significant advance in our understanding of social evolution, simply because the excavators have been asking themselves the same kinds of question that we are facing in this volume. Some of the publications are no longer recent, but all alike bear on one or more of the problems that I listed just now.

For the growth of the idea of citizenship, Claude Bérard (a member of the Greco-Swiss excavation team at Eretria) has shown that archaeology can at least in certain circumstances make a contribution. He has interpreted a funerary monument, put up in the early seventh century by one of the city's gates around a group of burials, one of them a very rich one, of about a generation earlier, as a kind of memorial to the founding heroes of Eretria, killed perhaps in a vital battle to confirm ownership of the site. His view has proved controversial, as witness his embattled defence of it in a recent volume of the excavation report (Bérard 1978): the arguments centre around the stratigraphic relationship of the monument to other domestic buildings and indeed to the fortification-wall of the city just beside it. Difficulties of a quite different kind may now arise from a remarkable and in some ways comparable discovery just made (March 1981) at a site a mere five miles away, but some 200 years earlier in date: I mean the temple, or more probably heroon, with its rich associated burials, found in the cemetery area of Lefkandi. What function can such a monument have served, at a date as early as c. 950 BC? What group's interests did it promote? If this represents a precocious step in state-formation, then one can only point to the desertion of Lefkandi around 700 BC and the apparent loss of the ancient name of the site, as prima facie evidence that the experiment was a failure. Yet the possibility - surely much enhanced by the new find - that Lefkandi marks the site of the 'Old Eretria' mentioned by Strabo and others in latter times, and that the centre of the city-state of Eretria was transferred, perhaps during the eighth century, to the new site along the coast where the Classical and modern town stands, does lend the Lefkandi find a new dimension. One might then arguably point to the main **difference** between the two cases - the extra-mural location of the Lefkandi monument - as conferring a new significance on the Eretria find. But at the very least the later case shows an excavator looking for the kind of evidence which could document physically the vital step of the establishment of a city, on which our later historical sources are so thin as to be almost worthless.

In a more general way, the second and third problems of Greek social evolution, the growth of urbanism and of chattel-slavery, are illustrated by some excavations of later town and country sites. As long ago as 1951, R.S. Young and Margaret Crosby published their important report on 'An industrial district of ancient Athens'. More recent work has been done on another Athenian industrial area, but this time a semi-rural one well away from the city: the lead and silver mines of Laurion, where the steady flow of reports from the Belgian excavation of the town of Thorikos is now backed up by investigation of the outlying installations (see Konophagos 1980). On the agricultural side, a landmark for brief, small scale yet productive digging and publication was set up by Ellis Jones, Sackett and Graham's investigation of two Athenian farmhouses in 1960 and 1966 (Jones et al. 1962, 1973). But to return to an earlier point, can even such work as this excel, for the rural sector, the contribution which can be made by a close survey of a square kilometre or two of agricultural land? Only, I would think, if it were possible to repeat it ten or twenty times over, and it is very doubtful whether preserved Classical farmhouses will prove sufficiently thick on the ground to make that possible.

A peculiarly Greek approach to these same problems of the nature of urban and rural society is available thanks to the existence of sculpted grave stones. It is hard to decide whether to classify this approach as applied art-history or as a special application of grave-archaeology, but this hardly matters. The identification of the sculptors, when combined with the locations of their works, tell us something about the relations between town and country; the incidence of the sculptured stones, together with their internal evidence for the status, occupation and family connections of the deceased, tell us about the pattern of settlement. More clearly assignable to grave-archaeology is the recent paper on 'Family tombs ... in ancient Athens' by Sally Humphreys (1980). This anthropologist, who has done so much to try to rouse Classical archaeology from its traditional trance-like contemplation of truth and beauty to a more serious social concern, has now produced a study drawing on the full range of archaeological evidence (together, admittedly, with epigraphy and other documentary sources) for the social attitudes displayed in Athenian family burials of the Classical period. Some of her most important conclusions relate to kinship, a question which I did not list in its own right among my chosen aspects of social evolution, but which plays an integral part in the first of our problems, the transition from tribesman to citizen.

At this point I may mention a general inference arising from grave-archaeology which is especially highlighted by Humphreys's paper. When one considers the funerary evidence from Greece as a whole, throughout the ancient period, and compares it with the kind of evidence so interestingly used in Susan Frankenstein and Mike Rowlands' paper of 1978 on Iron Age society in southwestern Germany, then what strikes one is the egalitarian appearance of Greek burials of most periods. There is simply nothing in Greece proper, at any rate south of Macedonia, to correspond with the tombs of paramount chief, vassal-chief, sub-chief status and so on which they discern in west-central Europe. Of all the hundreds of burials of the earliest Iron Age in Greece (roughly the eleventh and tenth centuries BC), most of them single graves, there is not one that can really be called rich. In the ninth and eighth centuries when the quantities are greater (I have counted 682 closely dated graves of this period from Attica alone), there are one or two whose contents are moderately impressive (say a few pieces of gold jewellery or a dozen bronze fibulae), but still none which is in any way imposing in terms of architecture or even sheer size. By the fifth and fourth centuries, as the Humphreys paper shows, there is still a broadly uniform, but by now a rather higher, level to be seen, with sculpted gravestones a fairly frequent bonus. In between, however, there is a period of deviation from this egalitarian appearance: the Archaic age of the seventh and sixth centuries, when some effort is made to differentiate the graves of prominent people, usually by the use of a tumulus; while life-sized statues, bigger, more striking and much more expensive, fill the role later taken by the grave-stones. Can we explain either the long-term trend or the apparent Archaic exception to it? If we can, we may be on to an important factor in the social evolution of at least Classical Athens, from which the main evidence comes.

The obvious contrast with central Europe can however be refined, by pointing to the developments of the **later** Iron Age there (cf. Bintliff, Iron Age Chapter, this volume). Here we find, unexpectedly, a **reduction** in burial differentiation at a time when there is documentation of very pronounced social stratification in Celtic society. Clearly a change in burial ethos, rather than an egalitarian social or economic transformation, is the main factor indicated; and the same no doubt applies to Iron Age and Classical Greece. It is worth noting another quite different change in Greek burial practice which coincides with the temporary rise in funerary ostentation in the Archaic period: this is the discontinuation, permanent in this case, of burial with arms in the more advanced regions of Greece, and the concomitant (and surely connected) rise in dedications of arms at sanctuaries. This latter is a group-oriented activity: I would add it to the other evidence for the rise of the Greek state in these years around 700 BC, but would also see it as proof that the Greek aristocracies were indeed changing their attitudes to burial.

There is, however, a further possible inference to be drawn from the peaceful ostentation of these Archaic burials in Greece, especially in Athens: I should like to suggest a connection between this phenomenon and another mentioned earlier, the development in the role of the state - cf. earlier discussion. The graves of the pre-state era do nothing to suggest that the material wealth of the aristocrats was great: later, there is proof that it had reached a high level, since the costliness of the burials increases enormously even allowing for the diversion of arms-dedications to the sanctuaries. It looks, therefore, as though the upper classes may have prospered **materially** for a time as a result of state formation, even if we observe the earlier caveat on drawing any conclusions as to changes in their **status**. There is also documentary evidence that their political power was in some cases enhanced by the rise of the city-state; but again, only for a time. The process began to go wrong for them with the establishment of the first tyrants, almost all of them individually of aristocratic birth, but collectively deeply hostile to aristocratic interests. They were the first rulers positively to represent the interests of the state as a whole, and (negatively) to initiate policies that were not favoured by the upper classes. It was probably in ancient Greece that the aristocracies, having played as energetic a part in the foundation of the state as anywhere, lost out more speedily in the sequel than anywhere else: in several cases their supremacy was gone within 200 years or less. Their temporary aggrandisement had, however, lasted long enough to have accompanied, perhaps motivated, and certainly benefited from the foundation of the Greek form of state.

Next I should like to single out two pieces of applied art-history, unexpected perhaps in that they relate to two of the primarily economic questions which I listed a little earlier: one to the growth of slavery, the other to the changing relationship between the state and its most prominent citizens. First, the corpus of Greek works of art, and especially of painted vases, can be brought to bear on a vast range of questions, and one of them is slavery. A paper by Nikolaus Himmelmann (1971) represents a most interesting move in this direction; despite its title 'Archäologisches zum Problem der griechischen Sklaverei', it is the artistic rather than the archaeological evidence that is used. Himmelmann employs two approaches, the one deriving from the quite frequent illustration of slaves on Greek works of art, the other from the possibility (which in several documented cases is more than a mere possibility) that the works themselves were produced by slaves. He detects a number of changes of attitude towards slaves, expressed in the monuments; I think it is fair to say that these had not emerged clearly from the study of contemporary literary sources, so that the work can be accounted an independent contribution of archaeology. Secondly, there is a striking piece of recent work on Athenian sculpture of the Hellenistic period, Andrew Stewart's Attika (1979). Unlike so many earlier writers on sculpture, Stewart is actively concerned with the social implications of his material, and devotes his last two chapters to considerations of this kind. Since one of the most conspicuous features of Hellenistic society is the growth of what I earlier referred to as euergetism - the system whereby rich citizens made large contributions from their own pockets towards civic purposes (municipal works, financing of campaigns etc.), partly for their own propaganda purposes, partly because the state could no longer afford to operate without this - since there is almost no element more significant than this in the society of the period, it is really very illuminating that sculpture in general, and portraiture in particular, lies at the very heart of this element. As Stewart shows, private munificence in earlier periods (the fifth and earlier fourth centuries) had been thought to be adequately rewarded by votes of thanks, memorial inscriptions, grants of privileges and the like. In the Hellenistic period, this was no longer felt to be enough, and publicly-commissioned portraits were thrown into the scales; soon privately-funded portraiture was sharply on the increase too. In Athens at least, it seems to us (in Stewart's words) that anyone was prepared, virtually at the drop of a hat, to put up a portrait of almost anyone else (or of himself for that matter). This is remarkable, when one finds that the price of the most extravagant form of portrait, a full-length statue in bronze, was a sum equal to about ten year's wages for an unskilled artisan -something like £40,000 in today's terms. But from our point of view, perhaps the most interesting thing is that a material artifact, and one of which numerous examples are extant today, should turn out to be at the very centre of a society's exchange system, instead of being (as so often in archaeology) a kind of husk from which we attempt to infer the nature of the grain. The repercussions are wide: by studying changes in the style of portraiture we can learn of changes in that society's values, while the location and context of the sculptures give a quite different dimension; and once again that recurrent asset of archaeology in Greece, the possibility of attributing a list of works to the same artist, makes its own contribution.

I should like to illustrate, even more briefly, the application of the other archaeological approaches which I mentioned at the beginning. For example, distribution studies: it is clear that a high priority here should be given to the commodities which are recovered in the largest quantities, rather than those which best repay study of the traditional, qualitative kind. A new field has been opened up here, in what many would have called the exhausted terrain of Greek pottery-studies, by Alan Johnston (1979). Since there are certain kinds of mark found on Greek pots discovered in overseas locations, and **only** on the pots found there, it is clear that they will offer potentially valuable evidence on that newly revitalized question, the purpose and context of Greek pottery exports. The old, unthinking assumption that every Greek pot found abroad has got there by simple commercial enterprise, first questioned by anthropologists and historians, is now being belatedly re-examined even by Classical archaeologists, and Johnston's book will provide them with a whole new body of material. But really convincing answers will depend on combining this approach with others: can we, for example, always be sure of the location of the centre of production? Can we decode the marks themselves?

Next, what contribution can sanctuary- or cult-archaeology make? Once again, I would stress that outstanding quality of the Classical Greek evidence, its tremendous richness. Because excavators in Greece - for entirely different motives from ours in this volume - have concentrated so heavily on sanctuary sites for the last hundred years or more, we have a vast mass of published material from sanctuaries of every level of importance. At the top of the scale, there are the great inter-state centres which, combining many of the functions of the Vatican, the United Nations, Geneva, the City of London and the World Cup in our own days, almost alone provided the Greeks with the opportunity to remember that they belonged not only to their own city, but to a Greek people as a whole. For generations now we have had available the publications of Olympia, of Delphi or of Delos with its 32 volumes of finds. Then there are the chief sanctuaries of the individual states, like the Athenian Acropolis, the Argive Heraion or Artemis Orthia's temple at Sparta. Below them come the lesser state sanctuaries; and finally, a host of sanctuaries of mainly local significance, many of them without a temple, some located in natural features like caves. What use can we make of the innumerable reports, apart from using them as bran-tubs from which to pull out new or unrecognized artistic masterpieces? The answer has been a discouraging one. I myself have

recently tried (1977) to use the second range of sanctuaries, the chief centres of cult in each city, as an index of something for which it is otherwise very hard to find any sort of archaeological co-ordinates: the emergence of the Greek state, and the concept of citizenship. Since we can nearly always identify a posteriori, the location of the prime official cult of a Greek state (with the help of literary and epigraphical evidence), then surely a moment of some importance in the life of that site - some would say the most significant moment - is the point at which worship actually begins: or rather, at which **material** evidence of worship begins. This last distinction has generated a fundamental clash of views; when we find, as we sometimes do, that the site served as a cult centre at a much earlier period (usually in the Late Bronze Age), but that a gap of three or four hundred years in the material remains then follows - this is what sorts out the two schools of thought from each other. On the one side, that of the believers in continuity, there is talk of 'simple devotions', 'archaeology an unreliable guide to human behaviour', 'dearer to God are the prayers of the poor' and so on. On the other side , the reiterated question - 'why?'. Why should the same people, worshipping at the same sanctuary, stop giving any material manifestation of their worship, and then after a long lapse, resume doing so? Changes in material prosperity? But even in the dark age, people could spare the odd pin, fibula or pot to put in the grave of a dead relation. Changes in level of population? Yes, but not of that order (I give two of the more dramatic statistics, of pins and fibulae dedicated at Philia in Thessaly: eleventh/tenth centuries - 1; ninth/early eighth centuries - 6; late eighth/seventh centuries - 1,810; and at Lindos in Rhodes: eleventh/tenth centuries - 19: ninth/early eighth centuries - 260; late eighth/seventh centuries - 3,158). Surely the most convincing answer is one deriving from the status of the site. There were times when it was unimportant to the community at large, and times when it was suddenly of great importance. The clearest tribute to that importance was when a permanent temple building was put up, especially if the temple was of a higher architectural standard than any contemporary domestic structure. The actual sequence that we find, at the Argive Heraion and at many other sanctuaries, is first that the dedications show a sudden upsurge or even begin from scratch; secondly that a temple is built; thirdly that the sanctuary begins to attract the kind of offerings that had previously appeared in graves. This process, all three stages of which can in some cases appear within the space of a generation, is best linked with the emergence of the state, an event which could explain all the phenomena. Suddenly a spot which had retained the vague miasma of a 'holy place' and which perhaps had some material traces to show for its earlier significance, was pressed into filling a new role, one which had only come into existence because of a reorganization of the community. And in Greece there is almost always, as I have already said, the evidence of later documents: we know that the Argive Heraion **was** the Argive Heraion, the main centre of official ceremony for the city of Argos and we are simply looking for the likeliest moment for this function to have begun.

Let me take this opportunity also to reassert an argument which I have advanced elsewhere (Snodgrass 1977) that the appearance of fortifications is in no sense a positive guide to the emergence of the city-state in Greece, though in a few cases like that of Eretria (cf. above) it can accompany that process. I draw comfort from Potter's illustrations (this volume) of how fallible a guide it would be in Iron Age Italy, where it is a phenomenon of the sixth and especially of the fifth century, a relatively late point in the career of the Etruscan and other city-states. In Greece, it appears often at a comparably late date and stage, sometimes much earlier: in neither case does it seem to correspond with the critical stage in state-formation.

I touched fleetingly on the subject of demography above and I should like to devote a few closing words about it. We have to use different methods of estimating population at different periods of Greek history and there are very serious difficulties in trying to integrate them with each other, as we must eventually do. For the prehistoric period, the most convincing guide at present seems to be the estimated density per unit of area in a settlement whose overall size is approximately known. For the Hellenistic period, to take a total contrast, the survival of annual enrolment-lists giving the entire age-group of male citizens reaching military age in one year enables quite accurate computations of at least the citizen population. For the full classical period, looser calculations of the same kind are possible from the sporadic statements of ancient authors about the size of citizen armies. For the early historical period, none of these methods is available: we have neither the fully-excavated settlements nor the documents. At present I can see little basis for estimates of absolute population at this time, though calculations derived from the size and time-span of excavated cemeteries give some alarmingly low figures. I have however chanced my arm (Snodgrass 1977; 1980 pp.14-17) at some **relative** estimates of changes in population level, and found that the evidence of settlements, sanctuaries and graves alike points to an enormous upsurge of population, at least locally, in the two generations before 700 BC. Recent comparative work (see Cohen 1978, especially pp.39-43) has suggested that population growth and state formation are indeed linked, but not so simply   - with the former acting as a contributory cause and the latter as the effect - as was once held. In any case, the past year or so has seen the evidence of the eighth-century burials stood on its head (Camp 1979) to produce almost the opposite conclusion: a sudden upsurge in **mortality**, brought on by a severe (and in my own opinion unbelievably sustained) drought. But at least this may bear some fruit, by drawing attention to the possibilities of this method in Greek archaeology.

I have done no more than suggest a few principles, and point to a few case-studies, for the investigation of social evolution in Greece. I am very conscious, as I hinted at the beginning, that some of these methods and examples are not very widely applicable and may even be confined in their scope to the ancient Greek world. But if you feel that there are wider lessons to be learned from the experiences of Greek archaeology, then I shall be more than content; and at least I hope that I have done nothing to weaken further such faith in Classical archae-ology as you may still retain. What I have conspicuously failed to do is to isolate, in Greek social evolution, what Cliff Slaughter (this volume) referred to as a 'prime mover'. There are a lot of processes taking place simultaneously, within quite narrow limits of date; yet I do not find that either the general body of anthropological theory or the details of the archaeological evidence as yet provide clinching evidence as to which is the **primary** process. This is a cause for discouragement: if we cannot discern the priorities for historical Greece, then this would appear to reduce the chances of doing so for Palaeolithic Europe. But I hope that the theorists will take it as a reason for including the ancient Greek world within their purview in future.

NOTES

Note 1
Several authors now in Papenfuss and Strocka (Eds.) 1982 have dealt interestingly with these same problems: not-ably Robin Hägg, "Zur Stadtwerdung des dorischen Argos" (pp.297-307) and Carmine Ampolo "Die endgültige Stadt-werdung Roms in 7. und 6. Jh v. Chr." (pp.319-23).

BIBLIOGRAPHY

ANDREWES, A. 1977 - Greek Society, Allen Lane, London.

BAECHLER, J. 1980 - "Les origines de la démocratie grecque", Annales européennes de Sociologie vol. 21, pp.223-84.

BERARD, C. 1978 - "Topographie et Urbanisme de l'Erétrie archaique", in Eretria, Fouilles et Recherches VI, Francke, Berne, pp.89-94.

CAMP, J. McK. 1979 - "A drought in the late eighth century B.C.", Hesperia vol. 48, pp.397-411.

CHILDE, V.G. 1963 - Social Evolution (2nd. ed.), Fontana, London.

COHEN, B. 1978 - "State origins: a Reappraisal", in The Early State, Eds. H.J.M. Claessen and P. Skalnik (New Babylon: Studies in the Social Sciences, 32), Mouton, The Hague, pp.31-75.

FINLEY, M.I. 1973 - The Ancient Economy, Chatto and Windus, London.

HIMMELMANN, N. 1971 - "Archäologisches zum Problem der griechischen Sklaverei", Abhandlungen der Akademie der Wissenschaften und der Literatur, Mainz (Geistes-und Sozialwissenschaftliche Klasse) 1971, pp.615-59.

HUMPHREYS, S.C. 1980 - "Family tombs and tomb-cult in ancient Athens: tradition or traditionalism?", Journal of Hellenic Studies vol. 100, pp.96-126.

JAMESON, M.H. 1977/8 - "Agriculture and slavery in Classical Athens", The Classical Journal vol. 73, 2, pp.122-44.

JOHNSON, A.W. 1979 - Trademarks on Greek Vases, Aris and Phillips, Warminster.

JONES, J.E., SACKETT, L.H. and GRAHAM, A.J. 1962 and 1973 - "The Dema house in Attica", Annual of the British School at Athens vol. 57, pp.75-114; and "An Attic country house below the Cave of Pan at Vari", ibid, vol. 68, pp. 355-452.

KONOPHAGOS, G. 1980 - Le Laurion antique. Athens.

PAPENFUSS, D. and STROCKA, V.M. (Eds.) 1982 - Palast und Hütte (Symposium der Alexander von Humboldt-Stift-ung, Berlin, 1979). Von Zabern, Mainz.

233

ROUSSEL, D. 1976 - Tribu et Cité (Annales littéraires de l'Université de Besançcon193, Paris).

SARKADY, J. 1975 - "Outlines of the development of Greek society in the period between the 12th and 8th centuries B.C.", Acta Academiae Scientiarum Hungaricae vol. 23, pp.107-25.

SNODGRASS, A.M. 1971 - The Dark Age of Greece, Edinburgh University Press, Edinburgh.

SNODGRASS, A.M. 1977 - Archaeology and the rise of the Greek state, Inaugural Lecture, Cambridge University Press, Cambridge.

SNODGRASS, A.M. 1980 - Archaic Greece: the age of experiment, Dent, London.

STEWART, A.F. 1979 - Attika: studies in Athenian sculpture of the Hellenistic age, Society for the Promotion of Hellenic Studies, London.

YOUNG, R.S. and CROSBY, M. 1951 - "An industrial district of ancient Athens", Hesperia vol. 20, pp.135-288.

9

SOCIAL EVOLUTION
IN IRON AGE AND ROMAN ITALY:
AN APPRAISAL

Tim Potter

Introduction

Current thought, particularly amongst Italian scholars (e.g. Torelli 1974, Colonna 1974, Cristofani 1979a), relates many of the developments of Iron Age and Roman Italy to changes in the structure and the fabric of society. Out of socially undifferentiated groups of Bronze Age date (i.e. the second millennium BC) there gradually emerged specialized artisans, producing an ever-increasing variety of goods. While the south western part of Italy was, from the early eighth century BC, undergoing colonization by Greek settlers, the mineral-rich central region of the peninsula, bordering the Tyrrhenian Sea, witnessed the incipient stages in the creation of small city-states. A clear hierarchy of orders, controlled by rich aristocrats, was established, and is attested by a series of elaborate burials from Etruria, Latium and Campania. By the end of the seventh century BC, a sharp growth in trade (stimulated by Greeks and Phoenicians) promoted the evolution of an affluent middle class, especially in central and southern Etruria and in Latium. Before long, some settlements (such as Rome, Veii, Caere and Tarquinia) had acquired many of the characteristics of 'urban' centres, with strict controls over their territories (including foreign communities). The interstate hostility that in some areas ensued and internal social divisions are seen as a direct cause behind the creation of republican regimes in some cities in the late sixth century.

The fifth century saw the beginning of Rome's expansion and the decline of the Etruscan states, particularly as a result of a series of reverses at the hands of the Greeks. While Rome engaged in a series of small scale local wars, the Etruscan city-states came increasingly under the control of a new ruling class. This 'new landed nobility' (Torelli 1974, p.20) ensured the identity of their centres by providing city walls, and paved the way for what is seen as a cultural and economic revival from early in the fourth century BC. Only the steady encroachment by Rome upon the territories of first the Samnites and then, city by city, of the Etruscans, reversed this trend. The Etruscan nobiles, faced with deep social unrest amongst their slaves and a hostile Roman Republic, underwent a slow erosion of their power. Even though some attempted to integrate themselves with the patrician class of Rome, they were in the long term unable to resist the forces of change.

The expansion of Rome brought about severe dislocation in both town and countryside. Apart from the construction of a new long-distance road network, and the creation of colonies and other settlements, there was also a rapid influx of slave labour from the third century BC onwards. This, it is argued, resulted in the break-up of the traditional agricultural small-holding - particularly in central Italy - and the gradual spread of large slave-run estates, latifundia. War, especially the Hannibalic invasions, also played its part in the dispossession of the free peasantry and in the consolidation of large landholdings.

The availability of cheap labour also had profound consequences in the building trade (where a gradual rise in the population necessitated an expansion of housing and facilities such as the supply of water) and in the development of small-scale industry. Roman Italy became increasingly an exporting country. Augustus, the victor of the 'Roman Revolution', which saw the 'warrior society' (Hopkins 1978) of the late Republic replaced by a bureaucratic administration, consolidated these trends. From a region of small city-states, Rome had been transformed into the centre of a tightly controlled empire, governed by Augustus's 'new men', and backed by an efficient professional army.

The Empire remained essentially stable for nearly two centuries: indeed, crises such as that of AD 69 served more to demonstrate its strength in the face of political upheaval than its weaknesses. However, in Italy, the expansion of the economy lasted only until the end of the first century AD. The symptoms of the decline that ensued are variously defined, amongst them a gradual move away from exporting (of wine, oil, lamps, pottery etc.) towards large-scale importation of goods and produce. 'Modes of production' also began to change. The slave-run villa became increasingly less viable, many were abandoned during the second and early third centuries AD, and contractual arrangements between owner and tenant diversified (with crop-sharing as a conspicuous practice). Free tenants more-and-more took over the role of slaves as labourers, it is suggested. The division between the rich honestiores and the poor humiliores became ever sharper and, with social divisiveness, came discontent and trouble. The decline in the size of the rural population in many parts of Italy in the later Roman period is manifest from archaeological evidence and is commonly seen as a reason behind legislative attempts to tie coloni to the land. Thus it was that tenants became increasingly more like serfs and productive methods ever less effective; at the same time, the money supply entered a period of fluctuation and instability, encouraging exchange of goods rather than of coinage. Society in Italy and elsewhere underwent, therefore, a substantial transformation from the third century as the koine of Empire gradually broke down into a pattern of regional units.

236

Comment on the approach

In very broad outline and in a grossly over-simplified way, these preliminary remarks introduce some of the lines of thought that relate to central Italy's social history in the Iron Age and Roman periods. It will provide a rough and ready framework for more detailed discussion, although it should be said that no short paper could ever hope to do justice to questions which have inspired deep and wide-ranging debate. None of the issues is simple and an 'overview' is often more likely to disguise the complexities rather than to illuminate them: "however complex we make our categories" of the social framework "there seems to be room for doubt about the model and how it relates to actual behaviour" (Frederiksen 1975, p.165).

Until recently, much of the thinking upon social and economic topics has been developed by ancient historians, primarily from literary, epigraphic and numismatic sources. The cogent appraisals of this massive body of evidence such as those of Brunt (1971a, b), Finley (1973), Jones (1964, 1974) and Duncan-Jones (1974) - to cite but a few - will surely stand as obligatory starting-points for all studies of these questions. It is the wealth of written material (and here I would include coinage, amphora-, brick- and pottery-stamps) which provides both the framework and much of the detail for statements about the fabric and development of the social and economic structure of the Roman world (and, to a substantial extent, also that of the Etruscans). Attempts to construct models that portray these situations have proved - inevitably - contentious (and reflect a wide series of ideological bases, epitomized by the overtly Marxist approach of Rostovzeff (1957)). This probably explains why there has been increasing resort to other forms of evidence, such as excavation and field-survey, so as to test certain hypotheses. Sometimes the archaeological data have been found wanting in precision (e.g. Brunt 1971a, pp.352-3), but more often the tendency has been to invest it with greater certainty than is really justified (e.g. Hopkins 1980, fn. 13). It is hard to overemphasize how patchy and uneven is our archaeological information. Just as Iron Age studies have been almost exclusively those of cemeteries and religious sites (but see Cornell 1980 for the beginnings of settlement investigation in Latium), so Roman archaeology has done little to provide a historical dimension to the development and decay of the towns (although Luni (Frova et al. 1977) and Ostia (Carandini et al. 1977) provide notable exceptions). There is also a dearth of well-investigated villas (Rossiter 1978) although this too is beginning to change (Painter 1980). Field survey, currently very much in fashion in Italy, is, on the other hand, in a healthier state and, with the application of more precise pottery-dating and more sophisticated techniques (floral and faunal analysis, soil studies etc.), has great potential. In some areas, it is serving to transform our picture of settlement patterns as derived from historical sources (e.g. Barker 1977). Moreover, it also helps to underline the enormous degree of regional variability within the Italian peninsula (Delano Smith 1979). As Garnsey (1979) has emphasized, there is a considerable variety of peasant contractual arrangements in present-day Italy, a situation which is hardly likely to be novel (as Martin Frederiksen pointed out more than once). The survey of the Biferno valley and its tributaries, which has disclosed that farming arrangements and buildings in antiquity could differ quite markedly from one pedological zone to another, makes the point quite neatly (Barker et al. 1978). Even where settlement patterns appear archaeologically uniform, they may disguise a complex process of formation. South Etruria in the Medieval period is a case in point (Potter 1979, Wickham 1978, 1979). Stretching northwards from Rome is a remarkable series of defended castles and villages, occupying topographically very similar positions on prom-ontories on rocky spurs. The documentary sources imply that these sites came into being mainly in the tenth century, with the abandonment of the dispersed settlement pattern that dominated classical south Etruria. More detailed research - archaeological and archival - showed that this was a superficial judgement and that the sequence of events varied from one small region (such as the Ager Veientanus) to another (such as the Ager Faliscus): archaeologically, the end result, incastellamento, was the same but the processes that brought about its formation could and did vary sharply. Indeed, east of the Tiber yet a third model operated (Toubert 1973). Even within the 200kms.² or so of the Ager Veientanus, Wickham (1979, p.91) found a complex picture: "clearly we cannot find an answer to the process of incastellamento that is valid for the whole of our region" the Ager Veientanus "for the simple reason that we have not consistent settlement-patterns even across a region as small as ours ..." It "... is the reminder that we misrepresent the early medieval period if we suppose that its social structures were as simple as they are ill-documented. Social change was as complex then as it is now". Reduced to essentials, then, there is a need to stress (i) the partiality of our historical sources (which may at times misrepresent) (ii) the deficiences in our archaeological data and (iii) the dangers that over-simplistic modelling of complex issues may bring. Thus, with these caveats in mind, we may now examine some case-studies in more detail.

'Proto-urbanization': the Late Bronze Age and Early Iron Age

"Within Iron Age villages ... class differences came into being at an early stage, as a result of contacts with the Phoenicians and Greeks..." It is in certain southern sites of Etruria"... where different social classes first appear" (Cristofani 1979a p.30).

It is generally agreed that the archaeological record for large parts of the Italian peninsula demonstrates a marked demographic increase from the later second millennium BC onwards. Small villages became steadily more established over this period, with in the late Bronze Age the occasional funerary expression of "episodic and local emergence of socially pre-eminent groups" (Peroni 1969). In Apulia, several coastal settlements in contact with Mycenaeans in the thirteenth and early twelfth centuries BC seem to Whitehouse (1973) to qualify as 'townships' which "arose as a direct result of trade with the Aegean world"; if so, they were however an isolated phenomenon. While some late Bronze Age villages were to develop into urban centres of classical (and post-Roman Italy) - Rome and Bologna are good examples - it is the beginning of the Villanovan Iron Age that saw the first real emergence of the future 'city-states'. Even then, it was a process that was largely restricted to west-central Italy and to parts of the south (a trend that persisted into Republican times). Peroni, whose writings remain the most influential on this period (e.g. 1969), sees this 'stabilization' of so-called proto-urban centres as the result of a process of synoecism: "one might almost think that new forms of political power have appeared, strong enough to compel different groups and tribes to live together". While the symptom of violence that he cites for the 'extinguishing' of some Final Bronze Age sites are perhaps less than convincing - a burnt layer over a building at Luni-sul-Mignone is hardly 'certain' evidence for destruction at the hands of an enemy - nevertheless the cemeteries do begin to show increased differentiation of wealth. The phenomenon appears not to be marked before the eighth century, however, especially in the Villanovan cemeteries. At Veii, for example, where the Villanovan settlement seems to have comprised a number of small separate communities, dispersed over a large, naturally defended plateau

(Ward-Perkins 1961), the Quattro Fontanili necropolis yielded few conspicuously rich ninth-century graves (Close-Brooks 1965, QF 1963 f.). During the eighth century, however, there is not only a great diversification in the range of the artifacts but also a marked differentiation in their quantity, quality and type. Some burials, for instance, are clearly those of notable warrior-leaders (e.g. Potter 1979, Fig. 8), others of wealthy ladies. That trade with the Euboean Greek colony of Pithecusa (Ischia) was a catalyst in this process is abundantly clear from the presence of Greek objects in the tombs at Quattro Fontanili and from Villanovan objects at Pithecusa and from Greece itself (Ridgway 1973). Indeed, Veii, the most southerly Villanovan settlement, may well have been a pioneer in the development of these contacts.

Other Villanovan centres were also rapidly involved in trade with the Greek colonies, and there was soon diffusion of the commercial network to inland sites such as Bisenzio (Delpino 1977) and beyond. Etruria controlled rich sources of metal ores - particularly iron - that were coveted by these early Greek traders and craftsmen. Nevertheless, the prosperity that accrued was by no means confined to Etruria. North of the Apennines, Bologna shared to a considerable extent (especially after c.750) in the economic transformation of its southern neighbours; and both Latium and Campania also show evidence for widespread exposure to the Greek trading network. The cemeteries of Latium in particular, have disclosed a great deal of important new information in recent years, usefully summarised in CLP (1976) and by Cornell (1980). The early phases of the Latian culture have been strikingly illuminated by Bietti Sestieri's excavation at Osteria dell'Osa. In its first phase (c.900-830 BC) inhumations and cremations cluster side by side, the latter being confined to certain males, whose ashes were stored in so-called 'hut-urns'. There were usually weapons with these burials, hinting at some social differentiation. Both the rite of cremation and the practice of using weapons as grave-goods then disappears; however, during the third phase (c.770 - 720/30 BC), the range of objects (as in Etruria) diversifies sharply, the contacts with the Greek world become explicit in the form of imported vessels and some degree of social differentiation is implied by variations in the wealth and contents of the tombs (Bietti Sestieri 1979). That this is not an isolated pattern is borne out by the results of other recent excavations, most spectacularly at Castel di Decima. A possible cenotaph (? c.750-725 BC), four chariot burials (none later than the early seventh century) and ranking distinctions based on weapons, all anticipate the development of the great princely tombs which are so characteristic of Etruria, Latium and Campania in the 'Orientalizing' period.

To sum up the argument so far, the 'evolutionary' model postulates the development of a series of 'proto-urban' tribal or early state societies, particularly in western central Italy. Although the background is seen as egalitarian, social classes came slowly into focus. On the one hand were 'warrior leaders' (Stary (1979) emphasises the Near Eastern 'military contacts' of the Villanovans from the ninth century onwards) and, on the other, the artifacts imply the emergence of specialist craftsmen. The role of the Greeks (and presumably the Phoenicians) is seen as crucial, and as trade developed the accumulation of wealth achieved increasing expression in the funerary record.

The 'orientalizing' aristocracy

"It is probably premature to see these" princely "tombs as a **single** phenomenon, artistic or sociological; extending as they do from Vetulonia to Pontecagnano (or indeed further still ...), these tombs appear in a variety of social contexts ..." (Frederiksen 1979, p.292).

The great series of princely tombs (e.g. the Regolini-Galassi tomb at Caere) of the late eighth and early-mid seventh centuries BC are amongst the best-known monuments of the Orientalizing period. As indicated above, recent work especially in Latium is extending the number of known sites, and demonstrates a remarkable cultural <u>koine</u> down the western seaboard of central Italy. The objects themselves are essentially prestige items (both imported and local imitations) and are clearly intended as a display of capital and wealth rather than for functional purposes. Cristofani (1975) has argued that they were used in a form of gift-exchange between chieftains (a ritual supported by inscriptions from Etruscan cemeteries); alternatively, they may reflect what Frederiksen (1979, p.294) describes as 'a fundamental lesson by the Greeks in primitive capital accumulation' (cf. Homer). But, whatever the truth (and here one should emphasize that the archaeological indications are of many different **ranks** of tombs), the emergence of an autocratic aristocratic class is not in doubt. Moreover, its contacts lay far beyond the confines of central Italy (Rathje 1979), presupposing a fairly sustained foreign presence in Etruria itself. Whether Stary's observation that between the late eighth century and c.650, the number of warrior graves in Etruria rises from c.5-15% to 35-40% (Stary 1979, p.187), is an argument for an increased level of conflict is a matter for debate; but it is striking to see how Etruria rapidly integrated itself into the broader spectrum of Mediterranean trade. Writing, employing versions of the Euboean script, was adopted from 690 or so, and enables us to talk of 'Etruscans' rather than of 'Villanovan culture'; production and trade not just in metal ores and metalwork objects, but in wine and oil (Cristofani 1979a) and various types of pottery was substantially increased; and by the end of the seventh century, the distinctive Etruscan product, bucchero pottery, was being widely distributed, examples being found as far afield as Carthage and in the sixth-century Cap d'Antibes wreck.

That some of this expansion in production was due to the arrival of foreign craftsmen is clear enough both from literary sources and from archaeological evidence. The Demaratus legend, which tells how this Corinthian noble was forced to emigrate from his home city in the mid seventh century and settled at Tarquinia, bringing with him a number of craftsmen, has a ring of truth about it. 'Etrusco - Corinthian' pottery is likely to have been the outcome of just such a migration. Rather later, c.580 BC, Tarquinia's port, Gravisca, saw the founding of a sanctuary initially dedicated to the patron deity of sea-travel and harbours, the goddess Aphrodite. Epigraphy makes it quite clear that this was a community of Greeks, which was later expanded by an influx of people from Ionia, no doubt refugees from the expanding Persian empire (Torelli 1977). Torelli (1974, p.19) sees the evolution of a Greek centre at Gravisca as a measure intended to control the immigrant population and to levy appropriate taxes. It marks a consolidation of the urban status of some of the Etruscan cities by the 'Orientalizing aristocrats', a tendency which, it is argued, promoted drastic social change.

The sixth-century middle class and cities

'Sociolinguistic' studies by Cristofani (1979b) and others suggest on the basis of Etruscan inscriptions that the two-part name came into general use during the second half of the seventh century: "Since the function of a <u>gentilicium</u> is to link people who are related by blood, religion or common political or economic interest, it seems evident that their coming into general use ... must be associated with the contemporaneous development of large urban centres ...". Gentilical names had the effect of associating individuals and families with particular settlements and their territories, gradually ousting the one-name system that epigraphically is widely attested in the early part of the seventh century.

At the same time, the growth of production and trade seems to have promoted the rise of a strong and ultimately very influential middle class of merchants. They are best reflected by the funerary architecture of sixth-century cemeteries, where serried ranks of cube-like tombs (often with the family name on the lintel above the entrance) are conspicuous features at a number of sites. They can be also seen at Caere (and provide a vivid contrast with the monumental tumuli of the seventh-century 'aristocrats'), and at the Crocefisso del Tufo necropolis at Orvieto. Here the graves are laid out in neat rows, recalling contempory orthogonal planning in Greek towns, and underlining the widespread contacts of these nouveaux riches. Many may have made their money from the sale of wine and oil (thought, without as yet much floral proof, to have become widely diffused in Etruria in the seventh century); others must have prospered from controlling metal-working, pottery and other manufacturing industries. The steady expansion of the Etruscans at this time - to Campania, the Po Valley and overseas to islands like Corsica - must have owed much to the activities of these traders.

The settlements themselves have yet to disclose any very clear archaeological picture of what was happening at this time. This is mainly a reflection of a dearth of large-scale excavation upon the settlements, but it is also a comment upon the very real logistic problems that result from the overlay of Roman buildings at Vulci, Roselle and elsewhere. Nevertheless, there are hints from a number of sites that the seventh century saw something of a transformation in styles of domestic architecture. Mirroring the elaboration of funerary chambers, rectangular houses (often with stone footings) can be seen to replace the oval timber buildings of the early Iron Age. The process appears to apply equally to Latium (as the recent work at Ficana shows: Cornell 1980, pp.81-2)) as it does to Etruria, and some of the so-called private houses seem to have been very elaborate. At the medium-sized nucleated settlement of Acquarossa near Viterbo, for example, elegantly painted terracottas embellished certain domestic buildings from the late seventh century and there was widespread use of roofing tile and figured terracottas (Ostenberg 1975). Whilst there is no suggestion of any formalized layout either here or at any other town in Etruria (Ward-Perkins 1974), it is not difficult to interpret these architectural innovations as a sign of 'urbanization'. Planning both of towns and sometimes of their territory was already well-established practice in many of the Greek colonies of southern Italy and these concepts were to become embodied in the layout of Etruscan 'new towns' such as Marzabotto and in the arrangement of some 'middle-class' cemeteries as at Orvieto. Greek inspiration also probably lay behind the beginnings of monumental architecture -particularly religious buildings as at Murlo near Siena -and perhaps, too, behind the construction of artificial defences at some sites. Roselle provides a well-known instance from Etruria, and now Ficana in Latium can be shown to have been given a bank and ditch perhaps as early as c.700 BC (Cornell 1980).

If formal planning was not adopted at towns like Ficana, Acquarossa or San Giovenale - the buildings tend to be scattered in an unsystematic way across the settlement area - this is the only real indication that these sites (none of them in the first rank of importance) were not fully urbanized. It is by no means impossible that a rather more organized pattern may emerge at some of these

larger foci. Rome, on the other hand, is yielding evidence to show that there were significant architectural developments at this time. At S. Omobono, for example, the sanctuary appears to have been laid out by the end of the seventh century, preceding a temple of c.600 BC; the first Regia was built in this period; Coarelli would now assign the earliest paving of the Comitium to the late seventh century; and this is also the date of the paving of the forum. It looks then as if the reign of Tarquinius Priscus (traditionally 616-578) witnessed the beginnings of a major building-programme. Moreover, this policy was continued by his successor, Servius Tullius (578-535); he is noted for, among other things, the construction of a defensive curtain which, according to Torelli (1974, p.19), converted Rome from an 'open' to a 'closed' city. If so, it is an architectural manifestation of the political and social tensions that became steadily more pronounced during the sixth century. Something of the military struggles of the period is portrayed in the paintings of the François Tomb; while a late work, it seems to depict a war in which Servius Tullius and the Etruscan condottieri, Aulus and Caelius Vibenna and Mastarna, are at odds. Episodes such as this suggest that individual towns and cities were coming increasingly into conflict during this period. This, it is argued, explains why many of the medium-sized settlements such as Acquarossa and Murlo were abandoned around the end of the fifth century: indeed, the excavators of Acquarossa claim that the whole site was deliberately sacked most probably by a 'foreign' enemy but possibly as a result of internal divisions (Ostenberg 1975).

These internal conflicts are a crucial feature of this period (as they are in Athens, Corinth and elsewhere at this time). As Livy (5,1, 3f.) tells us, they led at many cities (Rome of course being amongst them) to the replacement of monarchic rule by oligarchic 'Republican' regimes. To what extent this was a process of evolution rather than of revolution is matter for debate, given the paucity of our sources. No doubt the sequence of events varied markedly from place to place. But the episode does seem to be one that is manifest in the archaeological record at some sites, even though some appraisals would seem to overstate the case: "minor towns ... often came to a violent end ... whole areas of inland territory were abandoned as entire aristocrat-dominated communities moved into the big cities" (Cristofani 1979a, p.35).

Rome and Etruria: the fifth-third centuries

The fifth century brought a series of military reverses for the Etruscans, which initiated a steady erosion of their power and influence. At the same time, the scale of trade was sharply reduced as a result of the Ionian revolt (494 BC), of the wars between the Greeks and Persians and by competition from emporia on the Adriatic coast such as Spina. To social difficulties which emanated from the political transformations of the late fifth century, there was thus also an economic 'crisis'. Cristofani (1979a) suggests that this is one reason why programmes of land-reclamation, a conspicuous feature of the territory of Veii, some Latian towns such as Ardea and,to a lesser extent, that of Caere, were initiated at this time. We may perhaps doubt that any simple explanation can very readily account for this widespread phenomenon - changes in crops and techniques of agriculture, some fluctuation of climate and increasing population pressure may all have played their part (Potter 1981) - but these drainage schemes do underline the way in which the city extended its control over the countryside in the fifth and fourth centuries.

About the same time, there was a remarkably widespread trend towards the erection of artificial defences around both the major and the minor settlements. Whilst there is an obvious temptation to see this as a response to military threat - in particular the expansion of Rome - others would see it more as a reflection of a need to consolidate the fragile and divided nature of Etruscan society. This is not just a comment upon social instability resulting from unrest amongst the apparently large slave population, attested by literary sources at Arezzo in the fourth century, at Volsinii in the early third century and at a number of other Etruscan cities. Not only did Etruscan society lack a strong free plebeian class (a source of conflict but also of strength in the social fabric of Republican Rome), but the ruling class in many cities was also unable to maintain a firm base. Torelli (1970-71), for example, has provided an absorbing study in which he traces the fortunes of the Tarquinian nobiles as demonstrated by their tombs. It is a remarkable essay in the manner in which political, social and economic fortunes can be reflected in the funerary record. While his observation (Torelli 1974, p.20) that the "plight" of the Etruscans "is reflected by cultural stagnation all over Etruscan territory" in the fifth century BC" would hardly seem to apply to the magnificent Tarquinian painted tombs of this period, it is significant to see the way in which new 'patrician-plebs' took over from about 380 BC. Between about 340 and 300 BC these families dominate the richest graves, which then gradually give way to the poorer, more modest chambers of so-called 'small proprietors'. These Republican farmers hold their own until the end of the second century BC, by which time new patterns of land-owning had emerged and Tarquinian families were little favoured. Torelli records that in the registers of late-Republican and early Imperial senators, only five gens appear, three being long-established noble families and two completely non-Etruscan. It is a telling picture of the eclipse of an upper class that, five centuries earlier, had ruled Rome herself.

The 'patrician-pleb' class which came to dominate the Tarquinian aristocracy in the fourth century, reflects a brief revival of Etruscan fortunes, based particularly on new or reinvigorated manufacturing industries. The painters who embellished the tombs of Tarquinia provide an obvious example, as do the bronzeworkers of Arezzo and Vulci. Plutarch's record of guilds in Rome, in his Life of Numa lists metalworkers, masons, dyers, shoemakers, tanners, leatherworkers and potters and even flautists (a favourite theme on the Tarquinian tombs): together with the development of the terracotta industry (for which there was a guild in Rome from 580), this variety of activities illustrates something of the way in which a wide range of trades arose.

However, despite this economic revival in certain Etruscan cities in the fourth century, it is the steady expansion of Rome that dominates the historical narrative in this period. Rome's military successes reflect both the divided nature of the opponents - the Etruscan cities in particular could never mount a united front - and the strength of the 'citizen army'. The soldiers themselves were drawn essentially from the plebeians - Rome's famous 'soldier-peasant' - a class that politically always held its own during the Republic. Despite the power of the aristocratic patrician families, by 366 the consulship had been opened to the lower orders and over the next two centuries nearly every high office was held at one time or another by plebeians (Brunt 1971b). Thus, the mid-late Republic did see a gradual increase in democratic control, although power always lay with the richer families and never with the poor plebeians.

Rome's policy towards its newly conquered territories is a highly complex matter which, as Harris (1971) has emphasised, varied both according to local conditions and over time. In Etruria, at many cities Rome sought to

bolster the ruling aristocracy, as is shown by a number of interventions on behalf of the nobiles in various slave-uprisings (e.g. Arezzo in 302, Volsinii in 265 and many areas in 196, Harris 1971, p.143). The point is underlined by field-surveys such as that of the territory of Veii: in 396 BC, the date of the conquest "there was a considerable measure of disruption and a number of Etruscan farms were abandoned or incorporated into other holdings ... On the other hand, for every farm that was given up, two more can be seen to have continued in occupation ..." (Ward-Perkins 1968, p.145). However, even at this early period, Rome was evolving what, in the long-term, emerged as a vital strategy: the planting of colonies. Comprised either of settlers without the right of citizenship (Latin colonies) or of Roman citizens, they were to become the decisive means by which 'Romanisation' was spread (Salmon 1969). Whilst by no means common in Republican Etruria (Harris 1971, p.197f.), for reasons mentioned above, there were a number of important early foundations such as Cosa (273 BC, refounded in 197 BC) and, by the second Punic War (218-201 BC), probably four in territory that formerly belonged to Caere. When taken together with the land allocated to the colonists, these new settlements inevitably meant the break up of existing farming units in these areas. Given that this process was to a greater or lesser extent being repeated in many parts of Italy, it is difficult not to see the third and second centuries BC as something of a watershed in the organization of the countryside.

Moreover, the construction of a system of new long-distance highways in the third and especially the second century also introduced pressures for change. Veii for instance was by-passed when the Via Cassia was constructed and therefore lapsed into obscurity, noted only for the dreadful quality of its wine (Martial 1, 103, 9). Many other cities and towns suffered a similar fate, a trend very clearly revealed archaeoogiclly in Apulia where settlements like Ordona, Arpi, Egnazio, M. Sannace and Gravina went into rapid decline from the third century BC. Similarly, in the Ager Faliscus, conquered in 241 BC, the archaeological picture is of severe disruption. Zonaras (8, 189) tells us that half the Faliscan territory was confiscated, a measure which seems to be reflected in the fact that nearly every Faliscan farmstead found by field survey was abandoned at this time (Potter, forthcoming). Moreover, the capital of the region, Falerii, evacuated in favour of a new site, Falerii Novi, and most other Faliscan towns were also deserted at this time.

Slaves and peasants

At the time when many regions of Italy were, as we have seen, undergoing a significant degree of dislocation and change in the pattern of settlement, an additional factor becomes of increasing importance: the question of slavery. While slaves were undoubtedly common before this period (and in Etruria there were individuals who seem to have been ranked between free men and slaves, called by Dionysus (9.5.4), penestai) there is no doubt that a consequence of war was a great expansion in their numbers (Finley 1973, p. 79). Moreover, although a contentious campaigning of the mid-late Republic make available both the slaves themselves and the wealth to buy and to keep them, but it also became fashionable. "Who has no slaves and no money-box" is how a Roman poet (Catullus) describes a penniless man, when we might say 'not a bean' ' (Finley 1973, p.79). Moreover, although a contentious issue both in antiquity and today, there can be little real doubt that estates and industries that used slave labour were on the whole profitable (cf. Varro, de Agric, 1,17; Finley 1973, p.83; Carandini and Settis 1979). Many slaves became highly skilled and influential people (which a high rate of manumission must have encouraged), and it would be difficult to deny that they played a part in the extraordinary economic growth of Italy during the late Republic and early Imperial period (Hopkins 1980). This point is underlined by the estimates of their numbers in second-first centuries BC, the consensus being that there may have been between 2-3 million slaves out of a total population in Italy of some 6-7.5 millions (Brunt 1971a, p.124; Beloch 1886, p.418).

The role of slaves in agriculture and particularly in the formation and spead of latifundia is, however, an especially thorny issue. While not all would agree with Finley's verdict (1973, p.69) that "in Rome and Italy from early in the third century BC to the third century AD, slavery effectively replaced other forms of dependent labour", there can be no doubt that latifundia did become widely diffused (although the term itself was not used at this time). This was a consequence of many factors. Partly responsible was the break-up of former 'units of production', as must have happened in areas such as the Ager Faliscus (cf. supra). Here, the rich must often have snapped up land, as being one of the safest - indeed, probably the safest - form of investment. Moreover, opportunities to expand estates often came about since peasant proprietors were frequently absent for long periods, fighting in the wars. While resettlement in coloniae was an answer, debt, dispossession and a deep sense of discontent became increasingly prevalent. "The rich came to cultivate vast tracts instead of single estates, using slaves as labourers and herdsmen in place of free men, who might be called away from the work on military service", (Appian, Bellum Civile, 1,7).

The invasion of Italy by Hannibal towards the end of the third century BC is also generally seen as an important factor in the formation of latifundia. Devastation brought about by the wars (Toynbee 1965) and the confiscation of land from pro-Carthaginian Apulians and Lucanians (Brunt 1971a) are both thought to be factors that contributed to the decline in small-holdings and the creation of large estates, particularly in the south of Italy. What Toynbee (1965, II, p.159) describes as a 'pastoral revolution' is thought, from literary sources, to have involved the creation of large ranches primarily devoted to sheep-raising. Certainly, a degree of depopulation took place in many parts of southern Italy during the second century BC (Small 1977, 1978), although archaeological evidence is lacking for a detailed evaluation. Ironically, one of the very few sites of this period whose animal bones have been studied, Monte d'Irsi (province of Matera), has shown a decline in sheep production at this time (Barker in Small 1977).

Nevertheless, a combination of literary and archaeological sources do confirm that in some regions of Italy at least large slave estates did become increasingly prevalent. This explains why the proposed Gracchan legislation of 133 BC was just one of some twenty attempts over a period of a century or so to render help to the dispossessed free peasantry (assidui) (Hopkins 1978). One area that Tiberius Gracchus must have passed through on his famous journey up the Via Aurelia through Etruria was the territory of the colony of Cosa. Here, field-survey and excavation have disclosed a remarkable picture of the formation of these large estates (Carandini and Settis 1979, Carandini and Tatton-Brown 1980). In the fertile land of the Valle d'Oro, for instance, a dozen large villas, farming territories of c. 125ha., gradually took over from the original colonial allocations during the second and early-mid first centuries BC. This accords well with Tiberius Gracchus' description of lands worked only by slaves and of many abandoned fields. At Sette Finestre, one of these villas is currently under study, and has already yielded a clear plan of a magnificent residence, side by side with a working farm. Here were facilities for the pressing of oil and the production of

wine, a complex of 27 pig-sties and quarters for the slaves. The villa as a whole appears to have been laid out in the first century BC and was continuously occupied into Antonine times.

While these large 'capitalist' estates and the social problems that they engendered have tended to monopolize discussion of agrarian problems in this period, (and sometimes give the impression that most of Italy was converted into large-scale holdings during Republican times), recent work has tended to present a corrective to this view. Some of the impetus has come from field-survey which, while disclosing nothing of patterns of ownership (it was common practice to possess a number of geographically scattered estates), nevertheless makes it quite clear that peasant small-holdings remained common well into Imperial times (e.g. Monte Forco: Jones 1963, p.147). This is as true of the environs of Rome as it is elsewhere and, as Garnsey (1979, 1980), Frederiksen (1975) and others have emphasized, is one indication of the complex agrarian matrix to be found in Republican Italy: "to search for a single ethos among landowners in ancient times is likely to be wrong" (Frederiksen 1975, p.169). Not only can we anticipate marked variations in the economic arrangements within quite small regions (e.g. the Biferno valley of Molise: Barker et al.1978), but in the great reclaimed areas of the Po Valley flats, settled mainly by colonists, the slave-run estate must have been rare. This is not to argue that various types of villas did not become widely diffused over many parts of the peninsula: the sheer density of these sites, as recorded by surface-survey in south and central Etruria, Campania, the lower part of the Biferno valley in Molise and elsewhere, underlines the point. But we must infer a wide variety in the **type** of villa, its size, its economy and its labour-arrangements - whether slaves, tenants, hired-labourers, debt-labourers or a combination of these. Whilst the slave-run villa and its social and economic complications may have captured the imagination of contemporary observers (and inspired a spate of farming manuals), there was no single 'mode of production' in Republican Italy (pace e.g. Carandini 1973). The **trend** may have been towards latifundia of different kinds (Duncan-Jones 1974, p.323 f; White 1967), but other evidence, both literary and archaeological, serves to demonstrate an enduring diversity in the Roman countryside.

Trade and industry

Roman Italy was never destined to become an industrial country (Finley 1973). Although the manufacture and export of goods achieved increasing importance during the later Republic and in the early Imperial period - for example, the production of black-glaze and, later, of Arretine (and related wares); of a variety of metalwork; of wine and oil amphorae; and of glass vessels and lamps (to name but a few products: cf Frank 1933) - none of these industries was on a particularly large scale. At Arezzo, for instance, although there were some 90 pottery firms, the average number of artisans was only between 10 and 20 and no 'factory' employed more than 60 (Pucci 1973). Most of these artisans at Arezzo appear to have been slaves and there is little doubt that the abundance of cheap labour did affect the scale of production (cf Hopkins 1980).

One example, recently studied by Coarelli (1977), must suffice: the building industry in Rome in the second century BC. As Vitruvius makes clear (2.8.17) the population rose steeply at this time, creating both an enormous demand for housing and a large body of unemployed poor. Some of this cheap labour was put to work on public monuments such as aqueducts (an improved water supply being of obvious importance), while others were engaged in the erection of tenement housing. The wars of conquest had brought in the wealth to finance much of this work (although property speculation was always endemic in the capital and elsewhere) and the pool of labour was there: the problem was to devise techniques of construction which could be employed by unskilled men. This is why, Coarelli argues, the use of concrete, faced with opus incertum, appears in Rome around the beginning of the second century BC. It was a relatively inexpensive and technically undemanding technique, well adapted to the circumstances and needs of the time. Later, probably c.100 BC, opus incertum gives way to the more regular and better made opus reticulatum; this, he suggests, is a reflection of a 'division of labour' whereby the standardized components (the facing stones) could be produced at the quarries by specialized craftsmen, for use by unskilled labour.

This neat and persuasive explanation illustrates something of the way in which a combination of population increase and greater wealth may have brought about what was to amount to a revolution in architecture and engineering, whose consequences can be measured all over Italy. Indeed, it presages a remarkable expansion of the building industry, in both the public and the private sector. Many of these were 'prestige' monuments, reflecting the pronounced tendency of the rich late Republican families to flaunt their wealth (Hopkins 1978): one thinks of the Pyramid tomb of Gaius Cestius, who died in 43 BC, or the bizarre 'oven-tomb' of Vergilius Eurysaces, the baker. These extravagant symbols of affluence serve to epitomise the sharp differences between rich and poor in the first century BC. No wonder then when the complex struggles of the period had run their course, and Octavian had become Augustus, that it was to be seen as the victory of the rural and urban poor.

The principate: a postscript

Augustan Italy, with its restructured, bureaucratic administration, its professional army, its resettlement and building schemes and its 'new men', saw the end of the Roman city-state and the creation of the Roman Empire. The time is hardly ripe, however, to attempt an archaeological appraisal of the complex weave of events over the next few centuries. If the matrix of evidence is thin and patchy for Italy in the first millennium BC, then in some senses it is even thinner for the first millennium AD. While the historical narrative is full, archaeology has yet to exploit fully the wealth of information contained in the mid to late Imperial deposits at most town and country sites. This position is changing but we should surely be chary of testing historically-derived models against results derived from a couple of towns (particularly Ostia and Luni) and a small sample of villas.

There is no shortage of theory to test. Carandini, for example, in a series of influential papers and books has defined three main phases: (i) a first period in which the mode of production is principally that of slave-run estates (ii) from the reign of Trajan, a diversification of the productive methods, with a decline in slave-estates and, by the Antonine period, the onset of recession and (iii) in the later Roman period the gradual reversion to the tied colonate, whose status approximates to that of serfs. His excavations at Sette Finestre might be said to support this model very effectively with (a) the blocking up of the oil and wine press-rooms in the early second century (possibly because of a change to cereal production) and the desertion of the villa by the reign of Marcus Aurelius. "This possibly indicates that a vast latifundium had taken over" (Carandini and Tatton-Brown 1980 p.11). They go on: "Recent excavations in Ostia (Carandini et al. 1977) suggest that the production of food-stuffs etc. in Italy for export was already in decline in the middle of the

second century AD ... The golden age of the Antonines, which is believed by many to have been so prosperous, was also in fact the last period of Roman expansion."

There is no doubt that the **archaeological** signs for a decline in production are clear in many fields (e.g. lamp production, metalwork, some amphorae, and various sorts of fine pottery). In many of these industries it was North Africa which captured the markets (as, for example, recent results from Luni (Frova et al. 1977) show very well). Moreover, most ancient historians postulate a gradual decline in slavery somewhere between the reign of Augustus and the mid second century AD (Garnsey 1980). "If the explanation ... is not to be found in the drying up of the slave supply or in decisions about efficiency, productivity and the like, then it must lie in a structural transformation of society as a whole" writes Finley (1973 p.86). As time went on, the division of society into the upper orders (honestiores) and the lower classes (humiliores) became increasingly apparent with tied tenants now providing most of the labour on such land that was being worked.

How was the land being worked in the later Roman period and how prevalent did agri deserti become? Does the diminution of the number of sites in occupation in the third-fifth centuries, as suggested by the evidence of field-survey, really mean that large tracts of countryside were being abandoned in the wake of the 'crisis of production' in the mid-late second century? Here, there are reasons for being sceptical, at any rate for some areas (Wickham 1979, p.84 f.); but a great deal of precisely collected evidence needs to be assembled, especially from excavation of certain critical sites, before any real perspective can be achieved. We may not entirely share Garnsey's conclusion (1980 p.41) that "any statement about 'trends' between the late Republic and the middle Empire ... will be so guarded and full of qualification as to be almost useless". But any model, social or economic, evolutionary or non-evolutionary, must be presented with all caution. Just as the web of argument for pre-Roman Italy can be seen to be almost bafflingly intricate: so is the evidence for the age of the Republic and the Empire. What is emerging is that archaeology can be said to be providing something of a new perspective.

BIBLIOGRAPHY

BARKER, G.W.W. 1977 - "The archaeology of Samnite settlement in Molise" Antiquity vol. 51, pp.20-4.

BARKER, G.W.W., LLOYD, J., WEBLEY, D. 1978 - "A classical landscape in Molise", PBSR vol. 46, pp.35-51.

BELOCH, K.J. 1886 - Die Bevölkerung der griechisch - römischen Welt. Leipzig.

BIETTI SESTIERI, A.M. 1979 - Ricerca su una comunità del Lazio protostorico. Rome.

BRUNT, P.A. 1971a - Italian manpower 225 BC - AD 14. Oxford.

BRUNT, P.A. 1971b - Social conflicts in the Roman Republic. London.

CARANDINI, A. 1973 - "Dibattito sull'edizione italiana della 'storia economica del'mondo antico' di F. Heichelheim". Dialoghi di Archeologia 7, pp.312 - 29.

CARANDINI, A. et al. 1977 - Ostia IV. Le Terme del

242

Nuotatore: scavi dell'ambiente xvi e dell' area xxv. Studi Miscellanei 23, Rome.

CARANDINI, A. and SETTIS, S. 1979 - Schiavi e padroni nell 'Etruria romana. La villa di Sette Finestre dallo scavo alla mostra. Bari.

CARANDINI, A. and TATTON-BROWN, T. 1980 -"Excavations at the Roman villa of Sette Finestre in Etruria, 1975-9. First interim report". In ed. Painter, K.S., Roman Villas in Italy, BM Occ. Pap., pp.9-44.

CLOSE - BROOKS, J. 1965 - "Veio: Quattro Fontanili. Proposta per una suddivisione in fase", Not. Scav. 1965, pp. 53-63. (Reprinted in Ridgway and Ridgway 1979, pp.95-107).

CLP 1976 - Civiltà del Lazio primitivo. Exhibition catalogue. Rome.

COARELLI, F. 1977 - "Public building in Rome between the Second Punic War and Sulla". PBSR vol. 45, pp.1-23.

COLONNA, G. 1974 - "Preistoria e protostoria di Roma e del Lazio", Popoli e civiltà dell'Italia antica 2, pp.275-346. Rome.

CORNELL, T.J. 1980 - "Rome and Latium vetus", JHS vol. 100, pp.71-89.

CRISTOFANI, M. 1975 - "Il 'dono' nell' Etruria arcaica", Parola del Passato vol. 30, pp.32-52.

CRISTOFANI, M. 1979a - The Etruscans. A new investigation. London.

CRISTOFANI, M. 1979b - "Recent advances in Etruscan epigraphy and language". In Ridgway and Ridgway 1979, pp.373-412.

DELANO SMITH 1979 - Western Mediterranean Europe. A historical geography of Italy, Spain and southern France since the Neolithic. London.

DELPINO, F. 1977 - "La prima età del ferro a Bisenzio: aspetti della cultura villanoviana nell' Etruria meridionale interna", Mea.Lincei, 8th series, vol. 21, pp.453-93.

DUNCAN-JONES, R.P. 1979 - The economy of the Roman Empire: quantitative studies. Cambridge.

FINLEY, M.I. 1973 - The ancient economy. London.

FRANK, TENNEY 1933 - An economic survey of ancient Rome. Baltimore.

FREDERIKSEN, M.W. 1975 - "Theory, evidence and the ancient economy", (review of M.I. Finley, The ancient economy). JRS vol. 65, pp.164-71.

FREDERIKSEN, M.W. 1979 - "The Etruscans in Campania". In Ridgway and Ridgway 1979, pp.277-311.

FROVA, A. et al. 1977 - Scavi di Luni II. Relazione delle campagne di scavo 1972-1973-1974. Rome.

GARNSEY, P.D.A. 1979 - "Where did Italian peasants live?" Proc. Cambs. Phil. Soc. vol. 25, pp.1-15.

GARNSEY, P.D.A. 1980 - Non-slave labour in the Graeco-Roman world. Cambridge Philosophical Society.

HARRIS, W.V. 1971 - Rome in Etruria and Umbria. Oxford.

HOPKINS, K. 1978 - Conquerors and slaves. Sociological studies in Roman History I. Cambridge.

HOPKINS, K. 1980 - "Taxes and trade in the Roman Empire (200 BC - AD 400)". JRS vol. 70, pp.101-25.

JONES, A.H.M. 1964 - The later Roman Empire. A social, economic and administrative survey. Oxford.

JONES, A.H.M. 1974 - The Roman economy: studies in ancient economic and administrative history. (ed. P.A. Brunt). Oxford.

JONES, G.D.B. 1963 - "Capena and the Ager Capenas, part II". PBSR vol. 31, pp.100-58.

OSTENBERG, C.E. 1975 - Case etrusche di Acquarossa. Rome.

PAINTER, K.S. (ed.) 1980 - Roman Villas in Italy. B.M. Occ. Pap.

PERONI, R. 1969 - "Per uno studio dell'economia di scambio in Italia nel quadro dell'ambiente culturale dei secoli intorno al mille a.c." Parola del Passato. 24, pp.134-60. (Reprinted in Ridgway and Ridgway 1979 pp. 7-30).

POTTER, T.W. 1979 - The changing landscape of South Etruria. London.

POTTER, T.W. 1981 - "Marshland and drainage in the classical world". In Rowley R.T. (Ed.). Marshland and drainage.

POTTER, T.W. (forthcoming) - "An archaeological survey of the central and southern Ager Faliscus". PBSR

PUCCI, G. 1973 - "La produzione della ceramica arretina", Dialoghi di Archeologia vol. 7, p. 255.

QF. 1963 f. - "Veio - scavi in una necropoli villanoviana in località 'Quattro Fontanili'". Not. Scav. 1963,77-279; 1965, 49-236; 1967, 87-286; 1970, 178-329; 1972, 195-384; 1975, 63-184.

RATHJE, A. 1979 - "Oriental imports in Etruria in the eighth and seventh centuries BC: their origins and implications". In Ridgway and Ridgway 1979, pp.145-83.

RIDGWAY, D. 1973 - "The first western Greeks: Campanian coasts and southern Etruria". In (ed.) Hawkes C.F.C. and S., Greeks, Celts and Romans (London), pp.5-38.

RIDGWAY, D. and RIDGWAY F.R. (eds.) 1979 - Italy before the Romans. The Iron Age, Orientalising and Etruscan periods. London.

ROSSITER, J.J. 1978 - Roman farm buildings in Italy. BAR. S52.

ROSTOVTZEFF, M. 1957 - The social and economic history of the Roman Empire. Oxford.

SALMON, E.T. 1969 - Roman colonisation under the Republic. London.

SMALL, A.M. 1977 - Monte Irsi, southern Italy. BAR, S20.

SMALL, A.M. 1978 - The villa rustica of the Hellenistic period in south Italy. In (eds) Blake, H.M., Potter, T.W. and Whitehouse, D.B., Papers in Italian Archaeology. BAR, S41, pp.197-201.

STARY, P.F. 1979 - "Foreign elements in Etruscan arms and armour, eighth - third centuries BC", PPS vol. 45, pp.179-206.

TORELLI, M. 1970-71 - "Contributo dell' archeologia alla storia sociale: I. - L'Etruria e l'Apulia". Dialoghi di Archeologia vol. 4-5, pp.431-42.

TORELLI, M 1974 - "Introduction". In (Ed.) Coarelli, F., Etruscan Cities. London, pp.11-28.

TORELLI, M. 1977 - "Il santuario greco di Gravisca", Parola del Passato 32, pp.398-458.

TOUBERT, P. 1973 - Les structures du Latium mediéval. Bibliothèque des Ecoles françaises d'Athènes et de Rome, 221.

TOYNBEE, A.J. 1965 - Hannibal's Legacy. Oxford.

WARD-PERKINS, J.B. 1961 - "Veii. The historical topography of the ancient city". PBSR vol. 29, pp.1-123.

WARD-PERKINS, J.B. (with Kahane A. and Murray-Threipland, L.)1968 - "The Ager Veientanus north and east of Veii". PBSR vol. 36, pp.1-218.

WARD-PERKINS, J.B. 1974 - Cities of ancient Greece and Italy: planning in classical antiquity. New York.

WICKHAM, C.J. 1978 - "Historical and topographical notes on early medieval south Etruria (Part I)." PBSR vol. 46, pp.132-79.

WICKHAM, C.J. 1979 - Idem, part II. PBSR vol. 47, pp.66-95.

WHITE, K.D. 1967 - "Latifundia." Bulletin of London Institute of Classical Studies 14, pp.62-79.

WHITEHOUSE, R.D. 1973 - The earliest towns in peninsular Italy". In (ed.) Renfrew, C., The explanation of culture change: models in prehistory (London), pp. 617-24.

10

SOCIAL EVOLUTION
AND THE WESTERN PROVINCES
OF THE ROMAN EMPIRE

Rick Jones

Introduction

In examining the changes society underwent during the Roman Empire, it is necessary to deal with many complex themes which are familiar today: imperialism, acculturation, economic decline. Western Europe in the first half of the first millennium AD was first integrated into a world Empire which had contacts as far away as India and China (Fig. 1). Yet by AD 500 it had more or less fallen away from that Empire and begun a new phase, even though the rest of the Empire was to survive for another millennium. The turbulent five centuries of the Roman Empire in the west involved rapid change in social, political, economic and religious terms. They were also crucial to the formation of institutions which have been with us ever since, notably Christianity. This paper will deal firstly with the establishment of Romanized forms of behaviour and of buildings under the early Empire, since the later changes can only be understood in the context of what went before.

Social history and social archaeology

To prehistoric archaeologists the quantity of written evidence available for the Roman Empire might seem at worst to make the archaeology superfluous to any study of social developments, or at best to offer the opportunity to check the archaeology against the historical evidence. However, those who seek to emerge from prehistoric doubts into some kind of historical certainty for the Roman Empire are set for disappointment. There are widely recognized limitations on the written evidence for this period: the texts we have were essentially written by, for, and often about the educated classes. Their contribution to the study of any wider concept of Roman provincial society must be circumscribed. The proximity of interest between archaeologists and historians of the Roman provinces often persuades them that they are studying exactly the same things. Yet the natures of their evidence are fundamentally different. They may be attempting to deal with the same abstract 'reality', in the same period of the past, but their perspectives differ because the intellectual constructs which they make as their approximations to that 'reality' are made from different materials and therefore give different perspectives. The various models of 'reality' stand equal chances of validity within their own terms of reference, but a valid archaeological model of social change need not necessarily fit precisely with a valid historical one, although some consistency might be expected. Neither kind of model need be accorded a higher merit. It is clear that much of the interest and attraction of studying these historical or protohistoric periods lies in the opportunity

to compare the results of historical and archaeological analysis; what I am trying to stress is the need to see the archaeological evidence as distinct and interesting in its own right, and not as mere illustration for historians' theories. The study of the Roman army of the early Empire exemplifies some of these points. Excavations of auxiliary forts of this period normally reveal three main types of living accommodation: the commander's house, detached and often an elaborate courtyard house; the centurions' quarters, suites of rooms at one end of each barrack block; and the contubernia, the troopers' rooms, each holding eight or ten men in two small adjoining rooms. The difference in scale of space allotted is obvious, but does not seem to relate precisely to the much more complex system of ranks recorded in the literary evidence. The models derived from the evidence for ranks and grades and from the archaeological remains are consistent in general but not in detail. The archaeology demonstrates what living conditions were actually like for the different ranks: documentary study shows how the finer points of ranking were worked out by the soldiers themselves. To put the same point another way, the archaeologist can expect to excavate and recognize the homes of the rich man and the poor man, but not usually to distinguish the senator or the slave. Neither the archaeology nor the history is wrong, but they are not producing exactly the same conclusions.

However, it has been the historians who have been more willing to synthesize at the general level appropriate to this paper. Archaeologists have tended to deserve the criticisms made by Hopkins (1978a, p.71), that they have been more concerned with accumulating more data in the field than with trying to understand it. Although close acquaintance with the Roman archaeology of western Europe does reveal a frightening amount of very basic research still needing to be done, in this paper the attempt is made to offer a synthesis. Many historians have examined social issues in the Roman Empire in recent years. The various works of Finley (1973; 1974; 1977), MacMullen (1963; 1966; 1974), A.H.M. Jones (1964; 1966; 1974), Brown (1971; 1978), Hopkins (1978a; 1978b), and Garnsey (1970) have been particularly relevant. Yet many of these papers have dealt with topics such as elite mobility, social mobility for Imperial freedmen and slaves, or legal privilege. These are hardly susceptible to archaeological investigation. They often concern what was happening at the heart of the Imperial system, rather than in the provinces. They provide an important framework of ideas for the Roman world as a whole, but are difficult to apply in detail with any confidence in the western provinces, where the written evidence generally survives poorly. So much so that MacMullen's book Roman

246

Social Relations specifically excludes Spain, Gaul and Britain on grounds of the lack of suitable evidence (MacMullen 1974, p.vii).

Even when historians do attempt to use the archaeological evidence, they can often be grudging in accepting its relevance, or simplistic in its interpretation (cf. Garnsey 1979, pp.2-4). The author of a recent historical discussion of rural labour found it necessary to go to some lengths to point out that Gaul was not peopled exclusively by wild savages before the Roman conquest, which should hardly have been required for a modern archaeological readership (Whittaker 1980). Such apparent unfamiliarity with the archaeology is a serious weakness for any student of the western Roman provinces. For these regions in particular, archaeology alone has a potential for dynamic expansion of the available data. Although lacking the greatly increased quantity and quality of modern evidence, earlier attempts at generalization which have taken the archaeology prominently into account, such as those by Rostovtzeff (1957) and Haverfield (1912), did point to the essential theme of 'Romanization'. How far did the people of the western provinces become 'Roman', in the sense of the adoption of a set of manners and ideas developed in the Mediterranean? How great were the internal changes as the Empire grew and eventually collapsed, at least in political and military terms? What were the forces behind any changes that we can identify? Our understanding of these questions in western Europe rests on processes of inference and implication from the material archaeological evidence.

Roman economic systems

The nature of the Imperial economic systems has direct bearing on the development of social systems. The Roman economy of the late Republic and early Empire was one of conquest and imperialism. The central parts of the Empire and the central government were able to exploit the newly conquered territories in a wide variety of ways. The new provinces provided a rich mixture of slaves, taxes and raw materials, particularly metals. In return, the developed Greco-Roman world of the Mediterranean provided supplies of luxury goods which marked its culture, as well as capital investment and skills to enable the provincials to build their own versions of the Mediterranean (cf. Hopkins 1978b, p.1 ff.). Hopkins has argued that taxes stimulated trade and thereby increased production for sale, leading in due course to an economy monetized to a significant level (1980). The expressions of this process at work are to be found in the archaeology of the western provinces, not only in terms of imported artifacts, but more significantly in the building of towns and villas.

It is hard to deny that economic growth took place in western Europe in the early Roman Empire, even if it is difficult to quantify. In terms of the range and quantity of goods traded, the wealth invested in public monuments and private houses, and the increased division of labour implied by all that, the greater complexity of the Roman system is apparent. Ian Hodder (1979) has applied the theories of Polanyi and others to Iron Age and Roman Britain to argue that the pre-Roman economy was rooted essentially in gift-exchange: it was embedded in the social system rather than being a full-scale market economy. Integral to this concept are sites such as Hengistbury Head, defined as a port-of-trade, controlling long-distance trade, essentially with the Iron Age British tribal elites. This model can easily be extended to other parts of western Europe where coastal sites flourished in the last centuries BC as entrepôts dealing in Greco-Roman luxury goods and raw materials from the tribal hinterland. The clearest examples are Marseille and Ampurias. It has long been recognised that Marseille controlled trade into central Europe from the Mediterranean before the Roman

conquest spread under Julius Caesar (cf. Wells 1980). The same role for northern Spain was played by another Greek foundation at Ampurias. The later fortunes of both cities show a relative decline in their importance, as economic expansion took hold in their hinterlands. Marseille gave way as the dominant city at the mouth of the Rhône to Arles (cf. Février 1973). At Ampurias, excavation has produced clear evidence of a decline in activity from the second century AD (Ripoll 1973). It was succeeded in importance locally by Gerona (Nolla 1978), and on a regional scale for north eastern Spain by Tarragona and then Barcelona. It is significant that all the major cities which prospered later combined harbour facilities with improved road communications. The decline of the ports-of-trade and the rise of centres more firmly rooted in a developed hinterland in Britain and the western Mediterranean coincided with the development of manufactures in the new provinces. The outward movement of centres of pottery fine ware production from Arrezzo in Italy to Gaul and Spain was noted by Rostovtzeff (1957, pp.172ff.). Although the importance of this as industry has been scorned by Finley (1973, p.137), it remains the case that one of the few products made on a large scale which we can examine archaeologically saw its main centres of production shift from Italy to the provinces. The samian industries of successively southern, central and eastern Gaul are well known; that of Spain followed a similar pattern (cf. Beltrán Lloris 1978, p.109ff.). Although its shortcomings as data are well appreciated, pottery has to serve as a proxy for other items of trade, because it is so often the main evidence surviving (an argument accepted for example by Hopkins 1978a, p.58). Pottery studies can demonstrate the continuing process whereby fine ware production became much more locally based, so that by the early third century we can see the products of particular industries being traded over much shorter distances than previously. By the late third century and in the fourth, the pattern was of regional centres of production, dominating their own areas, but not reaching much further afield. It may be reasonably assumed that local production became the norm with many classes of goods, with the result that most trade in the later Empire was at a regional or provincial level. Yet even if the distance that goods were moved became less, there is no reason to suppose that the intensity of the trade diminished. Indeed the general growth in the local economies witnessed in town and country suggests that the volume of trade probably increased: an increase in volume was probably an essential requirement for the growth of local production. Such generalizations cannot at present be substantiated by many detailed cases, but more work on the quantities and sources of pottery and other items found in excavations should provide relevant information.

The nature of economic growth in the Greco-Roman world has been much discussed. While recognizing distinctions between aggregate and per capita growth, Hopkins has argued that the total wealth in the lands that formed the Roman western provinces must have been much greater under the Empire than before (1978a, pp.35-6). The physical manifestations of rural and urban life in the provinces seem to require a degree of economic growth compared to earlier times, and within the Roman period. Despite this apparently increased wealth in the provinces, the Imperial administration suffered a contrasting crisis of financial difficulty. The full discussion of these problems is beyond the scope of this paper, but it can be seen that there was a crucial failure to change the Imperial financial system from that of the era of conquest to one more suited to an era of developed provinces. The result was an inability to transform the wealth present in the provinces to make it useful for the needs of the state, essentially for paying the army. The Imperial state responded by increased taxation, often in kind, which still did not succeed in providing an army capable of resisting invasion and preserving the pax Romana (cf. Hopkins 1980). During the third century there was a considerable dislocation of the economic structures of the Empire (cf. various papers in King and Henig 1981). From the third to the fifth century there was a gradual evolution of local regional and provincial loyalties, parallel to developments in the economic and trading systems. Political, military, economic and social factors were closely intertwined.

The Roman urbanization of western Europe

In the archaeological study of social change in the western Roman Empire, central issues are the development of the town and its relationship to the countryside, with the light they shed on the structure of society and changing power relations within it. Other aspects must be seen at a more personal level, such as religion and burial. The spread of urban centres throughout western Europe in the Roman period was so dramatic that it demands first attention. Even where recognizing that the city was rooted in wider settlement patterns, as well as wider social, economic and political systems, most students of the Classical world have agreed on the primacy of the city, if only because of the way all those systems were most sharply expressed in the city itself. Finley has described "the growth of towns as the regular and relentless accompaniment to the spread of Greco-Roman civilisation" (1977, p.305). The nature of the Classical city as a type has been discussed for many years. Finley's argument hung on the role of the city in its relation to its hinterland and thus on the model of the 'consumer-city' (1977). This ideal type must first be considered in relation to the early Empire and the first adoption of the Classical urban form.

A provincial Roman town could be established in a variety of ways. It could have been a Roman imposition, founded as a colony for retired legionaries on a new site, or the site of a former legionary fortress. It could have been a natural evolution, simply developing from a pre-existing settlement without dramatic change. In practice the former extreme was more common than the latter, though most places experienced something in between them. New colonies could be established on the sites of former fortresses, like Lincoln or Gloucester, but even here there may well have been some existing civilian settlement already. In many parts of southern Gaul, and probably Spain, there were existing native settlements when Roman colonies were founded. Most common were the cities that underwent radical change in re-planning, or possibly re-siting, so as better to conform to the ideal of the Greco-Roman town. Few major cities in the west were not transformed in such a way. The native origins of urbanisation are beginning to emerge in most parts of western Europe. Iron Age archaeologists have argued that pre-Roman urban settlement was true urbanism in northern Europe, although not on the Greco-Roman model. Nucleated settlements on quite a large scale had developed in much of north-west Europe in the later part of the first millennium BC (cf. Collis 1979; Cunliffe and Rowley 1976; 1978). This was the beginning of western Europe's urban revolution. It happened rather earlier in the Mediterranean than further north and west, but both areas share many points of similarity. The very earliest urban centres were in southern Spain, under Carthaginian influence. Cadiz seems to have been a true city in the ancient sense by the middle of the first millennium BC (Blázquez 1975). The areas under Punic influence seem to have been further advanced than the Greek-dominated coasts. Stimulated by its mineral wealth, the area of southern Spain that became the Roman province of Baetica was already deeply involved in the most advanced Mediterranean culture before formal Roman conquest. This background enabled Baetica to become the most Italian of western

provinces, and incidentally to provide the first non-Italian Emperors, Trajan and Hadrian (cf. Thouvenot 1973). Sites in southern France, such as Entremont (Benoit 1975) or Ensérune (Jannoray 1955) flourished before Roman conquest, developing street systems and becoming recognisable as urban centres imitating the Greco-Roman model. The same sort of pattern may be found on several Iberian sites (Nicolini 1974). Ullastret in Catalunya shared many of the characteristics of Entremont and Ensérune. It had streets, defences, and a system of water cisterns similar to the contemporary Greek town of Ampurias on the coast nearby. It also shared in wider Mediterranean trade: excavation has produced Etruscan and Punic amphorae as well as Greek, and a figure of the Egyptian god Bes (Martin 1979). Ullastret flourished from the sixth century into the third BC, when it declined. It had no immediately obvious successor close by, but its role as the dominant centre of its region seems to have been taken over by the Iberian town of Indika which lay immediately alongside the Greek Neapolis at Ampurias, some 20kms. from Ullastret. In this respect Ullastret was similar to Ensérune, which seems to have been succeeded by Narbonne, again some 20kms. away, but differed from Entremont, which was moved under direct Roman influence from its hilltop to the nearby lowland site that became Aix-en-Provence. These sites formed only parts of the intense development of the region in the later part of the first millennium BC. Its importance has been recognized by Février: "the density and variety of the Roman cities, like their surroundings, did not derive from an act of colonisation, or were not simply the result of socio-economic changes themselves created by political changes; they grew out of a past which is shown to be more and more complex as research advances." (1973, p.15). Yet it is clear that the native tribes of southern Gaul were influenced by the Greek trading centre of Marseille in some way. The exact statuses of such sites as Saint-Blaise and Glanum remain uncertain, but they had at the very least strong Hellenic leanings in their architecture and their trade.

Ward-Perkins (1970) has pointed out that there was little sign of direct Roman influence in town-planning and architecture in the west until the mid-first century BC. Despite the growth of Roman political and economic power, the settlements, particularly in southern Gaul, retained their traditional aspects, whether native or Hellenized in style. In the mid-first century there came a sharp revolution in fashion, partly sparked off by the founding of veteran colonies in southern Gaul, which gave the opportunity for the latest Roman or Italian ideas to be put into practice, even where there had been an existing settlement before the colony. The basis for continuity and stability was transformed under the new régime of the Empire.

What happened in the north western provinces was very similar. Whatever the functions of the pre-Roman oppida had been, few sites survived unchanged into the Roman period. A colony was established at the most important oppidum in Britain, Camulodunum. At Silchester, the Roman town was planned with a grid-system on the existing site. At Verulamium the planned Roman city was laid out next to the pre-Roman nucleus of settlement (Wacher 1975). The Roman army has often been cited as a crucial influence on the origins of Romano-British towns (Rivet 1977) and also possibly for the towns of northern Gaul (Wightman 1977a). The classic illustration of the army's role is the case of Cirencester. The army's fort was sited not at the pre-Roman centre of Bagendon, but some 6kms. away on the main Roman road, the Fosse Way. Towards the end of the first century AD, when the fort had been given up and the area turned over to civilian rule, the tribal capital became the former fort site at Cirencester, rather than Bagendon (cf. Reece

1976) (Fig. 2). The new site had enjoyed for a generation the political and economic attractions offered by the army to the local population, and it retained an advantageous position in the road system. By the time of the decision to lay out a Roman style town in the late first century, the tribal leaders who made the decision concluded that it was the Cirencester site which fulfilled their new requirements better than the traditional centre of Bagendon. Even though Cirencester must have taken over the 'central place' functions of Bagendon, the move demonstrated a real change in the local population's expectations of what an urban centre should be like. In this process the army had been a catalyst, but had not been the main force at work. Similar shifts of site are known from Gaul and Spain. In Spain some towns moved from hilltop sites, such as Zaragoza, Mérida and Ilici; in other places the centres of the towns moved from hilltops into what had been lower-lying suburbs, as at Italica and Cadiz. Some towns even continued on their hilltops: Cástulo, Carmona, Uxama, Termes and Conimbriga (cf. Balil 1973, p.253ff.). Despite the earlier progress towards urbanization, it was the recognition of the new conditions of the Empire that crucially determined the formation of new Romanized towns. The new lay-outs demonstrated the acceptance of the idea of the Roman town. Whether the new towns' relationships with their hinterlands differed significantly from those of their predecessors is a separate issue.

Although they made up only a minority of towns, the foundation of the coloniae for legionary veterans was important for all the western provinces up to the beginning of the second century. In some areas they provided models of what Roman towns should be; almost always they acted as stimuli for innovation among their neighbours. Yet archaeologically, if new sites were chosen for both, the colonia and the locally-inspired city would be difficult to distinguish. The great surge of new foundations of both types of city in the early Empire meant that many places were characterized by a grid-plan lay-out (cf. Frere 1979). The significance of town-planning can be overstressed, since at its simplest it need have been no more than a convenient way of organizing a new settlement. However, ancient planners were interested in more than laying out the street grids. They were making conscious schemes for what they thought should be in a town: where the administrative buildings should be, where the theatre, baths and other public monuments were best placed, and where private housing should be. These were partly routine administrative decisions, but they were also the effective expression of the common idea of what a town should comprise. In that respect they are more significant than the frequently quoted remarks of the Greek travel writer Pausanias in the second century AD, about the aspirations of a small town in Greece for recognition as a city: "no government buildings, no theatre, no agora, no water conducted to a fountain, and ... the people live in hovels like mountain cabins on the edge of a ravine" (10.4.1).

Its monumental public buildings were among the most striking characteristics of the Roman town. They included theatres, amphitheatres, temples, markets and baths, but the most important was the forum and basilica. This expressed the political style of the town. Here took place the essential processes of Romanized political life: law courts, council meetings and religious dedications. In addition the forum was the commercial centre of the town for larger scale transactions, but also in some cases the site for an open market with stalls selling household goods. All of these activities could have been carried on in other buildings, had there been no forum-basilica. But it was more convenient to have them all together, and it expressed the civic identity of the community in a tangible way and in a Roman way. It was this that was most

significant. There was no formal pressure from the Roman government on the provincial cities to construct such buildings. As long as taxes were raised and order kept, the government would have been satisfied. It was not Imperial edict which spread the particular architectural form of the forum and basilica throughout the newly conquered western provinces, so that, whatever variations in detail there were, the forum in Silchester or Cirencester in Britain was demonstrably the same sort of thing as the one at Conimbriga in Portugal, or the one at Augst in Switzerland. Despite their conformity, they were erected by local initiative and at local expense, expressing local ideas. Presumably the initiatives, the expenses and the ideas were all those of the local ruling elite (Fig. 3)

The details of the plans of fora are surprisingly rarely known. It seems to have been normal that once it was built it remained a feature of the town for most of the Roman period. This generalization may be modified by excavation. In London and in Conimbriga, early forum-style buildings were demolished to make way for much grander structures in the later first century AD (Philp 1977; Alarcão and Etienne 1977). At Conimbriga this involved wholesale remodelling of the urban centre, with a similar extension in scale and grandeur being made to the baths shortly after. The rebuilding of the forum has been dated to the Flavian period; the excavators have interpreted it as a response to the grant of high status to the towns of Spain by the Emperor Vespasian. The two developments may have been coincidental, but it does seem more likely that the ruling elite of Conimbriga felt that their newly elevated status as a municipium required rather more impressive public monuments. As such, the rebuilding was a very clear expression of their feelings of civic pride. Sited in the forum was the main temple of the city, dedicated to the Imperial cult. At Conimbriga, like many towns, the forum housed the presence of the Imperial power as well as the local power, both reinforced by religion. Here was reflected a difference between the two fora at Conimbriga other than mere scale. Alarcão and Etienne have described how the earlier, Augustan forum was closely integrated with the existing developments. It was open to movement from the streets and houses around it. The Flavian construction changed the idea of an open forum where the routes in the town converged, into that of a closed space. There was only one monumental entrance to the Flavian forum. The complex was much more dominated by the temple of the Imperial cult: it had become "un forum impérial" (Alarcão and Etienne 1977, p.265).

It should be noted that the new buildings at both Conimbriga and London were erected still in the earlier stages of urbanization in the west as a whole. By the last quarter of the first century many towns were only just completing their first civic building programme. It was inevitable that the forms in fashion at that time should have become fixed. The same kind of phenomenon was seen in the industrial towns of northern England in the nineteenth century (cf. Cunningham 1981). The town halls of that period lasted with little substantial change for a century or more, until the relatively recent expansion of civic building which has happened in connection with an expansion of the functions of local government. Just as the town halls of the nineteenth century expressed one particular type of organization, now superseded so that the modern civic offices are difficult to distinguish from any other office block, the Roman forum-basilica represented the typical style of the early Imperial period. It is becoming clear that at some places in Britain at least the forum became outdated in its original concept, so that it became used for a range of activities that would have been inconceivable in earlier times. At Silchester in the third century the forum piazza was being used for metal-working hearths (Fulford 1982). The forum-basilica at

Wroxeter was not rebuilt after destruction in the third century (Atkinson 1942). These examples show real changes in attitudes to public buildings, and thereby to the political functioning of the community.

Of the other types of public building, theatres and amphitheatres have survived most dramatically and revealingly. Their size is most striking: the amphitheatre at Mérida has been estimated to have held 18,000 people seated, plus 6,000 more standing; that at Italica 25,000 to 27,000 people; that at Tarragona 15,000 (Balil 1973, p.263). Like the fora, these were outstanding monuments of civic display, in which the western provinces were in no way left behind by their eastern neighbours, at least in questions of scale. Many of the largest amphitheatres in the Empire were in Gaul, including northern Gaul (cf. Deman 1975,p.8). The west enjoyed the opportunities presented by the rapid expansion of towns to use all the latest ideas in building. Although many of the grandest surviving monuments still await modern publication, in many ways it is the simple existence of the monuments that matters most. These theatres and amphitheatres were places of mass entertainment. Even if they had to be built by the rich and powerful, to continue to prosper they needed wide popular approval. Even if the performances were put on at the expense of the rich and powerful, to achieve its purpose such munificence had to appeal to the population on a large scale. The size of the amphitheatres at Mérida or Italica was not so important as is shown by the theatre at Canterbury. The initial size of a theatre could have proved too ambitious, but at Canterbury there is clear evidence that the theatre was redeveloped on a larger scale (Frere 1970). The evident popularity of theatres and amphitheatres illustrates the acceptance of Roman manners in the urban population's tastes in entertainment, whether in the theatre or the coarser pleasures of the amphitheatre.

The same kind of process happened with public bath buildings. They were clearly used regularly and normally by the urban populations. It is difficult to understand otherwise not only the massive baths of the major cities of the Empire like Trier, but also the extended baths at Conimbriga, or those in Britain (Wightman 1970, p.82ff.; Alarcão and Etienne 1977; Wacher 1975, 48ff.) The habit of bathing seems to have had as strong a hold on the urban populace as had the amphitheatre. It required the essential urban amenity of a public water supply. The aqueducts and water systems of the Roman towns were hailed by Frontinus as an achievement greater than the pyramids or the masterpieces of Greek art (The Water Supply of Rome, I, vi). To the modest town dweller this was undoubtedly the case. The water supply system did not have to be as grand as to need great structures like the Pont du Gard, or the aqueducts for Mérida, Tarragona or Segovia, but adequate water supply and efficient drains were essential to the functioning of the town, and were one of the prime duties of the municipal administration. It is a mark of the workmanlike efficiency of the Roman system that these services were provided so widely. The system that did it was not the Imperial government but the local community. Urban life required that these local socio-political systems should continue to work, simply to maintain the basic services such as water and streets. They were central to the development and survival of Roman urbanism. It had to have substantial local organization, performing functions to the benefit of the community as a whole rather than the profit of individuals. This concept of community may have been little more than enlightened self-interest for an urbanized society, but it was necessary. It had to be expressed by the decisions of the local rulers, the rich and powerful. It was crucial to the success of Roman urbanism that under the system of the early Empire at least, competition by members of the elite and display of wealth by them was channeled into projects that benefited the community as a whole, such as town planning and public buildings.

Private houses and shops represent a different aspect of the town. It is astonishing to discover how few private houses have been excavated to modern standards. Only rarely are we aware of the buildings which housed the earliest inhabitants of a Roman town. In Britain, discoveries in the coloniae at Colchester and Gloucester have shown how the first colonists in both places retained essentially the same kind of buildings as the barracks of the preceding legionary fortresses (Crummy 1977; Hurst 1972). The precise details await full publication, but the impression is clear. The first stage of the coloniae did not involve wholesale replanning of their sites and the accommodation at first was modest. At Gloucester it was about half a century before the early buildings were replaced by a substantial town house. Unfortunately we cannot be confident about the processes behind this change. The mid-second century house was built over an earlier street, as well as two of the barrack-like buildings. Was the new house made possible by wealth acquired by one family, enabling it to buy out the people living where they wanted to build? Or were they able to build on land of relatively low value because the original allotment holders had died or had moved from the town? Without more information on what was happening elsewhere in the town we cannot understand the meaning of these changes, but they were real changes. Starting from relatively even allotments and generally modest housing, within two generations it was possible to build a much more impressive house in the Roman tradition of fine houses. The new layout did not necessarily mean that fewer people lived in the area, but it did mean a change in their social organization, as the later house presumably accommodated not just its owners, but also their servants and slaves. Verulamium too has produced evidence of its earliest Roman buildings. In Insula XIV, fronting on the main street of the town, Frere excavated a sequence of timber-built shops and workshops of the first and second centuries (Frere 1972). Later the area was apparently left open for about a century, after which, in the third century, some more shops were built, in stone. This part of the city remained much the same in function throughout its Roman life.

Recent work in Gaul has yielded important new information on the development of private houses. At Alésia in central Gaul, the early properties consisted of large courtyards with relatively small house areas. About the mid-second century the house area was greatly extended at the expense of the courtyard, with the standard of comfort improved as well (Benard 1976). Further south, at Fréjus excavations have shown houses considerably extended and elaborated around the end of the first century and the beginning of the second (Février et al. 1972). At Vaison-la-Romaine, Goudineau (1979) has shown how one large house grew from a relatively simple, but substantial, peristyle house into a much larger complex, more similar to an Italian town house, with the street frontage used for shops (Fig. 4). It is evidence for the infilling of space in the city, alongside the increasing elaboration of the homes of the rich. What all these examples show is that the pattern of housing was continually changing. It is likely that such changes were closely linked with social developments, but the evidence so far available does not provide us even with a reasonable sample of any one town's changes through its Roman life.

Some idea of the scales of rich and poor comes from the houses of Conimbriga in Portugal. The houses of the pre-Roman town survived in use alongside the Augustan forum. They were swept away and the street system changed with the Flavian redevelopment of the forum. The insulae between the forum and the baths were densely occupied, but the properties were modest. The plans of the buildings reveal a labyrinth of properties, the biggest with nine rooms, some with only one. Over time some rooms were taken over from one property to another. Yet throughout these buildings remained essentially an artisan quarter. They contrast sharply with the houses on a grand scale in the eastern part of Conimbriga. These were the elaborate mansions of the rich. The largest of them, the 'House of Cantaber', occupied almost as great an area as the Flavian forum. Four such mansions have been discovered. Whatever may one day be found in the rest of Conimbriga, it is clear that these were not the normal town houses for the mass of the population. The insulae were their homes. It is notable that there is little sign of any type of house between the two extremes - the mansion or a couple of rooms crammed into an insula. The only other choice offered a group of more rooms, but still in the insula (cf. Alarcão and Etienne 1977) (Fig. 5)

These housing distinctions seem to have been normal in the western Roman town, reflecting social distinctions, (cf. Balil 1972a; 1972b; 1974). Even if the pressure of space was less in the north west, the general pattern was the same. The more humble dwellings provided very simple accommodation, usually closely associated with a place of work, and sharply contrasted with a handful of large rich houses. Nevertheless the identification of a real urban poor presents some problems. Despite MacMullen's jibe that "no-one has sought fame through the excavation of a slum" (1974, p.93), humble houses have been investigated. Yet the distinction between the homes of the 'respectable poor', perhaps to be defined as an artisan class, and true slums has proved difficult for archaeology. Part of the problem lies in finding out exactly what was going on inside a house at any one time, so that we cannot tell for example how many people were living there. But it may also have been that the imagined slum-dwellers, perhaps those who could hope at best for casual labouring work, or beggars or cripples, were only a small part of the urban population. Anyway the poor and the homeless could hardly be expected to have left much archaeological trace. What town housing confirms is that there were very distant extremes of wealth and poverty. Most of the townspeople lived in quite restricted spaces, with few amenities, but apparently significantly above the level of destitution. A few families in each town lived in well-appointed town houses, often decorated with mosaics and provided with private bath-suites. These families were the 'big fish' in the relatively small pond of the local provincial town. Even though they were far removed from the poor of their town in wealth and power, they themselves were equally far from the levels of wealth and power enjoyed by the men who were 'big fish' in the Empire as a whole. Such people may elude us in the archaeology of any particular town, since they had estates scattered in many areas and in the territories of many cities. It was therefore perfectly possible that one of the largest landowners in the territory of a city might not have had a personal house there, even if his tenants did have. He might have trodden almost as lightly on the archaeological record of the city as the beggar at the other extreme of society.

How far can our understanding of the buildings of the cities help in deciding the role of the Classical city? The ideal type of the 'consumer-city' as defined most recently by Finley (1977) has much to commend it. There is little evidence for urban industry on the medieval pattern. Finley was right to point out the absence from the Greco-Roman city of the medieval Guild Halls of north west Europe. Yet, as discussed already, the Greco-Roman city had more than its share of public monuments. Its amenities were considerably more advanced than those of most medieval towns, in terms of public hygiene and water supply, streets and places of entertainment. It

therefore seems paradoxical to argue that the ancient city was less economically developed than the medieval. At the very least, the prosperity of the Greco-Roman town was used in different ways from that of the medieval, so that those amenities could be provided. Finley has pinpointed as the key question on the consumer-city model "whether and how far the economy and the power relations within the town rested on wealth generated by rents and taxes flowing to, and circulating among, town dwellers" (1977, p.326). It is therefore neither aggregate wealth nor the level of civic amenity that is of central importance. It is where the wealth of the cities was derived from. Despite the views of such writers as Rostovtzeff (1957), there is not sufficient archaeological evidence for industrial production in towns to overturn the model of the consumer city, nor to support the idea that the ancient city was simply smaller than the modern city, with fewer people, less commerce and less manufacture. However, we must realise the difficulty of defining an industry in archaeological terms, from excavated remains. Extensive commerce in textiles or foodstuffs is always hard to find (cf. Wild 1978). We know little of what was going on in the shops and workshops of Conimbriga or Verulamium, unless we find remains such as slags pointing to glass or metal working. These limitations should impose some caution on our acceptance of the consumer-city model. Something was thriving at Conimbriga. There was an active commercial class in the town. They were presumably catering for markets provided by the townspeople themselves as well as for the country dwellers. The very existence of the town population inevitably required servicing and so provided occupations for people in the towns. The question of scale is important here. A settlement of 500 people must have been fundamentally different from one of 5,000. Estimates of the size of Roman towns have varied from a few hundred to many thousands (cf. M.E. Jones 1979; Duncan-Jones 1974, p.259ff). If no exact figures are possible, there is a degree of agreement among modern writers that a modest provincial town might have had a population of between 2,000 and 5,000 people, while the bigger centres might have had in the order of 20,000 or 30,000. As Peter Brown has pointed out, the ancient town was nearly always small (Brown 1978, p.3). The level of opportunity for servicing the urban population was obviously greater with a total of 25,000; also the amount of industry was likely to have been greater in total and in proportion. Yet large size in itself was no obstacle to the consumer city: Rome itself was by far the biggest of ancient cities and was also a prime example of a consumer city, living off rents and taxes rather than its own production. However much industrial production there may have been, the land cannot be denied its predominant position as the source of wealth in the Greco-Roman world. There is little to show that the division of labour in the Roman west produced "the separation of industrial and commercial from agricultural labour, and hence to the separation of town and country and a clash of interests between them" (Marx and Engels 1938, p.8). The political and economic unity of town and country in the Classical system meant that the ruling elite of the town were also the rulers of the countryside. There were therefore real restrictions on the growth of a distinct urban commercial interest in any strength. Merchants and traders found it difficult to rival the wealth and power of the landowners, and anyway they were likely to invest what wealth they accumulated themselves in land (cf. Hopkins 1978a, p.74).

The impact of Rome on rural settlement

It is now becoming evident that in the Roman west, rural settlement underwent radical change from the Iron Age pattern. Archaeological work in many different areas is now showing astonishingly dense settlement in the Roman period. In southern Spain surface survey by French arch-aeologists under Michel Ponsich has revealed many substantial Roman farms (Ponsich 1974; 1979). The contrast in the distribution maps for the Roman and pre-Roman periods is remarkable around Lora del Rio and Carmona (Fig. 6) (Ponsich 1974, Figs. 41, 42, 85, 86, 88). As with all such surface survey, there is likely to be a bias in this work towards Classical period sites, because of the good survival qualities of the pottery and building materials. Nevertheless the order of magnitude of the increase in the number of sites of the Classical period in the Guadalquivir valley surely points to a genuine and substantial intensification of settlement there. In Catalunya in north east Spain, a recent study based on existing records rather than new field survey has suggested that the initial Roman political control of the area in the second century BC saw little change in the settlement pattern, but that from the mid-first century BC the Romanization of the countryside became rapid with the growth of developed villas and more intensive settlement (Nolla and Nieto 1976).

It may be argued that in both these areas intensive and prosperous rural settlement was only to be expected. The Guadalquivir valley was already thoroughly penetrated by Punic influence, it benefited from the nearby mines, and has long been known to have been very fertile, producing wine, oil and cereals. Ponsich has shown the scale of this production, which reached the level of production for an Empire-wide market. Catalunya had early contacts with the Greeks and was rich agriculturally. Both areas were firmly in the Mediterranean zone, in what can be seen as the original Greco-Roman world. However, sceptics about the size of Roman agricultural production now have to reckon with evidence from northern and central Gaul and Britain. The most remarkable comes from the aerial photography of the Somme valley by Roger Agache (1978). Conditions there have allowed him to reveal a pattern of closely packed villa settlement. If the map of the whole area is astonishing enough (Fig. 7) (Agache 1978, Fig. 42), closer scrutiny shows that in many places the villas are grouped very close together - at Warfusée-Abancourt there are six villas within less than 2kms. of the modern village (Fig. 8) (Agache 1978, Fig. 40). Furthermore these are very large farms. The buildings of Warfusée-sud and of Warfusée-nord each cover some 5ha. (Fig. 9) (Agache 1978, Figs. 15, 24). It is unfortunate that at the moment we have little more knowledge of these villas than their existence and their outline plans. Their relationships with Iron Age sites and their development during the Roman period still await the results of much more extensive excavation (cf. Agache 1978, pp. 366-82). The great profusion of such large villas in this region has been ascribed to the influence of the market for food provided by the army on the Rhine frontier. This argument has less force in view of the picture beginning to emerge from surveys in other parts of Gaul, inspired by the findings of Agache. Leday has presented an early publication on the territory of the Bituriges Cubi, around modern Bourges and the valley of the Cher in central France. His results show "a densely populated countryside and all the land in use" (Leday 1980,p.431). Many of these sites were substantial villas. Similar evidence may now be expected from other parts of central Gaul (cf. Agache 1978,p.466). In Britain aerial photography and such schemes as motorway construction have yielded enormous numbers of new Roman period sites (e.g. Fowler 1979). These recent discoveries, with the promise of more to come, give the lie to the idea of most of Gaul and Britain having been underdeveloped, with much forest uncleared (cf A.H.M. Jones 1966, p. 363).

Much of this great increase in the quantity of rural evidence still remains to be digested and fully understood.

Wightman has pointed out that several large villas in widely distant parts of Gaul seem to have started at about the same time in the mid-first century AD (Wightman 1975, pp.626-8). Two of them at least, Montmaurin in the south-west and Saint-Ulrich in Lorraine, began as elaborate Greco-Roman style buildings with baths. They developed into even larger and more impressive establishments later. The origins of other villas were more modest. However for all villas, there has been a continuing dispute about who actually lived in them. Were they merchants involved in capitalistic agriculture, (cf. Rostovtzeff 1957, p.223) were they veteran soldiers, or were they the continuing tribal aristocracy? (cf. Wightman 1975, 645-6, n.174). It is obviously difficult to be sure of the social origins of the owner from the excavation of a house and farm, but some hints may be taken from the evidence of gradual evolution from an Iron Age house into a Roman one. In Germany the type-site is still Mayen, where the commonly recognized villa form grew up in clear stages (Oelmann 1928). Extensive excavation on villa sites in Britain has now shown very frequent cases of Iron Age farm buildings underlying the Roman ones (e.g. at Gorhambury: Neal 1978). What they suggest, even if they cannot prove it, is that the Roman farmer was a direct descendant of the Iron Age one. That must now be taken as the normal interpretation of villa proprietorship, unless strong evidence is found to the contrary.

There was a distinct hierarchy in the size and wealth of farm sites, however they may have related to tenurial patterns. The classes of site can be defined in three groups: the large, mansion-style villas, with rich decorations and extensive buildings; the medium-size farms, with a substantial house and some outbuildings; and the small farms or farmsteads, probably with no more than one or two buildings, and often retaining pre-Roman styles. It has been tempting to try to fit such classes of site into known tenurial arrangements. In southern Spain very large estates or latifundia have been suggested, but Ponsich's work has shown very dense distributions of farms. To explain this, Blázquez has argued for small properties, but with a highly organized oil trade controlling their produce (Blázquez 1979). The problems of the relationships between sites are particularly pronounced with the unromanized rural settlements. Although the villa system is crucial to our understanding of the countryside in the Roman period, it has long been recognised in Britain and now increasingly elsewhere that there was also a substantial rural population living away from the Romanised sites (cf. Thomas 1966; M. Jones and Miles 1979; O'Brien 1979; Wightman 1975, p.646ff; Miles 1982). Were these people free labourers on villa estates, some kind of serf or bond-slave, tenants of large estates, or free farmers on their own land? Was their apparent poverty the result of purely economic forces, or were they socially constrained in some way? These questions may be asked, if not yet answered, in frontier zones, where settlement was dense, but where the numbers of sites turning into villas are very few (Higham and Jones 1975; Higham 1980). They may also be asked of parts of southern England where there were intense occupation, but no villas (M. Jones and Miles 1979; Millett 1982). What fieldwork can demonstrate is the way in which different types of settlement related to each other in the landscape, which should lead to a better understanding of other relationships between them.

The more general question of the role of slavery in the western provinces is something of a diversion. It seems clear that slaves obtained from wars of conquest had an important effect on the organization of agriculture in Italy, with consequential changes in society in general (cf. Hopkins 1978b). It was this aspect of a society in late Republican and early Imperial Italy based on slaves obtained from outside that has excited most interest, partly

252

because the changes could have been sudden and disruptive. There can be no doubt that the large villas of the
western provinces were run by a dependent work force. It
is hard to prove the exact nature of that dependence,
much harder still to show that the people involved were
slaves won in war. Most of the largest villas developed at
the earliest in the second and early third centuries,
significantly later than the main wars of conquest. There
are sites where 'slave quarters' can be claimed, as at
Liédena in Navarre in northern Spain, but there they are
fourth century in date (Gorges 1979, pp.323-4; cf. also
pp.147-8). The phenomenon illustrated is not so much
slavery, or even dependence, as the growth of large villas,
presumably run by dominant magnates. It seems most
probable that the forms of dependence which they
exploited were derived from existing forms of links in
their local societies, even if they developed them far
beyond their original scale.

Rural settlement and villas in Britain and Gaul have
provided the basis for attempts to identify Celtic social
and legal forms through the archaeology. Smith (1978a)
has noted different forms of villa plan, with different
distributions. Widely spread in Britain, but also in the
Somme valley, Belgium and Germany, are his unit-system
villas, in which he interprets symmetrical arrangements in
the plan as reflections of joint proprietorship. Despite the
shortcomings of many of the excavation plans on which
the theory is based and unsolved questions of chronology
at many sites, Smith has presented a case that awaits
serious challenge. At present we must accept that many
villas display a most curious duality in their planning,
which is difficult to explain more satisfactorily than by
Smith's ideas. He has further argued for a different kind
of social structure embodied in the hall-type villa,
common in Germany and parts of Britain (cf. Smith
1978b). Smith sees the system of joint proprietorship
eroded in the later Roman period, with wealth and ownership becoming more concentrated in individual hands, as
later changes in the villa plan saw the integration of what
had been separate units into one. These ideas are closely
related to those of C.E. Stevens, who proposed that land
tenure patterns in Roman Britain were similar to forms
known from tenth-century Welsh law codes (Stevens
1966). More recently links have been suggested between
Roman villa estates and early medieval tenurial patterns
in south east Wales (Davies 1979). The foundation of such
discussions lies in the idea that the Roman villa system
remained firmly embedded in the preceding Celtic social
structure, and that in some areas at least there was a
direct evolution into post-Roman forms. Much has been
made of the possible survival of Roman estate-names into
medieval and modern place-names in Gaul (cf. Percival
1976, p.118ff; Wightman 1975, p.642ff.). They may well
help to define something of the structure of tenurial
relationships, but they are of limited use. Smaller villas
existed within the orbit of large villas, whether or not
they formed part of the large estate. We cannot normally
tell who lived in the main house of a Roman villa; he
could have been a freeholder or a tenant, or some other
kind of dependant specified in Celtic law. If such legal
questions about the occupant of the main house of a villa
are not within the archaeologist's grasp, it is clear that
that occupant was as sharply distinguished by his style of
house from his farm workers as the rich man was from the
poor in the towns. The labourers and their families lived
in the working buildings, with the animals and the equipment. In the case of the larger villas of the Somme, there
may well have been a sizeable population living in these
farm buildings. It has been tempting to see the origins of
the local medieval villages there too (Agache 1978).

Town and country

The revelation of the high development of the Roman

countryside in the west has altered our focus on the
Roman period. Leday has argued that Gallo-Roman
civilization was not characteristically urban and that the
process of Romanization should be sought primarily in the
countryside rather than in the towns (Leday 1980, p.431).
This seems compatible with the agrarian nature of the
Roman economy, but somewhat out of keeping with the
prominence given to cities in both ancient and modern
writers. The difficulty can partly be resolved in Finley's
description of the city as "the pivotal institution in the
Greco-Roman world" (Finley 1977, p.325). The city was
not the driving force of the ancient socio-economic
system; it was the pivot on which the system moved. It
provided the administrative focus for the services embodied in the pax Romana - the collection of taxes, but
also law and religion, ceremonial and entertainment.
Economically, even if the towns were not involved in
major manufacture, they were the centres of trade.
Necessities and luxuries could be bought there by the
countryman (cf. Hopkins 1978a, p.75). Without the towns
the provision of these services would have been less
convenient, and impossible in some cases. Most important, the town ultimately provided the farmer with the
market to which he could sell his surplus, in order to buy
goods and pay taxes. Without that non-food producing
population conveniently to hand, the economic growth
that the density of rural settlement demonstrates would
have been much less likely. Roman agriculture has been
criticised for not generating spectacular breakthroughs in
crops, animal husbandry or farming technique. Yet what
mattered most was the application of techniques already
known, as a result of the stimulus of demand for surplus
production. It has been shown in central Africa recently
that subsistence cultivators could be expected to produce
a 'normal surplus', to ensure enough food even in difficult
seasons. There a change in the external marketing
conditions, without any corresponding change in agricultural technology, produced a massive and rapid increase in
surplus production (Allan 1965, p.38ff.). Recent work on
Iron Age agriculture now suggests that productivity often
was above the subsistence level (e.g. Reynolds 1979).
However, there can be little doubt that the Roman régime
brought a sudden expansion in the opportunities for the
disposal of farming surplus production, if in the first place
only to feed the Roman army. This model of an
expanding agriculture, with farmers participating to a
greater or lesser extent in a market economy, seems to
fit well the early Roman period in many parts of the west.
It is probable that such a limited scale market economy
developed alongside surviving earlier forms of economic
organization that may have been more socially controlled.
This is not to revive the idea of full-scale capitalistic
production on villa estates, geared entirely to producing
for the market rather than for consumption (cf.
Rostovtzeff 1957, p.223ff.). It seems most probable that
estate owners normally aimed to satisfy most of their
requirements from the estates themselves. However their
houses alone bear witness to the production and use of
surplus. The mosaics and bath-suites, found in even quite
small villas, are only the conspicuous part for us of what
must have been much greater consumption. The wealth
behind that must have come from the disposal of surplus.
That was also necessary for the investment in the farms
represented by the outbuildings. These were presumably
erected to shelter animals and equipment as well as
labourers, all of them together standing for resources
created through surplus production. That surplus production required the existence of the local town, at least in
the early Empire.

Religion, burial and personal life

It need not cause too much surprise that the provincials
became actively involved in the Roman socio-economic
system, since it offered an improved material culture in

many respects. Yet that does not necessarily tell us much about the process of Romanization at an individual level. If a provincial dressed in a Roman way and had a Roman-style house, did that mean a change in his personal attitudes? Some changes at this personal level resulted from changes in housing. The introduction of generally more durable materials for houses meant that there was more permanence about a building, over several generations. That applied to the wider urban or rural landscape as well. Such attitudes can hardly be quantified, but should not be ignored.

Changes in religion are a little easier to grasp. The introduction of official religions, especially the Imperial cult, has been mentioned already. The political importance of adherence to such cults was very great, as was demonstrated by the results of the Christians' refusal to participate. Yet the nature of Classical polytheism left ample room for other religions too. Local religions thrived in the Celtic provinces. The buildings in the centre of Verulamium show the co-existence of 'official' and Celtic religions (Fig. 10). In the forum the city's official cult had its temple. Only a block away was a temple in Romano-Celtic form, with a precinct of similar size to the forum piazza. At Trier and Silchester there were groups of Romano-Celtic temples in the towns (Wightman 1970; Boon 1974). These buildings were substantial structures, as is shown by the surviving structures at Autun and Périgueux. They could be associated with Roman theatres, as at Verulamium, Colchester or Ribemont-sur-Ancre in the Somme, which was a massive cult centre in the countryside (Wacher 1975; Agache 1978). Many inscriptions record the identification of a local deity with one of the Greco-Roman pantheon - Sulis Minerva, Mars Cocidius. The temples show a similar grafting of the Roman monumental style on to the Celtic shrine. Recent excavations at Romano-Celtic temple sites in Britain, at Hayling Island, Uley and Springhead, have discovered evidence of pre-Roman cult sites (Downey, King & Soffe 1980; Ellison 1980; Harker 1980). They suggest a direct continuity of sacred site and of the actual shrine. Whether there was a similar direct continuity in ritual is more difficult to say. The historians record a degree of tidying-up of practices regarded as barbaric by the Roman government. Yet, according to the excavations, the cults retained their popularity, and presumably therefore, their essential elements. Clandestine rituals may well escape the archaeologist, as they may have escaped Roman officialdom, but such possibilities seem to be outweighed by the positive evidence for the flourishing of Romano-Celtic religion. The new régime succeeded in assimilating the various local religions into acceptable forms, while maintaining their essential identities and their prominence.

The spread of the so-called Oriental mystery religions demonstrates the intellectual and religious integration of the Empire. Cults such as those of Mithras, Isis, Serapis and Cybele were often restricted in their attraction to the wealthiest classes and especially to their more cosmopolitan members. Their appeal in the western provinces was not to the mass of the population, but was nevertheless very widespread. Temples for these cults were frequently dedicated in the major cities and along the frontiers (cf. Vermaseren 1963). They are evidence for the creation of an elite to be found throughout the Empire which effectively controlled the Empire and shared a common culture. Religion was used as an instrument of Romanization. Local cults transformed, and those with an Empire-wide following, both moved people in the same direction of integration. These processes prepared the way for Christianity, which eventually gave them their fullest expression. At first Christianity spread through channels similar to those of other religions from the East; at the very first through Jewish communities and then beyond. It is hard to assess the degree of adherence to Christianity in the west before the conversion of Constantine. The archaeological evidence is patchy -moveable objects, Christian scenes in mosaics or sculpture, occasionally buildings. It is a matter of individual judgement whether the catalogue of Christian evidence constitutes a lot or a little (cf. Thomas 1981). As its following grew, Christianity had two main effects on society. Part of its appeal was that it welcomed everybody as believers, rich and poor, men and women, as well as offering spiritual comfort and hopes of eternal life. This reinforced feelings of a single community. Its institutional importance was something of a contrast. After the Roman state took over Christianity under Constantine the Great, the men who became bishops and provided the religion with its organization were the same group who had controlled pagan religions and who still held secular power (cf. A.H.M. Jones 1964). Despite the popular appeal of Christianity in its doctrines, its success as an official religion defused any real impact it might have had on the social structure. If anything it reinforced the powers of the powerful.

The study of Roman burial presents different opportunities. There is a set of data increasing rapidly in size and improving in quality. The potential for palaeopathological and demographic work is enormous, even if not fully realised. However most cemetery excavations almost certainly miss the extremes of Roman society. The richest often had elaborate above-ground tombs which have not survived; the burials of the poorest may have left little trace. Most work done therefore concerns a middle group of society and usually of urban society. The single most striking trend in Roman burial practice is its homogeneity across the western provinces. According to Roman tradition, cemeteries were always outside the city limits. In the early Empire, whatever the previous local customs had been, most people were cremated, their ashes collected and placed in a container in the ground, often with grave goods associated. Between the mid-second and mid-third centuries, more or less throughout the western Empire, the practice changed to inhumation, most commonly without grave goods. The process can be seen at most cities in the western provinces, such as Winchester (Clarke 1979) or Ampurias (Almagro 1955). The pattern of course has variations. There were always some inhumations in the early Empire and some cremations in the fourth century (cf. Clarke 1979, p.350ff.; van Doorselaer 1967,pp.50-2 fig.6). These were exceptions to a general rule. The change from cremation to inhumation seems not to have been the result of specific religious development such as the rise of Christianity. It spread through the west from Italy, essentially as a change in fashion. Whatever feelings caused people to adopt a different burial rite from their parents, the results of those feelings were the same throughout the western provinces, whether or not the feelings were the same. Also they applied throughout the population, urban and rural. The phenomenon suggests a bond of common culture much wider in society than just a privileged elite (cf. Nock 1932; R.F.J. Jones 1981).

Within these broad similarities of practice, there were many variations in detail. It is remarkable how rarely the rich mausolea of the rich are found related to mass urban cemeteries. At Carmona in southern Spain, many such tombs are known within a large cemetery, but only small parts have been adequately published (Bendala 1976). More commonly, small tomb monuments have been found, as at Ampurias (Almagro 1955). Even inscribed tombstones have only rarely been excavated in situ, despite their frequency as casual finds. Amongst one group excavated at Lattes in southern France, none of the tombstones mentioned a magistrate of the town, suggesting that the members of the ruling elite were buried

254

elsewhere (Demougeot 1972). I have discussed elsewhere some of the difficulties of working with the variations actually found in excavation, chiefly in grave type and grave goods (R.F.J. Jones 1977; 1980). Too often we lack such basic detail as the date of the burial, the age and sex of the deceased, or even the position of the grave in the cemetery. These are the most elementary variables which need examining first in relation to any pattern found in grave goods or grave forms. Practice has been shown to have changed over time in the cemetery at Blicquy in Belgium; over a period of about a century, the later graves tended to have more grave goods and the main burial area moved (de Laet et al. 1972; R.F.J. Jones 1980). At Ampurias some parts of the town's cemeteries were characterized by rich graves, others by poor (R.F.J. Jones 1984). The very distinctive Germanic-style burials at Lankhills, Winchester, suggest an intrusive community living in the fourth century town (Clarke 1979). There is evidence therefore that Roman burial forms offer information on society, if we can extract it. To say that there were some people who favoured more elaborate burials than others in early Imperial Ampurias is in itself saying very little. Even if we accept the assumption that elaborate graves should be equated with wealth in life, we can argue little more from Ampurias alone than that there were some richer and some poorer people there. Some confirmation of some genuine relationship between burial form and living wealth and social position may be taken from the correlations noted by Härke at Neuss in Germany between elaboration of grave form, in particular grave depth, and number of grave goods provided (Härke 1980 and pers. comm.). Investment of effort and material went together. However neither at Ampurias nor at Neuss is there any more than an indication of a spectrum of wealth and social prominence. The nature of the spectrum in terms of the proportions of rich and poor or the manner of definition of any social groupings still eludes us. If the present state of knowledge in these respects is disappointing, the burial evidence does show a remarkable consistency of tradition within burial areas, such as in the single cemetery of Blicquy or the several of Ampurias. In each area the community followed a regular practice, in which change came gradually. These were consistent practices in detail, within the overall similarities shared across the provinces (cf. R.F.J. Jones 1982).

In considering the levels of integration of the people in the western provinces into the Roman cultural system, language deserves a mention. The question of the level of literacy in the Roman period has not been fashionable in recent times. It is not susceptible to rigorous testing, but archaeology does point to proficiency in written Latin in surprising places. The number of graffiti on pots is enormous in all provinces, but even more significant is the writing done on tiles before they were fired. From Britain from towns such as London, Leicester and Silchester come examples of sometimes quite complex sentences doodled on tiles, presumably while the tiles were laid out to dry before firing (Frere 1974, pp.351, 374 n.8). It is hard to avoid the conclusion that there were labourers in tile yards who could write good Latin. The sheer quantity of occasional inscriptions shows that the Roman provincials were literate to a surprising degree. Also, literacy was not confined to the elite, but reached to lower levels of society on a larger scale than was the case again in Europe until early modern times (cf. Laslett 1971, pp.205-9).

The army: force, social mobility and structural differentiation

The army was the instrument of force in the Roman Empire. The security of the frontiers was essential to the peaceful development of the interior, for only through that peace could the economic system flourish. The army's abilities are demonstrated by their great forts and frontier works. These remain impressive, even if they have to be regarded primarily as 'displacement activities' for an army deprived of campaigns of conquest (Mann 1974). Fixed frontiers were the expression of the abandonment of the policies of expansion followed under the Republic and early Empire. I have already touched on the economic effects generally, which put an end to supplies of booty and other new resources. Yet the economic power of the army itself is shown by the growth of settlements alongside army posts on the frontiers. These were not just small villages beside auxiliary forts. Cities such as York or Carnuntum on the Danube owed their prosperity essentially to the army garrisoned there (R.C.H.M. 1962; Vorbeck and Beckel 1973). The army generated demand wherever it was, with striking effects on rural as well as urban settlement (G.D.B. Jones 1979). In new provinces the army's needs stimulated agricultural and industrial production. It also provided a new power structure: it represented the Empire and a new system of power relations on a quite different base from the pre-existing tribal arrangements. When local administration became civilian, the new schemes integrated the Imperial and the native, building on the army's legacy.

The army's position in the Empire was supreme. In the early Empire, it institutionalized force, using it to protect the frontiers and allowing the interior provinces to be disarmed. The army was therefore the key to internal and external peace. Also military service offered the most direct route to social advancement. For the young man in a new province, service in an auxiliary regiment gave him not only pay and high status while he served, but, if he survived, also the continuing status of a Roman citizen at the end, which could be passed on to his descendants. The separation of the army from civilian society opened up a way of escape from the community men were born into. There were other forms of social mobility, especially in the early Empire. Most were involved with the urban and commercial expansion. Greater craft specialization provided new opportunities for people to do something different from their peasant parents. Yet no other course brought so clearly defined rewards as army service.

After the first period of rapid expansion the opportunities for mobility became less again. Even the army was getting most of its recruits from the sons of soldiers or veterans, often living in the communities grown up outside the army posts. Nevertheless, at least until the middle of the third century, the army remained explicitly an Empire-wide system, with command structures clearly established and leading ultimately to the Emperor. The commands of auxiliary units and posts in the legions were specific stages in the careers of provincial aristocrats in the Imperial service (cf. Webster 1969). These were the men who effectively ran the Empire. This system of military command seems to have failed in the mid-third century (cf. Wilkes 1966, p.123). In the forts of northern England the later third century saw a lack of attention to the maintenance of the official buildings, suggesting a weakening in the traditional military discipline (R.F.J. Jones 1981b). The loyalties of the soldiers were in practice becoming stronger to their locality than to the Imperial system. Such a process was recognized in the military reforms of Diocletian and Constantine, which gave frontier troops a lower status than the main fighting forces. The result in late Roman northern Britain was a series of settlements which had earlier been clearly identified as forts or small civilian towns becoming practically indistinguishable (cf. Ferris and Jones 1980, pp.247-8; MacMullen 1963). Such places demonstrate the breakdown of the differentiated military system of the early

Empire. Parts of it remained recognizable, parts survived in a debased form, but as a whole the institution had collapsed.

The dynamics of change

All contributors to this volume have found it easy to describe substantial change which occurred during their chosen periods. It has proved more difficult to explain convincingly the dynamics behind such change; I can claim no comprehensive solution, but can offer some ideas. The complexity of the Roman period permits no oversimplified answer. The first characteristic to be identified is the nature of the Roman Empire itself. Roman imperialism was distinguished by the integration of the conquered peoples into a cultural unity. Conquered territories became provinces, not colonies. Power relations within the provincial communities were therefore of great importance, but they were also in constant interaction with the central power of the Empire itself. Within the Roman period there were distinct phases. The earliest was of conquest and acculturation. The two processes did not necessarily happen at the same time. It seems that the impetus to adopt obviously Roman ways did not arise until a century or two after the first conquest of Catalunya and Provence. What began there during the first century BC continued across western Europe to about the end of the first century AD. In little more than a century and a half the pattern of Roman-style towns and villas was laid down. Their buildings demonstrated not only full acceptance of Roman material culture, but also of political ways and of more general culture. Existing local power relationships were transformed through being expressed in Roman constitutional forms. The civic unit became the dominant arena within which power relations were exercised. Municipal life was sustained by the institution whereby local elites competed to provide buildings and facilities for their towns. Alongside political change, the development of new provinces stimulated quick economic growth, offering new opportunities for merchants and artisans, who traded with the new territories and established themselves in the growing towns (cf. Smith 1972). These people became important to the running of the newly commercialized economies, but never important enough to create their own power bases to rival those of the landowners. The general expansion also involved the smaller rural sites, which became more prosperous and increased in numbers. It is hard to escape the conclusion that throughout western Europe there was a substantial rise in population during this surge of Roman expansion and development. How far it was a cause and how far an effect of that expansion is difficult to say. The evidence for a population rise rests crucially on the great increase in the number of rural sites, but at present it is impossible to be sure when that increase began. It is most probable that here cause and effect are inextricably intertwined. The settlement evidence also suggests that by about the mid-second century the population rise had stabilized and that the population had fallen to some extent by the fourth century. Although these are impressions of the evidence rather than firm conclusions, the effects of a rapidly falling population are easy to imagine for the later Empire. Yet the poor state of knowledge of demographic change means that we can do little more than bear it in mind, while looking elsewhere for other forces at work which may have brought about change.

The developed provincial system which emerged in the second century was put under strain almost immediately. The end of new conquests and the development of the new provinces refashioned the patterns of long-distance trade which had supplied that development. Some towns declined in importance, like London, apparently (cf. Reece 1980; 1981); but more common was an overall increase in prosperity. The shift on the frontiers from attack to defence coincided with there being more to defend in the interior. The crucial period of adjustment was the third century. In a collection of papers recently devoted to this period many themes central to understanding the Empire as a whole are examined (King & Henig 1981). While old ideas of widespread destruction from barbarian raids are proving untenable, a new orthodoxy is beginning to emerge which encompasses the decline of towns to a pre-Roman scale and the growth of large villas which were functionally direct antecedents of medieval manors. Although there is much to commend this view, some of the evidence has been seriously overstated, in particular in relation to towns. Some towns clearly declined in importance and in size, but others such as Barcelona, Lincoln or York retained or enhanced their positions. As Blagg (1981) has pointed out, Gallic town walls of the late Empire were normally carefully built, presumably to protect something worthwhile. However, many town walls in Gaul enclosed very much smaller areas than the extents of the second century towns, (cf. Butler 1959; Roblin 1965; Galinié and Randoin 1979). They may have defended only small parts of the contemporary town, but it seems unlikely. In Gaul and in Spain there is however widespread evidence for very significant changes in the pattern of rural settlement in the course of the third century (Galliou 1981; Wightman 1981; Walker 1981; Buckley 1981; Keay 1981). Although there are important differences in chronology, with the process beginning in the late second century in some places but not until the later third in others, there is a general trend of decline in the numbers of smaller farms and small agricultural settlements, with a complementary flourishing of large villas in the fourth century. The larger landowners prospered at the expense of the smaller units.

These changes in settlement pattern were undoubtedly linked to political change. The course of the third century saw a decline in the importance of the civic institutions, as the rich withdrew their support for the towns and concentrated their wealth more directly in their own hands. The towns were forced to rely more centrally on their own economic bases, with varying success (cf. Février 1977; Wightman 1976). These changes in the towns were part of a weakening of the integrated system of Imperial government. We have already seen how much of the strength of the early Roman town was drawn from the commitment to them in terms of building and other ways that survive less tangibly. By concentrating their energies into their own estates and their prosperity, the powerful local elites opted out of Empire-wide structures like military careers. Local social structures were affected by this, as the rich grew richer in their villas, while almost everybody else grew poorer. The basis of the dominance enjoyed by such magnates seems to have become essentially economic, as municipal and tribal forms of authority withered, even though these same people still controlled offices like the bishoprics and the important magistracies.

The developed Empire of the fourth century was still Roman, despite the prevalence of regionalism and locally based power. The evidence of burial and religion demonstrates the essential cultural unity which existed, especially with the official adoption of Christianity. Haverfield put it neatly: "As the importance of the city of Rome declined, as the world became Romeless, a large part of the world grew to be Roman" (1912, p.11). Even if the functions of settlements came to resemble pre-Roman forms again, there can be no serious suggestion that there was a direct reversion to Iron Age ways of life. The passage of fifteen generations or more rules out any idea that people shrugged off a vain attempt to be Romans and gratefully returned to Iron Age ways (cf. Reece 1979). Too much had happened over too long a period.

Through all this, the pyramid of power can have changed remarkably little. There were always extremes of wealth and poverty. Wealth and power remained closely tied to the land. Although the early Empire saw expansion in commercial activities, the commercial classes failed to achieve real power. The provincial land-owning aristocracy expressed their power in local terms through civic institutions and in Empire terms in careers in the Imperial government. Their gradual withdrawal from both these areas left them freer of institutional controls and with more personal power, derived essentially from wealth. The dynamic of the early Empire owed much to aggression and greed, seeking to exploit more and more new territory. It also involved a more attractive enthusiasm for the benefits of peace and settled life within the Empire. These motives underlay the growth of the municipal system. Yet the rich were concerned with the immediate problems of getting richer, as well as the welfare of the cities. When the pressures of adjusting to the developed Imperial economy from one of conquest came to bear in the provinces, the rich withdrew from what had been their civic responsibilities in favour of their own direct power. The process was gradual, but its results led directly to the Medieval period.

BIBLIOGRAPHY

AGACHE, R. 1978 - La Somme pré-Romaine et Romaine. Amiens.

ALARCÃO, J. and R. ETIENNE 1977 - Fouilles de Conimbriga I: L'Architecture. Paris.

ALLAN, W. 1965 - The African Husbandman. Edinburgh and London.

ALMAGRO, M 1955 - Las Necrópolis de Ampurias II: Necropolis Romanas y Necrópolis Indigenas. Barcelona.

ATKINSON, D. 1942 - Report on Excavations at Wroxeter 1923-1927. Birmingham Archaeol. Soc.; Oxford.

BALIL, A. 1972a - "Arquitectura y sociedad en la España romana", Archivo de Prehistoria Levantina (Valencia) vol. 13, pp.139-47.

BALIL, A 1972b - Casa y Urbanismo en la España Antigua III. Studia Archaeologica 20, Univ. de Valladolid.

BALIL, A. 1973 - "El imperio romano hasta la crisis del siglo III", in V. Vázquez de Prada (Ed.), Historia Economica y Social de España I: La Antiguedad. Madrid, pp.245-328.

BALIL, A. 1974 - Casa y Urbanismo en la España Antigua IV. Studia Archaeologica 28, Univ. de Valladolid.

BELTRAN LLORIS, M. 1978 - Ceramica Romana: Tipología y Clasificación. Zaragoza.

BENARD, J. 1976 - "Un exemple de maison urbaine à Alésia", Revue Archéologique de l'Est et du Centre-Est vol. 27, pp.523-38.

BENDALA GALAN, M. 1976 - La Necrópolis Romana de Carmona (Sevilla). Publ. de la Excma. Diputación Provincial de Sevilla, historia, ser. Ia, XI, 2 vols. Sevilla.

BENOIT, F. 1975 - "The Celtic oppidum of Entremont, Provence", in R. Bruce-Mitford (Ed.) Recent Archaeological Excavations in Europe. London, pp.227-59.

BLAGG, T.F.C. 1981 - "Architectural patronage in the western provinces of the Roman Empire in the third century", in King & Henig 1981, pp.167-88.

BLAZQUEZ MARTINEZ, J.M. 1975 - "Aspectos económicos y demográficos en la colonización fénica", paper delivered to XIV international Congress of Historical Sciences. San Francisco.

BLAZQUEZ MARTINEZ, J.M. 1979 - "Gran latifundia o pequeña propiedad en la Bética (Hispania) en época imperial?", in Miscellanea in Onore di Eugenio Manni, AVAS XAPIV. Rome: Bretschneider, pp.245-55.

BOON, G.C. 1974 - Silchester: the Roman Town of Calleva. Newton Abbott.

BROWN, P. 1971 - The World of Late Antiquity. London.

BROWN, P. 1978 - The Making of Late Antiquity. Harvard.

BUCKLEY, B. 1981 - "The Aeduan area in the third century", in King & Henig 1981, pp.287-315.

BURNHAM, B.C. and H.B. JOHNSON (Eds.) 1979 -Invasion and Response: The Case of Roman Britain Brit. Archaeol. Rpt. 73. Oxford.

BUTLER, R.M. 1959 - "Late Roman town walls in Gaul", Archaol. J. vol. 116, pp.25-50.

CASEY, P.J. (Ed.) 1979 - The End of Roman Britain. Brit. Archaeol. Rpt. 71. Oxford.

CLARKE, G. 1979 - The Roman Cemetery at Lankhills. Winchester Studies 3: Pre-Roman and Roman Winchester, part II; Ed. by Martin Biddle. Oxford.

COLLIS, J.R. 1979 - "City and state in pre-Roman Britain", in Burnham & Johnson 1979, pp.231-40.

CRUMMY, P. 1977 - "Colchester, Fortress and Colonia", Britannia vol. 8, pp.65-106.

CUNLIFFE, B.W. and R.T. ROWLEY (Eds.) 1976 - Oppida in Barbarian Europe. Brit. Archaeol. Rpt. SII. Oxford.

CUNLIFFE, B.W. and R.T. ROWLEY (Eds.) 1978 - Lowland Iron Age Communities in Europe. Brit. Archaeol. Rpt. S48. Oxford.

CUNNINGHAM, C. 1981 - Victorian and Edwardian Town Halls. London.

DAVIES, W. 1979 - "Roman settlements and post-Roman estates in south-east Wales" in Casey 1979, pp.153-73.

DE LAET, S.J., A. VAN DOORSELAER, P. SPITAELS and H. THOEN 1972 - La Nécropole Gallo-Romaine de Blicquy. Dissertationes Archaeologicae Gandenses, 14. Bruges.

DEMAN, A. 1975 - "Matériaux et réflexions pour servir à une étude du développement et du sous-développement dans les provinces de l'empire romain" in H. Temporini (Ed.) Aufstieg und Niedergang der römischen Welt II(3) Berlin and New York, pp.3-97.

DEMOUGEOT, E. 1972 - "Stèles funéraires d'une nécropole de Lattes" Revue Archéologique de Narbonnaise vol. V, pp.49-116.

DOWNEY, R., A. KING. and G. SOFFE. 1980 - "The Hayling Island temple and religious connections across the

Channel", in Rodwell 1980, pp.289ff.

DUNCAN-JONES, R.P. 1974 - The Economy of the Roman Empire: Quantitative Studies. Cambridge.

ELLISON, A. 1980 - "Natives, Romans and Christians on West Hill, Uley", in Rodwell 1980, pp.305ff.

FERRIS, I.M. and R.F.J. JONES 1980 - "Excavations at Binchester 1976-9", in W.S. Hanson and L.J.F. Keppie (Eds.), Roman Frontier Studies 1979, Brit. Archaeol. Rpt. S71, Oxford, pp.233-254.

FEVRIER, P.-A. 1973 - "Cities of southern Gaul", J. Rom. St. vol. 63, pp.1-28.

FEVRIER, P.-A 1977 - "Towns in the western Mediterranean", in M. Barley (Ed.), European Towns, London, pp.315-42.

FEVRIER, P.-A., M. JANON, and Cl. VAROQUEAUX 1972 - "Fouilles au Clos du Chapitre à Fréjus (Var)", Comptes Rendus de l'Académie des Inscriptions et Belles Lettres (1972), pp.355-81.

FINLEY, M.I. 1973 - The Ancient Economy. London.

FINLEY, M.I. (Ed.) 1974 - Studies in Ancient Society. London.

FINLEY, M.I. 1977 - "The Ancient City: from Fustel de Coulanges to Max Weber and beyond", Comp. Studies in Society and History, vol. 19, pp.305-27.

FOWLER, P.J. 1979 - "Archaeology and the M4 and M5 motorways 1965-78", Archaeol. J. vol. 136, pp.12-26.

FRERE, S.S. 1970 - "The Roman theatre at Canterbury", Britannia vol. 1, pp.83-113.

FRERE, S.S. 1972 - Verulamium Excavations I. London.

FRERE, S.S. 1974 - Britannia. 2nd. ed. London.

FRERE, S.S. 1979 - "Town planning in the western provinces", in Festschrift zum 75 jährigen Bestehen Römisch-Germanischen Kommission. Beiheft zum Bericht der Römisch-Germanischen Kommission 58, 1977, Mainz-am-Rhein, pp.87-103.

FULFORD, M. 1982 - "Silchester", Current Archaeol. 82, pp.326-31.

GALINIE, H. and B. RANDOIN 1979 - Les archives du sol à Tours - survie et avenir de l'archéologie de la ville. Tours.

GALLIOU, P. 1981 - "Western Gaul in the third century", in King & Henig 1981, pp.259-86.

GARNSEY, P. 1970 - Social Status and Legal Privilege. Oxford.

GARNSEY, P. 1979 - "Where did Italian peasants live?", Proc. Camb. Philol. Soc. vol. 25, pp.1-25.

GORGES, J.-G. 1979 - Les Villas Hispano-Romaines: Inventaire et problematique archéologiques. Publ. du Centre Pierre Paris 4. Paris.

GOUDINEAU, C. 1979 - Les Fouilles de la Maison du Dauphin: Recherches sur la romanisation de Vaison-la-Romain. Suppl. à Gallia xxxvii. Paris.

HARKE, H. 1980 - "Die Grabung de Jahres 1976 auf dem Münsterplatz in Neuss", Bonner Jahrb. vol. 180, pp.493-587.

HARKER, S. 1980 - "Springhead: a brief reappraisal", in Rodwell 1980, pp.285ff.

HAVERFIELD, F. 1912 - The Romanisation of Britain 2nd ed. Oxford.

HIGHAM, N.J. 1980 - "Native settlements west of the Pennines", in K. Branigan (ed.), Rome and the Brigantes. Sheffield, pp.41-7.

HIGHAM, N.J. and G.D.B. JONES, 1975 - "Frontiers, forts and farmers", Archaeol. J. vol. 132, pp.16-53.

HODDER, I. 1979 - "Pre-Roman and Romano-British tribal economies", in Burnham & Johnson 1979, pp.189-96.

HOPKINS, K. 1978a - "Economic growth and towns in Classical Antiquity", in P. Abrams & E.A. Wrigley (Eds.), Towns in Societies. London, pp.35-77.

HOPKINS, K. 1978b - Conquerors and Slaves. Cambridge.

HOPKINS, K. 1980 - "Taxes and trade in the Roman Empire", J. Rom. St. vol. 70, pp.101-25.

HURST, H. 1972 - "Excavations at Gloucester 1968-71: first interim report", Antiq. J. vol. 52, pp.24-69.

JANNORAY, J. 1955 - Ensérune: Contribution à l'étude des civilisations pré-romaines de la Gaule méridionale. Paris.

JONES, A.H.M. 1964 - The Later Roman Empire 284-602. Oxford.

JONES, A.H.M. 1966 - The Decline of the Ancient World. London.

JONES, A.H.M. 1974 - The Roman Economy. London.

JONES, G.D.B. 1979 - "Invasion and response in Roman Britain", in Burnham and Johnson 1979, pp.57-79.

JONES, M., and D. MILES 1979 - "Celt and Roman in the Thames valley: approaches to culture change", in Burnham and Johnson 1979, pp.315-25.

JONES, M.E. 1979 - "Climate, nutrition and disease", in Casey 1979, pp.231-51.

JONES, R.F.J. 1977 - "A quantitative approach to Roman burial", in R. Reece (Ed.) Burial in the Roman World. CBA Res. Rpt. 22, London, pp.20-25.

JONES, R.F.J. 1980 - "Computers and cemeteries -opportunities and limitations", in P. Rahtz et al. (Eds.), Anglo-Saxon Cemeteries 1979. Brit. Archaeol. Rpt. 82, Oxford, pp.179-95.

JONES, R.F.J. 1981 - "Cremation and inhumation - change in the third century", in King & Henig 1981, pp.15-19.

JONES, R.F.J. 1982 - Cemeteries and burial practices in the western provinces of the Roman Empire to AD 300. Unpubl. Ph.D. thesis, London. University.

JONES, R.F.J. 1984 - "The Roman cemeteries of Ampurias reconsidered", in T.F.C. Blagg, R.F.J. Jones and S.J. Keay (Eds.) Papers in Iberian Archaeology. BAR Internat. Ser. 193, Oxford, pp.237-65.

KEAY, S.J. 1981 - "The Conventus Tarraconesis in the

258

third century A.D.: crisis or change?", in King and Henig 1981, pp.451-86.

KING, A. and M. HENIG. (Eds.) 1981 - The Roman West in the Third Century. Brit. Archaeol. Rpt. S109. Oxford.

LASLETT, P. 1971 - The World We Have Lost. 2nd. ed. London.

LEDAY, A. 1980 - La Campagne à l'époque romaine dans la Centre de la Gaule. Brit. Archaeol. Rpt. S73. Oxford.

MacMULLEN, R. 1963 - Soldier and Civilian in the Later Roman Empire. Harvard.

MacMULLEN, R. 1966 - Enemies of the Roman Order. Harvard.

MacMULLEN, R. 1974 - Roman Social Relations 50 B.C. - A.D. 284. Yale.

MANN, J.C. 1974 - "The frontiers of the Principate", in H. Temporini (Ed.), Aufstieg und Niedergang der römischen Welt II (I), Berlin, pp.508-33.

MARTIN ORTEGA, A. 1979 - Ullastret. Guía de las excavaciones y su museo. 4a. ed. Girona.

MARX, K. and F. ENGELS. 1938 - The German Ideology. English Ed. of Parts 1 & 3 by R. Pascal. London.

MILES, D. (Ed) 1982 - The Romano - British Countryside. Brit. Archaeol. Rpt. 103. Oxford.

MILLETT, M. 1982 - "Town and country : a review of some material evidence", in Miles 1982, pp.421-31.

NEAL, D.S. 1978 - "The growth and decline of villas in the Verulamium area", in Todd 1978, pp.33-58.

NICOLINI, G. 1974 - The Ancient Spaniards. Farnborough.

NOCK, A.D. 1932 - "Cremation and burial in the Roman Empire", Harvard Theol. Rev. vol. 25, pp.321-67.

NOLLA, J.M. 1978 - La Ciudad Romana de Gerunda. Tesis doctoral, Universidad Autónoma de Barcelona.

NOLLA, J.M. and F.J. NIETO 1976 - "Alguns aspectes de la Romanització al Nord-Est de Catalunya", in Els Pobles Pre-Romans del Pirineu, 2 Colloqui Internacional d'Arqueologia de Puigcerdà, pp.235-44.

O'BRIEN, C. 1979 - "Iron Age and Romano-British settlement in the Trent Basin", in Burnham and Johnson 1979, pp.299-313.

OELMANN, F. 1928 - "Ein Gallorömischer Bauernhof bei Mayern", Bonner Jahrb. vol. 133, pp.51-140.

PERCIVAL, J. 1976 - The Roman Villa. London.

PHILP, B. 1977 - "The Forum of Roman London", Britannia vol. 8, pp.1-64.

PONSICH, M. 1974 - Implantantion rurale antique sur le bas-Guadalquivir. Publ. de la Casa de Velázquez, série archéologie, fasc. II. Madrid and Paris.

PONSICH, M. 1979 - Implantation rurale antique sur le bas-Guadalquivir II. Publ. de la Casa de Velázquez, série archéologie, fasc. III. Paris.

RCHM 1962 - Royal Commission on Historical Monuments (England), Eburacum : Roman York. London.

REECE, R. 1976 - "From Corinion to Cirencester", in A. McWhirr (Ed.) Archaeology and History of Cirencester. Brit. Archaeol. Rpt. 30, Oxford, pp.61-79.

REECE, R. 1979 - "Romano-British interaction", in B.C. Burnham & J. Kingsbury (Eds.) Space, Hierarchy and Society. Brit. Archaeol. Rpt. S59, Oxford, pp.229-40.

REECE, R. 1980 - "Town and country: the end of Roman Britain", World Archaeol. vol. 12, (I), pp.77-92.

REECE, R. 1981 - "The third century : crisis or change?", in King & Henig 1981, pp.27-38.

REYNOLDS, P. 1979 - Iron Age Farm. London.

RIPOLL PERELLO, E. 1973 - Ampurias. Guide, 3a. ed., Barcelona.

RIVET, A.L.F. 1977 - "The origins of the cities of Roman Britain", in P.M. Duval & E. Frézouls (Eds.), Thèmes de recherches sur les villes antiques d'occident. Colloques internationaux du CNRS, No. 542, Strasbourg 1971, CNRS Paris, pp.161-72.

ROBLIN, M. 1965 - "Cités ou citadelles?", Revue des Etudes Anciennes vol. 67. (3/4), pp.368-91.

RODWELL, W. (Ed.) 1980 - Temples, Churches and Religion in Roman Britain Brit. Archaeol. Rpt. 77. Oxford.

ROSTOVTZEFF, M. 1957 - The Social and Economic History of the Roman Empire. 2nd ed., rev. by P.M. Fraser, Oxford.

SMITH, J.T. 1978a - "Villas as a key to social structure", in Todd 1978, pp.149-8.

SMITH, J.T. 1978b - "Halls or Yards?" Britannia vol. 9, pp.351-8.

SMITH, M.G. 1972 - "Complexity, size and urbanisation", in P. Ucko, R. Tringham and G. Dimbleby (Eds.), Man, Settlement and Urbanism. London. pp.567-74.

STEVENS, C.E. 1966 - "The social and economic aspects of rural settlement", in Thomas 1966, pp.108-28.

THOMAS, C. (Ed.) 1966 - Rural Settlement in Roman Britain, CBA Res. Rpt. 6. London.

THOMAS, C. 1981 - Christianity in Roman Britain to A.D. 500. London.

THOUVENOT, R. 1973 - Essai sur la province romaine de Bétique. 2e. ed. Paris.

TODD, M. (Ed.) 1978 - Studies in the Romano-British Villa. Leicester.

VAN DOORSELAER, A. 1967 - Les nécropoles d'époque romaine en Gaule septentrionale. Dissertationes Archaeologicae Gandenses, 10. Bruges.

VERMASEREN, M.J. 1963 - Mithras, the Secret God.

VORBECK, E. and L. BECKEL 1973 - Carnuntum: Rom an der Donau. Salzburg.

WACHER, J. 1975 - The Towns of Roman Britain. London.

WALKER, S. 1981 - "The third century in the Lyon region", in King and Henig 1981, pp.317-42.

WARD-PERKINS, J.B. 1970 - "From Republic to Empire - reflections on the early provincial architecture of the Roman West", J. Rom. St. vol. 60, pp.1-19.

WEBSTER, G. 1969 - The Roman Imperial Army. London.

WELLS, P.S. 1980 - "Contact and change: an example on the fringes of the Classical World", World Archaeol. vol. 12(1), pp.1-10.

WHITTAKER, C.R. 1980 - "Rural labour in three Roman provinces", in P. Garnsey (Ed.), Non-Slave Labour in the Greco-Roman World. Camb. Philol. Soc., Suppl. vol. 6, pp.73-99.

WIGHTMAN, E.M. 1970 - Roman Trier and the Treveri. London.

WIGHTMAN, E.M. 1975 - "The pattern of rural settlement in Roman Gaul", in H. Temporini and W. Haase (Eds.), Aufstieg und Niedergang der römischen Welt. II (4), Berlin, pp.584-657.

WIGHTMAN, E.M. 1977a - "Military arrangements, native settlements and related developments in early Roman Gaul", Helinium vol. 17, pp.105-26.

WIGHTMAN, E.M. 1977b - "The towns of Gaul, with special reference to the North-East", in M. Barley (Ed.), European Towns, London, pp.303-14.

WIGHTMAN, E.M. 1981 - "The fate of Gallo-Roman villages in the third century", in King and Henig 1981, pp.235-43.

WILD, J.P. 1978 - "Cross-Channel trade and the textile industry", in H. Cleere and J. du Plat Taylor (Eds.), Roman Shipping and Trade. CBA Res. Rpt. 24. London, pp.79-81.

WILKES, J.J. 1966 - "Early fourth century rebuilding in Hadrian's Wall forts", in M.G. Jarrett and B. Dobson (Eds.), Britain and Rome. Kendal, pp.114-38.

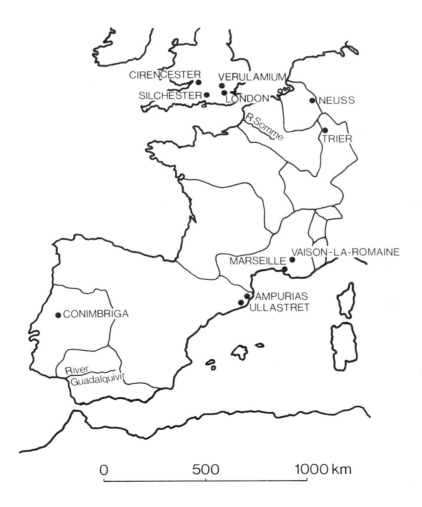

Fig 1
The western Roman Empire, showing the major sites discussed and provincial boundaries.

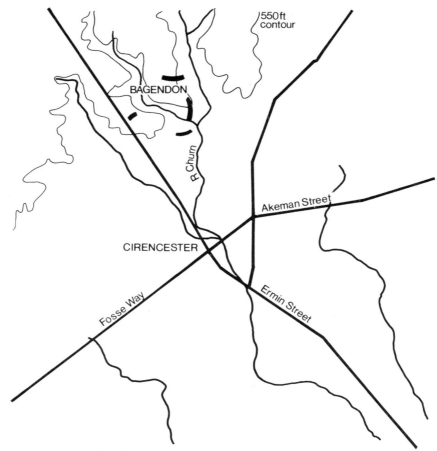

Fig 2
Bagendon and Cirencester (after Wacher 1975).

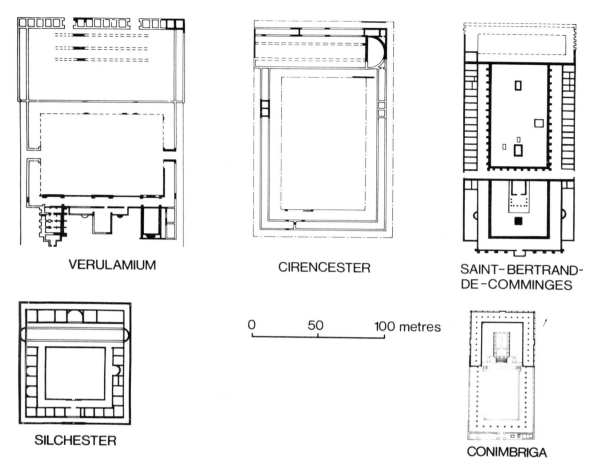

VERULAMIUM

CIRENCESTER

SAINT-BERTRAND-
DE-COMMINGES

SILCHESTER

0   50   100 metres

CONIMBRIGA

Fig 3
Early Imperial fora (after Wacher 1975; Alarcao and Etienne 1977; Ward-Perkins 1970).

262

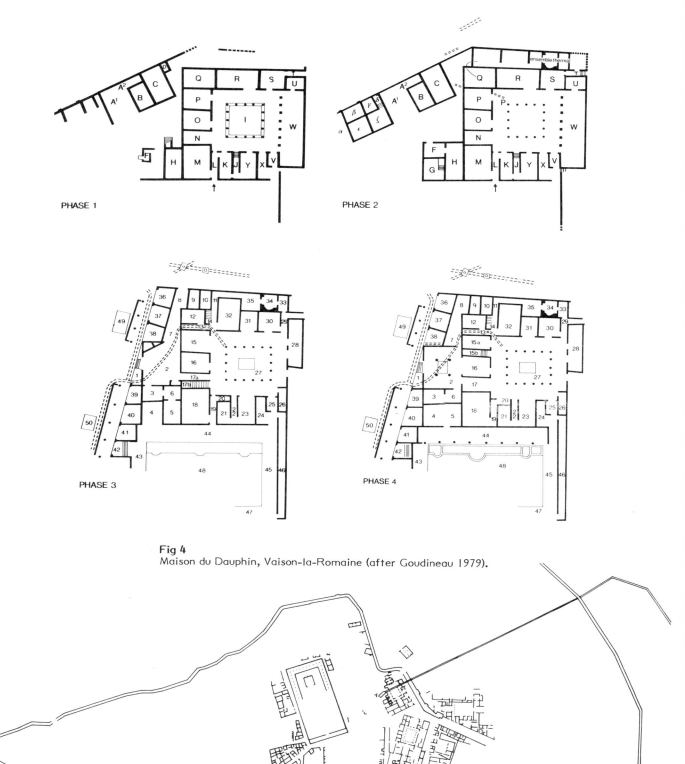

PHASE 1

PHASE 2

PHASE 3

PHASE 4

Fig 4
Maison du Dauphin, Vaison-la-Romaine (after Goudineau 1979).

0   50   100m

Fig 5
Conimbriga (after Alarcao and Etienne 1977).

263

a) LORA DEL RIO - Roman settlement

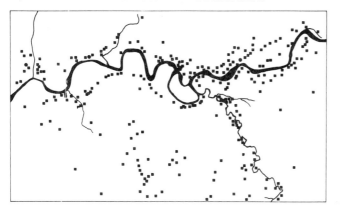

b) CARMONA - Iberio-punic settlement

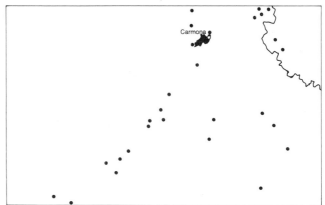

c) CARMONA - Roman period settlement

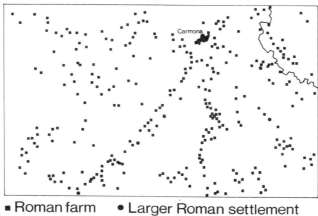

■ Roman farm ● Larger Roman settlement

Fig 6
Ancient settlement around Lora del Rio and Carmona, in the Guadalquivir valley (after Ponsich 1974). Scale 1cm. = 2kms.

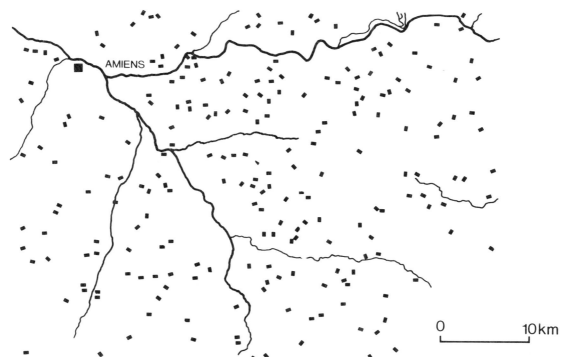

0   10km

Fig 7
Roman settlement in the Somme valley (after Agache 1978).

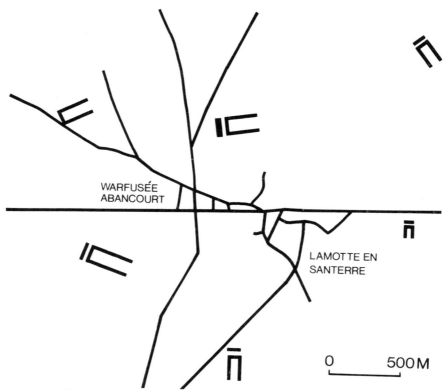

Fig 8
Villas at Warfusée-Abancourt (after Agache 1978).

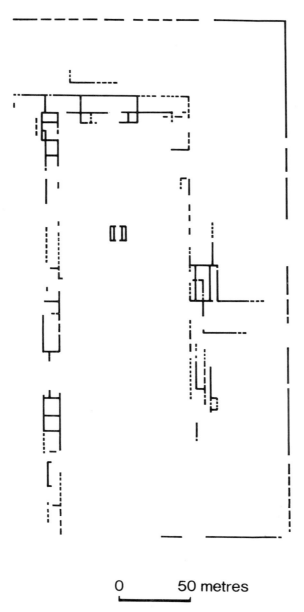

0   50 metres

Fig 9
The villa of Warufsée-Sud (after Agache 1978).

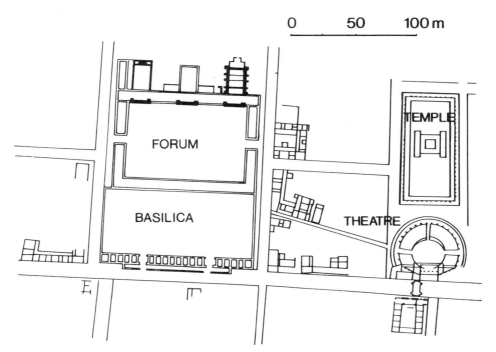

Fig 10
Verulamium – the central area (after Frere 1972).

11

CITIES AND SOCIAL EVOLUTION IN ROMAN AND BYZANTINE SOUTH EAST EUROPE

Timothy Gregory

As a serious approach to the Balkans in Roman and Byzantine times, social evolution has been generally ignored. It is curious and paradoxical, however, that a kind of nearly thoughtless evolutionism has been an unconscious basis of much modern historical analysis on the subject. Previous scholarship in the area has been dominated by a philological and legalistic approach that stressed the particular and dealt little with the dynamics of social change, let alone placing this in any kind of theoretical framework - except as individual historians wrote from the point of view of their own preconceptions. Examples of this tradition are the prestigious Cambridge Ancient History (Vols. 11 and 12, 1936, 1939) and Cambridge Medieval History (Vols. 1 and 4, 1924, 1966-67), the relevant chapters in Tenney Frank, Ed., An Economic Survey of Ancient Rome (1933-40), and the other standard handbooks of Roman and Byzantine history. Further, those few studies that have taken a more dynamic, diachronic, approach have focused largely on the imperial state and its attendant institutions, with little attention to local or regional developments.

Thus, the issue of the 'rise and fall of the Roman empire' (for this is essentially what we are discussing here) has been painted on the broadest canvas and it has exercised historians from Polybius and Gibbon to Toynbee and Eisenstadt. Broad explanations have been many and varied, ranging from an appeal to the invariable repetition of historical cycles to the growth of elites and specialized bureaucracies. Thus, for example, Polybius saw the growth of Roman power as a result of the excellence of the Roman constitution, with its balance among the various forms developed by earlier Greek experience (Book 6, 11-18; Walbank 1957, pp.617, 673-97), while he and many other Roman historians saw the seeds of the empire's demise in its very success and the elimination of viable international competition (Livy 39.6.7; cf. Brink and Walbank 1954).

Modern historians have focused on different factors as historiographic fashions have changed. Thus, Gibbon praised Roman moderation and enlightenment and characterized the fall as "the natural and inevitable effect of immoderate greatness" (Gibbon 1909, 4 p.173). Political and military explanations have always been most popular, but historians have frequently looked at changes in Roman society as underlying causes for the rise and fall of the empire. In this, of course, they were following the precedent set by the Roman moralist historians who saw the sturdy Roman peasantry and the duty-bound aristocracy as the strength behind the empire, while the disappearance of the former and the dilution and corruption of the latter were the causes of the collapse. Thus, the views of Tenney Frank (1915), Otto Seeck (1920-22), and A.E.R. Boak (1955) can be seen as more elaborate and sophisticated versions of a common ancient theme.

The issue of class conflict, however, represents a significant departure from the explanations espoused by the ancient sources and one of the few discussions which rests on an apparently consistent theoretical base. Thus, Marxist historians (e.g. Oliva 1962, Seyfarth 1963) explain the problems of late antiquity by reference to class conflict arising from the built-in contradictions of a slave economy: when the imperialism necessary to support such a system became impossible the system collapsed amid much turmoil, and feudalism became the characteristic means of social and economic organization. Thus, in this context the collapse of ancient Mediterranean civilization represented a crucial stage in the evolution of major social forms (cf. Weber 1976). Among western scholars there has been a tendency to downplay the importance of slaveholding in the ancient economic system (e.g. Finley 1973), although some recent work calls for a reassessment even in western historiographic terms (Hopkins 1978). Unique in this regard are the views of M.I. Rostovtzeff (1957 pp.523-41), who argued that the ancient world collapsed because of the 'class warfare' between the urban middle class, who represented the traditions of classical civilization, and an alliance of the rural 'proletariat' and the army, which represented the forces of barbarism and chaos. Although Rostovtzeff's ideas have never been fully accepted, they provide an interesting example of a great Roman social historian's attempt to understand the underlying factors which led to the collapse of the ancient world. Based on a less impressive display of ancient evidence and therefore far less influential were the views of F. W. Walbank (1969), who argued that the Roman world was all but doomed to collapse because of the weakness of its economic system which did not have a mass market for industrial products and could not, therefore, transform itself through economies of scale, but instead became decentralized and required the intervention of a centralized authoritarian state. More recently Keith Hopkins (1980) has examined the Roman tax structure and concluded that the low rate of taxation was not such as to encourage economic development and this, ultimately, contributed to the economic and social problems that characterized the later empire.

While obviously based on Roman and Byzantine experience, the great theoretical explanations of historical change have generally failed to deal satisfactorily with the historical reality. Thus, Arnold Toynbee was greatly influenced by the fall of Rome in the development of his paradigm for the stages through which civilizations pass (1954, 1: 51-181). Yet, Toynbee was probably least successful when dealing with the collapse of Rome and the issue of its 'internal and external proletariats': "By the time when" the barbarians "overran the Roman Empire, the Hellenic Society was already moribund - a suicide slowly dying of wounds self-inflicted during a 'Time of Troubles' centuries before" (1954, 1 p.62).

Eisenstadt, of course (1969), went beyond Toynbee and earlier theorists in that he employed the concepts of sociology, particularly those of Edward Shills, to historical societies, and he focused on the process of change through the combination of external and internal pressures and exigencies. What one notes in Eisenstadt, however, is a certain remove from the specific historical reality and a curious hesitance to deal fully with the transition from ancient to medieval society. Thus, traditional historians seem to have missed the general and theoretical in their examination of the particular, while the theoreticians have been criticized for their lack of depth and errors of fact on which the entire edifice is built.

What most general historical analyses fail to stress is obviously of crucial importance for the present study: regional differentiation and, particularly, the situation in the eastern part of the empire. Indeed, most considerations of the fall of the Roman empire are made from the point of view of the west, and social change in the east is inadequately studied in its own right, especially in anything resembling synthetic form (Baynes 1943). Exceptions to this are the numerous but highly particularistic works on Roman and Byzantine Egypt based on the papyri and the more synthetic recent work on northern Syria (Tchalenko 1953, Liebeschietz 1972). It is, unfortunately, often assumed that while western society changed, and thus declined, the east remained the same and thus survived the collapse that befell the western provinces. In this view, the study of social change in the East is unnecessary because there **was** no substantial change.

An indication of this 'fossil thesis' is the role that the Byzantine empire plays in most theoretical treatments: it is seen as an historical anomaly or at best a 'dead end' civilization that could not make the transformation from ancient to medieval on the historically praiseworthy road toward modernity. Thus, for Toynbee Byzantium was the 'ghost' of the dead Roman empire (1954, 1 p.64, n. 3; 4 p.19), while W. C. Bark (1958 p.66) could write that "A thousand years of Byzantium produced extinction; a thousand years of medieval effort produced the Renaissance, the modern state, and, ultimately the free world." With such blatantly modernist and probably unconscious evolutionist assumptions underlying much of modern historical thinking, it is no wonder that the question of social change in the Roman and Byzantine East has not received the thoughtful attention it deserves.

All of these considerations require that the present essay attempt only a few tentative observations, all the more since much of the fundamental research still remains to be accomplished. They also suggest that local society is the proper theoretical level for investigation. To do otherwise would require an examination of ideas and institutions that go far beyond the boundaries of southeastern Europe. More importantly, it seems to me that such regional investigations - as long as they continue to consider the larger questions - are likely to produce particularly interesting results simply because they do not blur regional social distinctions that ultimately underlay the great imperial structures. We have, I think, come a long way from a simplistic study of empires only 'from the top' and generally realize that they are frequently only shadowy and ephemeral structures that take advantage of serendipitous events to siphon off economic and political profit while leaving the underlying social fabric reasonably unaffected.

Of all the myriad problems that could be attacked in this paper, I have chosen what is perhaps the most critical: the survival of essentially ancient urban forms and institutions in south east Europe in the late Roman and early Byzantine age. The problem is broader than it might at first sight appear, for it involves a whole set of issues ranging from the continuation of a monetary economy to the social and economic differentiations that characterized and supported classical urban life. Cities were, after all, the primary characteristic of classical civilization and their survival or disappearance will mark a crucial stage in the evolution of society at least within the larger western tradition.

The question of the fate of the city in late antiquity has been vigorously debated in the scholarly literature, but no common view has yet emerged, in part because the literary sources are few and the archaeological evidence has not been fully utilized in a systematic and thoughtful manner. Fundamental as background, yet without any theoretical framework, are the books by A. H. M. Jones (1940, 1964, 1971), although they have all too little to say about conditions in south eastern Europe. All authorities agree that east Roman urban society underwent severe shocks in the fourth through the seventh centuries. Some scholars (e.g. Ostrogorsky 1959, Lipschitz 1963, Vryonis 1963), however, stress the fundamental continuity of urban life through this period, while others (e.g. Kazhdan 1960, Foss 1977, Mango 1980) emphasize the collapse of the cities and a fundamental break between the ancient and the medieval worlds, in the east as well as the west.

This paper represents an exploration of these themes, particularly from an archaeological perspective, although consideration will consistently be given to historical questions, something that is all but inevitable given the scholarly development of the field. In the discussion that follows considerable attention will be paid to the relationship between city and country and to the place of the city in individual societies. The reason for this is simple and derived only in part from the historiography of the problem: as we have said, ancient (classical) civilization was by definition and in origin urban in character, and the health and vitality of the city is probably the best gauge of the state of classical civilization. The question, however, is difficult, for how do we know whether the city in a specific period is 'healthy' or not? Even the biological metaphor is potentially misleading unless one accepts a specific, perhaps even biological, view of social evolution. I would argue that the city should be defined in economic or social, and thus perhaps functional, terms rather than political or cultural ones: thus, there is little reason to speak of the peculiar political forms of the classical Greek polis as normative - a city need not have a particular political organization and it need not, also, be politically independent in any sense whatsoever. What is crucial, it seems, is that the city serve as a complex economic center for the exchange of goods and services; there must be considerable division of labor and therefore a reasonable economic surplus. Further, the city must be a social centre in the sense that the economic surplus must be substantially concentrated and spent in the city; in other words, there must normally be considerable economic differentiation and the economic elite must either reside in the city or focus much of its attention on the urban centre. Almost always, such attention must involve expenditure of wealth not only for individual gratification, but also to reflect a kind of corporate existence, normally involving civic phenomena such as public display and monumental, frequently commemorative, architecture (Ganghoffer 1963, Claude 1969).

Great care needs to be taken in the theoretical delimitation of this problem since we are attempting to isolate factors which seem to have been determinative. Thus, there is always the danger of selecting factors which are symptomatic rather than causative. On the other hand isolation of even symptomatic factors should represent a step forward in our understanding of social transformations in late antiquity. What is more difficult to assess is the role that certain factors may have played in society and the degree to which that role may have changed over time. This, of course, is very much akin to the difficulty experienced by those who investigate the 'birth' and growth of civilization, except that here we are examining the collapse, or at least the transformation, of civilization.

Thus, in our investigation we will focus our attention on the urban aristocracy which represented the basis of classical civilization and the assumption will be that as long as we can identify such a group in society then classical civilization will still, in some form, be present - or, perhaps better, that social change will be characterized more by transformation than by radical change. This is not an unreasonable assumption and it is apparently borne out by a glance at the differences between the aristocratic society of the Byzantine Empire and that of the medieval West (Ganghoffer 1963, Février 1974). Nevertheless, there are obvious theoretical problems. Thus, it is possible to see the city of high antiquity with its flourishing range of classes and roles in mechanical interdependence yielding to something more approaching an organic system, with far more dependence on local nobles - still urban in orientation - as protectors and sources of much trade and industry. In this view, the city of late antiquity and the early Byzantine period would have become something like a cluster of manors in an urban environment. In Constantinople and Thessalonika and probably also in Thebes and Korinth during the middle Byzantine period this appears not to have been the case: society was highly regimented but there is ample evidence for complex differentiation. Whether this was true in all, or even most, Byzantine cities is a matter of considerable dispute, as is the question of the continuity between these middle Byzantine cities and their late classical predecessors. Nevertheless, a beginning has to be made somewhere, and with this theoretical caveat in mind, we may proceed with our investigation, realizing that the aristocracy, which we will treat as a simple social unit, is likely to have been extremely complex, both in composition and overall function.

One of the foremost difficulties in dealing with a topic of this dimension is the considerable geographical diversity of the area to be studied: the alternately mountainous and flat interior of the Balkan Peninsula is very different from its Mediterranean coastline, both in physiognomy and historical development (Obolensky 1971 pp.5-41). This very difference, however, is likely to provide an interesting comparative approach to the study of social evolution, since it will allow a contrast and a more empirical test for the evidence to be presented. Perhaps the most obvious and important difference between the two areas is that the interior of the peninsula remained longer outside the control of the various empires, maintaining its traditional forms of social and political organization, while the coast was intimately connected with pan-Mediterranean historical developments. Similarly, when the Roman empire began to collapse, the interior 'reverted' to earlier tribal and village systems, while the coastline generally remained an integral part of the imperial system. Indeed, the phenomenon of the political and cultural penetration of the interior of the Balkans by a coastal imperial regime repeated itself in the ninth and tenth centuries, as the newly-reconstituted Byzantine empire extended its influence among the Slavs (Obolensky 1971 pp.69-133). This phenomenon, in fact, has been characteristic of the Balkans from an early time until fairly recently, when the establishment of strong inland powers in central and eastern Europe and, more importantly, the disappearance of a powerful coastal empire in the eastern Mediterranean changed the situation completely (Braudel 1976).

Until the first tentative expansion of the Macedonian kings in the fourth century B.C. there were essentially no cities in the Balkan hinterlands except along the Adriatic and Black Sea coasts (Pârvan 1923; Hoddinott 1975 p.28). Further, large-scale urbanization and the involvement of the area in Mediterranean civilization came only with the expansion of Roman power and its stabilization after the conquest of Dacia in the early second century AD (Rostovtzeff 1957, pp.246-53). The second and early third centuries, then, represented a period of peace and prosperity for the Balkans and Romanization spread far into the countryside. The emperors acted to found cities and to embellish them with all the refinements of urban life; the social origins of these cities is, however, a matter of some debate. According to Ivanov (1969), for example, the cities were built on the social structure of the pre-Roman indigenous villages, while Condurachi (1969) argues that the cities were essentially imports from other parts of the empire.

There were other peculiarities of social evolution in this area, reflecting both the direction of Roman Imperial policy and the persistence of local traditions. Thus, throughout the Balkans, Romanization spread largely through the presence of the legions, the result being that the northern part of the peninsula - the Danube frontier - was brought more quickly and more fully into the mainstream of Mediterranean civilization than was the area farther south and closer, geographically, to the ancient centres (Hoddinott 1975, p.111). Further, many pre-Roman practices continued in both city and country, including the famous chariot burials and the widespread cult of the Thracian horseman (Rostovtzeff 1957 pp.252-53, 649-50).

In any case, whatever the origin of these cities, it is clear that society in the Balkan interior underwent important transformations as a result of the Roman conquest. These went far beyond cultural manifestations, although the importation of Roman culture may be a good measure of these changes (Mòcsy 1970). Thus, before the arrival of the Romans, society was essentially tribal and relatively undifferentiated. Excavation of wealthy burials from the pre-Roman period throughout the Balkan interior demonstrates the existence of aristocratic groups with widespread connections (e.g. Stripcević 1977). These were the burials of chiefs, head-men, or local political and economic leaders. Below this highest stratum of society the burials do not suggest great differentiation, as most other individuals were buried simply and with relatively uniform grave goods (Duknić and Jovanović 1965).

With the advance of the legions much of this seems to have changed as cities gave rise to a more complex society, complete with distinctions not always based on kinship (Mócsy 1970 pp.161-98). Epigraphy provides our best evidence for these changes, as the inscriptions frequently give the deceased's occupation and some evidence about his social status and origin, but literary sources (e.g. Livy and Pliny the Elder) and the study of burial practices also contribute some information.

Even more significant is the discovery of some large numbers of rural villas in the Balkan interior, many of them with extensive fortifications even in the early Roman period (Thomas 1964; Dremsizova-Nelcinova 1969;

Biro 1974; Lengyel and Radan 1980 pp.275-321). No thorough survey of the Roman villas of the Balkans has yet been made but they are encountered in every region. Thus, for example, in the area around Serdica (modern Sofia), six such villas have been identified (Stanceva 1969; Hoddinott 1975 pp.175-78), while near Pautalia three Roman villas have come to light (Hoddinott 1975 p.182). At Chatalka, 18km. southwest of Stara Zagora in Bulgaria, an enormous villa complex has recently been explored (Nikolov 1969; Hoddinott 1975 pp.209-12), and this allows some interesting observations about society in the area during the early Roman period. The villa was constructed in the first century AD and underwent several modifications over the years. The villa's owners, even at this early date, were apparently Romanized Thracians, since fragments of votive tablets dedicated to the Thracian Horsemen were found in a destroyed household shrine in the villa, and the nearby tumuli revealed various rich objects of Thracian work, along with imported goods from both Italy and Asia Minor. The living quarters of the main complex at Chatalka were especially luxurious and they were constructed in two storeys, but the villa was enclosed by a defensive wall some 2m. thick, a graphic reminder of the danger that was present in this part of the empire. Whether the villa owners were afraid of barbarians (Nikolov 1969) or latrones (Tudor 1969) remains unclear.

Besides the domestic accommodation and various farm buildings, the villa at Chatalka had two or three baths and a large pottery establishment which the excavators thought must have produced goods for sale outside the estate. The villa obviously 'employed' a large number of people, and a nearby cemetery has been suggested as the final resting place for some of these workers. Indeed, in many ways a villa such as this must be seen, along with the 'Mediterranean type' cities, as the successor of the earlier pre-Roman Balkan villages and in some ways as the precursor - already in the imperial age -of the later medieval manor. To the extent that the villa produced goods for sale, it resembled contemporary Italian capitalistic estates, but in other respects it was a self-contained rural establishment (Percival 1969). There is no evidence to allow us to establish the social and legal status of the Chatalka workers, whether they were slave or semi-free, but a variety of inscriptions testify to the contemporaneous existence of independent peasant villages in the area, side by side with the more exploitative form of labor that must have characterized the villa.

Clearly, the owners of the estate were, culturally at least, members of an empire-wide elite, as the grave goods from other areas demonstrate. In addition, there were apparently no heating facilities in the villa and the owners may have been forced to leave during the cold winter months. Nevertheless, the tie of these wealthy and important individuals to the land and to the rural countryside is an obvious conclusion to be drawn from Chatalka and similar villas in the Balkan hinterland.

Toward the end of antiquity - in the fourth through sixth centuries - the phenomenon of huge rural estates seems to have become even more widespread in the Balkan provinces (Velkov 1962, Wilkes 1969, Mócsy 1974). Mócsy connects this with a change in imperial policy and the decline in importance of the frontier legions vis à vis the new mobile comitatenses. In the earlier period, he argues, military pay had supplemented agricultural income and kept many small farms and estates in business, encouraging also the vitality of a money economy in the rural areas (1974 p.307). To the degree that he is correct, this represents an interesting example of how decisions made at the central, imperial level had an effect on the evolution of local society. Further, the curial class, which had been the backbone of the cities everywhere,

suffered by the preference given to the new imperial aristocracy. These latter were essentially exempt from the heavy municipal burdens which fell upon the curiales and they were, accordingly, able to build up large land holdings from their base in far-off Constantinople. The result was economic pressure on the Balkan cities and the local aristocracy (Velkov 1962, 1977; Lengyel and Radan 1980 pp.397-416).

Thus, in the Balkan interior as elsewhere within the empire, the period of late antiquity witnessed considerable social and economic polarization: wealthy houses and burials became even richer, but at the same time the gulf between these and the properties of the poor increased enormously (Mócsy 1974 pp.319-20). The prosperity that is evident in the form of rich mosaics, jewelry, and elaborate houses is thus probably misleading; wealth was much more concentrated and, perhaps more significantly, the proceeds of the land were ever increasingly carried off to the imperial capital, not so much in the form of taxes but as rents acquired by the absentee landlords. Even where the landowners were local in origin they purchased their immunity from financial burdens (munera) either by associating themselves with the imperial aristocracy or by building independent and perhaps separately fortified establishments where they could resist both the barbarians and the imperial tax collectors. In any case, the revenues of the land were divorced from the support of local civic institutions and the landowners lost whatever interest they had had in the local urban centers.

If such an analysis is in any way correct, it will obviously help to explain the weakness of the social fabric when it was subjected to the strains of barbarian invasions. The Germanic and Hunnic inroads of the third, fourth, and fifth centuries had been devastating and perhaps they exacerbated the social difficulties described above (Moss 1937, Lemerle 1954). But it was the Slavic invasions of the late sixth and seventh centuries that forever changed the ethnic make-up of the central Balkans and put an end to the institutions and urban forms that had characterized ancient civilization in that part of the empire. These invasions began in the early years of the sixth century but increased in intensity toward the end of the century when the Danube frontier effectively collapsed and the cities were without imperial military support (Lemerle 1954; Obolensky 1971 pp.52-55; Gomolka 1976). City after city was destroyed by the barbarians and their sites virtually abandoned; unlike the period of earlier invasions, there was no effective urban response. The literary sources for this period are notoriously weak and confused and the archaeological evidence is only just now beginning to be exploited. The conclusion of all research carried out to date seems, however, to be the same: the late sixth or early seventh century witnessed the virtual loss of the central Balkans to Mediterranean civilization.

In Greece the situation seems to have been considerably different; in the south the degree of cultural continuity was obviously greater and the fact that the inhabitants of Greece today speak Greek rather than a Slavic language is a significant indicator that conditions in the two parts of the Balkan peninsula were historically different. The rest of this paper, accordingly, will be devoted to an analysis of social developments in Greece, with a particular view toward the 'dark age' of early Byzantine Greece (cf. Bon 1951, Charanis 1972).

In the Roman imperial age Greece appears not to have been particularly prosperous; indeed, it is frequently described as something of a political and economic backwater (Whittaker 1976), especially in contrast with the more flourishing areas of the eastern Mediterranean, or in contrast with the glory of Greece's classical past, something which has always been a particularly difficult burden for the country to support (Larsen 1938).

A case in point is Pausanius' description of Greece, written about the middle of the second century after Christ. Although obviously excited by the antiquities and their historical and mythological associations, Pausanias was generally disappointed with contemporary Greece that had lost much of the splendor of the classical past: temples lay abandoned or in need of repair and cities which had once been great were nothing more than miserable villages. Nevertheless, a closer reading of Pausanias and an examination of the epigraphic and archaeological evidence shows that the cities of Greece in the imperial age - while perhaps not as glorious or 'noble' as Pausanias had expected - were frequently at least fully viable urban centers whose institutions seemed adequate to the needs of the day. In fact, basing their analysis largely on the epigraphic evidence that is abundant until the mid-third century, historians have been able to carry out a reasonably detailed analysis of Greek urban, particularly political, life (e.g. Geagan 1979). Changes accompanied the disasters of the third century, but archaeological evidence suggests considerable recovery in the fourth and fifth centuries, and some of the cities which Pausanias described as ruined in the second century were apparently flourishing in the fifth (Thompson 1959).

What is less clear is the economic and social bases on which this apparent urban prosperity must have been built. Important in this regard was the long tradition of essentially aristocratic urban life to which Greece was heir. Thus, in marked contrast to the interior of the Balkans, in Greece the emperors did not have to create new cities nor populate them with an aristocracy that was little removed from its village or tribal origins. The foundation of Roman colonies at Nikopolis, Patras, and Corinth did not affect the underlying social fabric and the Italian merchants who established themselves in Greece soon were assimilated into the local aristocracies (Jones 1970). For better or for worse, the Greek aristocracies which had long been fully tied to the cities and the amenities of urban life, survived and apparently prospered well into the Roman imperial age.

In contrast to the relative wealth of information about Greek cities in the imperial period, we have almost no evidence about the situation in the countryside, which must ultimately have provided the wealth to support the urban social structure. The poverty and rustic backwardness of the Greek countryside were proverbial in the Roman world and this in itself provides a particularly interesting paradox: how can Greece have had a strong urban economy without an equally strong rural economy?

In late antiquity we have a little evidence about Greek agricultural and industrial production and some of this may be useful here. For example, in the fifth century Paulinus of Pella (Eucharistikion 414-19) tells us that there were many estates in Greece owned by absentee landlords and farmed by coloni, a situation that can be paralleled in practically every province in the empire. Paulinus' mother had presumably been a Greek and, although he lived in Gaul, he owned estates in Epiros and Greece proper. The farms, he noted, were divided into many parcels, but these were not far separated from each other, and they would have provided sustenance even for an extravagant owner. Greece had recently been devastated by Alaric and the Visigoths, about twenty years before the events described in the poem, but Paulinus thought that he would be better off there than in Gaul, perhaps evidence that the Greek agricultural recovery had been rapid - in any case an indication that large-scale agricultural activity could be profitable in Greece at the time.

That Paulinus was not the only member of the imperial aristocracy to have estates in Greece is shown by a law of A.D. 357 (C.Th. 4.4.11) which ordered that senators who had fled Rome to reside in Achaia, Macedonia, or any other part of Illyricum should be sought out and compelled to return. The codes, however, generally paint a dismal picture of agricultural activity in Greece during late antiquity. Perhaps confirming the fate of owners like Paulinus, a law of 435 (C.Th. 10.8.5) discusses procedures for the confiscation of ownerless and delinquent land in Achaia. Although the purpose of the law was to regulate such sales to protect the rights of the landowners, it is clear that some land was being sold for delinquent taxes and that it had become a problem for the state. A few years earlier a delegation of Greek landowners had petitioned the emperor for tax relief and in 424 (C.Th. 11.1.33) the state formally agreed to an arrangement allowing the Greeks to pay only one-third of the taxes that had formerly been demanded of them. Undoubtedly there were similar pressures elsewhere, but it is surely significant that the taxes of Macedonia were reduced by only one-half, presumably reflecting the better financial condition of that area.

A similar view of the contemporary Greek economy is provided by Synesius of Cyrene who visited Athens at the very end of the fourth century (Ep. 13) Perhaps influenced by the devastation wrought by Alaric, Synesius compared the city to a burned sacrificial offering and said that the city which had once been famous for philosophers was now famous only for its bee-keepers (cf. Thompson 1959). Likewise, the Expositio totius mundi, written in AD 359/60, described Greece in the following words: "After Thessaly (comes) the land of Achaia, Greece, and Lakonika. Though it contains centers of higher learning, it cannot be equally self-sufficient in other things, for it is a small and mountainous region and cannot be so productive. True, it brings forth a little olive oil and Attic honey, and it can even glory in the fame of its teachings and orations, with more reason, for in other respects it is by no means so famous. It has, however, these cities: Corinth and Athens. Corinth is very active in commerce and has an outstanding structure of an amphitheatre. Athens has the centers of higher learning and ancient historical monuments ...".

So far, then, the situation does not look very promising and there is little correlation between the apparent vitality of the cities and the state of the Greek economy. From Paulinus, however, it will be remembered that the estates of the Greek landlords were apparently often broken up into large numbers of small plots. This same situation is suggested by several inscribed tax registers from the Aegean area (Jones 1953) which show that an individual's holdings might be divided into as many as twenty separate plots, each of them with its own family of coloni. These tax registers further confirm the phenomenon of absentee landlords in Greece, but it is significant that many of the landowners were local in the sense that they were citizens of nearby cities. More importantly, the registers suggest that the formation of large contiguous estates was apparently rare in Greece in this period. An individual's holdings might be scattered among several villages and even in several city territories. This would not, of course, absolutely prevent a landowner from constructing a villa or manorhouse on the largest of his holdings, but the texts of the inscriptions rather suggest a practice whereby the coloni lived more by themselves, or perhaps in peasant villages, owing only certain services and payments to the landowners (cf. Percival 1969).

Of obvious importance in this regard is the geographical location of villas of Roman date in Greece; but it is a sad commentary on the state of Byzantine studies in general, and the perceived importance of the Roman

272

period in Greece, that there is not even a preliminary catalogue of these villas, so we are rather in the dark on this score. Many villas have, of course, been discovered in Greece, but the vast majority of these were either inside or on the outskirts of cities (e.g. Shear 1930, Akerstrom-Hougen 1974). The exceptions known to me can be counted on one hand: they include two villas belonging to or connected with Herodes Atticus, one at Marathon, the other near Argos, and two villas in the southern Argolid, one at Halieis (Rudolf 1979 p.304), the other on the coast at Phourkari (Frost 1977). Perhaps because of the reasonably sheltered position of Greece, at least until the mid-third century, neither the urban nor the rural villas were apparently fortified, and they lay open to any invader who might happen upon them. Future archaeological exploration, particularly detailed field surveys, will probably turn up more examples of rural villas, and I suspect that some previously urban sites may have been transformed into villas in late antiquity -Epidauros Limera in the southeast Peloponnesos is a possible case in point - but only detailed and careful examination will tell for certain. And in this case it will be particularly important to lay down specific criteria to distinguish villas from other habitation sites and, perhaps, to classify different kinds of villas.

In this regard, it will be particularly difficult to distinguish an aristocratic 'manor' or villa from a large working farm, although the presence of mosaics and elaborate bathing facilities will probably be indicative. Further, it is probably impossible to tell, on the basis of archaeological evidence, whether an isolated farmhouse belonged to an independent farmer or to a colonus who worked for a large landowner. Survey data on the scattering of rural habitation sites in late Roman Greece is beginning to accumulate and this may well contribute to our understanding of the situation, but the primary consideration here is, in any case, the identification of large concentrations of property where a wealthy individual might virtually declare himself independent both of the central state of urban civilization. In this regard it would matter little whether the farmers were independent peasants or coloni (Dyson 1979).

In any case, by contrast with the rural villas, the number of urban villas in Greece is enormous and growing larger every year as modern building activities have their inevitable effect. Such luxurious private houses have been identified in Athens, Sparta, Corinth, Argos, and many other locations. The presence of these urban villas, coupled with the apparent scarcity of similar rural complexes suggests that the aristocracy of Roman Greece, unlike that of the Balkan interior, identified closely with the cities and, even in the later period, preferred to make their homes in the urban centers rather than in the rural countryside. This fact reflects or perhaps even partly explains the greater urban vitality which Greece displayed in the face of the barbarian invasions.

A specific example of this phenomenon is documented by an inscription from Corinth (Kent 1966, no. 502) set up to honor Memmius Pontius Ptolemaeus, also known as Parnasius, in the middle of the fourth century. Parnasius was apparently a native of Patras who had risen to high rank in the imperial service and became a governor of Egypt. From this exalted position he remembered the province of his origin and contributed lavishly to its capital city. Patras also must have benefitted from Parsanius's generosity and Parsanius cannot have been unique. A further indication of the continued urban identification of the aristocracy, from the opposite end of the Dark Ages, is the case of Michael II Rangabe, who in the early ninth century was the first Byzantine emperor with an attested surname. Modern scholarship is unanimous in connecting the appearance of last names with the rise of local aristocracies within the Byzantine empire, and it is therefore significant that the Rangabe family came from Athens and that their home was not in the country but on the flanks of the Akropolis. This is a single example and we do not know how representative the Rangabe family was, but it is tempting to suggest that the Greek aristocracy maintained its allegiance to urban life throughout the difficulties of the Dark Ages.

Funerary evidence from this area has received little attention and it is not presently possible to assess its possible contribution to the study of late Roman and early Byzantine society. Most work to date (Davidson 1937; Lengyel and Radan 1980 pp.397-416) has focussed on the introduction of new ethnic groups, particularly Avars and Slavs, into the peninsula and it has generally neglected evidence for social change. The spread of Christianity and the diminution (but not elimination) of grave goods also make discussion of social distinctions quite difficult (Wiseman 1967; 1969). Nevertheless, there is abundant material available for analysis and it is to be hoped that archaeologists and historians will make full use of it in years to come.

The survival of the east Mediterranean city through the crisis of the seventh and eighth centuries is one of the most vexed and hotly debated problems of early Byzantine history. Again largely because of the paucity of the literary evidence, archaeological material has come to play a leading role in the discussion, although it has not been used either very carefully or very imaginatively: the problem has usually been discussed either by historians who are not aware of the limitations and proper use of the archaeological evidence or by archaeologists who are ignorant of the period (or, worse, who accept historians' reconstructions and then use them as a datum point for their own analysis).

In this regard it is illustrative to look briefly at the fuss that the study of the numismatic material has occasioned (Charanis 1955; Vryonis 1963). In general the evidence is more or less clear. The standard procedure has been to count the number of coins discovered during excavation and range these over time, the expectation being that a prosperous money economy would produce a high yearly average of coins while a poor economy would produce substantially fewer. From this point of view the picture in Athens and Corinth is reasonably similar: considerable prosperity in the fourth through mid-sixth centuries, followed by a collapse in the late sixth, recovery in the early seventh, and a final collapse after c. 668. Thus, for the 143-year interval between AD 668 and 811, for example, only 19 coins were excavated at Corinth, for an average of 0.132 coins per year. This contrasts strikingly with the period between AD 491 and 578, when over a thousand coins were found, for a yearly average of 11.540, some 87 times greater!

The interpretation of this evidence, however, is not as clear-cut as it might initially seem, particularly in that we want to understand regional variation rather than change at the imperial level. Thus, everyone would agree that the empire as a whole weathered the storm of the Dark Ages and that Constantinople remained a city. Nevertheless, the fall-off of excavation coins in Greece seems to reflect, not local conditions, but an empire-wide phenomenon: a general decline in the money economy and in particular a decline in the number of coins that circulated in the provinces. This will certainly have affected Greece, but that effect is not simple to measure nor is the sequence of events nor the cause-and-effect relationship at all clear.

The general absence of Dark Age coins from excavated contexts has had another interesting result: lacking evidence for numismatic dating, excavators have simply assumed that there was no activity on their sites in the seventh and eighth centuries, something which careful examination of the ceramic evidence is slowly proving to be incorrect: the previous report of the death of various sites has been seriously exaggerated.

And there is more - most of which can only be mentioned here. For example, a striking observation about the period of late antiquity in Greece is the apparent multiplication of sites, many of them of considerable size. For example, on the basis of documentary evidence (the Synekdemos of Hierokles, early sixth century) it is possible to assign civic status to approximately eighty places in the province of Achaia, apparently making Greece one of the most highly urbanized areas of the eastern Mediterranean. Most of these cities cannot have been very large and the situation is in part undoubtedly a distant reflection of the multiplication of poleis in the classical period. The number is nevertheless significant, and a selective archaeological survey of these sites reveals evidence of habitation at every single one. That is, the documents which suggest a high degree of urbanization in Greece in late antiquity were not merely archaizing records; instead, they bore some resemblance to contemporary reality. Further, preliminary analysis of material from twenty-six sites examined in 1980 by the Cambridge/Bradford Boeotia Expedition has shown the late Roman period to be the most frequently represented, with habitation attested at eighteen of the twenty-six sites. Indeed, archaeological survey in Greece frequently notes late Roman material on sites which were occupied only during that period or on a few other occasions throughout the past. The reasons for this are not yet entirely clear and they may be connected either with the circumstances of archaeological deposit or possibly the displacement of population caused by historical circumstances (Hood 1970), but the phenomenon is certainly worth noting.

There is also the interesting circumstance of the introduction of burial into the center of cities such as Athens and Corinth (Weinberg 1974, Williams 1975). At Corinth, for example, burial begins to intrude even into the forum area, suggesting the decline of this critical region as a civic center (Scranton 1957).

Close analysis, however, suggests not the abandonment of the area but its shifting within the center of city and a probable change in the conception of what an agora should be. Further, several of the tombs were quite monumental, with vaulted roofs, several chambers, and one apparently with two storeys. These were thus perhaps monuments in the classical sense and the argument about their introduction can thus cut two ways: on the one hand, something had clearly changed in that it would previously have been unthinkable to bury people in the agora; nevertheless some of these tombs were also monuments to commemorate the dead (and possibly also places of assembly and cult) which demonstrate a mind-set that would have been completely at home in the classical world.

Finally, one might mention the importance of the cities as centers for the reconquest and full re-Hellenization of the Greek peninsula in the ninth century and after. Here we are not on very strong ground, since the weight of scholarship suggests that the impetus for this movement came from the emperor in Constantinople (Charanis 1946). Nevertheless, there is now ample evidence to show that cities like Athens, Corinth, Sparta, and Patras survived the barbarian onslaught and that many of the cultural phenomena of middle Byzantine Greece (e.g. the form of churches) were based on local early Byzantine prototypes which had been kept alive

somehow through the Dark Ages. This is naturally not to claim that the cities survived the crisis with all of their classical institutions intact; clearly they had not - and many of these classical institutions had been long gone by the fourth century AD in any case. But, in Greece the process of the Hellenization of the Slavs appears to have gone remarkably smoothly: one suspects either that the movement began at a very early date, probably immediately after the arrival of the new settlers -perhaps without the direct assistance of the central government - or that the number and effect of the Slavic invaders has been greatly exaggerated. I suspect that both factors are operating here and that the survival of reasonably strong and vibrant urban centers is the key to the continued existence of Hellenic culture in the southern Balkans. Clearly it is not enough to point simply to the 'obvious superiority' of Greek civilization since even that needs institutions and vehicles for its maintenance and transformation (Vryonis 1971). The cities, with their municipal and ecclesiastical institutions, seem to have been best equipped to meet the challenge of the invasions. In Greece the cities remained viable, while in the Balkan interior they were not - and this was in large measure responsible for the cultural and historical difference in these two areas in subsequent years.

In summary, I should probably attempt to suggest reasons, or even hypotheses, to explain the social changes that we seem, dimly, to perceive. Thus, if we are correct in seeing the survival of the city in the south and its disappearance (or possibly its non-appearance) in the north, how are we to explain **this** phenomenon? As mentioned above, it is probably not enough simply to document the survival of the urban aristocracy, since we then need to inquire into the reasons for its survival. But I fear that the evidence is presently far too fragmentary for such larger speculation, and I have already speculated far too much as it is. More detailed fundamental research, much of it archaeological, still needs to be done, but the possibilities are, I think, promising. Interesting lines for future investigation will be the analysis of environmental relationships (intensive agricultural exploitation leading to collapse?), population changes particularly at the mid-sixth century, and the importance of industry and sea-borne trade in Greece.

In the past it has been common simply to point to the historical development of both areas and to note that the Balkan interior never really developed anything more than a veneer of classical urban culture which then was unable to survive the strain of the barbarian invasions, while the Mediterranean coastline had centuries of experience with classical civilization which thus struck deeper roots. Such an analysis, while not patently false, seems to assume that a new social order cannot become entrenched within a period of several centuries, the time during which Roman rule held sway in the Balkan interior (from at least the second through the fourth century AD). What is more reasonable is to suggest that the kind of society long established on the Mediterranean coast was never fully introduced into the heartland of the Balkans. Thus, it was not merely a matter of time, but a matter of difference in substance, and the barbarian invasions in the south came up against a very different society from what they encountered in the north. As a possibly ironic variant on this theme, we might suggest that the very backwardness of Greece during the height of the Roman period may well have been a factor. Thus outside the main current of events, Greece may have maintained a society, based on Hellenistic lines, that was relatively little affected by the monumental changes going on in the world outside. When the shock of the invasions struck, Greece was ironically better prepared and we should not be overly surprised to learn that one of Athens' leading literary figures led a group of two thousand local youths against the barbarians who had attacked the city and helped to expel them from the country.

What does all of this have to do with the broader theories of social evolution? If we could explain the phenomena - naturally after identifying them - it would obviously contribute a great deal. The Roman and Byzantine periods in southeastern Europe present a fascinating spectacle of complexity and apparent social disintegration that is similar but strikingly different from what occurred in the West at the same time. It is easy to see why previous theorists were both fascinated and put off by the phenomena of the Byzantine Empire, an entity that seems to defy definition and neat classification. There is a curious sameness and resistance to evolution, and yet many things, such as the vast multiplication of archaeological sites in the period, to show that change was taking place. But was that change "upward" or "downward"? Perhaps we are simply using the wrong models or the wrong sets of evolutionary expectations. Or perhaps we are selecting the wrong sets of the sample for analysis. I would hate to think of the millennium-long Byzantine Empire simply dismissed as a kindly old Neanderthal, interesting and peculiar, but essentially outside the mainstream and therefore irrelevant.

BIBLIOGRAPHY

Actes - (cf. Condurachi, E. 1969).

AKERSTROM-HOUGEN, G. 1974 - The Calendar and Hunting Mosaics of the Villa of the Falconer in Argos. Stockholm. Swedish Institute in Athens.

BARK, W.C. 1958 - Origins of the Medieval World. Stanford, California. Stanford University Press.

BAYNES, N.H. 1943 - "The Decline of Roman Power in Western Europe. Some Modern Explanations", JRS vol. 33 pp.29-35.

BIRO, M. 1974 - "Roman Villas in Pannonia", Acta Archaeol. Ac. Scient. Hung. vol. 26 pp.23-57.

BOAK, A.E.R. 1955 - Manpower Shortage and the Fall of the Roman Empire in the West. Ann Arbor. University of Michigan Press.

BON, A. 1951 - Le Péloponnèse byzantin jusqu'en 1204. Paris. Presses universitaires de France.

BRAUDEL, F. 1976 - La Mediterranée et le monde mediterranéen à l'époque de Philippe II;2. Paris. Armand Colin.

BRINK, C.O. and WALBANK, F.W. 1954 - "The Construction of the Sixth Book of Polybius", CQ n.s. vol. 4 pp.97-122.

CAMBRIDGE ANCIENT HISTORY 1936, 1939 - vols XI and XII. Cambridge. Cambridge University Press.

CAMBRIDGE MEDIEVAL HISTORY 1924, 1966-67 - vols. I and IV. Cambridge. Cambridge University Press.

CLAUDE, D. 1969 - Die Byzantinische Stadt in 6. Jahrhundert. Munich. Byzantinische Archiv.

CHARANIS, P. 1946 - "Nicephorus I, the Saviour of Greece from the Slavs", Byzantina-Metabyzantina vol. I pp.75-92.

CHARANIS, P. 1955 - "The Significance of Coins as Evidence for the History of Athens and Corinth in the Seventh and Eighth Centuries", Historia vol. 4 pp.163-72.

CHARANIS, P. 1972 - Studies on the Demography of the Byzantine Empire. London. Variorum.

CONDURACHI, E. 1969 - In Actes de Ier Congrès international des études balkaniques et sud-est européennes. Sofia. Academy of Arts and Sciences. Vol. II pp.539-41.

DAVIDSON, G.R. 1937 - "The Avar Invasion of Corinth", Hesperia vol. 6 pp.227-39.

DREMISISOVA-NELCINOVA, T. 1969 - "La villa romaine en Bulgarie", Actes vol. II pp.503-12.

DUKNIC, M. and JOVANOVIC, B. 1965 - "Illyrian Princely Necropolis at Atenica", Archaeologia Iugoslavica vol. 6 pp.1-35.

DYSON, S.L. 1979 - "New Methods and Models in the Study of Roman Town-Country Systems", The Ancient World vol. 2 p.91-95.

EISENSTADT, S.N. 1963 - The Political Systems of Empires. London. Macmillan.

FEVRIER, A.P. 1974 - "Permanence et heritages de l'antiquité dans la topographie des villes de l'occident", Settimane di Studi sull'Alto Medio Evo 21.1. Spoleto. pp.41-138.

FINLEY M.I. 1973 - The Ancient Economy. London. Chatto and Windus.

FINLEY, M.I. 1980 - Ancient Slavery and Modern Ideology. London. Chatto and Windus.

FOSS, C. 1977 - "Archaeology and the 'Twenty Cities' of Byzantine Asia", AJA vol 81 pp.469-86.

FRANK, T. 1915-16 - "Race Mixture in the Roman Empire", AHR vol. 21 pp.689-708.

FRANK, T. 1933-40 - An Economic Survey of Ancient Rome. 4 vols. Baltimore. Johns Hopkins University Press.

FROST, F.J. 1977 - "Phourkari. A Villa Complex in the Argolis Greece", International Journal of Nautical Archaeology and Underwater Exploration vol. 6 pp.233-38.

GANGHOFFER, R 1963 - L'évolution des institutions municipales en occident et en orient au bas-empire. Paris. Librarie générale de droit et de jurisprudence.

GEAGEN, D.J. 1979 - "Roman Athens: Some Aspects of Life and Culture. I. 86 B.C. - A.D. 267", Aufstieg und Niedergang II.7.1. Berlin. De Gruyter. pp.371-437.

GIBBON, E. 1909 - The History of the Decline and Fall of the Roman Empire, Ed. J.B. Bury. 7 vols. London. Methuen.

GOMOLKA, G. 1976 - "Bemerkungen zur Situation der spätantiken Städte und Siedlungen in Nordbulgarien und ihrem Weiterleben am Ende des 6. Jahrhunderts", Studien zum 7. Jahrhunderts in Byzanz. Berlin. Akad. Verlag. pp.35-42.

HAMMOND, M. 1974 - "The Emergence of Medieval Towns: Independence or Continuity?" HSCP vol. 78 pp.1-34.

HODDINOTT, R.F. 1975 - Bulgaria in Antiquity. London. Benn.

HOOD, S, 1970 - "Isles of Refuge in the Early Byzantine

Period", BSA 65, pp.37-45.

HOPKINS, K. 1978 - Conquerors and Slaves. Cambridge. Cambridge University Press.

HOPKINS, K. 1980 - "Taxes and Trade in the Roman Empire (200 B.C. - A.D. 400)", JRS vol. 70 pp.101-25.

IVANOV, T. 1969 - "Der Stadtbau und Ober- in Untermösien und Thrakien in der Römerzeit und der Spätantike", Actes vol II pp.491-502.

JONES, A.H.M. 1940 - The Greek City from Alexander to Justinian. Oxford. Clarendon Press.

JONES, A.H.M. 1953 - "Census Records of the Later Roman Empire", JRS vol. 43 pp.49-64.

JONES, A.H.M. 1964 - The Later Roman Empire, 284-602. A Social, Economic and Administrative Survey. 3 vols. Oxford. Blackwell.

JONES, A.H.M. 1971 - Cities of the Eastern Roman Provinces.[2] Oxford. Clarendon Press.

JONES, C.P. 1970 - "A Leading Family of Roman Thespiae", HSCP vol. 74 pp.223-55.

KAZHDAN, A.P. 1960 - Derevnia i gorod v Vizantii IX-X vv, Moscow.

KAZHDAN, A. and CUTLER, A. 1982 - "Continuity and Discontinuity in Byzantine History" Byzantion Vol. 52 pp.429-78.

KENT, J.H. 1966 - Corinth VIII.3. The Inscriptions 1926-1950. Princeton. American School of Classical Studies.

KIRSTEN, E. 1958 - "Die Byzantinische Stadt", Berichte zum XI. Internationalen Byzantinisten-Kongress. Munich.

LARSEN, J.A.O. 1938 - "Roman Greece", in Frank 1938, vol. 4 pp.258-498.

LEMERLE, P. 1954 - "Invasions et migrations dans les Balkans depuis la fin de l'époque romaine' jusqu'au VIIIe siècle", Revue historique vol. 211 pp.265-305.

LENGYEL, A. and RADAN, G.T.B. 1980 - The Archaeology of Roman Pannonia. Lexington. University of Kentucky Press.

LIEBESCHIETZ, J.H.W.G. 1972 - Antioch. City and Imperial Administration in the Later Roman Empire. Oxford. Oxford University Press.

LIPSCHITZ, E.E. 1963 - "Gorod i derevnya v Vizantii v VI-pervoi IX v", Actes du XIIIe congrès international d'études byzantines. vol. 1. Belgrade. pp.9-20.

MANGO, C. 1980 - Byzantium. The Empire of New Rome. London. Weidenfield and Nicolson.

McKAY, A.G. 1975 - Houses, Villas and Palaces in the Roman World. London. Thames and Hudson.

MOCSY, A. 1970 - Gesellschaft und Romanisation in der römischen Provinz Moesia Superior. Budapest. Akademiai Kiado.

MOCSY, A. 1974 - Pannonia and Upper Moesia. London. Routledge and Kegan Paul.

MOSS, H. St. L.B. 1937 - "The Economic Consequences of the Barbarian Invasions", EHR vol. 7 pp.209-16.

NICOLOV, D. 1969 - "Une Villa rustica Thrace près de Stara Zagora", Actes vol II pp.513-25.

OBOLENSKY, D. 1971 - The Byzantine Commonwealth. London. Weidenfield and Nicolson.

OLIVA, P. 1962 - Pannonia and the Onset of Crisis in the Roman Empire. Prague. Ceskoslovenske Akademie Ved.

OSTROGORSKY, G. 1959 - "Byzantine Cities in the Early Middle Ages", DOP vol. 13 pp.47-66.

OSTROGORSKY, G. 1971 - "Observations on the Aristocracy in Byzantium", DOP vol. 25, pp.3-12.

PARVAN, V. 1923 - "La Pénétration héllenique et héllénistique dans la vallée du Danube", Bulletin de la Section Historique de l'Academie Roumaine, vol. 10.

PERCIVAL, J. 1969 - "Seigneurial Aspects of Late Roman Estate Management", EHR vol. 84 pp.449-73.

PERCIVAL, J. 1976 - The Roman Villa. London. Batsford.

ROSTOVTZEFF, M.I. 1957 - The Social and Economic History of the Roman Empire.[2] Oxford. Clarendon Press.

RUDOLF, W.W. 1979 - "Excavations at Porto Cheli and Vicinity. Preliminary Report V: The Early Byzantine Remains", Hesperia vol. 48 pp.295-320.

SCRANTON, R.L. 1957 - Corinth XVI. Medieval Architecture. Princeton. American School of Classical Studies.

SEECK, O. 1921 - Geschichte des Untergangs der antiken Welt.[4] 6 vols. Stuttgart. J.B. Metzler.

SEYFARTH, W. 1963 - Soziale Fragen der spätrömischen Kaiserzeit im Spiegel des Theodosianus. Berlin. Akademie Verlag.

SHEAR, T.L. 1930 - Corinth V. The Roman Villa. Cambridge, Mass. Harvard University Press.

SJUJUMOV, M.J. 1973 - "Nekotorye problemy istoriceskogo razvitija Vizantii i Zapada" Viz Vrem vol. 35 pp.3-18.

STANCEVA, M. 1969 - "Epanouissement et disparition de deux villae rusticae près de Serdica", Actes vol. II pp.535-41.

STOOB, H. 1977 - Die mittelalterliche Stadtbildung im südostlichen Europa. Köln. Bohlau.

STRIPCEVIC, A. 1977 - The Illyrians. Park Ridge, N.J. Noyes Press.

TCHALENKO, G. 1953 - Villages antiques de la Syrie de Nord. Paris. P. Geuthner.

THOMAS, E.B. 1964 - Römische Villen in Pannonien. Budapest.

THOMPSON, H.A. 1959 - "Athenian Twilight: A.D. 267-600", JRS vol. 49 pp.61-72.

TINNEFIELD, F. 1977 - Die frühbyzantinische Gesellschaft. Strukturen. Gegensätze, Spannungen. Munich. W. Fink.

TOYNBEE, A.J. 1954 - A Study of History. 12 vols. London. Oxford University Press.

TUDOR, D. 1969 - In Actes vol II p.541.

VELKOV, V. 1962 - "Les campagnes et la populations rurale en Thrace aux IVe-VIe siècles", Byzantinobulgarica, vol. I pp.31-66.

VELKOV V. 1977 - Cities in Thrace and Dacia in Late Antiquity. Amsterdam.

VRYONIS, S. 1963 - "An Attic Hoard of Byzantine Gold Coins (668-741) from the Thomas Whittemore Collection and the Numismatic Evidence for the Urban History of Byzantium", Zbornik radova vizantoloshkog instituta vol. 8 pp.291-300.

VRYONIS, S. 1971 - The Decline of Medieval Hellenism in Asia Minor. Berkeley. University of California Press.

WALBANK, F. 1957-79 - A Historical Commentary on Polybius. 3 vols. Oxford. Clarendon Press.

WALBANK, F. 1969 - The Awful Revolution. Liverpool.

WEBER, M. 1976 - The Agrarian Sociology of Ancient Civilizations. London. NLB (1909).

WEINBERG, G. 1974 - "A Wandering Soldier's Grave in Corinth", Hesperia vol. 43 pp.512-21.

WEISS, G. 1977 - "Antike und Byzanz. Die Kontinuität der gesellschaftsstruktur", Hist. Zeitschrift vol. 224 pp.529-60.

WHITTAKER, C.R. 1976 - "Agri Deserti", in M.I. Finley Ed. Studies in Roman Property. Cambridge. Cambridge University Press. pp.137-65.

WILKES, J.J. 1969 - Dalmatia. London. Routledge and Kegan Paul.

WILLIAMS, C.K II 1975 - "Corinth 1974: Forum Southwest", Hesperia vol. 44 pp. 1-15.

WISEMAN, J. 1967 - "Excavations at Corinth: The Gymnasium Area, 1966", Hesperia vol. 36 pp.402-28 (esp. 417-20).

WISEMAN, J. 1969 - "Excavations at Corinth. The Gymnasium Area, 1967-68" Hesperia vol. 38 pp.64-106 (esp. 79-80).

SOCIAL EVOLUTION
IN POST—ROMAN WESTERN EUROPE

Chris Arnold

Summary

In north west Europe the Germanic tribes were a powerful force who gradually won territory from the Western Empire and from the third century onwards were restructured both socially and economically. The economic stimulus provided by the Empire and its social developments were seriously disrupted by the migrations that followed. Gradual political consolidation in north west Europe led to the formation of petty kingdoms amongst the Celts, Germans and Slavs, perhaps influenced by Byzantine policies, although to an extent which is difficult to gauge. Distinct areas of political power and wealth emerge, based especially on agricultural potential and the quality of communication, areas that were later to be powerful forces in Medieval Europe. Formerly populations were tribally based, if we are to accept the descriptions of Tacitus, in c. AD 100, in the Germania. There, the impression is given of a society based on the family unit and groups of inter-connected families or kindreds (Thompson 1965). The majority of the members of a tribe (civitas) were men of free will and from whom was drawn a tribal assembly which took major decisions. There is little evidence of rigid class divisions, but in a society geared (it seems) to warfare, certain individuals and families would have the means and opportunity of acquiring more wealth and thus a higher social position than others. The tribal groups gradually evolved into national states, with a more formalized social stratification, whose hierarchies were eventually dominated by warriors and kings. The powers acquired by such groups were eventually diffused by the development of magnates who levied taxes and defended their districts for the king. The growing power of the magnates was consolidated as a result of the extensive raids by land and sea into western Europe from the late eighth to the tenth century.

....

The early development of ranked societies in north west Europe represents a period of transition, a movement towards the formation of states; the prerequisites for those states were being established, a stage that has been described as inchoate (Claessen and Skalnik 1978, pp.22-3). Service has argued that in the examination of the formation of states our concern should be with two main areas, conflict and integration (1975). Conflict theories are concerned with friction between individuals, between societies in the form of conquest, or within societies in the form of class or kin group struggle. Integrative theories are those where controls are placed by geographical or military barriers, or in terms of the organizational benefits of redistribution, war organization and public works. Service sees development of the state as an **inevitable** result of the growth in power of a few members of society. Others see four main factors having a formative influence: population growth and/or pressure; war, the threat of war or conquest and raids; conquest; and the influence of previously existing states (Claessen and Skalnik 1978, p.642). The early undeveloped state is viewed as a society in which: "kinship, family and community ties still dominate relations in the political field; where full-time specialists are rare; where taxation systems are only primitive and ad hoc taxes are frequent; and where such differences are offset by reciprocity and close contacts between the rulers and the ruled." (ibid. p.23).

Claessen views the early state as: "a centralised socio-political organization for the regularization of social relations in a complex, stratified society divided into at least two basic strata, or emergent social classes -viz. the rulers and the ruled - whose relations are characterized by political dominance of the former and tributary obligations of the latter, legitimized by a common ideology of which reciprocity is the basic principle." (1978, p.640).

Such conclusions, based on a wide range of data, are particularly appropriate in this context, in tracing the social evolution of the Germanic groups in the last century of the Roman Empire, and the growth of more complex societies following the migrations. In north Germany and Denmark towards the end of the third century a series of rich graves appears, widely distributed although lacking uniformity, for instance a group in the Elbe-Saale basin dated AD 270-310. It is noted for the richness of Roman imports which have been interpreted as the spoils of raiding, but the limited range of goods would suggest otherwise (Todd 1977, p.40). Hedeager's analysis of the distribution of such objects (1979a) suggests three zones: firstly the Roman Empire characterized by money and market economy; secondly a buffer-zone, lacking independent coinage, but maintaining a limited market economy, perhaps including markets and a merchant class; thirdly, Free Germany, using money without a monetary economy, perhaps moneyless markets. The distribution suggests that the political and economic power of distant areas may strongly influence this distribution, creating a curve that increases with distance, up to 800kms. from the source, and then gradually falls away between 800 - 1200kms. There appears to be a relationship between an increased influx of Roman imports and the development of political centralization in at least one local Germanic area (Hedeager 1980).

The settlements over this area during the period included the isolated farmstead, the hamlet or group of two or three farms, and the larger agglomeration of farmsteads. Some, like Wijster and Barhorst, suggest a degree of planning (van Es 1967). Occasionally, as at Feddersen Wierde and Fochteloo, there is the possibility of social stratification (Parker 1965, Haarnagel 1961), but the territorial power of leaders was only rarely expressed by the construction of defensive structures.

The history of the Germanic peoples in the fourth and fifth centuries is inextricably bound up with the declining Roman provinces, some of which were occupied after they had been ceded by Rome, where others exemplify an admixture of barbaric settlers. Along with the possible factors of overpopulation and ecological degeneration as possible causes of the migrations, the new military and political state of affairs which established, may in several cases have stimulated tribes to migrate, as for example in east Denmark where the formation of the first 'kingdom' or 'state' unified the area for a period of some generations (Hedeager 1979b).

England also provides a useful laboratory for the study of social evolution in the centuries after the migrations. Following the collapse of Roman civilization, the early Anglo-Saxon period, AD 400-700, takes us from the initial fifth-century merger of the Romano-British and the immigrant, Germanic, populations, to the development of the seven principal 'kingdoms'. These were Kent, the East, South and West Saxons, the East Angles, Mercia and Northumbria, often referred to as the Heptarchy. In anthropological terms such societies should be described as chiefdoms, and it was not until the eighth or ninth century that true state societies emerge (Hodges 1982a, p.185ff; Renfrew 1982, pp.113-6). The rate of change during these centuries rapidly accelerated as groups consolidated their position; the seventh century in England is a particularly remarkable period of change, which has been viewed in terms of endogenous factors (Arnold 1982).

The development of the Anglo-Saxon kingdoms may be considered in terms of a number of related themes: changes in the structure of society; levels and distribution of wealth; administrative organization; aggression between groups. Levels of decision-making may manifest themselves in settlement patterns and such an organization has implications for the economy, especially in terms of exchange and subsistence. Certain aspects have tended to figure large in the literature concerned with the formation and development of the kingdoms, especially the role of central places concerned with the exchange of goods, and the provision of services including administration. What is most important here is the change from exchange between kins and territories to that of a market economy. However, a broader perspective is needed to understand fully the development of the kingdoms.

The change in the type and size of settlements in early Anglo-Saxon England, to which population density is a related question, is an important theme. In the late fifth and sixth centuries the only known settlements are rural. The quality of the evidence has improved considerably in recent years, yet excavation has rarely been complete or in conditions with good preservation, making the sequence of structures, their date, and an analysis of their functions difficult. The quantity has increased and it is possible to identify two main building types, the large rectangular timber buildings, often referred to collectively as 'halls', and smaller structures with sunken floors. They are found together in varying proportions in different areas of the countryside. The buildings are often arranged in groups associated with enclosures. At West Stow each of the six halls was the centre of a cluster of sunken buildings and an animal pen (West 1969, 1978). At Cowdery's Down and Chalton the halls are attached to fenced enclosures which contain smaller timber buildings (Millett 1980, 1981; Champion 1977), whereas at Catholme the buildings are contained within ditched enclosures (Losco-Bradley 1977). While the arrangement and building types may vary regionally the concept is the same. These farm modules are found either singly, as at Cowdery's Down, or in groups, as at West Stow and Chalton, although survival of features on such sites is generally poor and phasing difficult (Fig. 1).

The distribution of such settlements is wide (Fig. 2) although there are glaring gaps in our knowledge. Added to this, there are very few rural settlements of the eighth century which have even been excavated, yet alone published in a form which allows generalization or comparison with the earlier settlements. One, Maxey, did not reveal the type of module visible in the early Anglo-Saxon settlements (Addyman 1961), although such a unit may have continued in use at Catholme, and at St. Neots enclosures were associated with the site (Addyman 1972). Where extensive fieldwork has been carried out, eighth-century settlements tend to occur on new sites or on sites of existing villages (Arnold and Wardle 1981). At the same time there is evidence of widespread desertion of settlements occupied in the sixth and seventh centuries and changes in the agrarian economy indicating an intensification. None of the 'early' Anglo-Saxon settlements has produced definite evidence for a church.

Another significant change that takes place around AD 700 is the development of a greater range of settlement types. In addition to rural settlements, the seventh and eighth centuries witness the appearance of centralized places of exchange and royal sites, acting as stimuli to urban growth. Only one of each has been extensively excavated, the royal administrative centre at Yeavering (Hope-Taylor 1977) and the West Saxon port of Hamwic, Saxon Southampton (Addyman and Hill 1968, 1969, Holdsworth 1976, 1980). Other settlements of these types are known from more limited excavations, inference or documentary evidence.

A four-step road to the state has been suggested in terms of economic development by Hodges (1977, 1982a). The first step consists of the 'early state module' (Renfrew 1975), groups of territories which form early state civilizations when unified. Such territories would have an incipient trading site, a central person, with kin-exchange and tribal exchange. The second stage is described as the polity, with large, spasmodically used trading sites with trade as before, with the addition of long-distance prestige trade. Thirdly, the proto-state, which is associated with the first markets and market exchange, and a defined bureaucracy. The final step is the state with its hierarchy of markets and a more developed market exchange.

The development of long-distance exchange, however, is in evidence well before the appearance of even 'incipient trading sites'. The interpretation of the small-scale movement of metalwork in the fifth to seventh centuries remains difficult but the importation of raw materials during the period can easily be traced. This is particularly the case in Kent from the early sixth century onwards, seen in both the distribution of raw materials amongst certain ranks in society and their exchange with other territorial groups (Arnold 1980, pp.96-9). It may seem more probable that leaders gained control of imports because of their local eminence, based on powers created locally, which serve to reinforce their position. Geographic location, as is the case with Kent, may be an important factor in an argument for powers being created by preferential access to imports. For an individual to achieve this preferential position implies, as do the later ports of trade, that a surplus was being produced by the working population, but to what extent leaders were provided with a surplus through the allegiance of a population or by a slave class is not known. The observable commodities of this prestige exchange include amber, gold, glass, garnet, cowrie shells, mercury, wine jars, ivory, rock-crystal, amethyst. That many of these materials were necessary pre-requisites for established manufacturing processes as in the case of jewellery, suggests this was a more regular activity than the haphazard payment of tribute, ransoms, etc. (Grierson 1959). There is also a marked patterning in their distributions; those from Mediterranean and other eastern sources have a concentrated distribution in England, those from Scandinavia are dispersed. Detailed studies have yet to be made of many of these commodities, but they are most commonly found in graves with a greater overall wealth. Of the imported materials in evidence by the eighth century, finished metalwork, ceramics and quernstones are amongst those virtually absent in the sixth century, emphasizing the different nature of exchange at these times.

Hodges has suggested that incipient trading settlements might be identified, but the archaeological evidence used to argue for such sites are sets of weights and scales, dated to the late sixth and seventh centuries, which have been found in cemeteries close to the sites suggested, but also elsewhere in England (Arnold 1980, pp.90-91). Their distribution certainly implies exchange in luxury goods but need not be taken to indicate that this was carried out at a fixed trading site at this time, as opposed to a point of entry and/or the presence of a local power base. More importantly, the regular unit of weight used in the sets implies a level of agreement between traders and/or administrators in each area, the kingdom of Kent playing a major role.

The earliest occupation of the south coast port of Hamwic is dated to the period AD 700-750 on the basis of a silver coinage, the secondary series of sceattas. This series of coins has a lower silver content than the primary series found particularly in Kent (Rigold 1977). Hamwic is characterized by houses laid out along the spine of the Southampton peninsula, beside gravel streets. The settlement may not have originated as a single large unit, rather a series of dispersed clusters of buildings, as is apparent on contemporary continental sites and at London (Hodges 1977, p.193). The imported pottery is from a variety of regions in north France, probably connected with a trade in wine, just as the earlier evidence for exchange between Kent and the continent is in part involved with wheel-turned bottles which may have served to carry wine (Evison 1979). This phase of Hamwic's occupation 'terminates' towards the middle years of the eighth century, followed by a hiatus in coin production and occupation. The major crafts represented on the site are metalworking, carpentry, textiles and boneworking, and a similar range of activities are represented at Ipswich where the rapidly accumulating evidence can demonstrate the production of pottery, and bone, metal and textile industries. Like Hamwic the imported material includes glass, pottery and quernstones from the continent.

Hodges takes the relationship between the origins of the medieval market and the formation of the state as his central theme, and sees exogenous activities, particularly trade, as the principal stimulus to change (Hodges 1982a, 1982b). Settlements such as Hamwic may originate as inlets for international trade directed towards a central person in a territory and its existence would, therefore, be affected if the role of that central person were to change. An increase in wergeld payments for the king by the early eighth century is taken to indicate the growth in power of the central person, a development which underlines the new and distant role of kingship in a larger territory. By the ninth century, Hodges believes that kingship "was no longer concerned with prestige items previously so important in upholding the king's delicately balanced relationship with the community". Important here is the later development of markets: "... the changing distribution of wealth and the birth of the market system which necessarily means that coinage is no longer primarily confined to coastal regions as media in long-distance trade. Coinage is no longer bullion, but clearly integrated to the growth of the market as the proliferation of mints in the later-tenth century indicates." (Hodges 1977, pp.207-8).

Hamwic and other eighth-century ports are viewed as being dependent on a rural surplus "but whether the surplus 'came first' and was therefore available to the traders from other territories bringing prestigious items, or vice versa, is unclear" (ibid. p.209).

Royal centres have been indicated using a variety of evidence, at Eastry (Hawkes 1979), Canterbury, Dorchester-on-Thames (Dickinson 1974), York, Goodmanham, Rendlesham, Hatton Rock (Rahtz 1970), and Winchester, at least four of which have a close relationship with an early port of trade (Fig. 2). The documentary sources reveal how such centres display some of the elements seen earlier in the sixth century rural settlements. The burh at Merantun whose features are deducible from the Anglo-Saxon Chronicler's account of the death of Cynewulf in AD 755, had an outer enclosure with a gate, a hall and small separate buildings, the bowers, which provided night quarters for those of rank, and storage. The only royal palace that has been examined extensively is Yeavering, although others have been discussed on the basis of air photographs. At Yeavering, beside a large timber enclosure of the late sixth century, stood a massive rectangular hall, and subsidiary buildings, some with associated fenced areas, and a timber grandstand (Hope-Taylor 1977).

Whatever their precise role, by the eighth century there were at least three levels of settlement in England: rural settlements presumably principally concerned with food production and supporting, to an increasing extent, the resident population of the ports and the royal centres; food production, commerce and administration. This development emphasizes the self-sufficiency of the rural settlements of fifth- and sixth-century date, with craft production at a local level (e.g. pottery manufacture, cf. Arnold 1981, 1983), except for some prestige trade in luxuries. Movement of products was through a system of redistribution between kin and a limited interchange between territories. By the eighth century such rural settlements may have lost their 'central persons'. Such are Service's 'governors', some of whom have removed themselves to royal sites, and some of the craft specialists have been relocated, and centralized, at the ports of trade. Thus the small rural settlements of the sixth century were largely self-contained, the 'lord' with his 'retainers', with a redistributive form of economy which, at least, becomes dismembered during the seventh to eighth centuries. Is this also a reflection of a move away from the rarity of private ownership of land to the growth of state control? Sawyer has indicated how prior to the eighth century "land held by individuals was thought to belong either to their families or to their lords". Individuals could not make grants of land having only a life interest (1978, p.155). A change appears to have taken place from the seventh century onwards, partly because of a need to give churches permanent rights over land through royal charters. At least, certain sections of the population were gradually freed for full-time specialization, be it craft/industry or administration. Such a redistribution of the population may be reflected in the distribution of wealth. One way in which societies are able, or desire, to accumulate and store wealth, is in the hoarding of precious metal. It is one of the surprising aspects of the period that there is no hoarding until the middle of the seventh century, except in the form of grave-goods which were not intended to be recovered. Hoards, especially of silver coinage, become more frequent from the late seventh century onwards which may be a reflection of the role of the new silver coinage. The removal of the ruling minority from rural settlements to administrative tasks in central places also implies a centralized accumulation of capital and the imposition of taxation or tribute on a more formal basis. The seventh century also sees the start towards the codification of laws and punishment, although kinship as a local institution may have remained immensely strong in ordinary social life. While forms of the kinship structures are visible in late Saxon England, Loyn has argued that the kinship system never fully developed in Anglo-Saxon England (1974).

The centralization of wealth and the wealthier can be seen more directly in the rich graves which are found associated with the royal administrative centres; Cuddesdon with Dorchester-on-Thames, Sutton Hoo with Rendlesham, Winchester, Eastry and the royal Christian graves at Canterbury, and those probably of high rank at such sites as St Paul-in-the Bail, Lincoln. Others are known, principally in Wessex, such as Coombe, Swallowcliffe, Lowbury, Taplow, Broomfield, Asthall. The majority are burials with conspicuous wealth displayed in their grave-goods under large earthen monuments (Vierck 1972; Arnold 1980, p.135; 1982). The role of Christianity in the changes that are being observed is difficult to gauge. The new religion not only caused the redirection of wealth into an alternative system. The construction of churches, at least the sees at Dorchester, Winchester and Canterbury, minster churches, and the earliest rural churches identified at such sites as Wharram Percy, are the first public monumental buildings known in the post-Roman period (except possibly for the numerous post-Roman, but otherwise imprecisely dated, linear earthworks), and are therefore yet another reflection of the centralization of resources and the control of manpower. Inevitably, with their need for patronage, property and protection, churches erected in the seventh century are closely associated with royal centres.

Certain structural changes have been observed in rural settlements over the seventh and eighth centuries; the increasing rarity of the hall-enclosure module as the norm, and the abandonment of many rural settlements at about the same time; an intensification of agriculture in the use of new soil types and possibly new field systems (Arnold and Wardle 1981). Such changes should be reflected in the structure of the pagan cemeteries. Analyses have been published which demonstrate the extent to which the distribution of wealth in early Anglo-Saxon society was markedly disproportionate and was changing through the period (Arnold 1980, 1982). The sixth-century cemeteries suggest increasing wealth and the polarization of levels of wealth; luxury imports may be seen to represent, in social terms, the growing extent of regional control. In the late sixth and early seventh centuries there is a marked reduction in the range and value of grave-goods, and in the overall number of graves in the seventh century. The richest classes of graves in the sixth century are found in the communal cemeteries, but in the seventh century are found isolated from the remainder of the population and contain far greater wealth. Such are the graves, both pagan and Christian, associated spatially with royal sites, symbolizing the growing control over larger territories.

Attempts have been made to relate the evidence of the early cemeteries to the later documented ranks in society, by scholars in England and on the continent (Alcock 1981, Hubener 1977). The methods of analysis, however, have been flexible. Alcock takes the social ranking of early Anglo-Saxon England to have been at three levels, thegns, coerls and free warriors, and links them to three classes of grave identified in the cemeteries of northern England, although ignoring 'rare' graves with many grave-goods. An objective approach to the distribution of wealth in graves reveals a more complex pattern and the rigidness of the social stratification revealed in the earliest law-codes need not have been so apparent in life or directly correlated with wealth (Shephard 1979, Arnold 1980).

The limited number of sources, especially laws and charters, are often difficult to reconcile with each other (Chadwick 1905, Seebohm 1911, Bullough 1965). From the Anglo-Saxon laws, especially those of King Ethelbert of Kent, it would appear that there were a number of classes of person, ranging from the 'slave' (theow) to the unfree or half-free cottagers, freedmen occupying farms and rent-paying tenants (gafolgelda), and also the free farmer (frigman) and landed nobleman (gesith). As a relative scale of position this is probably as close as it can be defined, being based especially on the fines paid by each rank for specific crimes. It is important to note that, by the time the laws were committed to parchment, the distinctions between the ranks were normally made in terms of property holding. The problems encountered in trying to relate wealth grades from pagan cemeteries to the documented rankings may in part be due to the difference in date of the two forms of evidence and the assumption that the Anglo-Saxon society is hierarchical as opposed to continuously stratified. The hierarchical system described by Sawyer (1978, pp.168-9) may have developed out of a less clearly defined system of the fifth to seventh centuries.

To understand the changes that have been observed between the sixth and eighth centuries in more detail, a different form of analysis can be undertaken. It has often been suggested, given the strong kinship ties in early English society, that certain graves in the pagan cemeteries distinguished by their grave furniture and/or structure, may act as a focus for the poorer, less elaborate, graves. Hawkes, for instance, has argued that the cemetery of Finglesham, Kent, began with the burial of an "aristocratic family, and their adherents" represented by "founder's burials, four with exceptionally rich jewellery and weapons" (1977, p.33) ... "We seem to have the principal family, their retainers and servants, but not the whole work-force required to support such an establishment' (ibid. p.35). While this ascribes, perhaps, too small a size and too great a status to the settlement associated with the cemetery, which was not located, it is suggested that: "By c. 600 at latest our upper class family had abandoned the site. Perhaps, they were early converts to Christianity in 596-7 and were therefore buried elsewhere, possibly in the seventh-century Christian cemetery at Eastry itself ... the more numerous graves of the seventh century, though by no means impoverished, tell us that the community was now dominated by a family of lesser wealth and status." (ibid. pp.35-7)

Therein may lie a more general change, the disappearance of the wealthier section of society from rural cemeteries; but is the changing structure of society visible in other cemeteries? That regular patterns may be produced physically in the cemeteries implies a regularity in the way people died or that areas of cemeteries were allocated to groups at an early stage. While there are obvious practical problems such an hypothesis can be examined. The isolation of clusters of graves can be carried out on the basis of the range of types of object in the graves (Fig. 3), and the structure of such groups can thereby be studied. In the predominantly sixth-century cemeteries examined (Figs. 4-8) the groups reveal the wide disparity in wealth distribution with small membership of the many groups, while the majority have few grave-goods. The range of wealth possibly argues against these being family groups. In the seventh century the pattern changes. The overall levels of wealth are much lower, there is far less differentiation on that basis, and the groups are very small (Figs. 9-10). This can hardly be the result of an overall reduction in population as only certain classes are absent. Are we to believe that society was becoming more egalitarian on this road to statehood? The alternative may be to view this as the result of the isolation of the rich and the removal of craftsmen to the central places, leaving subsistence farmers in the countryside. We have seen that the rich graves of the seventh century are found associated with royal sites, which are in close association with ports of trade and where the debris from the activities of craftsmen is to be found in profusion (Fig. 11). Such ports, however, need be no more than a centralization, or formalization of the processes of exchange that had existed earlier.

The implication of this change would be the formation of a politically organized society based on territorial principles as opposed to the earlier one based on kin ties. The establishment of such territories may in part be seen as the result of recurring aggression documented between the various 'kingdoms'. This activity was most commonly carried out by the kingdoms of Mercia and Wessex, taking the form of either the annexation of smaller groups, or frequent attacks on the stronger groups. Such aggression shows signs of giving way to statesmanship in the late seventh century. Thus the integration of early state modules in early Anglo-Saxon England takes place as the result of aggression for the control of access to resources. The details of this process are not clear, as the Anglo-Saxon Chronicle and Bede concentrated on the major groups whose relationship to the smallest groups is unclear. But we should not expect the process of integration to proceed uniformly.

A glimpse of the complexity of the social organization of middle Saxon England is given by the document known as the Tribal Hidage, in which a variety of groups are distinguished even when they are recorded elsewhere as having already been annexed (Davies and Vierck 1974).

A synthetic approach to the matter of state formation is most successful in establishing effects; causes may continue to elude us. The role of a growing population is hard to assess but may be crucial. The two most apparent elements in the data are wealth and power, whose importance grows with centralization and specialization. It was perhaps inevitable in early Anglo-Saxon England that social change would be brought about by the increasing wealth of a minority, a wealth that could only be achieved with power. We lack the catalyst. A growth in population would have necessitated an intensification in agriculture and in technology, and any moves towards mass-production and commercial activity would have required control and administration, emphasizing the role of kingship. The wealthy class's desire for luxuries must have been a major incentive for the regularization of international trade; intensification and specialization ultimately require a market to maximize efficiency. The maintenance of power implies the production of surplus and a change that it is suggested took place was from the self-contained rural settlement in which a surplus was produced for the maintenance of leaders, to that of a system of taxation in which a surplus was provided more formally.

The establishment of the Germanic states in western and central continental Europe on the ruins of the Roman Empire marked the beginnings of a new social order. This still contained elements of tribal structure, but there was an increasing emphasis on class hierarchy which was to lead eventually to aristocracy and feudalism. The developments on the Continent are very similar to those traced for Anglo-Saxon England, albeit within a stronger framework of 'Romanitas'.

The prosperity of many of the Roman towns in the Frankish kingdom was ultimately due to the presence of early Merovingian kings, whose presence is emphasized by the Merovingian basilicas with cemeteries for the nobility which date from the beginning of the sixth century. During the Roman period the forts and urban settlements served as centres for large rural areas which were the source of the food supply, but in the Frankish period the manor developed as the basis of economic and social life. The structure of surviving Roman towns was greatly changed in consequence (Janssen 1976). Great royal palaces developed in Paris and Mainz, and in their respective nearby manors of St. Denys and Ingelheim. Manors were also built within surviving Roman towns (which might also serve as a model for Canterbury) and determined the further development of the Medieval towns.

On the Continent also, developments in the settlement hierarchy can be paralleled with changes in the composition of cemeteries. The complete structure of Frankish society is indicated by the range of grave-goods in accompaniment, and Hubener has attempted to link such structure with that which is documented (1977). In many cemeteries, as at Krefeld-Gellep, the oldest grave in particular areas of a cemetery is very rich, such wealth being equated with high social rank. That successors buried in the cemeteries are accorded the same burial ritual, suggests that small groups of people retained the role of chieftain within a settlement or region for several generations. The common pattern, therefore, in Frankish cemeteries, as at Rubenach and Schretzheim, is of wealthier graves distributed about the cemeteries representing the various phases of its use. This ruling elite is most clearly separated from the rest of society where its graves are not in the communal cemetery, but form either a group on their edge or are totally removed, as with the well known royal graves of Childeric at Tournai, Morken, and those of Cologne and St. Denys. In Frankia, therefore, the graves of the 'governors' are distinguished by the range and quality of the grave-goods and by the location and structure of the grave itself.

The role of the towns in the Frankish kingdom during the fourth to sixth centuries depended on the survival of important ancient 'projects' in preserving some central functions. It is not possible to consider the urban layouts inherited from antiquity as having an absolute character (Roslanowski 1976). At Trier, for instance, only ten per cent of the walled area was utilized at this time, and the inhabitants from the social and legal point of view did not differ in any essential detail from their country neighbours (Schindler 1976).

The important changes which occurred in Frankish towns were brought about by the church, particularly the cathedral and also by the residences of the royal palatia or lay dignitaries. To these political and religious functions were added economic ones, both in terms of trade and production, and being organized on dominial principles did not absolutely need the agency of markets. They made possible, however, considerable surpluses of agricultural produce and craft manufactures which were introduced into trade, and this stimulated the emergence and functioning of markets. This economic development was coupled with the general maturing of feudal-type structures and the accompanying political transformation. Under the Carolingians such factors were favourable to the consolidation of the control authority, but also strengthened the role of the residences of various intermediary ranks. Later there was a tendency towards decentralization which in practice meant the forming of seigneurial authorities and with them, of numerous centres fulfilling central functions of a lower rank. The additional pressures of the ninth-tenth centuries, Viking and Hungarian raids, became an important though not autonomous catalyst of these spatial mutations. They stimulated at least some extension of the threatened urban centres, especially defence facilities and thus contributed to the creation of compact settlements also in areas previously weakly urbanized.

On the other hand, the trading emporia on the North Sea and Baltic had different socio-topographical characteristics, comparable to those on the English Channel. They had many craftsmen as residents and their socio-economic functions clearly dominated the less developed layout.

At whatever time states can be said to have existed in north west Europe, the process of change as society moved in that direction, is becoming clearer. A few of the more relevant changes can be isolated: increasing differentiation by wealth closely associated with the control of the movement of exotic luxuries, made possible by the growing need for decision-making by a minority; the emergence of royal power and administration in areas successful in acquiring luxury goods and with a sound subsistence base, and latterly in areas acting aggressively against their neighbours; increasing stratification in society with the appearance of agriculturalists, craftsmen and administrators as distinct groups and a settlement pattern which reflects this stratification; this phase broke down with the growth in power of officials, whose increasing properties developed into lordships, territorial principalities. Such independent lords began to exercise the rights of owners of land as well as the right to command and punish. Thus, taking over from public authorities and collecting the revenues, they became territorial lords.

BIBLIOGRAPHY

ADDYMAN, P.V. 1964 - "A Dark-Age settlement at Maxey, Northants", Medieval Archaeology vol. 7, pp.20-73.

ADDYMAN, P.V. 1972 - "Late Saxon settlements in the St. Neots area: III. The village or township at St. Neots", Proceedings of the Cambridge Antiquarian Society vol. 64, pp.45-100.

ADDYMAN, P.V. and HILL, D.H. 1968 - "Saxon Southampton: a review of the evidence", Proceedings of the Hampshire Field Club and Archaeological Society vol. 25, pp.61-93.

ADDYMAN, P.V. and HILL, D.H. 1969 - "Saxon Southampton: a review of the evidence Pt. 2", Proceedings of the Hampshire Field Club and Archaeological Society vol. 26, pp.61-96.

ALCOCK, L. 1981 - "Quantity or quality: the Anglian graves of Bernicia" in Angles, Saxons and Jutes (Ed.) V.I. Evison, Oxford, pp.168-86.

ARNOLD, C.J. 1980 - "Wealth and social structure: a

matter of life and death" in Anglo-Saxon Cemeteries 1979 (Eds.) P. Rahtz, T. Dickinson and L. Watts (BAR 82), Oxford, pp.81-142.

ARNOLD, C.J. 1981 - "Early Anglo-Saxon Pottery: production and distribution" in Production and Distribution: a Ceramic Viewpoint (Eds.) H. Howard and E.L. Morris (BAR International Ser. 120), Oxford, pp.243-255.

ARNOLD, C.J. 1982 - "Stress as a stimulus for socioeconomic change: Anglo-Saxon England in the seventh century" in Ranking, Resource and Exchange (Eds.) S. Shennan and C. Renfrew, Cambridge, pp.124-31.

ARNOLD, C.J. 1983 - "The Sancton-Baston Potter", Scottish Archaeological Review, 1983, pp.17-30.

ARNOLD, C.J. and WARDLE, P. 1981 - "Early Anglo-Saxon settlement patterns in England", Medieval Archaeology vol. 25, pp.145-49.

BULLOUGH, R.A. 1965 - "Anglo-Saxon Institutions and Early English society" Annali della Fondazione Italiana per la Storia Administrativa vol. 2, pp.647-59.

CHADWICK, H.M. 1905 - Studies in Anglo-Saxon Institutions. Cambridge.

CHAMPION, T.C. 1977 - "Chalton", Current Archaeology, vol. 59, pp.364-69.

CLAESSEN, H.J.M. 1978 - "The Early State: a structural approach" in The Early State (Eds.) H.J.M. Claessen and P. Skalnik, The Hague, pp.533-96.

CLAESSEN, H.J.M. and SKALNIK, P. 1978 - - The Early State. The Hague.

DAVIES, W. and VIERCK, H. 1974 - "The contexts of Tribal Hidage: social aggregates and settlement patterns" Fruhmittelalterliche Studien vol. 8, pp.223-93.

DICKINSON, T. 1974 - Cuddesdon and Dorchester-on-Thames (BAR 1). Oxford.

EVISON, V.I. 1979 - Wheel-thrown pottery in Anglo-Saxon graves. London.

GRIERSON, P. 1959 - "Commerce in the Dark Ages: a critique of the evidence" Transactions of the Royal Historical Society (5th Ser.) vol. 9, pp.123-40.

HAARNAGEL, VAN W. 1961 - "Zur Grabung auf der Feddersen Wierde 1955-1959" Germania vol. 39, pp.42-69.

HAWKES, S.C. 1977 - "Orientation at Finglesham: sunrise dating of death and burial in an Anglo-Saxon cemetery in East Kent" Archaeologia Cantiana vol. 92, pp.33-51.

HAWKES, S.C. 1979 - "Eastry in Anglo-Saxon Kent: its importance and a newly found grave" in Anglo-Saxon Studies vol. 1 (BAR 72). Oxford, pp.81-114.

HEDEAGER, L. 1979a - "A quantitative analysis of Roman imports in Europe north of the Limes (0-400 AD), and the question of Roman-Germanic exchange" Studies in Scandinavian Prehistory and Early History vol. 1, pp.191-216.

HEDEAGER, L. 1979b - "Processes towards state formation in early Iron Age Denmark" Studies in Scandinavian Prehistory anbd Early History vol. 1, pp.217-23.

HEDEAGER, L. 1980 - "Besiedlung, soziale Struktur und politische Organisation in der alteren und jungeren römischen Kaiserzeit Ostdänemarks" Präehistorische Zeitschrift vol. 55, pp.38-109.

HODGES, R. 1977 - "Trade and urban origins in Dark Age England" Bericht der Rijksdienst Oudheidkundig Bodemonderz 27, pp.191-215.

HODGES, R. 1978 - "State formation and the role of trade in Middle Saxon England" in Social Organization and Settlement (Eds.) D. Green, C. Haselgrove and M. Spriggs (BAR International Ser. 47, ii). Oxford, pp.439-53.

HODGES, R. 1982a - Dark Age Trade: the origins of towns and trade A.D. 600-1000. London.

HODGES, R. 1982b - "The evolution of gateway communities: their socio-economic implications" in Ranking, resource and exchange (Eds.) S. Shennan and C. Renfrew. Cambridge, pp.117-23.

HOLDSWORTH, P. 1977 - "Saxon Southampton: a new review" Medieval Archaeology vol. 20, pp.26-61.

HOLDSWORTH, P. 1980 - Excavations at Melbourne Street, Southampton 1971-76 (CBA Res. Rep. 33) London.

HOPE-TAYLOR, B. 1977 - Yeavering: an Anglo-British centre of early Northumbria. London.

HUBENER, W. 1977 - "Waffenarmen und Bewaffnungstypen der Frühen Merowingerzeit" Fundberichte Aus Baden-Württemberg vol. 3, pp.62-88.

JANSSEN, W. 1976 - "Some major aspects of Frankish and Medieval settlement in the Rhineland" in Medieval Settlement (Ed.) P. Sawyer. London, pp.41-60.

LOSCO-BRADLEY, P. 1977 - "Catholme" Current Archaeology vol. 59, p.358-63.

LOYN, H.R. 1974 - "Kinship in Anglo-Saxon England" Anglo-Saxon England vol. 3, pp.197-209.

MILLETT, M. 1980 - Excavations at Cowdery's Down, Basingstoke: Interim Report. Basingstoke.

MILLETT, M. 1981 - Excavations at Cowdery's Down, Basingstoke: Interim Report. Basingstoke.

PARKER, H. 1965 - "Feddersen Wierde and Vallhager: a contrast in settlements" Medieval Archaeology vol. 9. pp.1-10.

RAHTZ, P. 1970 - "A possible Saxon palace near Stratford-on-Avon" Antiquity vol. 44, pp.137-43.

RENFREW, A.C. 1975 - "Trade as action at a distance: questions of integration and communication" in Ancient Civilization and Trade (Eds.) J.A. Sabloff and C.C. Lamberg-Karlovsky. Albuquerque, pp.3-60.

RENFREW, A.C. 1982 - "Post-collapse resurgence: culture process in the Dark Ages" in Ranking, Resource and exchange (Eds.) S. Shennan and C. Renfrew. Cambridge, pp.113-6.

RIGOLD, S.E. 1977 - "The principal series of English Sceattas" British Numismatic Journal vol. 47, pp.21-30.

ROSLANOWSKI, T. 1976 - "Comparative Sociotopography on the example of early medieval towns in central Europe" Acta Poloniae Historica vol. 34, pp.7-28.

SAWYER, P.H. 1978 - From Roman Britain to Norman England. London.

SCHINDLER, R. 1976 - Trier in merowingischer Zeit. Berlin.

SEEBOHM, F. 1911 - Tribal Customs in Anglo-Saxon Law. London.

SERVICE, E.R. 1978 - "Classical and Modern theories of the origins of government" in Origins of the State (Eds.) R. Cohen and E.R. Service, Philadelphia, pp.21-34.

SHEPHARD, J.F. 1979 - "The social identity of the individual in isolated barrows and barrow cemeteries in Anglo-Saxon England" in Space, Hierarchy and Society (Eds.) B.C. Burnham and J. Kingsbury (BAR International Ser. 59) Oxford, pp. 47-80.

THOMPSON, E.A. 1965 - The Early Germans. Oxford.

TODD, M. 1977 - "Germanic burials in the Roman Iron Age" in Burial in the Roman World (Ed.) R. Reece. London, pp.39-43.

VAN ES, W.A. 1967 - "Wijster: a native village beyond the Imperial frontier 150-425 AD" Palaeohistoria vol. 11.

VIERCK, H. 1972 - "Redwalds Asche" Offa vol. 29, pp.2-49.

WEST, S.E. 1969 - "The Anglo-Saxon Village of West Stow: an interim report of the excavations" Medieval Archaeology vol. 13, pp.1-20.

WEST, S.E. 1978 - "Die Siedlung West Stow in Suffolk" in Sachsen und Angel-sachsen (Ed.) C. Ahrens. Hamburg, pp.395-412.

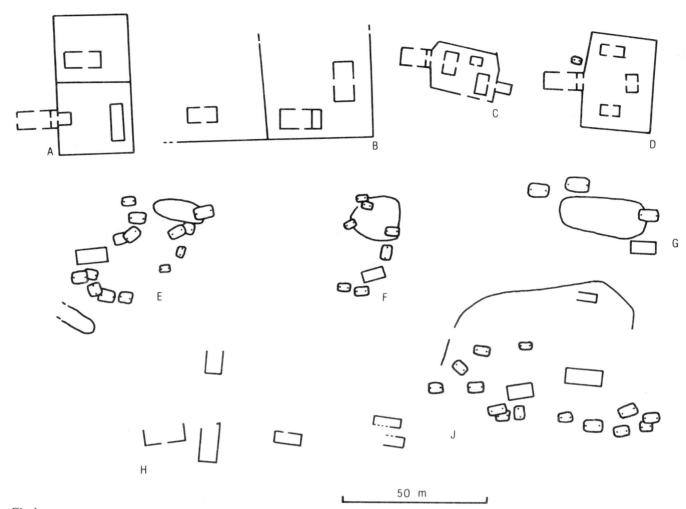

Fig 1
Plans of early Anglo-Saxon farm modules isolated from settlement plans. A, B Cowdery's Down, Hampshire; C, D Chalton, Hampshire; E, F, G, J West Stow, Suffolk; H Maxey.

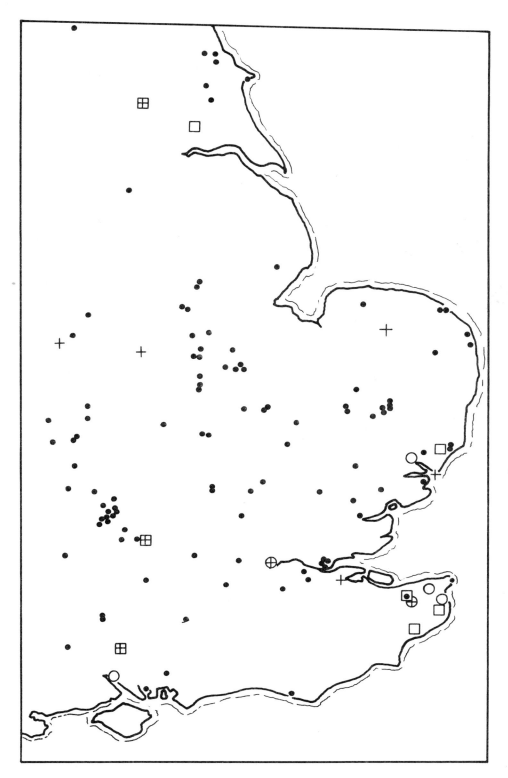

Fig 2
Distribution of early Anglo-Saxon settlement types. Black dots, rural settlements. Open Squares, royal 'palaces'. Open circles, ports of trade. Crosses, episcopal sees.

286

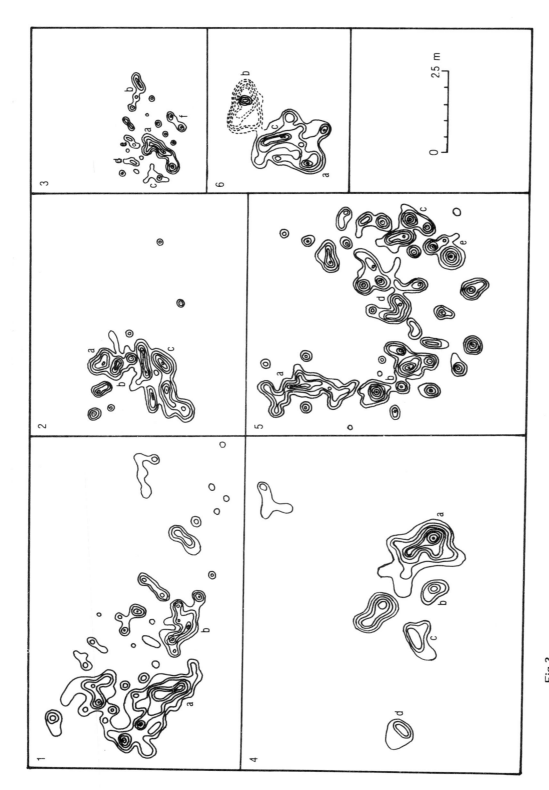

Fig 3
Clusters of graves in early Anglo-Saxon cemeteries established by range of types of objects. 1 Polhill, Kent; 2 Petersfinger, Wiltshire; 3 Winnall II, Hampshire; 4 Collingbourne Ducis, Wiltshire; 5 Alfriston, Sussex; 6 Lyminge, Kent. For details of lettered clusters, see Figs 4-10.

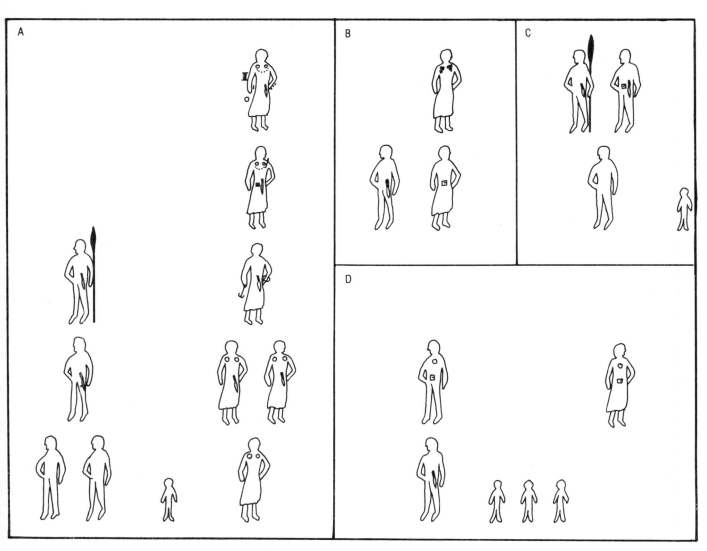

287

Fig 4
Colllingbourne Ducis, Wiltshire.

288

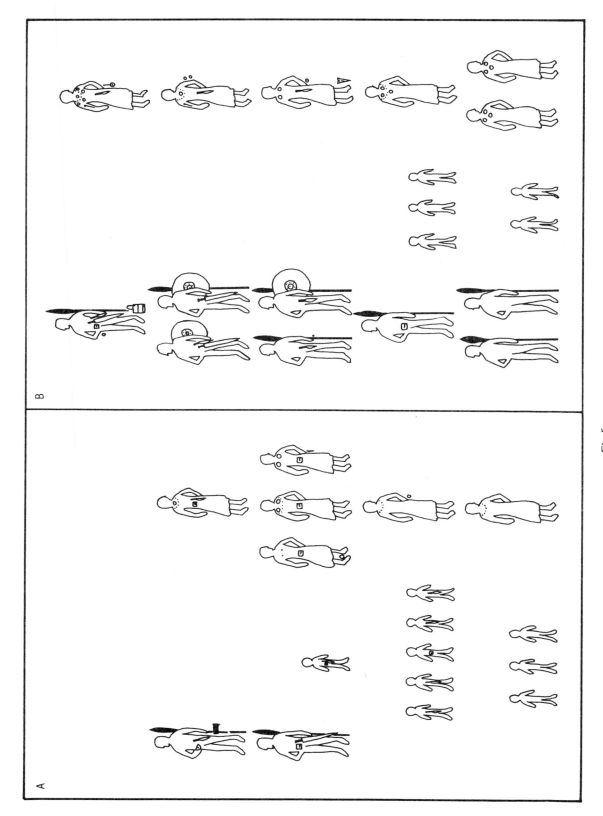

Fig 5
Alfriston, Sussex.

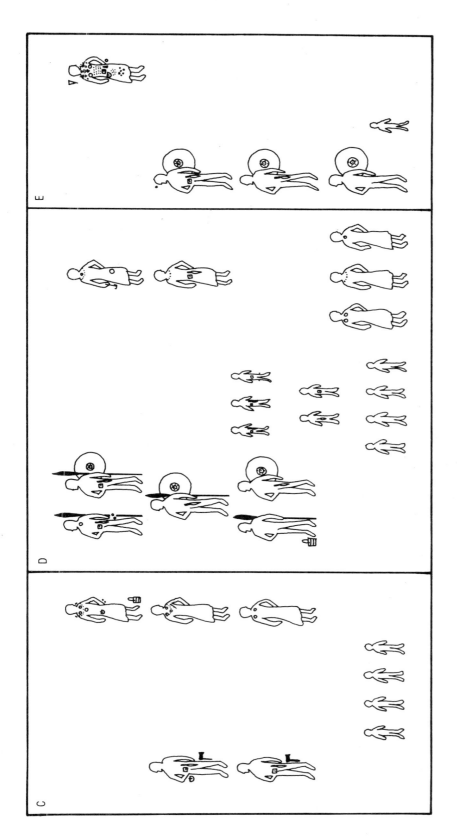

Fig 6
Alfriston, Sussex.

290

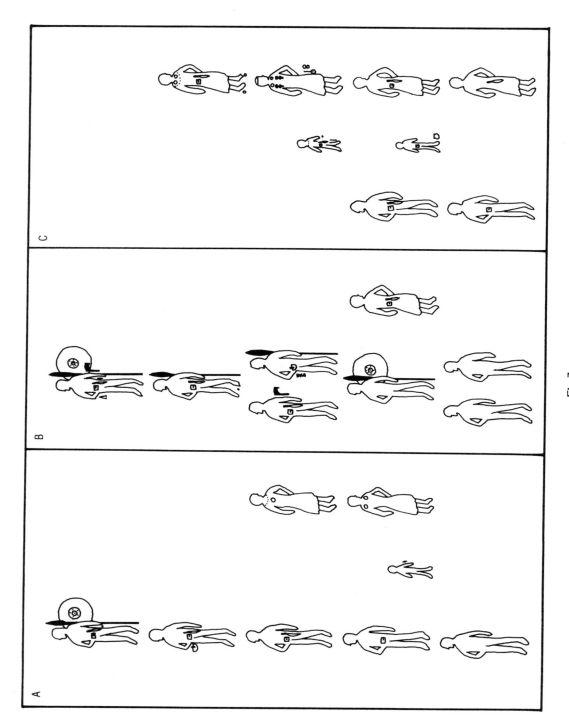

Fig 7
Lyminge, Kent.

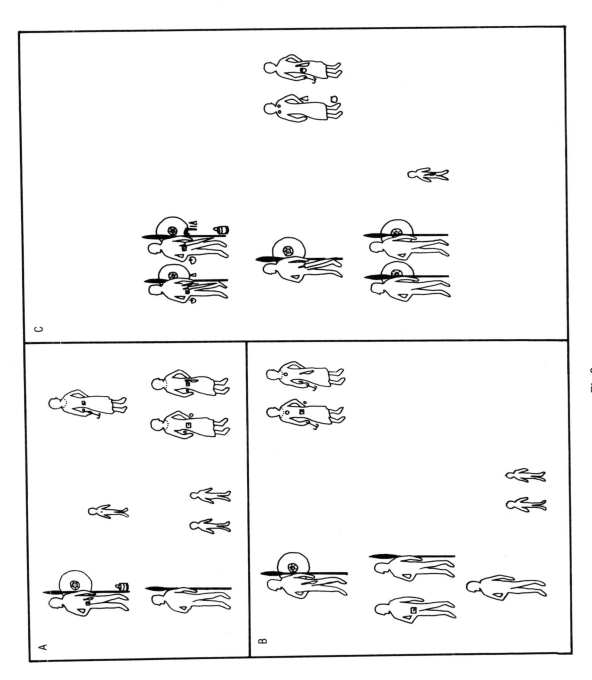

Fig 8
Petersfinger, Wiltshire.

292

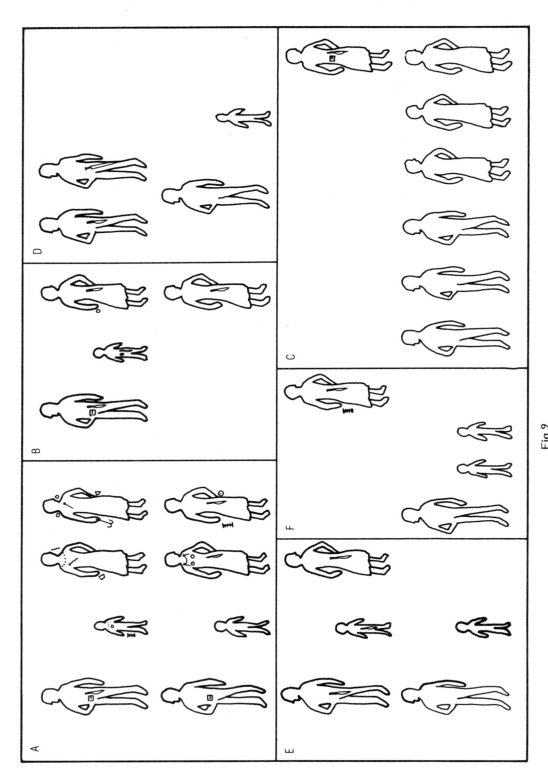

Fig 9
Winnall II, Hampshire.

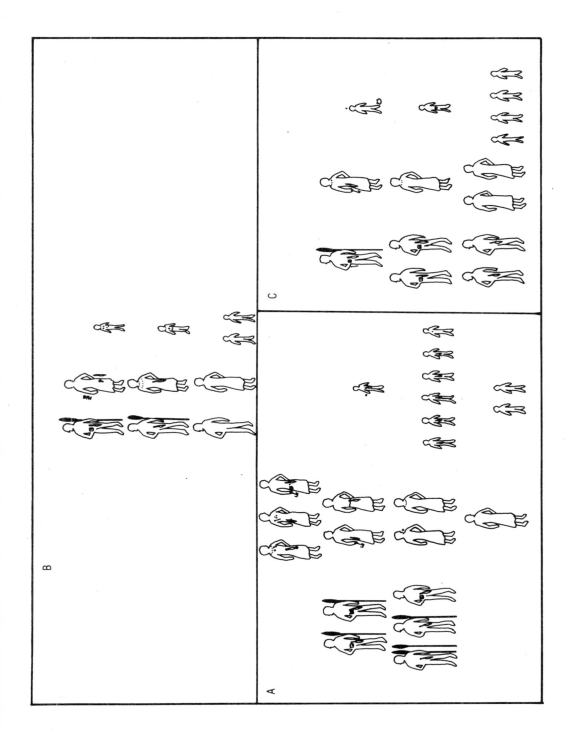

Fig 10
Polhill, Kent.

293

294

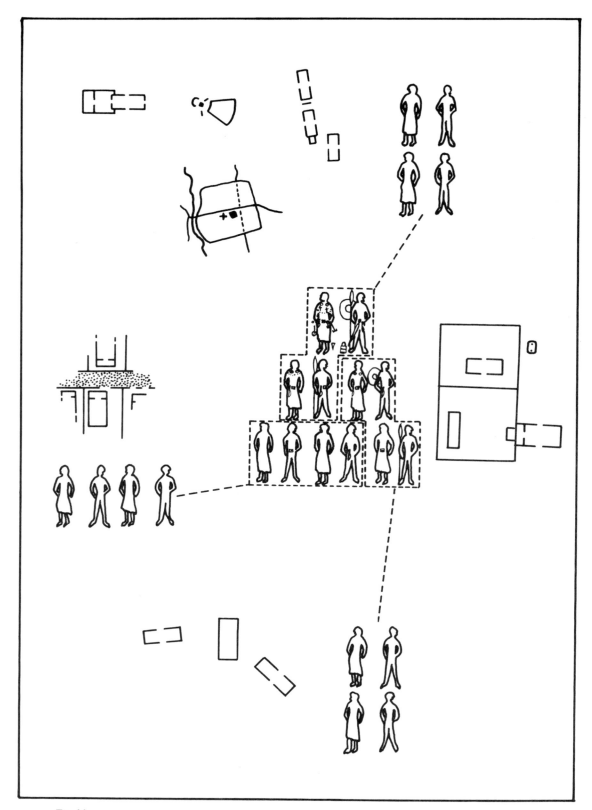

Fig 11
Diagram illustrating proposed evolution in early Anglo-Saxon social and settlement hierarchies.

VIKING SOCIETY: CHANGES ON THE FRINGES OF EUROPE

Klavs Randsborg

The study of the Vikings

The study of the Vikings in their Scandinavian homelands was originally a purely historical occupation.[1] The written historical data about the Vikings 'at home' are scant, however, as far as contemporary sources are concerned. The manifest idea that we possess a detailed knowledge is due to the Norse sagas which were written down in the high Middle Ages, several hundred years after the Viking Age, and based on an oral tradition given a novel-like character. In addition, the sagas mainly deal with Iceland, a marginal Scandinavian area where the economic and social development did not correspond to the profound transformations that Danish society, for instance, was undergoing during the Viking Age (about AD 800-1050). The contemporary texts of the Viking Age are all foreign, in the main West European, and only in the lapidaric inscriptions of Scandinavian runestones, which are memorials to high ranking personages, do we meet the Vikings directly.

Traditional research on the Vikings has drawn heavily on the historical sources while archaeology, in spite of its growing role - and data - has rather supplied the 'illustrations' as in Sawyer (1971). Characteristically the general studies of the age have concentrated on political and cultural issues like kingship, the role of the Vikings in Russia, Scandinavian placenames, or arts and ornaments. In particular, the Viking Age and its institutions are seen in retrospect from the Middle Ages, and usually an integrated socio-economic view is lacking (e.g. Foote et al. 1970). Where the latter is present, as in a number of Marxist works, (e.g. Anderson 1974), only disjunctive historical sources are applied. In the past one hundred years, and especially during the last decades, archaeology has added considerably to our factual knowledge and the field has moved towards a study of social dynamics from that of culture. A modern appraisal of the Vikings, from subsistence and social structure to trade, raids and colonization, must therefore bring the archaeological data into focus and relate these, and the other information to a body of theory about society dealing with structural relationships and changes. However, theories of society are only guidelines for thought and it is logically possible to view the same data from several angles. An inherent danger when discussing single cases, like the Viking Age, is the temptation of reifying findings if a relation is established between a particular explanation and the data. In the present context an evolutionary approach is, after all, found appropriate and may serve to illuminate some of the major economic and social changes that the Viking Age experienced, especially in the areas closest to the more developed societies in Western Europe. It is exactly in the interface between a local development and changing relations to the outside world that the conspicuous events of the Viking Age should be seen. To survey the entire Scandinavian area plus the Atlantic 'colonies' and the areas in England and other places under Viking rule or influence, would be too difficult and therefore Denmark, with its significant development and central geographical position, is chosen to pilot this paper. This does reduce our horizon. However, the social evolution of Danish society exemplifies well the Scandinavian transformation and its archaeological vestiges. At the end of the paper we shall briefly consider the 'Viking phenomenon' in general.

Social transformations of the Viking Age in Denmark

In Denmark the Early Iron Age (500 BC to AD 400) by and large corresponds to a climatic optimum phase of relatively warm (and dry) weather (Randsborg 1980, p.45 ff.). In the third century AD, however, there begins a phase of cooling, culminating around AD 500, while at the beginning of the Viking Age proper, at around AD 800, warm weather is back, lasting until the fourteenth century AD where the Late Medieval climatic and agrarian crisis starts. Periods of good weather see expansion of settlement and a relatively large population, while periods of poorer weather conditions correspond to population decline due to insufficient nutrition and diseases like the Black Death. The recession periods also witness a return to more extensive forms of subsistence with, for instance, heavier stress on the raising of cattle. However, the population was overall on a track of general increase causing a sharp rise in the growing of cereals at the end of the first millennium AD where animal husbandry lost in importance; the domesticated animals actually grew smaller due to poorer nutrition except for horses which were kept for military purposes and, especially, for drawing the new types of ploughs, (among them perhaps, the mould-board plough), which were becoming common during the Viking Age. This shift to a labour-intensive landed economy would, in itself, lead to stricter norms of inheritance and more interference on the local level by the larger socio-political and judicial system. To accommodate such needs the society will turn more complex, which is exactly what happened during the Viking Age in Denmark. Also in the regulation of settlements and in the expansion of private property rights we detect the influence and the politics of the Viking kings and magnates. The interest of the rulers in subsistence is exemplified by the cache of high quality rye found in the tenth-century royal fortress at Fyrkat in north Jutland (Helbaek 1977).

The rye came from south Poland or the Ukraine and was possibly seed-corn.

Early Iron Age villages are often large but the farmsteads are identical in layout in spite of differences in size (e.g. Hvass 1975; Randsborg 1980, p.59 ff.; 1982). Towards the end of the Early Iron Age small farms seem to disappear while the remaining farmsteads grow considerably in size. The main long-houses are now divided into several rooms with different functions and the very size of the units implies the existence of a number of servants or, perhaps, an extended family. (Earlier farms seem to have been occupied by nucleated families). This picture is still valid at the beginning of the Viking Age although we can clearly recognize both large and normal sized farms. In the late Viking Age, however, there are a number of very large farmsteads alongside the ones of standard size (Hvass 1979; Nielsen 1979; Stoumann 1979; Jørgensen and Skov 1979). These magnate farms occur in the same settlements as the other farms and thus reveal a difference in access to land, and in living standards, not seen earlier among the primary producers. Along the perimeter of the fenced crofts lie a number of buildings with different functions, stables, workshops, living quarters etc. In the middle of the croft is a splendid hall, primarily the living quarters of the owner, rivalled only by the royal fortresses. From this period onwards the memorial runestones speak of bailiffs, agents or managers of land, indicating the developed form of private ownership of land. We are now dealing with a true social stratification in terms of access to the primary resources.

But it would be unfortunate to consider the social developments of the Danish Viking Age exclusively in the framework of the landed economy and its organization. The transformation of society was more than a question of the mentioned changes which in part are broadly dated to the Viking period, in part started at the time of the first true state and continued into the High Middle Ages as for example the alterations of the settlement system (Grøngard Jeppesen 1981). In fact, some of the characteristics and institutions making up the first state - founded in western Denmark in the tenth century - and certainly present in the corporate state of Denmark at AD 1000 predate the significant alterations of the settlement. I am referring in particular to intensive foreign relations, either in the form of long distance trade or warfare with concomitant establishment of ports and markets, cross-country defences and royal command of large military forces. The regulation of ports and towns was a royal prerogative securing large tax-incomes, and the ultimate spread of towns and cities (with regional markets) across the country is closely linked to the state-system of politics, rights and ownership (cf. Hodges 1982, p.162 ff.). The Christian church gradually entered this structure, especially after the royal acceptance of Christianity as the state religion in the mid-tenth century, and carefully linked up the bishoprics with the larger towns. At this stage Denmark was in its Middle Ages.

Two hundred or more years before, the country, still organized in a traditional way, witnessed the engulfing of its southern neighbours, the Saxons, by the Frankish Empire under Charlemagne who pushed its borders towards the Ejder river at the foot of Jutland (cf. Annales Francorum). A series of dangerous situations for the Danes, for example an assault by the Frankish land army was countered in various ways, including attacks on the Frankish allies among the western Slavs on the Baltic, raids on the coast of Franconia (which may have had other reasons also) and the construction of a wall of defence - one of the Danevirke walls (Andersen et al. 1976) - across Jutland to the north of the river Ejder, but to the south of the important emporium of Hedeby (Jankuhn 1976). Hedeby was a transit station between the North Sea area and the Baltic, brought under close Danish control by the wall system and in fact registered and regulated in those very years. According to the Frankish Annals King Godfred built the ruler-straight wall, with only one gate, probably to ease the collection of tolls, and was supported by Danes from both west and east in crucial situations. In this period Danish kings also exercised some power in southern Norway, among the north western Slavs (on the Baltic) and on the coast of Frisia. In the early ninth century the Franks had to use diplomacy and interference with dynastic politics in Denmark to cope with their northern neighbours. In the middle of the ninth century the Danes were raiding the coasts of France and England in increasing numbers (cf. Fig. 2). However, in the same decades Danish kings permitted the first mission churches to be built in the ports of Hedeby and Ribe (in south west Jutland). These events inform us of the existence of a number of magnates (including members of royal lineages) and of royal officials (army leaders, commanders of the border provinces, counts of towns etc.) and we find disclosed parts of the social infra-structure which archaeology alone could not have exposed.

The runestones of the ninth century, for instance, include a few examples of the usual type: 'X raised this monument over Y', significantly a male linked to another male person (Randsborg 1980, p.25 ff.). This supports the interpretation 'X inherited Y's property (or land)' which is sometimes mentioned specifically. The status of the deceased may, of course, also be inherited. Later this type becomes absolute but in the ninth century most stones carry only one name, probably that of an owner of property, and are otherwise characterized rather by magic elements in the texts. Before about AD 800 runestones are unknown in Denmark and their very appearance may signal changes in the social structure of the country. More important, the difference in text between earlier and later monuments clearly separates the early Viking Age from the later one which sees the coming of state-type societies. The early runestones of the ninth century supply titles like 'chief' (of a local area) and cluster, incidentally, in the population medians of the country which may have experienced more social stress than marginal areas.

Denying the early societies the status of 'state' we stress the lack of continuity between the political establishments of the ninth and of the tenth century. In the ninth century much dynastic fighting is reported while there is no indication of a permanent administration. This corresponds to the period of raids and other operations of a large number of Danish 'kings' in western Europe. The supreme kings or 'warlords' may, however, have been in the process of gaining new incomes from trade and taxation of trade at the same time as their military following was probably larger than earlier due to the severe pressures on the area.

In the tenth century the runestones were all of the succession or transfer of property type: 'X raised this monument over Y'. Geographically they cluster in western Denmark, the area of the Jelling dynasty that supplied rulers like Harald and his grandson Canute who at the beginning of the eleventh century conquered England. Jelling was a royal estate and burial ground in mid-Jutland. The most prominent of these runestones comes from Jelling proper, king Harald's stone over his parents, 'that Harald who' - according to the stone - 'won over himself all of Denmark and Norway and made the Danes Christians'. The control of Norway was hardly real and this casts a rather oblique light on the wording of the Danish supremacy. Considering the distribution of the runestones, and outlining the provinces with many non-traditional examples of transfer of property, and two significant types of burial, which can be related to the establishment of the Jelling dynasty, we propose that Harald's realm, in a strict sense, was only the western part of Denmark. This does not, however, preclude the possibility that, perhaps according to older norms, he was also hailed as supreme king by larger areas by AD 960, the approximate date of the stone.

The above mentioned two types of west Danish graves comprise a group of cavalry burials in a belt around Jelling, up to 150kms. from the centre (Randsborg 1980, p.126 ff.; 1981b) (Fig. 1). This belt also houses the large, excellently built fortresses of Trelleborg type and the Danevirke walls on the German frontier which were strengthened in the same period. The cavalry graves indicate new social positions, obviously of warrior type and related to the Jelling dynasty, since weapons traditionally were passed on to the heir at the death of their owner and for seven or eight hundred years now had not been common in the graves of Denmark. The other type of grave is female burial in a carriage (without wheels) (Randsborg 1980, p.129 ff.; 1981b). One of these appeared in the huge, so-called 'North Mound' at Jelling, probably holding Queen Thyra, the mother of Harald. A similar grave from Jutland was found beneath an early stave-church as a kind of founder's tomb, illustrating the words on King Harald's stone about the acceptance of Christianity (Krogh et al. 1961). By this acceptance the lords of the western part of Denmark separated themselves ideologically from the rest of Scandinavia but met some of the German pressures effectively. The German emperor had, for instance, nominated bishops for the Danish towns of Hedeby, Ribe and Arhus, all in Jutland, a few years earlier, in AD 948, and German military attacks are reported for the years AD 934 and 974 (a German nomination of a bishop for the town of Odense on the island of Funen is mentioned for AD 988).

Compared with the situation of the ninth century we are inclined to call King Harald's realm by c. AD 960 a 'state'. We have clear indications, for instance from titles on the runestones, of a firm royal establishment with a number of 'vassals' for lower level control, not only in towns and at the borders, but also settled among the general population. We have royal fortresses and fortifications, large bridges and other works to improve control and communication (Olsen et al. 1977, Roesdahl 1977, Andersen et al. 1976). (A two-lane bridge carrying the road to Jelling is almost one kilometre long; Ramskou 1980). By the year 1000, however, the Jelling dynasty had 'broken' its border belt and extended firm political control to the eastern parts of Denmark, exemplified by the spread of contemporary runestones (Randsborg 1980, p.30, Fig. 6). These late stones seem to denote a kind of military settlement and are perhaps also referrable to the late campaigns in England. Significantly, the minting of King Canute (the grandson of Harald) was in the main an eastern phenomenon (Randsborg 1980, p.74, Fig. 19).

By the beginning of the second millennium AD towns were found in all provinces and served as local centres at a time when long distance trade seems to have dwindled (cf. Randsborg 1980, p.71 ff.; Hodges 1982, p.177 ff.). This development took off with the royal founding of the towns of Aarhus in Jutland and Odense on Funen (an old pagan centre) in the tenth century. Roskilde on the island of Zealand and Lund in Scania were founded around AD 1000 and, in the eleventh century Viborg and Aalborg in Jutland were functioning in much the same way as the other cities to which should be added Hedeby (Slesvig) and Ribe, the ancient ports of trade from the period around AD 800. Also minor towns are known, but it is noteworthy, with the tenth-century situation in mind, that the political centre (Jelling) was lying, not in or near any of the towns, but like a spider, in an optimal position at the junction of the catchment-areas of a number of towns,

near the north-south highroad though Jutland (Fig. 1). To the west was the cattle and sheep land, to the east the heavy clay-soils and forested regions apt for pigs. The eastern provinces were to become central from the Viking Age onwards with their great potential for the growing of cereals. We will not, however return to the discussion of the subsistence economy, but turn to the world outside Viking Denmark to which the country, like other Scandinavian regions, was closely linked, first and foremost through trade and warfare.

The outside world

Viking warfare, apart from its archaeological expression (finds of weapons, fortifications etc.), is known in the main from written historical sources. They tell little about conditions in Scandinavia but record in detail the miseries that the Norsemen inflicted on the west. Viking long distance trade is also mentioned in the historical record but less detailed than the raids and campaigns that were politically more interesting. Archaeologically, trade and other kinds of exchange are manifested in finds of foreign artifacts, coins etc.; the silver hoards of Scandinavia have proved to be an especially rich source for tracing the fluctuations of trade abroad. The changes in silver and gold wealth are remarkable and we must reckon with strong pressures on the ruling elites during periods of recession, when payments for military and other services would have to cease or be found in other ways, like payment in kind.

The early ninth century sees much exchange and the silver stock is relatively large (Randsborg 1980, p.137 ff.). This is the period of the Frankish attacks on Denmark and the registration of the port of Hedeby where the first Nordic minting took place. The ports of Birka in Sweden (near Stockholm) and Kaupang in southern Norway start in this same period. On the grand international level, Scandinavia, previously a backwater, found itself at one end of a world economic trading system that stretched all the way from China. This led to a significant injection of cash into the economies of the north. Some time in the 780s a regular trade route was set up for the first time linking Scandinavia and the Near East (cf. Lombard 1971): Vikings bearing furs, slaves, iron weapons etc. travelled by boat along the broad rivers of central Russia, the Don, the Dnieper and, most important, the Volga to trading cities at the river mouths such as Sarkel, a gate to the Black Sea and the Byzantine Empire, and Itil on the Caspian. There the Vikings met merchants, notably Jewish ones, who opened up trade with the Near East and even with Africa, India, China and the Far East. Islamic, and some Byzantine silver flowed through Russia into Scandinavia and from there into Western Europe. The Scandinavians seemingly acquired silver (in the main Arabic) from the east and goods from the west. The petty Scandinavian courts also received exotic goods such as silk and peacocks from these distant lands along the trade routes, as did other rulers. Haroun-al-Raschid, for example, the Caliph of Bagdad of the 'Arabian Nights', sent an elephant to Charlemagne, the Frankish Emperor. (The elephant actually died of flu when brought north to participate in the fighting against the Danes).

Before the middle of the ninth century, however, the surplus silver stock drops drastically due to the decline in long-distance trade which affected many ports in Western Europe, like Dorestad and Hamwih (cf. Hodges 1982, p.151 ff.) and in Scandinavia knocked out Kaupang; at Hedeby, minting ceased. In contrast, the mid and late ninth century also sees a sharp rise in Danish raiding on Franconia and England which gradually involved the Danes in the political superstructure of these areas and was followed by Danish settlement (Fig. 2). In spite of the political gains little wealth was won for the home country by these events; according to the written sources the Franks paid enormous sums in silver to the Danes but hardly any Frankish coin of this period is known from Denmark. Seemingly the silver was spent abroad (if ever paid fully and in silver) and the Viking gangs in the West, for instance the so-called 'big army', had relatively little direct contact with their native countries. The departure of the 'armies' and their warrior-kings from Denmark must, however, be seen as a response to local disorder. No part of the country could afford to lose just a single manned longship, and raiding is probably never a sound alternative to trading although it may relieve stress due to lack of income in a traditional society.

Shortly before AD 900 we note a very strong increase in silver followed by a clear recession around AD 950 which knocked out the Swedish port of Birka (Fig. 2, cf. Fig. 3). Birka was much dependent on the eastern trade that supplied most of the silver of the early and middle Viking Age. The key to the whole system is the Samanid Empire in central Asia (cf. Lombard 1971). Based around the fabled cities of Samarkand and Bukhara in Turkestan, this dynasty occupied a position at the crossroads of international trade, including Teheran, the gateway to India and China, either via the Persian Gulf or, overland, by the Old Silk Road. The contact with Scandinavia travelled via Russia, whence Nordic traders went as far as Bagdad, and Muslims went north to market centres like Bulghar on the middle Volga. The Samanids lost control of the trade routes about AD 950 and so the second wave of eastern trade, and with it, the massive injection of Islamic silver collapsed.

In tune with the above we would have expected the recession at AD 950 to be followed by a renewed wave of raiding, but this is not the case (cf. Randsborg 1981a). Practically no raids are reported in the historical sources of England and France in the mentioned period. When Danish military activities in the west are reported again, and especially after the year AD 1000, they are directed only towards England and are well-executed campaigns rather than raids and migrations of hordes of warriors. Also in this period the silver stock is rising in Denmark, in part due to very many German coins, probably from the smaller Baltic trade, in part to the incomes from the English adventure, which, in contrast with the ninth-century Frankish payments, actually went back to the home land and to other Scandinavian regions that supplied some of the troops of the Danish fleets and armies. The reason for this 'Rückstrom' is, of course, that the Danish rulers in England and in Denmark at the beginning of the eleventh century belonged to the very same political establishment.

What is the cause of this change? The overall reason is most probably the transformation of the social infra-structure of Denmark which was well under way at AD 950, the period of King Harald's stone at Jelling. The late crisis in silver could be and was handled locally due to the state system of society described above. Payments in silver may have been partly substituted for by grants of land, which is in accordance with the rise in private rights that we have seen reflected in the texts of the rune-stones. These rights and the changes which were taking place in the subsistence economy would give the ruling echelons profitable ways of investing their prerogatives. The spread of towns and markets is, of course, another aspect of these changes. A number of enterprises spurred by the magnates and the kings, like the building of the Trelleborg fortresses and the new Danevirke walls, the bridges, churches etc. may, however, as well as the military establishment, have turned out to be so costly that extraordinary incomes were necessary. Actually, Norwegians were raiding the coasts of England in the 980s when the Danes entered the stage again.

It is significant that the eastern areas of Denmark, as well as non-Danish regions further to the east, like Gotland in the Baltic, in the late tenth century and in the eleventh century, saw more wealth than the growing state-society in west Denmark, nearest to Western Europe. Obviously, only the west was in a position, through various enterprises, to utilize wealth in the building up of the country, rather than keeping it as 'dead' capital in the hands of the magnates. One way of using silver is to trade it for materials and services, which as far as King Harald's early state was concerned may have been obtained from eastern Denmark. In fact the formation of the nation-state might have been started by a series of exchanges. In this context it is also significant that the Danes, when carrying out the take-over of England, paid Swedish troops for participating, as is evident from some runestone texts (Jansson 1976, p.76 f.). Royal payments may furthermore be exemplified by the above mentioned eastern distribution of the mints of King Canute of the early eleventh century. After minting was taken up anew at Hedeby in the earlier tenth century, parallel to the second peak in silver importation, and continued at this site for some period, it is not until the first half of the eleventh century that we find coins carrying the picture of the king along with his name (Randsborg 1980, p.149 f.). These coins were minted in great quantities but so were already the latest types of the Hedeby coins and contemporary 'anonymous' coins with a cross that most probably were minted by the newly Christianized King Harald. In fact, the intensity of royal minting seems to be a fine index for the Viking period of the size of the 'state budget', indeed, of the coming of such. Significantly the latest silver hoards were made up entirely of coins, while coins are rather few in the hoards from before c. 950 that in the main consisted of jewellery, complete or broken (for exchanges) (Fig. 4).

The Viking Phenomenon

The Danish example has, it is hoped, served to demonstrate some of the important variables of Scandinavian Viking societies and of the relations of these variables as they are expressed in 'real' historical situations and in finds of their material culture and other reflections of social processes. I am not claiming that this survey has exhausted the number of important factors. For instance, a sharp climatic recession in the ninth century may well have played a role in the dramatic events of a period which also saw Danish settlement in England and the beginning of the colonization of Iceland (Randsborg 1980, p.45 f.). Problems of feeding the growing populations of Scandinavia may have become very critical during periods of poor harvests and may have added to the social stress. I am neither claiming that the Danish study is a complete model of the development in all parts of Scandinavia, nor of the Viking component in, for instance, the British Isles, in Franconia, or in Russia. But I think it is safe to say, that much of the general social development in Norway, and later, in Sweden followed some of the same lines as in Denmark in spite of the differences in environment within Scandinavia that made Denmark a much more densely populated region than the rest (cf. Blom 1977). Exempted from this rule are, of course, the marginal areas to the extreme north where hunting and gathering coupled with nomadism was the main subsistence base. The general character of the presentation is also exemplified by the excursuses already made to Swedish and Norwegian circumstances. It is striking how many of the basic elements of technology and economy, as well as in social relationships and in ideology and use of symbols are recurrent in the various Scandinavian regions.

The arts, for instance, or at least those of the aristocracy, were highly abstract or ornamental, almost completely lacking in recognizable content. The Viking

North was pagan which meant belief in a number of gods whose behaviour resembled an idealized version of the life of the magnates: travelling, feasting, and seeking excitement. In addition the Vikings believed in lesser, often evil, supernatural beings, resembling the commoners. Also venerated were the forces of nature. As in Islam the death of a warrior could mean a ticket to Valhalla, the 'Hall of the slain', in Asgaard, the home of the gods.

Another characteristic trait is the skilfully made Viking long ship, equipped and manned by a group of men of similar standing, in most cases also from the same region. These ships are mentioned in runic inscriptions and seen on pictorial representations. The craft could enter even small rivers and withstand high waves on the open sea. They were very fast, whether under sail, or when being rowed by a crew of some 40 men. With the mast, prow and stern lowered the ships were easy to hide, yet could be moved out instantly.

But these phenomena must not of course lead us to think about the Vikings in a monolithic way, as there were great social differences from area to area and especially from period to period in the Viking age. The powerful Viking culture was even imposed upon different population groups, some of them unwilling; a study of the major blood-types among the population of Iceland has shown no relation with Norway (or Denmark) but identity with the 'Celtic' populations of Ireland, Wales and western Scotland (Frydenberg et al. 1963, p.145 f.). The 'Norwegian' settlement of Iceland was, in spite of the Scandinavian cultural patterns, and of Scandinavian leadership, seemingly carried out mainly by Irish and other slaves. This example is extreme, no doubt, but so were at some stages the social developments in Denmark which led to the introduction of 'modern' West European state-societies in Scandinavia.

The fierce 'Danes' met with some successes in their search for easy gains abroad exactly because they were undeveloped and less vulnerable that the western states they were dealing with. Even the Danish sway over England in the early eleventh century is a result of abnormal circumstances. Denmark had at this time just completed the first stage in its state-formation and had large military forces at hand, ready for other enterprises. Later in the same century and in the twelfth century, when Denmark had become a smaller, Christian, quasi-feudal, almost West European state with a developed market-economy, it was, ironically, pillaged by its barbarian neighbours, Norwegians and Slavs, among others.

In reality it was never possible for the Danes to administer both England and Denmark across wide stretches of sea. King Canute was more a king of England than of Denmark. In fact the Danish rulers were elected kings of England to stop their extraction of tribute under the threat of plundering, since payment of ordinary taxes was far cheaper than tributes exceeding even 80,000 pounds of silver at a time. Danish rule in England was based on military power and motivated by easy gain, but after the conquest it was no longer possible to extort tribute. It seems that the Danes had no plans for a continued political presence in England and may well have over-reached themselves. For instance, after the conquest they disbanded most of the army. This made the occupation much less onerous on the English, but the Danes lost a crucial instrument of power. From the point of view of social evolution it was the Nordic countries that changed upon contact rather than the more developed English one.

With this survey I have hoped to put the Viking phenomenon into the framework of contemporary rational analyses of society using and explaining all accessible information. Although the Vikings are still with us, with horned helmets and unshaved, but somewhat toothless, they are intelligible first and foremost in terms of social contacts, changes and development. The Vikings make up no crucial stage in the evolution of European society as a whole, being more of an epi-phenomenon. Their overall importance lies in the questions they raise about transformations of established political, and social forms and in the factors that allowed for such external instruments of change to appear.

NOTES

Note 1
A general reference can be given for the following to Randsborg 1980; Hodges 1982 excellently presents the north west European perspective. For the established views see e.g. Wilson 1980; for a recent historical view, Sawyer 1982.

BIBLIOGRAPHY

ALBRECTSEN, E. 1976 - Vikingerne i Franken, Odense, Odense Universitetetsforlag.

ANNALES FRANCORUM = Buchner, R. (Ed.) -Ausgewählte Quellen zur deutschen Geschichte des Mittelalters V-VII. Berlin 1955-60.

ANDERSEN, H.H. MADSEN, H.J. and VOSS, O. 1976 - Danevirke, Jysk Arkaeologisk Selskabs skrifter XIII. Aarhus.

ANDERSEN, P. 1974 - Passages from Antiquity to Feudalism, London (NLB).

ARBMAN, H. 1943 - Birka I. Die Gräber, Stockholm, Kungl. Vitterhets Historie och Antikvitets Akademien.

BLOM, G.A. (Ed.) 1977 - Urbaniseringsgrossen i Norden, Oslo, Universitetetsforlaget.

CHAPMAN B., KINNES, I. and RANDSBORG, K. (Eds.) 1981 - The Archaeology of Death, Cambridge, Cambridge University Press.

FOOTE, P.G. and WILSON, D.M. 1970 - The Viking Achievement. London, Sidgwick and Jackson.

FRYDENBERG, Aa and SPÄRK, J.V. 1963 - Arv og race hos mennesket, København. Berlingske.

GRØNGAARD JEPPESEN, T. 1981 - Middelalderbyens opstaen, Fynske Studier XI, Odense. Odense Bys Museer.

HARDH, B. 1976 - Wikingerzeitliche Depotfunde aus Südschweden, Acta Archeologica Lundensia, serie in 8to, no. 6 and serie in 4to, no. 9. Lund.

HELBAEK, H. 1977 - 'The Fyrkat grain' in Olsen et al., (1) -(4).

HODGES, R. 1982 - Dark Age Economics, The origins of towns and trade A.D. 600-1000, London, Duckworth.

HVASS, S, 1975 - 'Das eisenzeitliche Dorf bei Hodde, West Jütland', Acta Archaeologica, vol. 46, pp.142-58.

HVASS, S 1979 - 'Vorbasse, The Viking-age Settlement at

Vorbasse, Central Jutland', Acta Archaeologica, vol. 50, pp.137-72.

JANKUHN, H. 1976 - Haithabu, Ein Handelsplatz der Wikingerzeit, (6th ed.), Neumünster. Karl Wachholtz.

JANSSON, S.B.F. 1976 - Runinskrifter i Sverige, Uppsala. Almqvist och Wiksell.

JØRGENSEN, L.B. and SKOV, T. 1979 - 'Trabjerg, A Viking-age Settlement in North-west Jutland', Acta Archaeologica, vol. 50, pp.119-36.

KROGH, K.J. and VOSS. O. 1961 - 'Fra hedenskab til kristendom i Hørning', Nationalmuseets Arbejdsmark, pp.5-34.

LOMBARD, M. 1971 - L'Islam dans sa première grandeur, Paris. Flammarion et Cie.

NIELSEN, L.C. 1979 - 'Omgaard, A Settlement from the Late Iron Age and the Viking Period in West Jutland', Acta Archaeologica, vol. 50, pp.173-208.

OLSEN, O. and SCHMIDT, H. 1977 - Fyrkat, en jysk vikingeborg I. Borgen og bebyggelsen, Nordiske Fortidsminder serie 8, in 4to, no. 3 (København).

RAMSKOU, T. 1980 - 'Vikingebroen over Vejle aa-dal', Nationalmuseets Arbejdsmark, pp.25-32.

RANDSBORG, K. 1980 - The Viking Age in Denmark, The Formation of a State, London (Duckworth); New York (St. Martin's Press).

RANDSBORG, K. 1981a - 'Les activités internationales des Vikings: Raids ou Commerce?', Annales Economies Sociétés Civilisations 5, Sept.-Oct., pp.862-68.

RANDSBORG, K. 1981b - 'Burial, Succession and Early State Formation in Denmark' in Chapman et al., pp.105-21.

RANDSBORG, K. 1982 - 'Rank, rights and resources, an archaeological perspective from Denmark', in Renfrew et al., pp.132-39.

RENFREW, C., and SHENNAN, S. (Eds.) 1982 - Ranking, Resources and Exchange: Aspects of the Archaeology of Early European Society, Cambridge. Cambridge University Press.

ROESDAHL, E. 1977 - Fyrkat, en jysk vikingeborg II. Oldsagerne og gravpladsen, Nordiske Fortidsminder serie B, in 4to, no. 4 (København).

SAWYER, P.H. 1971 - The Age of the Vikings, London, Edward Arnold.

SAWYER, P.H. 1982 - Kings and Vikings, Scandinavia and Europe AD 700-1000, London, Methuen.

STOUMANN, I. 1979 - 'Saedding, A Viking-age Village near Esbjerg', Acta Archaeologica vol. 50, pp.95-118.

WHITELOCK, D. (Ed.) 1955 - English Historical Documents I, c. 500-1042, London. Eyre & Spottiswoode.

WILSON, D.M. (Ed.) 1980 - The Northern World, The history and heritage of Northern Europe A.D. 400-1100, London. Thames and Hudson.

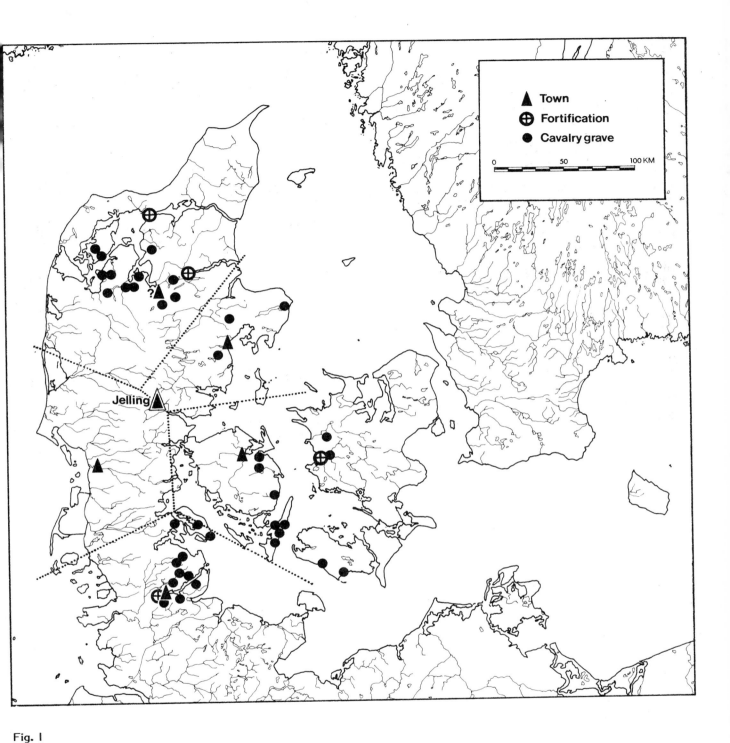

Fig. 1

Denmark at the time of King Harald (mid- to late tenth century). Cavalry graves after Randsborg 1980, Appendix VIII. Jelling = royal centre. 'Fortification' = fortresses of the Trelleborg type plus the Danvirke walls on the German frontier. Broken lines = borders of theoretical catchment areas of (larger) towns.

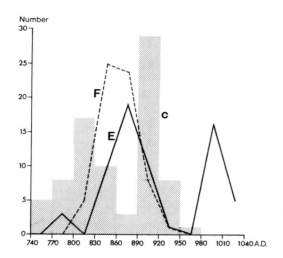

Fig 2

Frequencies of foreign (in the main Arabic) coins in the graves of the town of Birka (mid-Sweden) = C, contrasted with frequencies of years with Viking-attacks on England (E) and on the continent (Franconia = F). Coins after Arbman 1943. Historical information after Whitelock 1955 (the Anglo-Saxon Chronicle) and Albrechtsen 1976 (the continental sources). Note negative correlation between trade and raids in the ninth to early tenth centuries.

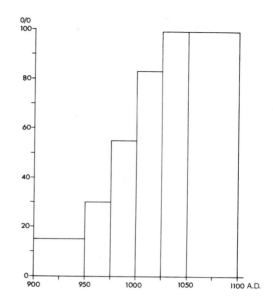

Fig 4

Percentage of coins (by weight) in a sample of silver hoards from east Denmark (data Haardh 1976). Note disappearance of silver jewellery as a medium of exchange.

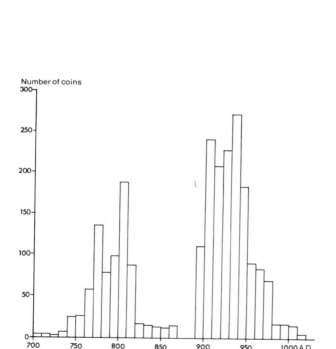

Fig. 3

Arabic coins in sample of north west Russian silver hoards. Note period of little trade in between phases of close contacts (cf. Randsborg 1980 p.154 f.).

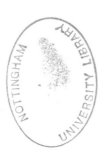